IMMUNOPHARMACOLOGY OF THE LUNG

LUNG BIOLOGY IN HEALTH AND DISEASE

Executive Editor: **Claude Lenfant**

Director, National Heart, Lung, and Blood Institute
National Institutes of Health
Bethesda, Maryland

Volume 1 IMMUNOLOGIC AND INFECTIOUS REACTIONS IN THE LUNG, *edited by Charles H. Kirkpatrick and Herbert Y. Reynolds*

Volume 2 THE BIOCHEMICAL BASIS OF PULMONARY FUNCTION, *edited by Ronald G. Crystal*

Volume 3 BIOENGINEERING ASPECTS OF THE LUNG, *edited by John B. West*

Volume 4 METABOLIC FUNCTIONS OF THE LUNG, *edited by Y. S. Bakhle and John R. Vane*

Volume 5 RESPIRATORY DEFENSE MECHANISMS (in two parts), *edited by Joseph D. Brain, Donald F. Proctor, and Lynne M. Reid*

Volume 6 DEVELOPMENT OF THE LUNG, *edited by W. Alan Hodson*

Volume 7 LUNG WATER AND SOLUTE EXCHANGE, *edited by Norman C. Staub*

Volume 8 EXTRAPULMONARY MANIFESTATIONS OF RESPIRATORY DISEASE, *edited by Eugene Debs Robin*

Volume 9 CHRONIC OBSTRUCTIVE PULMONARY DISEASE, *edited by Thomas L. Petty*

Volume 10 PATHOGENESIS AND THERAPY OF LUNG CANCER, *edited by Curtis C. Harris*

Volume 11 GENETIC DETERMINANTS OF PULMONARY DISEASE, *edited by Stephen D. Litwin*

Volume 12 THE LUNG IN THE TRANSITION BETWEEN HEALTH AND DISEASE, *edited by Peter T. Macklem and Solbert Permutt*

Volume 13 EVOLUTION OF RESPIRATORY PROCESSES: A COMPARATIVE APPROACH, *edited by Stephen C. Wood and Claude Lenfant*

Volume 14 PULMONARY VASCULAR DISEASES, *edited by Kenneth M. Moser*

Volume 15 PHYSIOLOGY AND PHARMACOLOGY OF THE AIRWAYS, *edited by Jay A. Nadel*

Volume 16 DIAGNOSTIC TECHNIQUES IN PULMONARY DISEASE (in two parts), *edited by Marvin A. Sackner*

Volume 17 REGULATION OF BREATHING (in two parts), *edited by Thomas F. Hornbein*

Volume 18 OCCUPATIONAL LUNG DISEASES: RESEARCH APPROACHES AND METHODS, *edited by Hans Weill and Margaret Turner-Warwick*

Volume 19 IMMUNOPHARMACOLOGY OF THE LUNG, *edited by Harold H. Newball*

Volume 20 SARCOIDOSIS AND OTHER GRANULOMATOUS DISEASES OF THE LUNG, *edited by Barry L. Fanburg*

Other volumes in preparation

IMMUNOPHARMACOLOGY OF THE LUNG

Edited by

Harold H. Newball

Physiology Division
Institute of Chemical Defense
Edgewood, Maryland

MARCEL DEKKER, INC. New York • Basel

Cover illustration: Human lung mast cells isolated by enzymatic digestion, countercurrent elutriation and IgE affinity column. (Compliments of A. Dvorak, K. Pyne, E. Shulman, D. MacGlaushen, L. Lichtenstein, and H. Newball.)

Library of Congress Cataloging in Publication Data
Main entry under title:

Immunopharmacology of the lung.

(Lung biology in health and disease ; v. 19)
Includes bibliographical references and indexes.
1. Lungs–Diseases–Immunological aspects.
2. Immunopharmacology. I. Newball, Harold H., [date]. II. Series. [DNLM: 1. Immunochemistry. 2. Lung–Immunology. 3. Anaphylaxis. 4. Lung diseases–Etiology. W1 LU62 v.19 / WF 600 I335]
RC756.L83 vol. 19 616.2'4s [616.2'4076] 8 83-1799
ISBN 0-8247-1827-5

MARCEL DEKKER, INC.
270 Madison Avenue, New York, New York 10016

Current printing (last digit):
10 9 8 7 6 5 4 3 2 1

PRINTED IN THE UNITED STATES OF AMERICA

This book is dedicated to my cherished children Kim, Kelli, and Kristi who have been my source of inspiration.

CONTRIBUTORS

N. Franklin Adkinson, Jr., M.D. Associate Professor, Department of Medicine, Division of Allergy and Clinical Immunology, The Johns Hopkins University School of Medicine, The Good Samaritan Hospital, Baltimore, Maryland

Tahir Ahmed, M.D.* Associate, Division of Pulmonary Disease, Mount Sinai Medical Center, Miami Beach, Florida

Michael J. Ansfield, M.D. Assistant Professor, Department of Medicine, University of California School of Medicine, San Francisco, California

K. Frank Austen, M.D. Professor, Department of Medicine, Harvard Medical School, and Department of Rheumatology/Immunology, Brigham and Women's Hospital, Boston, Massachusetts

Bradley J. Benson, Ph.D. Assistant Professor, Department of Biochemistry, Cardiovascular Research Institute, and Department of Biochemistry and Biophysics, University of California School of Medicine, San Francisco, California

Colin M. Bloor, M.D. Professor, Department of Pathology, University of California School of Medicine at San Diego, La Jolla, California

Harvey Carp, Ph.D.† Instructor, Department of Pathology, State University of New York, Stony Brook, New York

Leland G. Dobbs, M.D. Assistant Clinical Professor, Department of Medicine, Cardiovascular Research Institute, University of California School of Medicine, San Francisco, California

Haig Donabedian, M.D.‡ Clinical Associate, Bacterial Diseases Section, Laboratory of Clinical Investigation, National Institute of Allergy and Infectious Diseases, National Institutes of Health, Bethesda, Maryland

---

Present Affiliation

*Assistant Professor, Department of Medicine, University of Miami School of Medicine, Mount Sinai Medical Center, Miami Beach, Florida

†University of Miami School of Medicine, Miami, Florida

‡Assistant Professor, Department of Medicine, Medical College of Ohio, Toledo, Ohio

Jeffrey M. Drazen, M.D. Associate Professor, Department of Physiology, Harvard School of Public Health, Respiratory Disease Division, Brigham and Women's Hospital, and Associate Professor, Department of Medicine, Harvard Medical School, Boston, Massachusetts

Joseph C. Fantone, M.D. Assistant Professor, Department of Pathology, The University of Michigan Medical School, Ann Arbor, Michigan

James E. Fish, M.D. Assistant Professor, Department of Medicine, The Johns Hopkins University School of Medicine, The Good Samaritan Hospital, Baltimore, Maryland

John I. Gallin, M.D. Head, Bacterial Diseases Section, Laboratory of Clinical Investigation, National Institute of Allergy and Infectious Diseases, National Institutes of Health, Bethesda, Maryland

Marilyn Halonen, Ph.D. Adjunct Assistant Professor, Division of Respiratory Sciences, The University of Arizona College of Medicine, Tucson, Arizona

Donald J. Hanahan, Ph.D. Professor and Chairman, Department of Biochemistry, The University of Texas Health Science Center at San Antonio, San Antonio, Texas

Tony E. Hugli, Ph.D. Member, Department of Immunology, Scripps Clinic and Research Foundation, La Jolla, California

Aaron Janoff, Ph.D. Professor, Department of Pathology, State University of New York, Stony Brook, New York

Claude Lenfant, M.D. Director, National Heart, Lung and Blood Institute, National Institutes of Health, Bethesda, Maryland

Robert A. Lewis, M.D. Assistant Professor, Department of Medicine, Harvard Medical School, Boston, Massachusetts

Lawrence M. Lichtenstein, Ph.D., M.D. Professor, Department of Medicine, The Johns Hopkins University School of Medicine, The Good Samaritan Hospital, Baltimore, Maryland

Linda M. McManus, Ph.D. Assistant Professor, Department of Pathology, The University of Texas Health Science Center at San Antonio, San Antonio, Texas

Henry L. Meier, Ph.D.* Research Associate, The Johns Hopkins University School of Medicine, The Good Samaritan Hospital, Baltimore, Maryland

Jay A. Nadel, M.D. Chief, Section of Pulmonary Diseases and Professor, Departments of Medicine, Physiology, and Radiology, and Director, Multidisciplin-

Present Affiliation
*Research Chemist, Basic Pharmacology Branch, Institute of Chemical Defense, Edgewood, Maryland

ary Research Training Program in Lung Diseases, Cardiovascular Research Institute, University of California School of Medicine, San Francisco, California

Harold H. Newball, M.D.* Associate Professor, Department of Medicine, The Johns Hopkins University School of Medicine, The Good Samaritan Hospital, Baltimore, Maryland

Charles W. Parker, M.D. Professor, Departments of Medicine, Microbiology, and Immunology, Division of Allergy and Immunology, Howard Hughes Medical Institute, Washington University School of Medicine, St. Louis, Missouri

R. Neal Pinckard, Ph.D. Professor, Department of Pathology, The University of Texas Health Science Center at San Antonio, San Antonio, Texas

Edward S. Schulman, M.D.† Instructor, Department of Medicine, The Johns Hopkins University School of Medicine, The Good Samaritan Hospital, Baltimore, Maryland

Norma P. Stimler, Ph.D.‡ Postdoctoral Fellow, Department of Molecular Immunology, Scripps Clinic and Research Foundation, and Department of Pathology, University of California School of Medicine at San Diego, La Jolla, California

Adam Wanner, M.D. Chief, Division of Pulmonary Disease, Mount Sinai Medical Center, and University of Miami School of Medicine, Miami Beach, Florida

Peter A. Ward, M.D. Professor and Chairman, Department of Pathology, The University of Michigan Medical School, Ann Arbor, Michigan

---

Present Affiliation

*Chief, Physiology Division, Institute of Chemical Defense, Edgewood, Maryland

†Assistant Professor, Department of Medicine, Jefferson Medical College, Philadelphia, Pennsylvania

‡Assistant Professor, Department of Pathology, Loyola University Stritch School of Medicine, Maywood, Illinois

FOREWORD

Most of us who are asked to name how the great advances in modern medicine and surgery have come about, would probably respond by listing some Nobel laureates and the discoveries closely linked with their names: for example, Roentgen and X-rays; Koch and the tubercle bacillus; Fleming and penicillin; Enders and culture of polio virus; Banting and insulin. Yet, once in awhile, an event that is ineligible for a Nobel Prize has had just as important an impact on medical advance as one that was eligible and won an award. One such event was Abraham Flexner's 1910 report "Medical Education in the United States and Canada" that resulted in a considerable decrease in the number of American medical schools and a considerable increase in their quality and in the scientific content of their curricula. Another was the opening of the Johns Hopkins Medical School in 1893, staffed by four professors, each outstanding as a scientist in his specialty and each believing in joining scientific research, medical education, and patient care.

Sometimes a book or a series of books has had a strong influence on the advance of medical science. One such book was the first edition of Osler's *Medicine* (1892) because Osler's emphasis on how little physicians knew for sure led John Rockefeller's adviser on philanthropy to recommend the building of the great Institute for Medical Research, which opened in 1904 and for decades was the foremost institution for research in basic medical sciences in the United States. Another was the first (1941) edition of Goodman and Gilman's *Pharmacological Basis for Medical Practice* that revolutionized teaching and research on the action and use of drugs; as one professor of pharmacology stated in 1941, no professional pharmacologist could from then on teach at a lower level than that of the superb text used by his students!

In the field of respiration and the lungs, there are some classic monographs and a comprehensive *Handbook of Physiology* that have heightened the interest of scientists, students, and physicians in this subject and stimulated them to enter pulmonary research. One can safely predict that this new series of monographs, "Lung Biology in Health and Disease," will have an even greater impact on young (and older) researchers because it is the first truly comprehensive, monumental work in this field. It does not deal just with cellular processes or just with clinical problems but with the entire spectrum of basic sciences and of lung function, metabolic functions, and respiratory defense mechanisms. The series will also include volumes that apply modern biological knowledge to elucidate mechanisms of pulmonary and respiratory disorders (immunologic, infectious, and genetic disorders, physiology and pharmacology of airways, genesis and resolution of pulmonary edema, and abnormalities of respiratory regulation). Other volumes will deal with the biology of specific pulmonary diseases (e.g., cancer, chronic obstructive pulmonary disease, disorders of the pulmonary circulation, and abnormalities associated with occupational and environmental factors) and with early detection and specific diagnosis.

This series shows the lung as a challenging organ, with many problems calling for innovative research. If it attracts some imaginative, creative, and perceptive young scientists to attack these difficult problems, the tremendous effort in writing, editing, and publishing these volumes will be well worthwhile. The volumes cannot win the Nobel Prize, but someone may who was challenged by them.

Julius H. Comroe, Jr.
San Francisco, California

PREFACE

Most lung diseases involve inflammatory mechanisms in one fashion or another. The elements of inflammatory processes may include: mediators of immediate hypersensitivity reactions, lymphokines, and proteolytic enzymes from mast cells, neutrophils, and macrophages, all of which may induce pathologic manifestations of the inflammatory response.

The mediators of immediate hypersensitivity reactions are numerous, with an ever increasing number. Histamine, for many decades, was considered to be the predominant mediator of immediate hypersensitivity reactions. This assumption was primarily justified by the observation that antigen-challenged, sensitized guinea pigs die of acute bronchospasm, and that this response is completely ablated by antihistamines. Recent data, however, question the importance of histamine in immediate type hypersensitivity reactions, and indeed suggest that histamine is probably of little importance in generating the symptom complex observed during many IgE-mediated reactions. This experimental data is supported by our clinical acumen which shows that antihistamines are ineffective in the therapy of bronchial asthma.

The past several years have seen the discovery of a number of potent and fascinating molecules (e.g., leukotrienes, platelet activating factor) that on a molar basis are 1000-fold more potent than histamine. These exciting discoveries have increased our knowledge of the mediators that may be operative in immunopharmacologic lesions of the lung, such as bronchial asthma. In this monograph, we have attempted to place the role of these newly discovered mediators in perspective, and to point out some of the complexities arising from these data, thus emphasizing the many questions that remain to be resolved.

Perhaps the most exciting new data relate to the chemical definition of several mediators. In the case of the leukotrienes (SRS-A), many investigators provided data that led to the experiments by C. Parker (Chapter 2), and B. Samuelsson and his colleagues which indicate that leukotrienes are products of arachidonic acid via the lipoxygenase pathway. In the last two years, the structure of platelet activating factor has been delineated by Pinckard and Hanahan–it is likewise a lipid, acetyl glyceryl ether phosphorylcholine (AGEPC).

While much attention has been given to the possible role of these low molecular weight mediators (histamine, AGEPC, leukotrienes) in inflammatory processes, little data has been available pertaining to the possible role of high molecular weight mediators which are also actively secreted during IgE-mediated events. Recent studies with mast cells have shown that during secretory events high molecular weight mediators are actively secreted, and they do possess biological activities. Thus, during IgE-mediated events, heparin bound to a large molecular weight proteoglycan is secreted, and is biologically active. Our studies with the human lung mast cell model also show that biologically active molecules are secreted bound to large molecular weight complexes. We have described the IgE-mediated secretion of four high molecular weight mediators from human lung mast cells (Chapter 6): a lung Hageman factor activator (LHFA), a lung prekallikrein activator (LPKA), a lung kallikrein-like activity (LK-A), and a molecule exhibiting tosyl arginine methyl ester (TAMe) esterase activity. In vitro, these high molecular weight mediators are capable of generating kinins from plasma kininogen, and activating human Hageman factor. This was the first description of mediators, released by IgE mediated mechanisms, that are capable of interacting with the coagulation, and the kallikrein-kinin systems to generate biologically active peptides. In fact, this represents the only known immunologic pathway into the plasma cascade systems. These high molecular weight mediators may participate not only in immediate type inflammatory processes, but may also function in important aspects of the entire inflammatory response. While the role of these high molecular weight mediators in immediate hypersensitivity reactions and in other inflammatory processes is not clear, they do represent a first and important interface between IgE-mediated reactions and the Hageman factor dependent pathways of the inflammatory response.

The identification and characterization of several mediators of the inflammatory response provide the potential for the synthesis of antagonists and the definition of biochemical pathways; these in turn provide the potential for the development of pharmacological agents that can inhibit various aspects of the inflammatory process. Thus, the next decade of studies on the mechanisms and therapy of inflammatory processes will be fruitful. It must be recognized, however, that inflammatory disorders of the lung are extremely complex, and that we have only begun to understand the mechanisms by which inflammatory processes injure the lung.

The contributors to this book are recognized internationally as authorities on the topics that they have written. All of the authors are pioneers in their field of research, and their contributions to this volume are truly at the cutting edge of research. I highly commend the reader to this monograph.

Harold H. Newball

INTRODUCTION

> Healing is a matter of time, but it is sometimes also a matter of opportunity. However, knowing this, one must attend in medical practice not primarily to plausible theories, but to experience combined with reason. . .
>
> *Hippocrates, 5th Century B.C.*

During the last ten to fifteen years we have witnessed the birth and maturation of modern immunology. First it was a science limited to molecular biology—today it is a clinical and therapeutic instrument which has revolutionized many concepts of, and approaches to clinical medicine. In the 5th Century B.C. Hippocrates, the founder of medicine, was speaking about a matter of opportunity, medical practice, plausible theories, and reason. No other words could apply more appropriately to immunology today.

A fallout of the many advances has been the evolution of a new discipline: immunopharmacology. Because the lung is such a unique organ with regard to immune reactions, it was only natural that immunopharmacology should be applied to that organ.

This volume, edited by Harold Newball, gives us the state of the art of immunopharmacology of the lung. But it does more than that: it takes us into the future. By asking questions, it points to new research directions which will pave the way to new observations. The authorship of this volume is truly remarkable: it brings together foremost researchers and clinicians who are at the cutting edge of their field. That such an authorship could be assembled is a tribute to the editor of this monograph, and, in turn, the volume is one more asset of the series "Lung Biology in Health and Disease."

Undoubtedly, this volume will contribute greatly to the goals of the series. Hence, it is with great pleasure that I express my appreciation to all who made this book possible.

Claude Lenfant, M.D.
Bethesda, Maryland

CONTENTS

IMMUNOPHARMACOLOGY OF THE LUNG

1

Pharmacologic Modulation of the Immune Release of Mediators from Mast Cells and Basophils

HAROLD H. NEWBALL*
and LAWRENCE M. LICHTENSTEIN

The Johns Hopkins University School of Medicine
The Good Samaritan Hospital
Baltimore, Maryland

I. Introduction

All lung diseases, with the possible exception of direct trauma, involve inflammatory processes in one fashion or another. We can now classify these elements of inflammatory processes into rather simple categories: (a) they may involve immediate hypersensitivity reactions, the sequelae of IgE-mediated processes, and the release of mediators by mast cells and basophils; (b) they may involve the action of a variety of chemotactic stimuli that attract neutrophils and stimulate these cells and macrophages to release proteolytic enzymes which, over a period of time, have the potential for the destruction of almost every element that constitutes lung tissue; (c) they may involve lymphocytes capable of releasing destructive lymphokines with direct pathologic manifestations. There is, additionally, ample evidence that the plasma cascade systems, as illustrated by the activation of the Hageman factor-dependent pathways (kinin generation, and the

Present Affiliation
*Institute of Chemical Defense, Edgewood, Maryland

Supported in part by Grant No. 1392 from The Council for Tobacco Research–U.S.A., Inc., and N.I.H. Grant No. HL24210. We thank Ms. Judy Mason for her technical assistance.

activation of the complement, coagulation, and fibrinolytic pathways), play a role in each of these processes leading to inflammation and destruction of lung tissue.

Although the processes of inflammation can be outlined and many of the pathophysiologic mechanisms delineated when each of these systems is considered separately, little is known about their interaction, and it is this interaction that dictates whether disease or healing occurs. That the interactions take place is quite clear: for example, many of the mast cell products released in immediate hypersensitivity reactions serve to bring neutrophils or eosinophils to the site of a reactive process; other mast cell mediators activate the plasma cascade systems. Macrophages interact with lymphocytes in a facultative or obligative fashion in order to cause activation of effector cells and subsequent release of lymphokines; lymphocytes, in turn, release products that invoke a response from macrophages, neutrophils, and basophils. This chapter begins with a discussion of the most rapid or immediate-type response of lung inflammatory cells, namely those of mast cells and basophils. The direct function of other cell types in inflammatory processes will be considered in other chapters, but even there, the importance of mast cell mediators in eliciting and modulating other inflammatory processes will be evident.

II. Mediators

A. Low Molecular Weight Mediators

Histamine

Mast cells and basophils contain in their granules a variety of mediators of inflammation whose number is rapidly increasing. Many of these mediators are considered in detail in their own chapters; thus, what is required here is an overview.

The classic mediator of immediate hypersensitivity reactions and the one which, for many decades, was considered to be the sole cause of anaphylactic reactions, is histamine. If mediators are divided into two classes—those preformed in the granules of effector cells and those formed only after mast cell or basophil stimulation—then histamine is the paradigm of a preformed mediator. Each mast cell contains 2–10 pg histamine (Ishizaka and Tomioka, 1972; Peters et al., 1982), while basophils average about 1 pg per cell (Ishizaka et al., 1972). The effects of histamine are well appreciated. Thus, histamine may cause smooth muscle contraction and vasodilation leading to the efflux of plasma components and cells into an inflammatory focus. Histamine levels are known to be elevated in human anaphylaxis (Smith et al., 1980) and, indeed, this mediator can account for most of the pathophysiologic events observed; histamine alone can cause bronchospasm, cardiac arrhythmias, hypotension, and widespread cutaneous manifestations (Douglas, 1980). Indeed, a still unresolved question concerns the relative importance of histamine in the total response of an animal to antigen. It has long been known that antihistamines (of the H1 type), which have no major effect on any of the other mast cell mediators, completely prevent the fatal anaphylaxis that occurs due to bronchospasm in the guinea pig. Studies on isolated airway smooth muscle of the guinea pig and man, however, suggest that histamine has only a minor and transient role in antigen-induced bronchospasm: the leukotrienes seem to play the predominant role (Adams and Lichtenstein, 1979).

More recent data make it necessary to consider the anti-inflammatory effects of histamine that occur by its interaction on the histamine-2 (H2) receptor. Although discussed below, it is worth noting at this point that histamine can negatively modulate the inflammatory effects of basophils, neutrophils, and lymphocytes (Lichtenstein and Gillespie, 1973; Plaut et al., 1975), although the human lung mast cell does not appear to have an H_2 receptor (Peters et al., 1982). The confusion that still surrounds the role of histamine as a mediator provides an appropriate introduction to a consideration of the role of other mediators.

Leukotrienes

Historically, the next mediator described in the context of immediate-type hypersensitivity reactions was the slow-reacting substance of anaphylaxis (SRS-A) recently characterized as the leukotrienes (Kellaway and Trethewie, 1940; Murphy et al., 1979). SRS-A has been associated with immune and, particularly, IgE-mediated reactions for several decades and it serves as the prototype for the mediators that are not performed: if the cells that eventually generate this mediator are lysed before stimulation, no SRS-A is present (Austen, 1974). Perhaps the most exciting new data relate to the chemical structure of this mediator. Research on SRS-A was begun even before 1940 when Kellaway and Trethewie showed that this lipid mediator was involved in anaphylactic reactions. Many investigators provided data that led to the publication by Murphy et al. (1979), which indicates that the leukotrienes are products of arachidonic acid via the lipoxygenase pathway. The IgE-mediated release of several forms of biologically active leukotrienes (SRS-A) from human lung was first reported many years ago (Takahasi et al., 1976). However, it was only recently shown that the leukotrienes are derived from the lipoxygenase pathway of arachidonic acid metabolism and that there are at least three biologically active compounds (leukotrienes C, D, and E) (Parker et al., 1979; Orning et al., 1980). Another interesting observation is that a major source of the leukotrienes in inflammatory reactions may not be mast cells or basophils, but rather other cell types. Thus, Bach and Brashler (1978) have shown that SRS may be derived from rat peritoneal mononuclear cells, and we have demonstrated that SRS is readily derived from human polymorphonuclear leukocytes (Newball and Lichtenstein, 1981). The precise role of the leukotrienes in inflammatory disorders of the lung is not fully elucidated but, with respect to airway smooth muscle, the duration of its action is known to be much longer than that of histamine. The definition of the structure of the leukotrienes will, for the first time, allow the synthesis of a series of antagonists that may delineate the role of this mediator in inflammatory processes of the lung. (For a more detailed discussion of the immunopharmacology of the leukotrienes, see Chap. 2.)

Acetylglyceryl Ether Phosphorylcholine

A more recently discovered mediator, platelet-activating factor (PAF), was first described in 1971 (Siraganian and Osler, 1971). The structure of this mediator has been elucidated by Demopoulos et al. (1979): it is another lipid, acetylglyceryl ether phosphorylcholine (AGEPC). This latter name (AGEPC) seems more appropriate than its earlier name (PAF), because it is now known that AGEPC has effects not only on platelets but also on a wide variety of cells, thus, its original name was misleading. The effects of AGEPC on the human respiratory system are unknown. There have, however, been extensive studies of the physiological effects of AGEPC on rabbits and baboons. It has become evident that AGEPC is a very important mediator, with physiological effects being evident at the nonomolar level. In lower species, AGEPC is capable of increasing pulmonary resistance and decreasing pulmonary compliance. At a dose of 0.5 μg/kg, AGEPC was observed to produce physiological alterations in the lung that were both qualitatively and quantitatively indistinguishable from those characterizing IgE anaphylaxis in the rabbit (Halonen et al., 1980). If AGEPC participates in anaphylactic reactions in man, as it does in rabbits, the data of Pinckard and associates (see Chap. 4) provide strong evidence that AGEPC has the potential to be an important mediator of allergic and inflammatory responses in the human lung.

Chemotactic Mediators

There are a number of chemotactic mediators that have been reported to be derived from mast cells and basophils. Two of these have been characterized as tetrapeptides by Goetzl and Austen (1975); however, here as well there is the observation that eosinophil chemotactic factors may be readily obtained from polymorphonuclear leukocytes when they are challenged with the calcium ionophore or as a result of phagocytic stimuli (Konig et al., 1976). There is also recent evidence that arachidonic acid is the precursor of an important chemotactic factor. The studies by Goetzl and coworkers have shown that LTB_4 (5,12-dihydroxy-6,8,10,14-eicosatetraenoic acid [5,12-di-HETE]) is derived from arachidonic acid by the lipoxygenase pathway. Microgram quantities of 12-hydroxy-5,8,10,14-eicosatetraenoic acid (12-HETE) and 5-hydroxy-6,8,11,14-eicosatetraenoic acid (5-HETE), and nanogram quantities of 5,12-di-HETE

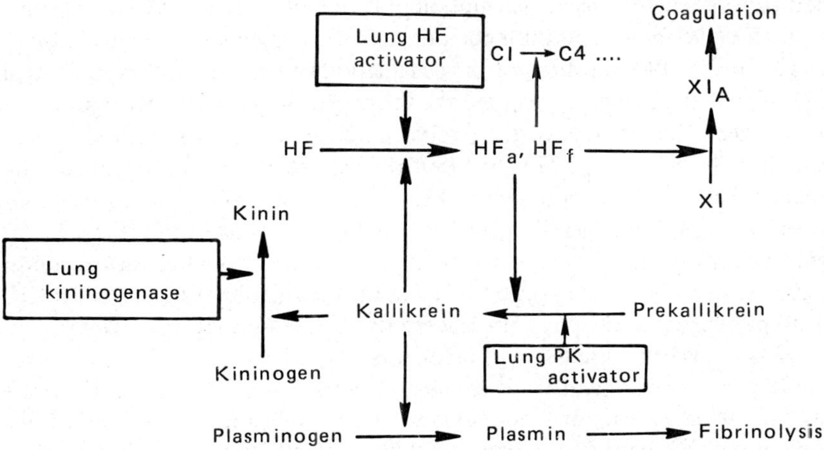

Figure 1 High molecular weight mediators from human lung. Partial outline of the Hageman factor-dependent pathways illustrating how the activation of these pathways could occur by the lung Hageman factor activator (LHFA) or the lung prekallikrein activator (LPKA). The lung kininogenase represents a third protease, which can directly generate kinins from high and low molecular weight kininogens. HF, Hageman factor; HF_a, activated Hageman factor; HF_f, Hageman factor fragment; C, complement; XI, coagulation factor XI. (From H. Newball (1981). Mast cells and basophils: Effector cells in inflammatory disorders in lung. *Thorax, 36*:721-725.)

(LTB_4) are capable of eliciting a rapid accumulation of eosinophils and a delayed accumulation of neutrophils (Goetzl, 1980). Thus, yet another important metabolite of arachidonic acid has been shown to have the potential of an important inflammatory mediator.

B. High Molecular Weight Mediators

It appears that the low molecular weight mediators described thus far (histamine, leukotrienes, AGEPC, chemotactic mediators) are responsible for but a part of the symptom complex observed during reactions of the lung, such as those observed during anaphylaxis and inflammatory disorders. Consider, for example, the least complex type of allergic reaction, anaphylaxis, which we have studied as part of our work on insect allergy. This reaction is solely caused by IgE antibody, and to a first approximation, the degree of hypotensive shock seems to parallel the plasma histamine level. A closer examination of physiological responses, however, indicates that many other events are probably occurring during anaphylaxis. We have recently published data which indicate that intravascular coagulation occurs during human anaphylaxis, with depletion of coagulation factors. There is also consumption of high molecular weight kininogen, C4, and C3 (the fourth and third components of complement). The mediators that account for the activation of the coagulation system have not been defined. We have recently, however, reported the IgE-mediated release of three proteases from antigen-challenged, passively sensitized human lung, and sensitized human basophils (Newball et al., 1979a,b; 1980; 1981). One of these proteases activates Hageman factor, another activates prekallikrein, and a third cleaves high and low molecular weight kininogens to generate a biologically active kinin (Fig. 1). Figure 1 illustrates how these newly described protease mediators may account for at least some of the changes observed in the coagulation proteins, which appear to participate in the physiological events observed during anaphylaxis.

While this brief discussion of mediators is by no means complete, it serves to indicate the breadth and scope of the molecules that are released as the result of an IgE-mediated reaction, and provides the first indication of the marked potential of such mediators for interacting with all elements of the inflammatory response.

III. Mechanisms of Mast Cell and Basophil Mediator Release

A. Desensitization

There have been extensive studies of the mechanism by which chemical mediators are released from mast cells and basophils. The cross-linking of IgE molecules on the surface of mast cells and basophils lead to the initiation of two distinct processes, the outcome of which determines the extent of mediator release. There is first an activation pathway that leads eventually to the exocytosis of mast cell and basophil granules. Simultaneously, however, a desensitization process which stops the release of mediators is set in motion. Recent work in our laboratories has shown that two different types of desensitization can occur. When a small number ($<10{,}000$) of cross-linked triggering units results from an antigenic stimulus, specific desensitization occurs. That is, the cells are rendered specifically unresponsive to a particular antigen but are able to respond to other antigens or to anti-IgE. Specific desensitization leads to inactivated triggering units, but the remaining units of other specificities remain fully operative. When, however, the number of cross-linked triggering units is higher ($>30{,}000$), nonspecific desensitization occurs, such that the cell is now unresponsive to any IgE-mediated stimulus (Sobotka et al., 1979). The mechanism for this nonspecific desensitization is not clear, but a variety of studies suggests that it involves the closing of calcium gates (the hypothetical structures that allow the influx of calcium) upon which release of mediators is totally dependent. If the desensitization process does not predominate, activation proceeds to histamine release through an extremely complex set of reactions that are only beginning to be appreciated. Control of the relative degree of activation versus desensitization can have an important influence on the extent of the inflammatory response.

B. Immunoglobulins in Mediator Release

Much of the information concerning release mechanisms has come, in both the mast cell and basophil studies, as a result of the use of pharmacologic agents as probes to individual steps of the release process. Thus, the evidence for the description which follows will be provided in Section IV of this chapter. More recently, some direct biochemical studies of the mechanism of release have been carried out in highly purified cell types (the rat peritoneal mast cell and a rat basophil leukemia cell line); these will be considered here.

The initiating event in mediator release is the exposure of the mast cell or basophil to antigen. The cells are responsive by virtue of having an occupied cell-surface receptor for the IgE antibody against the antigen in question. It is worth noting, parenthetically, that while IgG antibodies may exist on mast cells and basophils and may play a role in mediator release, this has, to date, been poorly documented. Highly purified anti-IgG is, like anti-IgE, capable of releasing mediators from human basophils; further, in most mammalian species, there exists a subclass of IgG (IgG_1 in the guinea pig [Ovary et al., 1963], IgG_A in the rat) that clearly fixes to mast cells and allows histamine release. Thus, it is anticipated that IgG antibodies that can mediate an allergic response in man will be found. It seems unlikely, however, that they will play a major role in human inflammatory disorders.

C. IgE Receptor

A number of laboratories are working to identify the IgE receptor on mast cells and basophils. It appears that the IgE receptor is a protein which is placed in, but does not transverse, the phospholipid cell membrane. The receptor appears to contain two components, one of approximately 60,000 daltons that binds IgE, and a second protein of approximately 30,000 daltons that is linked to the binding component, but does not, itself, bind IgE (Hempstead et al., 1979, 1981). This receptor complex seems to be the key element in initiating the release reaction. It has been demonstrated by a number of lines of evidence that it is necessary to cross-link two IgE molecules and or their receptors in order to initiate the release process (Ishizaka, 1981). Thus, univalent antigens are inactive and breaking the cross-links caused by a divalent antigen with a monovalent hapten immediately stops the release process (Dembo et al., 1979). Monovalent anti-IgE is ineffective in mediating release, but, if two such molecules are cross-linked by an antibody, this provides a signal for release (Ishizaka, 1981). Thus, the simple approximation of two IgE receptors serves as the unit signal for initiating release of mediators. In the basophil system, higher forms of complexes (i.e., trimeric or quadrameric) are not more effective releasers than are the bivalent complexes (Kagey-Sobotka et al., 1982). There is evidence that the IgE antibody's main function is to serve as a ligand to insure receptor approximation; anti-receptor antibody, in the absence of IgE, is a fully sufficient signal for initiating the release process, while the univalent anti-receptor antibody is completely ineffective (Ishizaka, 1981).

D. Phospholipid Metabolism

Following the cross-linking of IgE receptors, a number of perturbations rapidly occur in the phospholipids of the cell membrane. These include a series of transmethylation reactions which serves to transform phosphatidylserine to phosphatidylcholine and, additionally, provides a supply of the substrate, arachidonic acid. Arachidonic acid metabolites are then generated via both the cyclooxygenase and the lipoxygenase pathways (Ishizaka, 1981). These phospholipid alterations appear to be similar to the perturbations that are seen when a variety of cell types are stimulated (Hirata and Axelrod, 1978).

E. Influence of cAMP Agonists

The basophil release reaction can be divided into an antigen-dependent, calcium-independent first stage, and a calcium-dependent second stage (Lichtenstein, 1971). The first stage, which typically occurs in less than a minute, is completely inhibitable by agents that increase cAMP levels. More recent evidence (limited to the rat mast cell) has shown, paradoxically, that an early event in the release process is an increase in cAMP, rather than the expected decrease (Ishizaka, 1981). Further, the rat mast cell studies show that some agents that increase cAMP levels inhibit release, whereas other agents, which cause an increase in cAMP levels of the same magnitude, fail to affect the release process (Holgate et al., 1981). This suggests a compartmentalization of cAMP with only certain pools being responsible for the modulation of mediator release.

It is at these early stages in the release process that the cell-surface receptors for endogenous hormones, such as epinephrine, adenosine, histamine, and prostaglandins (to be considered below), can modulate the release process. The subsequent sequence of the steps involved in mediator release are less clear. It is universally agreed (without conclusive evidence) that the purpose of some of the early steps in the release process is to open a calcium "channel" or "gate," which allows the influx of calcium ions. Whether calcium is a necessary component of one of the enzymatic release steps or whether it interacts with cytoskeletal elements of the cell that are necessary for secretion is not clear. Colchicine and cytochalasin B, which affect microtubules and microfilaments, affect the release process in different ways (Gillespie and Lichtenstein, 1972), and suggest that these cytoskeletal elements are involved in the release process. Another major component of the release process involves arachidonic acid metabolism. The evi-

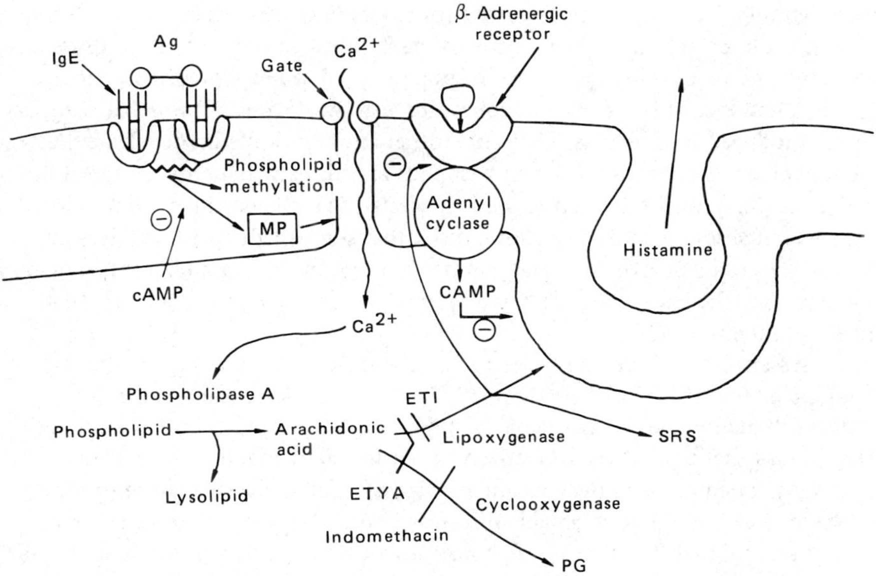

Figure 2 Model of the histamine release process. Cross-linking of cell-surface IgE (*top, left*) by antigen (Ag) or anti-IgE leads to activation of a serine esterase, phospholipid methylation, and, perhaps, a membrane protein (MP) involved in the opening of "calcium gates." The subsequent influx of calcium triggers a phospholipase A_2-catalyzed degradation of phospholipids to arachidonic acid. The arachidonic acid, thus derived, is apparently essential for the release process; inhibitors of its metabolism through the lipoxygenase pathway (ETI and ETYA) prevent histamine release. In the absence of inhibitors, the lipoxygenase pathway leads to the generation of leukotrienes (SRS-A) and, in concert with other as yet undetermined events, histamine release. IgE, immunoglobulin E; MP, membrane protein; Ag, antigen; ETYA, eicosatetraenoic acid; PG, prostaglandin; SRS, slow-reacting substance; ETI, eicosatriynoic.

dence for this will be delineated later, but may be summarized as suggesting that, at some stage in the release process, arachidonic acid is made available from phospholipids, and a product is generated through the lipoxygenase pathway which is required for the release process (Peters et al., 1981). What is known about the mechanism of release, without providing complete evidence at this time, is summarized in Figure 2.

F. Non-IgE Secretory Stimuli

In addition to mediator release induced by an antigen-IgE antibody interaction, an active, secretory, noncytotoxic release process can also be induced by many other stimuli. There are cogent reasons for examining these other stimuli. Perhaps most important is the conviction of many intestigators that mediator release plays a major role in a number of pulmonary diseases, notably bronchial asthma; however, it is the current consensus that most cases of bronchial asthma are not induced by allergens. Therefore, other stimuli for mediator release must be sought. Studies of the release of basophils in asthmatic patients, a subject beyond the purview of this chapter, have suggested that the pertinent stimuli in many asthmatics may not be antigen, but rather some of the peptide-releasing factors described below. An equally important reason for examining these other stimuli is for the insight that they may provide with respect to general mechanisms of mediator release.

An example of such a release stimulus is the calcium ionophore A23187 (Foreman et al., 1973; Lichtenstein, 1975). This complex organic molecule enters cell membranes by virtue of its lipophylic nature, and contains a moiety that binds calcium relatively selectively. Once in the membrane, the calcium ionophore opens a "window" for the passage of calcium down a concentration gradient. The ionophore is capable of causing noncytotoxic histamine release without additional stimuli, thus demonstrating that the influx of calcium, in and of itself, is a sufficient condition for mediator release. Furthermore, while the mechanisms of ionophore release are quite different from those of antigen-induced release, the two stimuli are synergistic, suggesting that calcium influx is also a part of the IgE-induced release process. There are many other nonphysiologic stimuli that have been used to explore the mechanism of mediator release. These include polycations such as 48/80, which has been extensively studied in the rodent mast cell, and polyarginine and ornithine, which have been used in studies of human basophils (Foreman and Lichtenstein, 1980). Hyperosmolarity, by itself, is also a stimulus for a noncytotoxic release process (Findlay et al., 1981). This may have relevance in reactions to contrast media, where transient conditions of hyperosmolarity may exist in vivo.

Of the potentially biologically relevant releasing stimuli, perhaps the most interesting are the anaphylatoxins (see Chap. 13). Serum, when exposed to immune complexes and certain types of biological particles, become activated, resulting in the enzymatic cleavage of certain components of the complement system. The major products resulting from such activation that are relevant to release processes are C3a, C4a, and C5a. In the last few years, these anaphylatoxins have been purified to homogeneity. The mechanism of release by the anaphylatoxins is quite different from that induced by antigen: the release of mediator is rapid, being over in 1 or 2 min rather than in 10–30 min as with antigens. Furthermore, many of the drugs that are capable of abolishing antigen-induced release have little or no effect on anaphylatoxin-induced release. That these two types of stimuli are distinct is demonstrated by the fact that a cell can be desensitized (rendered unresponsive) to antigen, while remaining completely responsive to the anaphylatoxins; the reverse is also true. Anaphylatoxins release by interacting with specific cell-surface receptors which are quite distinct for C3a and C5a. The latter statement is justified by the fact that there is no cross-desensitization between C3a and C5a.

Another interesting group of releasing agents are the formyl methylated peptides. These are a series of bi-, tri-, and higher oligopeptides that were synthesized because of their similarity to bacterial proteins (Schiffman et al., 1975). The first activity of these f-met peptides to be appreciated was neutrophil chemotaxis. Later, it was established that higher concentrations also caused neutrophils to release their granular enzymes. More recently, it has been shown that these peptides are also capable of inducing a noncytotoxic release of histamine from basophils (Hook et al., 1976). The release process is in many ways similar to that induced by the anaphylatoxins, being relatively rapid and more resistant to pharmacologic controls than is the release process observed with antigen. However, the pathways are quite distinct, as indicated by a lack of cross-desensitization between the anphylatoxic peptides and the f-met peptides.

One reason for an interest in these peptides relates to the fact that it has been found that basophils of asthmatic patients react normally to antigen, to anti-IgE, or to the ionophore, but are hyporesponsive to C5a and the f-met peptides (Findlay and Lichtenstein, 1980). This has been interpreted as being due to the fact that the cells are desensitized in vivo, as the result of interaction with these stimuli. This implies that, in vivo, these stimuli may be causing mediator release from the cells of asthmatic individuals.

Although not strictly a releasing agent, heavy water (D_2O) also has interesting effects on basophils of asthmatic individuals. D_2O was first described as an agent that enhanced antigen-induced release of mediators and whose mechanism of action appeared to involve microtubules (Gillespie and Lichtenstein, 1972b). While antigen-induced histamine release is uniformly enhanced by D_2O (Patterson et al., 1975), the cells of normal individuals show no response to D_2O in the absence of an additional stimulus. On the other hand, D_2O of itself does cause the release of histamine from about half of atopic individuals and from more than three-fourths of asthmatic individuals (Tung and Lichtenstein, 1982). While the mechanism of this release process is not clear, it represents a striking difference between the mediator-containing cells from normal and asthmatic individuals.

There are many other releasing agents which, at the present, have no obvious biological significance, although each has been used to shed some light on the mechanism of mediator release. Given the fact that there is some evidence that nonantigen-induced mediator release plays a role in diseases such as bronchial asthma or cold-induced urticaria, a search for the relevance of some of these releasing agents, as well as their potential role in elucidating release mechanisms, makes this an interesting and important avenue for future research.

IV. Modulation of Mediator Release

Since it is the underlying assumption of studies in this area that mediator release causes disease, it follows that the negative modulation of this process should prevent disease. There has, therefore, been considerable interest in the pharmacologic control of the release process. The prototype disease that is related to mediator release is bronchial asthma. A number of drugs have been utilized to treat this disorder, including β-adrenergic agonists and methylxanthine derivatives. While in many instances controlled studies demonstrating efficacy and relating to questions of dosage have not been carried out, these agents remain the mainstay of therapy. In recent years, since the development of scientific trials for drug efficacy, only one new agent, cromolyn, has been introduced (Altounyan, 1967). It is worth pointing out that this drug was discovered by sheer empiricism (self-trials by an asthmatic) and that in vitro or in vivo models played no role in its development. Since the introduction of cromolyn, a great effort has been mounted in both industry and academia to discover additional drugs useful in the treatment of bronchial asthma. Although many drugs have been found which stop mediator release in in vitro or in vivo animal models, no drug has yet emerged from these studies that has proven useful in the clinic. Therefore, in viewing the results which come from animal model systems, we must be aware that they may not have in vivo, clinical relevancy to man. Appropriate models must be utilized for drug development and, in our opinion, these models should primarily involve primate cells and tissues.

A. The Cyclic Nucleotide System

Before turning to specific drugs, a general comment on the role of the cyclic nucleotide system in mediator release is necessary. By the early 1960s, the work of Sutherland and his colleagues had established that cAMP played a central role in most secretory systems. Whatever the initial stimulus for secretion, cAMP seemed to be subsequently involved and it was therefore termed a "second messenger." At about the same time, data from a number of laboratories had demonstrated that mediator release from mast cells and basophils, rather than being a cytotoxic process as hypothesized by previous investigators, was rather an active secretory process. It, therefore, seemed reasonable to assess the role of cAMP in mediator release: this was accomplished in the late 1960s. In the other secretory systems that had been described at that time, the stimulus was followed by an increase in the intracellular cAMP level, which was linked intimately to secretion. In the basophil model, the reverse was observed. It was found that drugs which increased the cAMP levels, such as β-adrenergic agonists or methylxanthines, inhibited mediator release (Lichtenstein and Margolis, 1968). Over the ensuing decade, this negative modulation by increased cAMP levels was extended to a large variety of other inflammatory systems and cell types. These systems include the cytolytic or lymphokine-producing capabilities of lymphocytes (Plaut et al., 1975), the release of destructive enzymes from neutrophils, and the release of mediators from rodent and human mast cells (Austen, 1974; Johnson et al., 1974; Sullivan et al., 1975). By the middle 1970s, the concept of an inverse relationship between cAMP level and inflammatory processes dominated scientific thinking (Bourne et al., 1974). Shortly thereafter, however, as in other secretory systems, detailed investigation of different inflammatory cells and agonists began to show discrepancies between the cAMP level and function. At present, considerable confusion exists. In particular, the finding that, in antigen-stimulated rat mast cells, the cAMP levels are increased prior to, or at the same time of mediator release must be accounted for, as must the fact that some, but not all stimuli (e.g., PGD_2), that increase cAMP turn-off mediator release in the cell (Holgate et al., 1981). It should be noted, parenthetically, that the rat mast cell is rather unique, being different from the mast cells of most mammalian species in a number of ways.

B. Agents That Affect cAMP Levels

β-Adrenergic Agonists

Among the first drugs to be studied in the context of mediator release were the β-adrenergic agonists. Epinephrine inhibited human mast cell and basophil histamine release at pharmacologic concentrations, and an order of drug potency ranging from isoproterenol (which was highly effective) to phenylephrine or norepinephrine (which had only marginal effects) was established. Further, the potency of these drugs in inhibiting mediator release correlated well with their ability to increase the cAMP level of human leukocyte preparations. Propanolol, a β-adrenergic antagonist, was completely effective in blocking the inhibition of mediator release induced by epinephrine, whereas α-adrenergic blocking agents were ineffective. These studies were germane, since isoproterenol and epinephrine are extensively used in therapeutics. However, since, in addition to inhibiting mediator release, isoproterenol is a very potent bronchodilating agent, the question of whether the efficacy of isoproterenol in bronchial asthma is due to its effects on airway smooth muscle or on mediator-containing cells, remains unanswered.

Methylxanthines

The methylxanthines (theophylline, isobutylmethylxanthine, etc.) were also found to be effective inhibitors of mediator release (Lichtenstein and Margolis, 1968). Furthermore, as might be expected of agents that act to increase cAMP by blocking the phosphodiesterase system, their action was synergistic with the β-adrenergic agonists. Although direct inhibition of mediator release by methylxanthines was noted, rather high concentrations (millimolar levels) of drugs were required. Even though high concentrations of theophylline are required for in vivo therapeutic effects, the in vitro concentrations are at least an order of magnitude higher than the concentrations required for therapeutic effects. Attempts to establish that methylxanthines operate in vivo to stop mediator release have been disappointing. We have carried out studies in asthmatic subjects who have experienced antigen-induced bronchospasm, a model in which mediator release most likely plays a role. It was demonstrated that the dose of antigen required for a given fall in pulmonary function was the same, whether or not therapeutic blood levels of theophylline had been achieved (Bleecker et al., 1981). Furthermore, the bolus administration of theophylline during an episode of antigen-induced bronchospasm led to no more rapid a recovery than did placebo administration. It is evident, from these considerations, that the role of methylxanthines in the therapy of bronchial asthma must be given further consideration. It must be pointed out, however, that there are many types of phosphodiesterases and that a definition of those present in mast cells and basophils has not been achieved. Thus, the possibility of effective drugs having this mode of action should certainly not be dismissed.

cGMP

As noted above, it was postulated that the inhibitory effect of β-adrenergic agonists and methylxanthines was due to their ability to cause an increase in the intracellular level of cAMP. Experiments with dibutyryl cAMP and other stable cAMP derivatives seemed to confirm this hypothesis, since they were potent inhibitors of antigen-induced mediator release. At about the same time, there was speculation that cGMP played an inverse role: that is, that an increase in the intracellular level of cGMP potentiated mediator release, rather than causing inhibition. Some studies were carried out with cGMP derivatives that seemed to confirm this hypothesis. Additionally, cholinergic stimulation which, in a number of cell types caused an increase in cGMP, was reported to potentiate mediator release (Kaliner et al., 1972). More recently, this "ying-yang" concept, in which cAMP and cGMP play antagonistic roles, has fallen into disfavor as being an oversimplification. Currently, the role of cGMP in mediator release is unknown. In particular, careful studies have demonstrated that cholinergic stimulation has no effect on the release of mediators from basophils or rat mast cells (Lichtenstein et al., 1972).

H_2 Agonists

The next series of studies continued to focus on the role of the cAMP system but, rather than being pharmacologically oriented, these studies explored the role of receptors on mast cells and basophils that might exercise a homeostatic control of mediator release. The first agonist to be studied was histamine which, at micromolar concentrations, inhibited basophil histamine release (Bourne et al., 1971). This observation occurred before the discovery of the H2 antagonists, and it was observed that the standard H1 antagonists had no effect on this inhibitor. Just how histamine operated was not clear until the discovery of the H_2 antagonists, burimamide (Black et al., 1972). Burimamide and the more recently discovered H2 antagonists, such as metiamide and cimetidine (Ganellin, 1978), completely block histamine's ability to inhibit the release of histamine. Histamine and other H2 agonists, such as dimaprit (Parsons et al., 1977), also increase the cAMP level of leukocyte preparations, and it was assumed that histamine negatively modulated release by this mechanism. In this and the other receptor studies to be discussed, controls always revealed that a specific receptor was being defined, since the antagonist in question had no effect on agonists that increased cAMP by acting through other receptors. The question of whether H2 receptors also occur on human mast cells (in contrast to human basophils) has been more difficult to answer. Early experiments (Drazen et al., 1978; Chakrin et al., 1974) showed that H2 antagonists potentiated mediator release in several mammalian species. However, Kaliner (1978), using both histamine and specific H2 agonists, failed to find any effect on the release of histamine or SRS-A in chopped human lung tissue. More recently, it was reported that histamine inhibits histamine release and degranulation of human skin mast cells (Ting et al., 1981). Our data fail to demonstrate an H2 receptor on either human lung or skin mast cells (H. H. Newball, unpublished data). Thus, current evidence would suggest that neither the mast cell located in human lung tissue nor the skin mast cell contains a functional H2 receptor.

Prostaglandins

The cyclooxygenase products of arachidonic acid metabolism have been studied to establish their effects on mediator release. It was found that the E prostaglandins were potent inhibitors of mediator release (Newball et al., 1980). A series of prostaglandins have been studied for their effects on leukocyte cAMP levels, and it was found that those that increased cAMP levels most dramatically inhibited, while those that failed to increase cAMP levels, such as $PGF_{2\alpha}$, had little or no effect on histamine release. More recently, prostacyclin has also been shown to increase cAMP levels and to inhibit mediator release (L. M. Lichtenstein, unpublished data).

Adenosine

The dual effects of adenosine have also elicited recent interest, since this agonist has also been found to influence inflammatory systems. Just as there are α and β receptors for adrenergic agonists and H1 and H2 receptors for histamine, there are A1 and A2 receptors for adenosine that subserve opposite functions (Londos et al., 1980). An inhibitory adenosine receptor has been found on human basophils which, when stimulated, markedly decreased histamine release (Marone et al., 1979). This receptor is activated by micromolar concentrations of adenosine —concentrations that appear to obtain in vivo. Of interest is the fact that the methylxanthines and, in particular, theophylline, act as antagonists of the inhibitory adenosine receptor. This action of theophylline is observed at a concentration of 10 μM, far below the concentration required to increase cAMP or to inhibit histamine release. The in vivo consequences of this type of interaction are not clear, but it is at least worth noting that, at pharmacologic concentrations of theophylline, most inhibitory adenosine receptors would be blocked, thereby denying the body any of the homeostatic controls that this agent might have on mediator release. Recent studies in rat mast cells (Holgate et al., 1980) have defined both A1 and A2 receptors with competing effects.

Arachidonic Acid

One of the most interesting recent observations concerning release of chemical mediators from mast cells and basophils relates to the role of arachidonic acid metabolism. Eicosatetraenoic acid (ETYA), which blocks both the lipoxygenase and the cyclooxygenase pathways of arachodonic acid metabolism, completely inhibits the release of histamine from basophils. On the other hand, the nonsteroidal anti-inflammatory drugs, such as indomethacin, aspirin, and meclofenamic acid, which are selective inhibitors of the cyclooxygenase pathway of arachidonic metabolism, potentiate the release of basophil histamine. These observations suggest that a product of the lipoxygenase pathway is necessary for histamine release, and that the nonsteroidal anti-inflammatory drugs act by shunting arachidonic acid metabolism to the lipoxygenase pathway. In keeping with this suggestion is the fact that arachidonic acid, itself, also potentiates histamine release. A related observation, with respect to the above data, is that indomethacin and other nonsteroidal anti-inflammatory drugs selectively block the inhibition of histamine release caused by each of the agonists (isoproterenol, histamine, adenosine, prostaglandin) that acts through specific receptors to increase adenylate cyclase activity. Arachidonic acid has a similar activity. On the other hand, neither indomethacin nor arachidonic acid has any effects on the inhibition of histamine release caused by drugs or agents which increase cAMP by other mechanisms. Thus, indomethacin and arachidonic acid do not reverse the inhibition of histamine release caused by theophylline or isobutylmethylxanthine; similarly, they have little or no effect on the inhibition of histamine release caused by dibutyryl cAMP itself. These data strongly suggest that there must be subcompartments of cAMP that are differently affected by cyclase agonists and by other agents that increase cAMP levels. They further suggest that not only is there a product of the lipoxygenase pathway that is necessary for histamine release, but that another product of that pathway modulates the effects of endogenous hormones or pharmacological agents on the control of histamine release. We have recently investigated the influence of several lipoxygenase products on the release of histamine from suspensions of basophils. The data indicate that products of the 5-lipoxygenase pathway (5-HPETE [5-hydroperoxy-eicosatetraenoic acid] and, to a lesser extent 5-HETE) are selective enhancers of the release process. None of the other mono- or dihydroperoxy products of arachidonic acid metabolism, so far studied, share this property (Peters et al., 1981).

V. Conclusions

It is possible to summarize what is now known about the biochemical mechanism of mediator release in the following fashion, recognizing that this simply represents the present state of the art. The cross-linking of IgE receptors leads to a change in the intracellular activity of adenylate cyclase and an increase in membrane phospholipid transmethylation (Ishizaka et al., 1980). Through as yet unknown mechanisms, this is associated with or causes an increase in the permeability of the cell to calcium, perhaps via a modulatory protein which serves as the interface between receptor bridging and the opening of the postulated calcium channels. It is clear, at least in human cell types, that these processes can be antagonized by hormone-receptor interactions which lead to the stimulation of adenylate cyclase and an increase in intracellular cAMP. The above events occur early in the secretory process. Later on in the sequence of reactions are the changes in phospholipid biosynthesis and the release of arachidonic acid. It seems likely that the latter event follows the activation of phospholipase A_2, although other enzymes such as phospholipase C and diglyceride lipase have been implicated. Steroids, which inhibit histamine release with a time course reminiscent of their in vivo anti-inflammatory activity, may well act through the induction of a protein which blocks phospholipase-A activation. It appears clear that one of the products of arachidonic acid metabolism via the lipoxygenase pathway is necessary for histamine release. These data were obtained by the inhibition of histamine release by specific and nonspecific lipoxygenase inhibitors. Moreover, we have identified a product of the lipoxygenase pathway, 5-HPETE, which has this activity. Thus, the effects of indomethacin on histamine release are caused by the shifting of the metabolism of arachidonic acid from the cyclooxygenase to the lipoxygenase pathway. All of these biochemical changes lead, in a yet undefined way, to changes in the cytoskeletal elements of the cell which cause an energy-dependent exocytosis of mast cell and basophil granules and, thus, the release of mediators.

Both the identification of the mediators of allergic reactions, with the potential for the synthesis of antagonists, and the delineation of biochemical pathways, with the potential for developing pharmacological agents which block the entire release mechanism, suggest that the next decade of studies on the mechanism and therapy of bronchial asthma and other immune disorders, will be fruitful. It should be recognized, however, that immune disorders of the lung are extremely complex and that we have only just begun to understand the biochemical nature of mediators and the mechanism of their release.

References

Adams, G. K., III, and Lichtenstein, L. M. (1979). In vitro studies of antigen-induced bronchospasm: Effect of antihistamines and SRS-A antagonist on response of sensitized guinea pig and human airways to antigen. *J. Immunol., 122*:555-562.

Altounyan, R. E. C. (1967). Inhibition of experimental asthma with a new compound-Disodium cromoglycate, "Intal." *Acta Allerg. 22*:487-491.

Austen, K. F. (1974). Reaction mechanisms in the release of mediators of immediate hypersensitivity from human lung tissue. *Fed. Proc. 33*:2256-2262.

Bach, M. K., and Brashler, J. R. (1978). Ionophore A23184-induced production of slow reacting substance of anaphylaxis (SRS-A) by rat peritoneal cells in vitro: evidence for production by mononuclear cells. *J. Immunol. 120*: 998-1005.

Black, J. W., Duncan, W. A., Durant, C. J., Ganellin, C. R., and Parsons, E. M. (1972). Definition and antagonism of histamine H_2-receptors. *Nature 236*: 385-390.

Bleeker, E. R., Mason, P. L., Nissim, J. E., and Norman, P. S. (1981). The effect of chronic aminophylline therapy on methacholine and antigen airways reactivity in asthma. *Am. Rev. Respir. Dis., 123*:53.

Bourne, H. R., Melmon, K. L., and Lichtenstein, L. M. (1971). Histamine augments leukocyte adenosine 3′ 5′-monophosphate and blocks antigenic histamine release. *Science, 173*:743-745.

Bourne, H. R., Lichtenstein, L. M., Melmon, K. L., Henney, C. S., Weinstein, Y., and Shearer, G. M. (1974). Modulation of inflammation and immunity by cyclic AMP. Receptors for vasoactive hormones and mediators of inflammation regulate many leukocyte functions. *Science, 184*:19-28.

Chakrin, L. W., Krell, R. D., Mengel, J., Young, D., Zaher, C., and Wardell, J. R., Jr. (1974). Effect of a histamine H_2-receptor antagonist on immunologically induced mediator release in vitro. *Agents Actions, 4*:297-303.

Dembo, M., Goldstein, B., Sobotka, A. K., and Lichtenstein, L. M. (1979). Degranulation of human basophils: Quantitative analysis of histamine release and desensitization, due to a bivalent penicilloyl hapten. *J. Immunol., 123*:1864-1872.

Demopoulos, C. A., Pinckard, R. N., and Hanahan, D. J. (1979). Platelet-activating factor: evidence for 1-0-alkyl-2-acetyl-sn-glyceryl-3-phosphorylcholine as the active component (a new class of lipid chemical mediators). *J. Biol. Chem., 254*:9355-9358.

Douglas, W. W. (1980). Histamine and 5-hydroxytryptamine (serotonin) and their antagonists. In *The Pharmacological Basis of Therapeutics,* sixth edition. Edited by A. G. Gilman, L. S. Goodman, and A. Gilman. New York. MacMillan Publishing Co., pp. 609-646.

Drazen, J. M., Venugopalan, C. S., and Soter, N. A. (1978). H_2 receptor mediated inhibition of immediate type hypersensitivity reactions in vivo. *Am. Rev. Respir. Dis., 117*:479-484.

Findlay, S. R., and Lichtenstein, L. M. (1980). Basophil "releasability" in patients with asthma. *Am. Rev. Respir. Dis., 122*:53-59.

Findlay, S. R., Dvorak, A. M., Kagey-Sobotka, A., and Lichtenstein, L. M. (1981). Hyperosmolar triggering of histamine release from human basophils. *J. Clin. Invest., 67*:1604-1613.

Foreman, J. C., and Lichtenstein, L. M. (1980). Induction of histamine secretion by polycations. *Biochim. Biophys. Acta., 629*:587-603.

Foreman, J. C., Mongar, J. L., and Gemperts, B. D. (1973). Calcium ionophores and movement of calcium ions following the physiological stimulus to a secretory process. *Nature 245*:249-251.

Ganellin, C. R. (1978). Selectivity of the design of histamine H_2-receptor antagonists. *J. Appl. Chem. Biotechnol., 28*:183-200.

Gillespie, E., and Lichtenstein, L. M. (1972a). Heavy waters IgE-mediated histamine release from human leukocytes: evidence for microtubule involvement. *Proc. Soc. Exp. Biol. Med., 140*:1228-1230.

Gillespie, E., and Lichtenstein, L. M. (1972b). Histamine release from human leukocytes: Studies with deuterium oxide, colchicine, and cytochalasin B. *J. Clin. Invest., 51*:2941-2947.

Goetzl, E. J. (1980). Mediators of immediate hypersensitivity derived from arachidonic acid. *N. Engl. J. Med., 303*:822-825.

Goetzl, E. J., and Austen, F. K. (1975). Purification and synthesis of eosinophilotactic tetrapeptides of human lung tissue: Identification as eosinophil chemotactic factor of anaphylaxis. *Proc. Natl. Acad. Sci., 72*:4123-4127.

Halonen, M., Palmer, J. D., Lohman, I. C., McManus, L. M., and Pinckard, R. N. (1980). Respiratory and circulatory alterations induced by acetyl glyceryl ether phosphorylcholine, a mediator of IgE anaphylaxis in the rabbit. *Am. Rev. Respir. Dis., 122*:915-924.

Hempstead, B. L., Kulczycki, A., Jr., and Parker, C. W. (1981). Phosphorylation of the IgE receptor from ionophore A23187 stimulated intact rat mast cells. *Biochem. Biophys. Res. Comm., 98*:815-822.

Hempstead, B. L., Parker, C. W., and Kulczycki, A., Jr. (1979). Characterization of the IgE receptor isolated from human basophils. *J. Immunol., 123*: 2283-2291.

Hirata, F., and Axelrod, J. (1978). Enzymatic synthesis and rapid translocation of phosphatidylcholine by two methyltransferases in erythrocyte membranes. *Proc. Natl. Acad. Sci., 75*:2348-2351.

Holgate, S. T., Lewis, R. A., and Austen, K. R. (1980). Role of adenylate cyclase in immunologic release of mediators from rat mast cells: Agonist and antagonist effects of purine- and ribose-modified adenosine analogs. *Proc. Natol. Acad. Sci., 77*:6800-6804.

Holgate, S. T., Winslow, C. M., Lewis, R. A., and Austen, K. F. (1981). Effects of prostaglandin D_2 and theophylline on rat serosal mast cells: Discordance between increased cellular levels of cyclic AMP and activation of cyclic AMP-dependent protein kinase. *J. Immunol., 127*:1530-1533.

Hook, W. A., Schiffman, E., Aswanikumar, S., and Siraganian, R. P. (1976). Histamine release by chemotactic, formyl methionine-containing peptides. *J. Immunol., 117*:594-596.

Ishizaka, K., and Tomioka, H. (1972). The release of histamine and slow-reacting substance of anaphylaxis (SRS-A) by IgE and anti-IgE reactions on monkey mast cells. *J. Immunol., 108*:513-516.

Ishizaka, T. (1981). Analysis of triggering events in mast cells for immunoglobulin E-mediated histamine release. *J. Allergy Clin. Immunol., 67*:90-96.

Ishizaka, T., Hirata, F., Ishizaka, K., and Axelrod, J. (1980). Stimulation of phospholipid methylation, Ca^{2+} influx, and histamine release by bridging of IgE receptors on rat mast cells. *Proc. Natl. Acad. Sci., 77*:1903-1906.

Ishizaka, T., DeBernardo, R., Tomioka, H., Lichtenstein, L. M., and Ishizaka, K. (1972). Identification of basophil granulocytes as a site of allergic histamine release. *J. Immunol., 108*:1000-1008.

Johnson, A. R., Moran, N. C., and Mayer, S. E. (1974). Cyclic AMP content and histamine release in rat mast cells. *J. Immunol., 112*:511-519.

Kagey-Sobotka, A., Dembo, M., Goldstein, B., Metzger, H., and Lichtenstein, L. M. (1982). Qualitative characteristics of histamine release from human basophils by covalently crosslinked IgE. *J. Immunol.,* (In Press).

Kaliner, M. (1978). Human lung tissue and anaphylaxis: The effects of histamine on the immunologic release of mediators. *Am. Rev. Respir. Dis. 118*:1015-1022.

Kaliner, M., Orange, R. P., and Austen, K. F. (1972). Immunological release of histamine and slow reacting substance of anaphylaxis from human lung. IV. Enhancement by cholinergic and alpha adrenergic stimulation. *J. Exp. Med., 136*:556-567.

Kellaway, C. H., and Trethewie, E. R. (1940). Liberation of slow reacting smooth muscle stimulating substance in anaphylaxis. *Q. J. Exp. Physiol., 30*:121-145.

Konig, W., Czarnetzki, B. M., and Lichtenstein, L. M. (1976). Eosinophil chemotactic factor (ECF). II. Release from human polymorphonuclear leukocytes during phagocytosis. *J. Immunol., 117*:234-241.

Lichtenstein, L. M. (1971). The immediate allergic response: in vitro separation of antigen activation, decay and histamine release. *J. Immunol., 107*:1122-1130.

Lichtenstein, L. M. (1975). The mechanism of basophil histamine release induced by antigen and by the calcium ionophore A23187. *J. Immunol., 114*:1692-1699.

Lichtenstein, L. M., and Gillespie, E. (1973). Inhibition of histamine release by histamine controlled by H_2 receptor. *Nature, 244*:287-288.

Lichtenstein, L. M., and Margolis, S. (1968). Histamine release in vitro: Inhibition by catecholamines and methylxanthines. *Science, 161*:902-903.

Lichtenstein, L. M., Gillespie, E., and Bourne, H. (1972). Studies on the biochemical mechanisms of IgE-mediated histamine release. In *The Biological Role of the Immunoglobulin E System.* Edited by K. Ishizaka and D. Dayton, Jr. Washington, D.C., U.S. Government Printing Office, pp. 165-186.

Londos, C., Cooper, D., and Wolff, J. (1980). Subclasses of external adenosine receptors. *Proc. Natl. Acad. Sci., 77*:2551-2554.

Marone, G., Findlay, S., and Lichtenstein, L. M. (1979). Adenosine receptor on human basophils: modulation of histamine release. *J. Immunol., 123*: 1473-1477.

Murphy, R. C., Hammarstrom, S., and Samuelsson, B. (1979). Leukotriene C. A slow-reacting substance from murine mastocytoma cells. *Proc. Natl. Acad. Sci., 76*:4275-4279.

Newball, H. H., and Lichtenstein, L. M. (1981). Mast cells and basophils: effector cells of inflammatory disorders in the lungs. *Thorax, 36*:721-725.

Newball, H. H., Meier, H. L., and Lichtenstein, L. M. (1980). Basophil mediators and their release, with emphasis on BK-A. *J. Invest. Dermatol., 74*:344-348.

Newball, H. H., Talamo, R. C., and Lichtenstein, L. M. (1979). Anaphylactic release of a basophil kallikrein-like activity. II. A mediator of immediate hypersensitivity reactions. *J. Clin. Invest., 64*:466-475.

Newball, H. H., Berninger, R. W., Talamo, R. C., and Lichtenstein, L. M. (1979a). Anaphylactic release of a basophil kallikrein-like activity. I. Purification and characterization. *J. Clin. Invest., 64*:457-465.

Newball, H. H., Meier, H. L., Kaplan, A. P., Revak, S. D., Cochrane, C. G., and Lichtenstein, L. M. (1981). Activation of the Hageman factor dependent systems during IgE-mediated reactions of the human lung. *Int. Arch. Allergy Appl. Immunol., 66*:165-167.

Orning, L., Hammarstrom, S., and Samuelssson, B. (1980). Leukotriene D: A slow reacting substance from rat basophilic leukemia cells. *Proc. Natl. Acad. Sci., 77*:2014-2017.

Ovary, A., Benacerraf, B., and Bloch, K. J. (1963). Properties of guinea pig 7S antibodies. II. Identification of antibodies involved in passive cutaneous and systemic anaphylaxis. *J. Exp. Med. 117*:951-954.

Parker, C. W., Huber, M. M., Hoffman, M. K., and Falkenheim, S. F. (1979). Characterization of the two major species of slow reacting substance from rat basophilic leukemia cells as glutathionyl thioethers of eicosatetraenoic acids oxygenated at the 5 position: Evidence that peroxy groups are present and important for spasmogenic activity. *Prostaglandins 18*:673-686.

Parsons, M. E., Owen, D. A., Ganellin, C. R., and Durant, G. J. (1977). Dimaprit-*S*-3-(*N*,*N*-dimethylamino)propyl isothiourea–a highly specific histamine H_2-receptor agonist. Part 1. Pharmacology. *Agents Action 7*:31-37.

Patterson, R., Irons, J. S., and Harris, K. E. (1975). Potentiating effect of D_2O on the ascaris-induced, reagin-mediated model of asthma in the Rhesus monkey studied with a double aerosolized antigen challenge technique. *Int. Arch. Allergy Appl. Immunol., 48*:412-421.

Peters, S. P., Siegel, M. I., Kagey-Sobotka, A., and Lichtenstein, L. M. (1981). Lipoxygenase products modulate histamine release in human basophils. *Nature 292*:455-457.

Peters, S. P., Schulman, E. S., Schleimer, R. P., MacGlashan, D. W., Jr., Lichtenstein, L. M., and Newball, H. H. (1982). Dispersed human lung mast cell pharmacology. *Am. Rev. Respir. Dis.,* (In Press).

Plaut, M., Lichtenstein, L. M., and Henney, C. S. (1975). Properties of a subpopulation of T cells bearing histamine receptors. *J. Clin. Invest., 55*: 856-874.

Schiffman, E., Corcoran, B., and Wahl, S. M. (1975). N-formyl-methionyl peptides as chemoattractants for leukocytes. *Proc. Natl. Acad. Sci., 72*:1059-1062.

Siraganian, R. P., and Osler, A. G. (1971). Destruction of rabbit platelets in the allergic response of sensitized leukocytes. I. Demonstration of a fluid phase intermediate. *J. Immunol., 106*:1244-1251.

Smith, P. L., Kagey-Sobotka, A., Bleecker, E. R., Traystman, R., Kaplan, A. P., Gralnick, H., Valentine, M. D., Permutt, S., and Lichtenstein, L. M. (1980). Physiologic manifestations of human anaphylaxis. *J. Clin. Invest., 66*:1072-1080.

Sobotka, A. K., Dembo, M., Goldstein, B., and Lichtenstein, L. M. (1979). Antigen-specific desensitization of human basophils. *J. Immunol., 122*: 511-517.

Sullivan, T. J., Parker, K. L., Eisen, S. A., and Parker, C. W. (1975). Modulation of cyclic AMP in purified rat mast cells. II. Studies on the relationship between intracellular cyclic AMP concentrations and histamine release. *J. Immunol., 114*:480-485.

Takahasi, H., Webster, M. E., and Newball, H. H. (1976). Purifications of slow reacting substance of anaphylaxis (SRS-A) from human lung. *J. Immunol.* *117*:1039-1044.

Ting, S., Zweiman, B., Lavker, R., and Dunsky, E. (1981). Histamine suppression of in vivo eosinophil accumulation and histamine release in human allergic reactions. *J. Allergy Clin. Immunol.*, *68*:65-71.

Tung, R., and Lichtenstein, L. M. (1982). *In vitro* histamine release from basophils of asthmatic and atopic individuals in D_2O. *J. Immunol.*, (In Press).

2

Immunopharmacology of Slow-Reacting Substance of Anaphylaxis

CHARLES W. PARKER

Howard Hughes Medical Institute
Washington University School of Medicine
St. Louis, Missouri

I. Introduction

Bronchial asthma is a disease characterized by repeated episodes of rapidly reversible bronchoconstriction. While it has long been assumed that the bronchoconstriction is mediated by a soluble mediator(s), the identity of the mediator(s) has remained uncertain. One of the first candidates to be considered was histamine, which is present in lung and capable of producing marked constriction of bronchial smooth muscle, both in vitro or when administered by aerosol. However, when antihistamines became available for therapy it soon became clear that they were ineffective in bronchial asthma, thus casting doubt on the importance of histamine as a primary mediator of the increase in airway resistance. In the 1960s, attention began to center on possible roles of metabolites of long chain fatty acids such as the prostaglandins (PGs) in the control of airway smooth muscle function. A number of arachidonate (AA) metabolites, including PGE_2, PGA_2, and $PGF_{2\alpha}$, were shown to be present in human lung either under basal conditions or after immunologic or pharmacologic activation (reviewed in Mathe, 1976; Hyman et al., 1978; Newball et al., 1978; Parker, 1979; Adkinson et al., 1980). Later the thromboxanes and prostacyclin were also shown to be generated by human lung (Schulman et al., 1980a,b; 1981, 1982). Prostaglandin

E_2 and $PGF_{2\alpha}$ were found to exert opposing actions in isolated tracheal or bronchial smooth muscle preparations, with PGE_2 producing relaxation and $PGF_{2\alpha}$ producing contraction. These two substances were also demonstrated to be effective via the aerosol route with PGE_2 decreasing (usually) and $PGF_{2\alpha}$ increasing pulmonary resistance. Thromboxane A_2 and breakdown products of $PGF_{2\alpha}$ such as 15-keto-$PGF_{2\alpha}$ also contracted bronchial smooth muscle (Dawson et al., 1974). Not only were these various bronchoconstrictors and bronchodilators present in lung, but many of them were also formed in increased amounts during acute antigen challenge in sensitized lung fragments. In addition, individuals with asthma were found to be extremely sensitive to $PGF_{2\alpha}$ by inhalation suggesting, that $PGF_{2\alpha}$ might be an important mediator of asthmatic paroxysms (Mathe, 1976; Newball and Lenfant, 1977; Newball et al., 1980). However, no evidence was forthcoming to indicate that cycloxygenase inhibitors such as aspirin were effective in the control of asthmatic paroxysms, and, indeed, a subpopulation of asthmatic patients was identified in whom these drugs produced an acute deterioration of airway function. As with the antihistamines, the failure of the cyclooxygenase inhibitors to produce a beneficial response raised serious questions about the importance of cyclooxygenase products as primary mediators of bronchoconstriction. On the other hand, as our laboratory first reported in 1976, the other major pathway of AA metabolsim, the lipoxygenase pathway, is involved in the biosynthesis of slow-reacting substance (SRS), a bronchoconstrictor agent produced de novo in lung during actue immunologic activation. Since SRS is extremely potent as a constrictor of human bronchial smooth muscle (and probably peripheral airway smooth muscle as well), it is probably a key mediator in bronchial asthma, although this remains to be conclusively demonstrated.

II. Historical Background

A. Discovery of SRS

SRS was first described by Feldberg and Kellaway in 1938 as a smooth muscle contracting activity released during the perfusion of guinea pig lungs with cobra venom (reviewed in Parker, 1979). In 1940 Kellaway and Trethewie reported the production of a substance with similar properties during perfusion of sensitized guinea pig lungs with antigen. Using isolated guinea pig ileal smooth muscle strips as a bioassay system for SRS, Brocklehurst (1960) clearly differentiated the SRS activity from histamine by the failure of the contractile response to be inhibited by antihistamines and the characteristics of the contractile response itself, which developed slowly and was sustained for many minutes without tachyphylaxis. Subsequent progress was impeded by the marked lability of the SRS molecule and the inherent lack of precision and specificity of the bioassays required for its detection and measurement. Nonetheless, considerable information accumulated. SRS was shown to be produced by a variety of tissues including human, guinea pig, rabbit, monkey, calf and pig lung fragments, perfused guinea pig lungs, human and monkey bronchial lavage cells, human nasal polyps, perfused cat paws, mixed human peripheral blood leukocytes, human polymorphonuclear leukocytes, leukemic basophils and rat peritoneal mononuclear cells (Anggard et al., 1963; Patterson and Suszko, 1971; Strandberg and Uvnäs, 1971; Bach and Brashler, 1974; Grant and Lichtenstein, 1974; Lewis et al., 1974; Burka and Eyre, 1975; Takahashi et al., 1976; Parker, 1979). SRS responses were found to be initiated by IgE or IgG_1 antibodies as well as by a variety of nonimmunologic stimuli such as compound 48/80 (a polycation) and A23187 (a divalent cation ionophore) (Orange and Austen, 1969; Ishizaka et al., 1971).

Interest in the possible role of SRS in allergic bronchoconstriction in man was stimulated by Brocklehurst (1962) who showed that SRS contracts human tracheal-bronchial smooth muscle preparations and by similar observations by Collier and James (1966) in guinea pig respiratory muscle preparations. In addition, crude aerosolized preparations of SRS were observed to affect airway function in vivo in asthmatic patients although not in control subjects (Herxheimer and Stresemann, 1963). It was later shown that human lung fragments sensitized with serum containing reaginic antibodies produce SRS in response to environmental antigens (Lewis et al., 1974). Taken together with evidence that anti-IgE antibodies can generate SRS in sensitized human or monkey tissues (Ishizaka et al., 1971), this strongly suggested that SRS might well be produced during IgE-mediated allergic reactions in vivo.

Based on these and other studies, it became increasingly clear that SRS was probably important in the pathogenesis of bronchial asthma. However, in other respects the status of the SRS field was quite unsatisfactory in that after more than 3 decades of research the molecule had not been purified to homogeneity. Moreover, while SRS had been characterized as a labile acidic lipid more subject to inactivation at acid than at alkaline pH, no definitive information was available in regard to either its structure or mechanism of biosynthesis.

Our own involvement in the SRS field began in 1975. We felt that one of the reasons for the slow rate of progress was the limited quantities of material available and the heterogeneity of the tissues from which it was being purified. We therefore, sought to identify a cell line that could be maintained in tissue culture and from which SRS could be produced in relatively large quantities. Since SRS is produced during IgE-mediated reactions, we studied a line of rat basophilic leukemia cells (RBL-1) which has receptors for IgE immunoglobulins, (Kulczycki et al., 1974). While immunologic stimuli were ineffective, the divalent cation ionophore A23187 generated substantial amounts of SRS-like activity from these cells (Jakschik and Parker, 1976; Jakschik et al., 1977b). This activity was very similar to or identical with SRS from other sources with respect to all of the criteria then available, including chromatographic behavior as a relatively polar acidic lipid, the nature and spectrum of the smooth muscle-contracting activities, and susceptibility of the spasmogen to inhibition by either aryl sulfatase or the selective SRS antagonist, FPL-55712. Thus, it appeared that we were in fact studying a molecule that was very similar or identical to previously described SRSs and that RBL-1 cells would provide a better source of SRS than had previously been available. Indeed, it was in the RBL-1 cell line and its mouse mastocytosis cell variant (Siraganian and Metzger, 1978) that the structure of naturally occurring forms of SRS was later first defined (see below). Using the RBL-1 cell systems, we went on to show that SRS was a metabolite of AA produced through the lipoxygenase pathway and that it had a sulfur-containing side chain. Later studies by ourselves and other laboratories led to the recognition of the essential features of SRS structure. The structure was completely determined by comparing naturally occurring SRS's with candidate SRSs with various double-bond configurations prepared by organic synthesis. The first portion of this chapter will review the work leading to the elucidation of SRS structure. Later in the chapter, the biosynthesis, metabolism, and biologic activity of SRS will be discussed.

B. Identification of Arachidonate as an SRS Precursor

Once a convenient source of SRS had been identified, we next attempted to identify its biosynthetic precursors (reviewed in Parker, 1980d, 1981). Since the amounts of SRS produced are small, even in RBL-1 cells, the existing purification methods for SRS had to be improved before incorporation of radiolabel could be convincingly demonstrated. The work proceeded slowly and with considerable difficulty. Since SRS was thought to be an acidic lipid, considerable emphasis was given to the possible involvement of long-chain fatty acids in SRS synthesis. One approach was to add inhibitors of fatty acid metabolism at the time the SRS was generated and determine whether the yield of spasmogenic activity was altered. A second approach was to produce SRS in the presence of radiolabeled fatty acids, sugars, and amino acids and determine if radioactivity comigrated with SRS after extensive chormatographic purification. From this work, convincing evidence was obtained that AA was an SRS precursor (Jakschik et al., 1977a). Low concentrations of eicosatetraenoic acid (ETYA), a C_{20} analog of arachidonic acid that has triple bonds instead of double bonds at the 5, 8, 11, and 14 positions, almost completely inhibited SRS biosynthesis. AA itself, when added exogenously to the tissue culture medium at the same time as A23187, produced severalfold increases in SRS biosynthesis (Jakschik et al., 1977a). Other long-chain fatty acids–including dihomo-γ-linolenic acid (8,11,14,eicosatetraenoic acid), a C_{20} fatty acid which lacks only the 5 double bond of AA–were ineffective or inhibited SRS formation. In addition, incorporation of radioactive AA into SRS could be demonstrated. SRS was generated in

RBL-1 cells which had been preincubated either overnight or for much shorter time periods with ^3H- or ^{14}C-labeled AA (Jakschik et al., 1977a). The SRS was then extensively purified by column and preparative thin-layer chromatography (TLC). Regardless of the preincubation time, significant amounts of radioactivity still comigrated with SRS at the completion of the purification procedure. Comigration of spasmogenic activity and radioactivity was further demonstrated in a variety of chromatographic systems, establishing convincingly that SRS is derived from AA. The radiochemical purity of these preparations was later confirmed by high-pressure liquid chromatography (HPLC). In contrast to AA, other long chain fatty acids did not incorporate their radioactivity into SRS.

The evidence from our laboratory that AA is an SRS precursor in RBL-1 cells was reported originally in 1976 at the plenary session of the Central Society for Clinical Investigation in Chicago (Jakschik and Parker, 1976) and in March 1977 at the plenary session of the International Prostaglandin meetings in Vail, Colorado (Jakschik and Parker, 1977c). Detailed reports of the work appeared later in 1977 (Jakschik et al., 1977a; Jakschik et al., 1977b).

C. Identification of SRS as a Lipoxygenase Product

The lipoxygenase and the cyclooxygenase pathways are the two major pathways of AA metabolism in mammalian cells (Fig. 1). To determine which of these pathways is involved in SRS biosynthesis, the effect of indomethacin, a selective inhibitor of the cyclooxygenase pathway, was studied in A23187-stimulated RBL-1 cells.

The generation of SRS was unaffected or even enhanced by indomethacin (Jakschik et al., 1977a) under conditions in which PGD_2 formation could be shown to be markedly decreased. This strongly suggested that SRS was a product of the lipoxygenase pathway (Parker, 1977, 1979; Jakschik et al., 1977a). Moreover, when SRS biosynthesis was stimulated by A23187 with radiolabeled AA present, up to 5% of the radiolabel was incorporated into a product cochromatographing in a number of TLC systems with 5-hydroxy-6,8,11,14-eicosatetraenoic acid (5-HETE), a lipoxygenase product that had just been described in rabbit neutrophils (Borgeat et al., 1976). When A23187 was absent, very little or no 5-HETE was produced, indicating that the lipoxygenase pathway was being stimulated by this agent.

The production of 5-HETE by both RBL-1 cells and neutrophils was of considerable interest since neutrophils also produce SRS (Conroy et al., 1976). By contrast, the major lipoxygenase product in human platelets is 12-hydroxy-5,8,10,14-eicosatetraenoic acid (12-HETE), not 5-HETE, and these cells could not be shown to produce SRS in response to A23187. Finally, as already discussed, 8,11,14-eicosatrienoic acid, which is identical to AA structurally except for the absence of the 5 double bond, was apparently not an effective SRS precursor in RBL-1 cells (Jakschik et al., 1977a), indicating that the 5 double bond

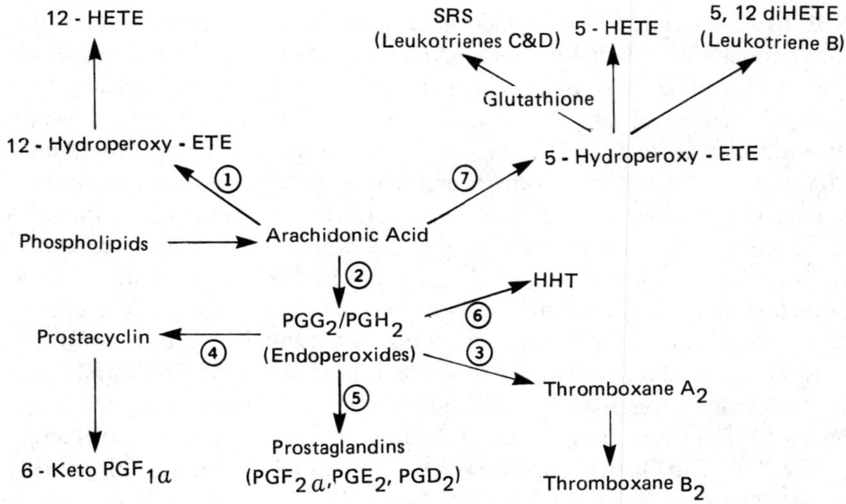

Figure 1 Pathways of arachidonate metabolism. (Modified from Parker, 1979c.)

is crucial for SRS biosynthesis. Taking these various lines of evidence together, in the Proceedings of the Second International Symposium on Bronchial Asthma in 1977, I indicated that SRS is a product of a 5-lipoxygenase (Fig. 1) (Parker, 1977). This was later verified by several additional lines of evidence, including direct structural studies of the SRS molecule.

Even though the evidence that SRS was a lipoxygenase product was convincing, the pathway involved was clearly a quantitatively minor one from the point of view of overall SRS metabolism (Parker, 1981). Only 0.1–0.5% of the radioactivity from [1-^{14}C] AA was recovered in chromatographically purified SRS in contrast to PGD_2 and 5-HETE, which together accounted for about 10% of the total AA radioactivity originally added to the cells. This low level of incorporation taken with the marked lability of the SRS molecule, and the difficulty in isolating SRS from heterogenous tissues such as lung, almost certainly explains why several laboratories were initially unable to confirm that AA is an SRS precursor. The first apparent confirmation was by Bach and his colleagues (Bach et al., 1977) who reported that SRS from rat peritoneal mononuclear cells could be radiolabeled with [^{14}C] AA. However, their observations were quite preliminary and they later reported that they were unable to confirm their own earlier observations in this system (Bach et al., 1979). They did find that ETYA inhibited SRS synthesis, as we had reported earlier for RBL-1 cells. However, based on studies with indomethacin and a newly developed thromboxane synthetase inhibitor, they suggested that the cyclooxygenase instead of the lipoxygenase pathway was involved (Bach et al., 1977).

D. Characterization of SRS as a Thioether

During our screening studies for possible SRS precursors with various radiolabeled compounds, [^{35}S] cysteine and [^{35}S] methionine were also shown to be incorporated into the SRS molecule. This result was reported briefly in 1978 (Parker, 1979) and in more detail in the spring of 1979, at meetings of the Federation of American Societies for Experimental Biology in Atlanta in April (Parker et al., 1979b) and the American Society for Clinical Investigation in Washington in early May (Parker et al., 1979a). Most of the basic information was summarized in our abstracts appearing before these meetings, although considerably more detail and some entirely new information was brought out in the presentations themselves. A more detailed report was published in the summer of 1979 (Parker et al., 1979d). RBL-1 cells were grown for 16 hr in tissue culture medium with [^{35}S] cysteine or [^{35}S] methionine, and SRS was generated with A23187. Using our usual chromatographic purification for SRS purification in combination with reverse-phase HPLC on C-18 reverse-phase columns, three distinct SRS species, each containing ^{35}S radioactivity, were obtained. This not only showed that the SRS molecule contains sulfur but also confirmed earlier evidence that SRS is heterogeneous (Takahashi et al., 1976; Jakschik et al., 1977a). The three SRS species were arbitrarily designed as types I, II, and III representing approximately 50%, 35%, and 15% (or less), respectively, of the total spasmogenic activity recovered (Parker et al., 1979b). When SRS preparations labeled with [^{14}C] AA or [^{35}C] cysteine were compared, their behavior on reverse-phase HPLC columns and other chromatographic systems was apparently identical. Moreover, when the spasmogenic activity of the SRS was inactivated by boiling in dilute acid the chromatographic behavior of the ^{35}S and ^{14}C radiolabels was altered in parallel, confirming that the labels were actually contained in the biologically active molecule (Parker, 1981). The overall yields of SRS activity during the SRS purification were as high as 50%, making it highly likely that the most active SRS species were being recovered.

The ^{35}S incorporation studies by our laboratory provided the first convincing evidence that the SRS molecule contains sulfur (Parker et al., 1979d; Parker, 1980d; Parker, 1981). Orange et al., (1974) had previously reported that the SRS molecule was susceptible to inactivation by aryl sulfatase B, suggesting the possible presence of a sulfate ester group in the molecule. However, as we later showed, the inactivation by aryl sulfatase is not due to cleavage of sulfate from the remainder of the SRS molecule but to degradation of its oligopeptide side chain by a contaminating protease present in commercial preparations of the enzyme as well as other still undefined changes in the SRS molecule probably involving its double-bond structure (Parker et al., 1980c). While microanalytical data also were presented as support for the presence of sulfur (Orange et al., 1974), it is clear in retrospect that samples did not even remotely resemble any of the presently known SRS species and must have been highly contaminated.

Later investigators also suggested that SRS might contain sulfur based on an ability of exogenous thiols added to the medium at the time of SRS biosynthesis to enhance the SRS response in human lung fragments and rat peritoneal mononuclear cells (Orange and Chang, 1975; Orange and Moore, 1976; Bach and Brashler, 1978). However, it is now clear that under the conditions of their experiments these exogenous thiols are not incorporated as such into the SRS molecule (Parker et al., 1979c). While the basis for the enhancing effect of thiols is still not completely clear, it appears that they may be acting to decrease SRS breakdown by peptidases (Sok et al., 1980). In any event, it is apparent that none of the reasons for originally suspecting that the SRS molecule might contain sulfur was valid.

Our ^{35}S incorporation studies demonstrating that each of the three SRS types contain sulfur, taken in conjunction with the earlier evidence that SRS is a lipoxygenase product (Jakschik et al., 1977a; Parker, 1977), was of considerable interest since Gardner and his colleagues had recently reported that analogs of cysteine form thioether adducts with lipid hydroperoxides (Gardner et al., 1977). However, to verify that a similar reaction was occuring during SRS biosynthesis, it was necessary that the purified SRS molecule be characterized structurally. Since our initial attempts at direct mass spectroscopy of purified SRS had been unsuccessful, we decided to degrade the SRS molecule chemically. In our presentation at the American Society for Clinical investigation in early May of 1979, in Washington, we reported that both of the two major SRS species could be degraded by chemicals that cleave thioether bonds, including Raney nickel, cyanogen bromide, and sodium metal in liquid ammonias, as indicated by dissociation of the ^{14}C and ^{35}S labels by TLC when the SRS was reacted with these reagents and then chromatographed (Parker et al., 1979a,b,c). The results with cyanogen bromide were of particular importance, since it is far more selective for thioether bonds than the other agents. Based on TLC and column chromatographic studies of the sodium metal cleavage product, the side chain was not cysteine itself but one of its metabolites.

During the same presentation in Washington, we also reported that when either of the major SRS species was labeled with ^{14}C from [1-^{14}C] AA and degraded with sodium metal in liquid ammonia the major radioactive product was an acidic lipid which migrated very similarly to 5-HETE in several TLC systems. An unsubstituted C-20 fatty acid was also present, apparently due to loss of the 5-OH group from the 5-HETE during or subsequent to cleavage. Since 5-lipoxygenases introduce oxygen at the 5-position of the AA molecule, the recovery of 5-HETE following SRS cleavage provided the first direct structural confirmation that SRS is a 5-lipoxygenase product. At the presentation in Washington, some information was also reported in regarded to the double bond structure of SRS. Each of the two major SRS species from RBL-1 cells had an ultraviolet absorbancy maximum at 280 nm before degradation as described for SRS isolated from guinea pig lungs perfused with antigen (Morris et al., 1978). Both acidic lipid cleavage products also had this ultraviolet absorbancy, indicating that the absorbancy was in the lipid portion of the SRS molecule which in turn suggested the presence of three conjugated double bonds. We later demonstrated that after further reduction of the cleavage products with hydrazine, and analysis by mass spectroscopy, 5-hydroxyarachidic acid could be identified, establishing conclusively that both of the major SRS species have a fatty acid core with 20 carbons and an oxygen group at the 5 position (Parker et al., 1979c).

About 1 month after this second oral presentation by our laboratory, our results were confirmed and significantly extended by Samuelsson and his colleagues in an oral presentation at the International Prostaglandin Meetings in Washington (Murphy et al., 1979; Samuelsson et al., 1979). SRS from mouse mastocytoma cells stimulated with A23187 was shown to incorporate radiolabel from AA and cysteine, in accord with our earlier results with SRS from RBL-1 cells reacted with the same reagent. After treatment of the SRS molecule with Raney nickel, a nonspecific reducing agent, 5-hydroxyarachidic acid was identified by mass spectroscopy. Digestion with soybean lipoxygenase, which had been reported previously to inactivate SRS (Sirois, 1979), produced an increase in ultraviolet absorbancy at 308 nm which taken together with the results of ozonolysis and the original 280-nm absorption maximum in undigested SRS, indicated that the double bonds were at the 7, 9, 11, and 14 positions and the sulfur-containing side chain was at the 6 position. Although important new information was provided in their presentation, several of their major observations were confirmatory and in a number of respects their data were more preliminary than our own (Parker, 1980d; Parker, 1981). The only thioether cleavage reagent that was used, Raney nickel, is highly nonspecific and therefore capable of cleaving a variety of sulfur-containing bonds, including sulfones and sulfoxides. The side chain was stated to be cysteine (Samuelson et al., 1979), which we had already shown to not be true as reported briefly in May and September 1979 and in more detail later that same year (Parker et al., 1979c; Parker 1980a). Moreover, no data were given on the critical issue of SRS yields during purification. Only a single SRS species was studied, and no attempt was made to show that as the SRS was inactivated, decreases of SRS spasmogenic activity were associated with an alteration in the chromatographic behavior of the radiolabel, thus verifying that the radioactivity was indeed present in the SRS molecule.

Amino acid composition and column and thin-layer chromatography studies which elucidated the true nature of the sulfur-containing side chains of SRS were first reported by our laboratory at the International Meeting on Prostaglandins in Paris in September 1979 (Parker, 1980a) and in more detail in the November 1979 issue of *Prostaglandins* (Parker et al., 1979c). The most polar form of SRS, type II, contained 0.91 mol of glutamic acid, 0.97 mol of glycine, and 0.21 mol of cysteine (as 1/2 cystine) per mole of SRS. Apart from the low yield of cysteine, presumably due to attachment of the fatty acid, the amino acid composition strongly suggested that the side chain of this form of SRS was glutathione, the predominant thiol inside cells, although no amino acid-sequencing studies were actually performed. This was confirmed by TLC and column chromatographic studies of the sulfur-containing side chain after its cleavage with sodium metal cleavage. Type I, the major nonpolar SRS species in RBL-1 cells (and the predominant form of SRS where these cells are stimulated with A23187 for 15 min at 37°C), contained 0.85 mol of glycine, 0.30 mol of glutamic acid, and 0.14 mol of cysteine (Parker et al., 1979c). Its side chain, therefore appeared to be a mixture of cysteinyl-glycine with smaller amounts of glutathione, although other interpretations also had to be considered. Subsequent studies confirmed that variable amounts of glutathionyl SRS were present in our type-I SRS preparations. With minor adjustments in the purification procedure, preparations with very little or no glutamic acid and approximately 1 mol of glycine/mole of SRS were obtained, confirming that this species of SRS has a cysteinyl-glycyl side chain (Parker, 1980b; Watanabe-Kohno and Parker, 1980; Parker, 1981). Based on the susceptibility of SRS to partial inactivation with mild reducing agents, we also suggested that SRS might contain a reducible function important for activity such as masked peroxy group (Parker et al., 1979c). However, the evidence was indirect, and because quantities of SRS were very small and no synthetic material was available for comparison, definitive studies were not feasible.

E. Complete Determination of SRS Structure and Its Preparation by Organic Synthesis

Subsequent studies by other laboratories confirmed the existence of the cysteinyl-glycine and glutathionyl forms of SRS by amino acid sequence and composition analysis and organic synthesis. Hammarström et al. (1979) reported that the major species of SRS from mouse mastocytoma cells has a glutathionyl side chain. The mouse mastocytoma SRS was compared with various synthetic products prepared in Corey's laboratory with respect to chromatographic behavior and spasmogenic activity on guinea pig ileal strips. It was concluded that the major SRS species from the mastocytoma cells was 6-*S*-glutathionyl-5-hydroxy-7,9(*trans*), 11, 14(*cis*)eicosatetraenoic acid. This was the first complete structural elucidation of an SRS molecule. After we had reported that one of the SRS species had a glutathionyl side chain in September 1979 (Parker 1980a), Rokasch and his colleagues at Merck had independently undertaken the synthesis of several SRS isomers with glutathionyl side chains. They also obtained evidence that glutathionyl SRS was indistinguishable from naturally occurring SRS as a spasmogen, and that the most active species had 7, 9(*trans*), 11, 14(*cis*) double bonds (Rokasch et al., 1980). Morris and his colleagues (1980) and

Örning et al. (1980) both concluded that the major species of SRS from RBL-1 cells has a cysteinyl-glycyl side chain. In the study by Morris et al. (1980), the first successful mass spectroscopy studies of an intact SRS molecule were presented. In addition, as we first reported at the Kroch Foundation Meetings in May 1980, there is still another form of SRS which has only cysteine in its side chain (Parker, 1980b; Parker et al., 1980a). This has been confirmed by Lewis et al. (1980b) and Sok et al. (1980). In addition to the three known SRS species, which differ in regard to their oligopeptide side chains, naturally occurring SRSs, which differ in their double bond numbers or configurations, have been identified. Included in this group is an SRS with an 11-*trans* instead of an 11-*cis* double bond (Clark et al., 1980) and an SRS with five instead of four double bonds (Hammarström, 1980). In addition SRSs with their sulfur-containing side chains at the 12 position instead of at the 6 position have been obtained biosynthetically in our laboratory, although they apparently have very little biologic activity. Whether there are active SRSs which differ in the oxidation state of their sulfur is less clear. Ohnish et al. (1980) have suggested that the major form of the SRS produced in sensitized guinea pig lungs is a sulfone, not a sulfide. On the other hand, their evidence is indirect and it is not clear that they have excluded the possibility of oxidation of their SRS during purification. Our own studies indicate that there are sulfone groups (or some other form of oxidized sulfur) present in some SRS preparations from RBL-1 cells, particularly in the glutathionyl form of SRS, but the SRS with oxidized sulfur is not the predominant product arising during purification of SRS (C. W. Parker, M. M. Huber, and S. F. Falkenhein, 1981, in preparation). We therefore continue to feel that the major SRS species are indeed sulfides. We have now found synthetic LTD^4 obtained from Dr. Rokasch is as susceptible to chemical reduction as our cysteinyl-glycyl SRS from RBL-1 cells, so there is probably no need to postulate an additional reducible function in the SRS molecule apart from the conjugated double-bond system itself. Nonetheless, the possibility of an unexpected rearrangement of the molecule probably still needs to be kept in mind (Parker, 1980d; Parker et al., 1980a; Parker, 1981).

It is apparent that there are a number of biologically active SRS species, raising the question of what the most appropriate and unambiguous nomenclature for these molecules is. Because leukocytes make SRS and the SRS molecules contain three conjugated double bonds, Samuelsson and Hammarström (1980) have proposed that the usual forms of glutathionyl, cysteinyl-glycyl, and cysteinyl SRS be termed leukotrienes C_4, D_4, and E_4 respectively (LTC_4, LTD_4, and LTE_4) with the number 4 denoting the total number of double bonds. SRSs with larger or smaller numbers of double bonds would be designated by a change in the number. Since mast cells also make SRS and the most active forms of SRS are tetraenes, not trienes, I personally feel that this nomenclature leaves something to be desired (Parker et al., 1980a), but it seems to be becoming ingrained to some extent in the literature and does have the virtue of brevity.

F. Further Evidence Linking SRS to the Lipoxygenase Pathway

The structural studies indicating that SRS contains an oxygen atom at the 5 position strongly supported a possible role of a 5-lipoxygenase in SRS synthesis. Nonetheless there are a variety of possible mechanisms for introducing oxygen into unsaturated fatty acids and more definitive evidence was needed (Parker et al., 1980e; Falkenhein et al., 1980; Parker, 1981). Since the oxygen introduced by lipoxygenase is from molecular oxygen, we produced SRS biosynthetically in the presence of $^{18}O_2$, and purified the SRS in the usual way. After degradation of the purified SRS with sodium metal and hydrazine, ^{18}O was identified by mass spectroscopy at the 5 position at an isotope abundance close to that of the O_2 on the original reaction mixture, demonstrating that the 5 oxygen in SRS is derived from molecular oxygen (Parker et al., 1979c). We also showed that the lipoxygenase inhibitors, nordihydroguaiaretic acid and pyrogallol, inhibited the formation of SRS and two known lipoxygenase products, 5-HETE and 5,12-dihydroxy-6,8,10,14-eicosatetraenoic acid (5,12-di-HETE, leukotriene B) to a similar extent (Falkenhein et al., 1980). Moreover, when the initial 5-lipoxygenase product, 5-hydroperoxy-eicosatetraenoic acid (5-HPETE), was synthesized and added to RBL-1 cell suspensions, SRS synthesis was markedly stimulated, even in the absence of A23187 (Falkenhein et al., 1980). Furthermore, RBL-1 cells incubated with [1-^{14}C] 5-HPETE incorporated a portion of their radioactivity into SRS as indicated by comigration of spasmogenic activity and radioactivity despite extensive chromatographic purification (Parker et al., 1980e). These observations provided strong additional evidence that SRS is a 5-lipoxygenase product. Since 5-HPETE stimulates SRS formation in the absence of A23187, it appears the major action of A23187 is to increase the availability of 5-HPETE rather than to promote its reaction with thiols. Based on chemical considerations Murphy et al. (1979) and Radmark et al. (1980) have suggested that the actual reactive fatty acid intermediate is the 5,6-epoxide (leukotriene A), an unstable but highly raactive product formed by rearrangement of the 5-hydroperoxide.

Since A23187 releases free AA from phospholipids in RBL-1 cells, one of its actions in stimulating SRS biosynthetesis is to increase the availability of nonesterified AA to the 5-lipoxygenase. However, when graded amounts of AA are added exogenously to RBL-1 cells in the absence of A23187, relatively little SRS and other lipoxygenase products are produced. This suggests that A23187 must also be activating the 5-lipoxygenase. Since A23187 promotes the transfer of divalent cations into and out of cells and Ca^{2+} must be present in the medium for stimulation of lipoxygenase product formation, this response may well be mediated by Ca^{2+}. In accord with this possibility, Jakschik et al. (1980) have presented evidence that the lipoxygenase in the cytosol of RBL-1 cells is markedly stimulated by Ca^{2+}. Our own data are very similar. It is not yet clear whether the Ca^{2+} is acting directly on the enzyme or indirectly through other proteins present in the cytosol, such as calmodulin.

III. Metabolism of SRS

We originally suggested that the cysteinyl-glycyl form of SRS (type I, LTD_4) might arise from the glutathionyl form (type II, LTC_4) by the action of γ-glutamyltranspeptidase, an enzyme that is widely distributed in tissue and cleaves the γ-glutamyl linkage in glutathione (Parker et al., 1979c; Parker et al., 1980a; Parker, 1981) (Fig. 2). Indeed, when the relative amounts of the cysteinyl-glycyl and glutathionyl forms of SRS were compared at various times after stimulation of RBL-1 cells with A23187, it was found that glutathionyl SRS was the most prominent species in the first few minutes of the reaction, whereas cysteinyl-glycyl SRS predominated at 10–20 min (Parker et al., 1980a). In addition, it was possible to show that purified LTC_4 was rapidly converted to LTD_4 by RBL-1 cells. It was also found that partially purified γ-glutamyl transpeptidase cleaves the γ-glutamyl group from glutathionyl SRS (Parker et al., 1980a) as shown independently by Örning et al. (1980).

In addition to enzymatic cleavage of the γ-glutamyl group of LTC_4, the glycyl residue of cysteinyl-glycyl SRS (and possibly glutathionyl SRS) can be removed, explaining the presence of cysteinyl SRS under natural conditions of SRS biosynthesis in vitro (see above), particularly when relatively long incubation times are used (Parker, 1980b; Parker et al., 1980a). Purified LTD_4 was found to be converted by RBL-1 cells to cysteinyl SRS (LTE_4), which has about 10% of the spasmogenic activity of LTD-4. This conversion took place over a period of many minutes, but by 60 min only the cysteinyl SRS was present. We have also found that human plasma converts glutathionyl and cysteinyl-glycyl SRS to cysteinyl SRS with changes occurring at high plasma dilutions as well as in undiluted plasma (Parker et al., 1980d). Commercial preparations of limpet type-B aryl sulfatase also remove the glycine residue from LTC_4 and LTD_4, apparently due to a contaminating peptidase. This, at least in part, explains the partial inactivation of SRS by this enzyme (Parker et al., 1980c), although apparently there is an additional action which may involve either an oxidation or double-bond isomerization of the SRS molecule. The peptidases involved in these various inactivations remain to be adequately defined.

While it is clear that degradation of the oligopeptide side chain of SRS is a major pathway for SRS degradation, other pathways need to be considered (Parker, 1981). It is already known that SRS is partially or completely inactivated by lipoxygenases (Sirois, 1979) and peroxidases (Henderson and Kaliner, 1979)

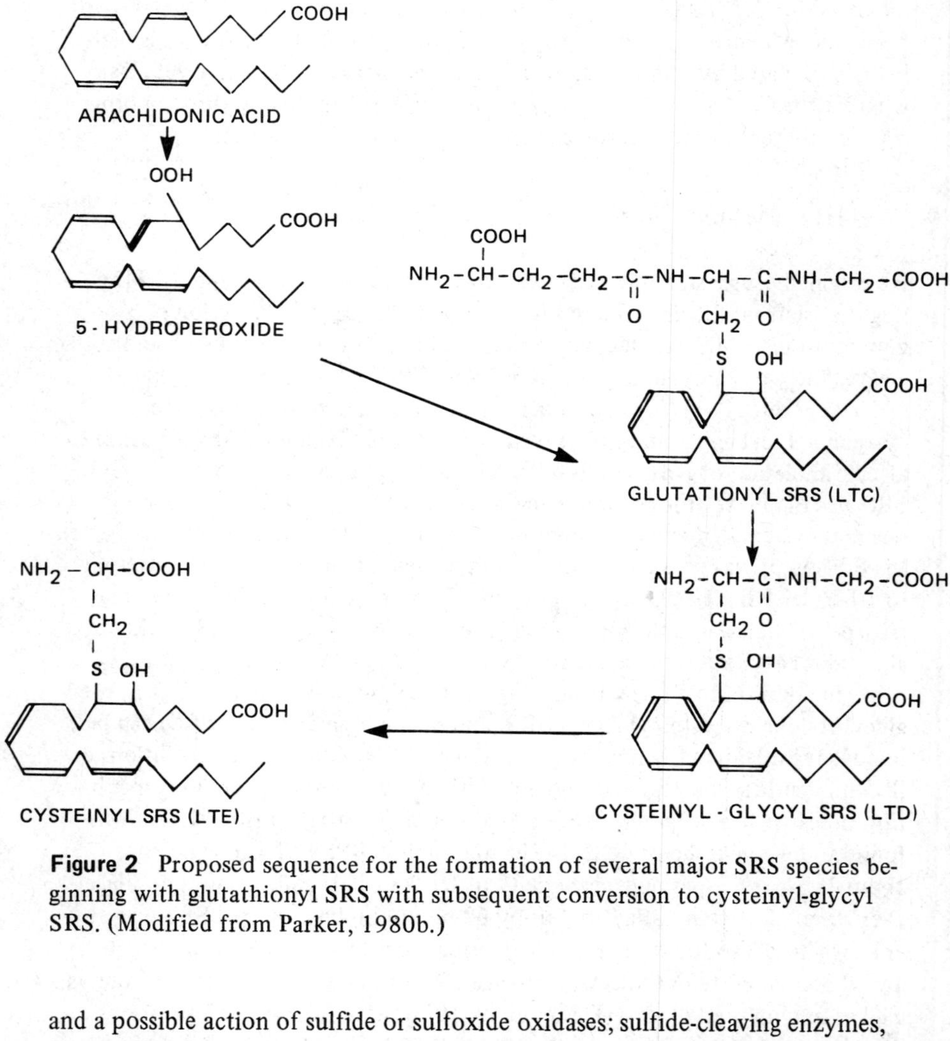

Figure 2 Proposed sequence for the formation of several major SRS species beginning with glutathionyl SRS with subsequent conversion to cysteinyl-glycyl SRS. (Modified from Parker, 1980b.)

and a possible action of sulfide or sulfoxide oxidases; sulfide-cleaving enzymes, fatty acid reductases, or isomerases also need to be considered. As far as possible sources of SRS-inactivating enzymes in vivo are concerned, it appears that RBL-1 cells (and therefore presumably basophils) (Parker et al., 1980a), macrophages (Paterson and Craig, 1979), eosinophils (Wasserman et al., 1975), and plasma (Parker et al., 1980d) all inactivate SRS. Since several of the enzymes that inactivate SRS are widely distributed, it seems likely that many tissues will turn out to have this capability.

IV. Generation of SRS

A. Immunologically Generated SRS from Lung

While the above studies provided structural information on nonimmunologically produced forms of SRS, it was still necessary to study the SRSs produced during allergic responses, since it was by no means certain that they would be identical or even closely related. This subject was investigated by Watanabe-Kohno and myself with SRS from antigen-stimulated, guinea pig lung fragments. Guinea pigs were immunized with bovine IgG in adjuvant and lung fragments were prepared after 4–6 weeks, stimulated with antigen for various time periods, and studied for SRS biosynthesis. When animals are immunized using this experimental protocol, the lung fragments undergo a typical anaphylactic reaction although the sensitizing antibody is an IgG_1 not an IgE antibody. As in the RBL-1 cell suspension system, SRS biosynthesis in the lung fragment system was enhanced by AA but not by other long-chain fatty acids (Watanabe-Kohno and Parker, 1980). Moreover, in accord with the previously published results of Hitchcock (1978) in the same species, ETYA was inhibitory although the inhibition was considerably less impressive than in RBL-1 cell suspensions possibly because of less effective penetration of the reagent. Another similarity to the RBL-1 cell system was that indomethacin enhanced SRS synthesis, as had been reported some years previously in lungs perfused with antigen (Walker 1973; Burka and Eyre, 1975a,b), although the explanation at that time was not apparent. Initially we were unable to demonstrate that radiolabel from radioactive AA was incorporated into the guinea pig lung SRS. However, with refinements in the original purification procedure of Watanabe and Koda (1979), we were eventually able to recover 50% of the original spasmogenic activity in the lung SRS purification and show unequivocally that a small percentage of the original AA radioactivity (0.03%) was incorporated into the molecule. By purifying batches of SRS from 100 or more animals, further characterization of the immunologically generated SRS was possible. It proved to be very similar or identical to the cys-gly SRS product (type I, LTD_4) from A23187-stimulated RBL-1 cells in regard to its behavior on C-18 reverse-phase HPLC columns, absorption spectrum in the presence and absence of soybean lipoxygenase, molar spasmogenic activity on guinea pig ileal smooth muscle strips, and amino acid composition (Watanabe-Kohno and Parker, 1980; Parker, 1981). Moreover, as with the RBL-1 cell SRS, 5-hydroxyarachidic acid could be identified by mass spectroscopy after cleavage with sodium metal and further reduction, indicating that their fatty acid cores were identical. Because of the excellent overall recovery of SRS activity during the purification, there was little doubt that the most active SRS species was being characterized. However, while the cysteinyl-glycyl form of SRS (LTD_4) was clearly the predominant form of SRS, only a single incubation time with antigen (20 min) was used in our structural characterization studies. Judging from the kinetic studies in RBL-1 cells described above, it seems likely that the glutathionyl or cysteinyl forms of SRS (LTC_4 and LTE_4) would have been more prominent if shorter or longer incubation times with antigen had been utilized.

While no overall recovery values were given, based primarily on mass spectroscopic studies of the purified SRS molecule Morris et al. (1980) also concluded that the SRS from guinea pig lungs perfused with antigen is predominantly in the cysteinyl-glycyl form. Lewis et al. (1980a) have reported the isolation of cysteinyl-glycyl SRS from antigen-stimulated human lung fragment suspensions, but the recovery of spasmogenic activity was only 6% and was only given subsequent to the Amberlite XAD-8 column purification step, so it may have been even lower. Moreover, the identification of the human SRS was based primarily on its HPLC behavior. No amino acid analysis or mass spectroscopic data were given. Indeed, when synthetic cysteinyl-glycyl SRS and the presumed cysteinyl-glycyl SRS from human lung were compared in regard to their spasmogenic activities in several bioassay systems, some puzzling inconsistencies were observed. In view of these inconsistencies and the very poor recovery of spasmogenic activity, further studies are needed.

B. SRS from Other Sources

Our laboratory has also studied the role of AA in SRS biosynthesis in A23187-stimulated rat peritoneal mast cells and human myelogenous leukemia cells rich in apparently mature basophils. In each system, ETYA inhibited and AA increased SRS release (Yecies et al., 1979a,b,c,d). Moreover, when either cell type was stimulated with A23187 in the presence of [^{14}C] or ^{3}H[AA] and the SRS was purified, incorporation of radioactivity into SRS could be shown. The behavior of these SRSs on HPLC columns was indistinguishable from that of the major RBL-1 cell SRS product. Thus, while the structure of these SRSs has not yet been evaluated by mass spectroscopy or amino acid analysis, there is good reason to believe that they are very similar or identical to other forms of SRS. Human polymorphonuclear leukocytes (Conroy et al., 1976) and murine peritoneal monocytes or macrophages (Bach et al., 1979; Rouzer et al., 1980) also make SRS. The major SRS species from rat peritoneal monocytes are apparently LTC_4 and LTD_4 (Bach et al., 1980a,b; Rouzer et al., 1980). Other organs such as the liver and kidney have also been reported to make SRS (Benveniste, 1980), but this may be due to their leukocyte or mast cell content and the SRS has not yet been adequately characterized in any case. We have preliminary evidence that lymphocytes probably make small amounts of SRS but further studies are needed. Lewis et al. (1980a) have reported that rats injected intraperitoneally with anti-IgGa antibody make both glutathionyl and cysteinyl-glycyl SRS, based primarily on chromatographic studies.

The cell source(s) of SRS in IgE-mediated reactions in human and animal lungs remains to be established. While mast cells and basophils (or at least the basophilic cell line, RBL-1) both make SRS in response to A23187, we and others have been unable to demonstrate convincingly an SRS response in immunologically stimulated rat peritoneal mast cells, even though these cells readily release histamine. While it is possible that some cofactor necessary for SRS generation is lacking after mast cells have been extensively purified, other cell types such as macrophages or even neutrophils need to be considered as possible sources, either alone or in collaboration with mast cells. In this connection, it is of interest that some macrophages apparently bear IgE receptors (Dessaint et al., 1979), so a direct IgE-mediated response of macrophages to antigen is theoretically possible.

V. Biologic Actions of SRS

Studies of crude SRS have usually been conducted on isolated guinea pig ileal muscle strips. SRS can usually be distinguished from other spasmogenic substances such as histamine and the prostaglandins in this system by use of an antihistamine and the selective SRS antagonist, FPL-55712, and by the character of the response itself. SRS also differs from the prostaglandins in its more limited spectrum or intensity of activity in other smooth muscle preparations such as the rat uterus and rat colon. Another useful approach has been to digest the SRS with aryl sulfatase (Orange et al., 1974) and show that much of the activity is lost. However, with the advent of reproducible chromatographic procedures for SRS purification, particularly HPLC, partial purification before bioassay clearly provides a more rigorous approach to the determination of SRS activity, since other spasmogenic products which might cause problems in interpretation can readily be eliminated.

Until recently, studies of SRS activity had involved impure material preventing final conclusions about its spectrum of biological activities and biological potency. Now that pure SRS is available, it is apparent that it has potent effects on smooth muscle of the intestine, large and small bronchi, and probably peripheral lung airways; lowers systemic blood pressure; alters vascular permeability and vessel tone in the skin; and affects nerve cell activity in the central nervous system. In isolated smooth muscle preparations from guinea pig intestine and guinea pig and human bronchi, SRS is much more potent that histamine-producing responses at subnanomolar concentrations (Jakschik et al., 1977a; Hammarström et al., 1979; Parker et al., 1979c; Lewis et al., 1980a). In contrast to the histamine response, the response to SRS is sustained for many minutes without tachyphylaxis. As a rule, cysteinyl-glycyl SRS has been more potent than glutathionyl SRS in these systems. The responses also differ qualitatively in that the contraction produced by glutathionyl SRS is slower in onset (Örning et al., 1980; Parker et al., 1980a). In our hands cysteinyl SRS is about 10% as active as cysteinyl-glycyl SRS, so even after the loss of two of the three amino acid residues from the original glutathione SRS molecule, considerable activity is still present (Parker et al., 1980a; Parker, 1980b). Moreover, once the cysteinyl SRS has been generated, it appears to be relatively stable to further degradation. Recent studies in collaboration with L. M. Lichtenstein and coworkers indicate that LTC_4 and LTD_4 are active in small as well as large bronchi. Drazen and his colleagues (Drazen et al., 1979, 1980) have reported preliminary data which may indicate that SRS is active even in peripheral lung airways. This conclusion was based in part on the demonstration of contractile responses in isolated peripheral lung preparations in vitro. The problem in these studies is to be certain that the contraction is really occurring in airway smooth muscle rather than small blood vessels (Parker, 1981a). However, since it appears that peripheral airway resistance is increased in vivo by the intravenous injection of SRS in guinea pigs (Drazen et al., 1979), the conclusion that peripheral airway contraction is occurring may be valid. If true, this observation is of considerable interest since it is well known that asthmatics may have peripheral as well as central airway dysfunction (Parker, 1980c). LTC_4 and LTD_4 have been reported, respectively, to constrict and dilate blood vessels in guinea pig skin as well as increase their permeability (Drazen et al., 1980). Studies by Hoffer and Murphy indicate that SRS also exerts an exceptionally sustained action on Purkinje nerve cell activity (Palmer et al., 1980a), raising the possibility of a regulatory action in the nervous system and conceivably in the reflex pathways that contribute to lung dysfunction in asthmatics.

VI. Pharmacologic Control of SRS Biosynthesis

According to our present state of knowledge, the biosynthesis of SRS requires that AA be released and converted to 5-HPETE. 5-HPETE is then conjugated to glutathione. Theoretically, SRS biosynthesis could be inhibited at any of these three levels. SRS release in lung fragment systems has been reported to be inhibited by ETYA, lipoxygenase inhibitors, cAMP-raising agents such as isoproterenol and theophylline, and disodium chromoglycate and to be enhanced by cholinergic agents, cytochalasins, cycloxygenase inhibitors, and α-adrenergic catecholamines. The site of the enhancing or inhibitory action is not clear for most of these agents. The two enzyme systems that have been implicated in AA release in mammalian tissues are phospholipase A_2 (van den Bosch, 1974) and diacylglycerol lipase (in combination with phospholipase C) (Kennerly et al., 1979). While truely selective inhibitors of these enzyme systems are not available, increases in cAMP have been found to be associated with reductions in AA release in a number of tissues. An action at this level might explain the inhibition of SRS release by cAMP agonists, although other sites of action are obviously possible. Based on studies in tissues that do not produce SRS, it is also possible that the beneficial effects of glucocorticoids in asthma are due in part to decreased release of AA. While the glucocorticoid levels generally required for direct effects on AA release are high, it is now common practice to administer very large glucocorticoid doses in the early phases of treatment of acute severe asthma, particularly when other measures have been ineffective. Moreover, even at more conventional glucocorticoid doses, delayed effects on AA release or an indirect action through an increase in the availability of a peptide that inhibits AA release appear possible. The biosynthesis of this inhibitory peptide is apparently increased by glucocorticoids (Flower and Blackwell, 1979).

Enhancement of SRS release by cycloxygenase inhibitors is demonstrable in a number of in vitro systems although the magnitude of the increase is usually less than two- to three-fold. Whether increased SRS synthesis is occuring in the subpopulation of asthmatics with the clinical syndrome called aspirin-sensitive asthma remains to be established, although this is an attractive possibility (Parker, 1977). In these individuals, various nonsteroidal anti-inflammatory agents with known cyclooxygenase inhibitory activity produce dramatic symptomatic exacerbations (reviewed in Parker, 1977, 1980c). Obviously, decreased metabolism of AA through the cyclooxygenase pathway would increase its availability to the competing lipoxygenase pathway, and presumably provide more 5-HPETE for SRS biosynthesis. In addition nonsteroidal anti-inflammatory agents have been recently reported to inhibit the long-chain fatty acid peroxidase that converts 12-HPETE to 12-HETE in platelets (Siegel et al., 1979). A similar effect in SRS-producing cells would tend to stabilize the 5-HPETE, increasing its availability and rate of conjugation with glutathione (Parker, 1980a). Moreover, since prostacyclin and PGE_2 considerably increase cAMP in most tissues and cAMP inhibits SRS synthesis, any decrease in PGE_2 and prostacyclin levels produced by the cyclooxygenase inhibitor might be expected to increase SRS biosynthesis, suggesting still another possible mechanism for the enhancing effects of aspirin and related agents.

SRS biosynthesis is inhibited by lipoxygenase inhibitors such as ETYA nor-dihydroguiaretic acid and pyrogallol as discussed above. However, it remains to be established that these or other recently identified lipoxygenase inhibitors are sufficiently nontoxic for long-term clinical use. Nonetheless the potential value of lipoxygenase inhibitors in the treatment of asthma deserves careful evaluation, particularly since the biosynthesis of the other 5-lipoxygenase products, 5-HETE and 5,12-di-HETE, would also be inhibited. These substances may contribute importantly to allergic inflammation through their effects on cell migration (both chemotaxis and chemokinesis) (Ford-Hutchinson et al., 1980; Palmer et al., 1980b; Goetzl and Pickett, 1980) and granule enzyme release (Stenson and Parker, 1980; Stenson et al., 1980). Moreover, since 5-HETE is incorporated covalently into membrane phospholipids and triglycerides (Stenson and Parker, 1979), it appears capable of producing long-term effects on cellular membrane function that might help to perpetuate the inflammatory response. The use of lipoxygenase inhibitors might also indirectly affect the formation of thromboxane A_2, which is a labile but highly potent bronchoconstrictor agent. Several laboratories have observed that SRS increases thromboxane A_2 fromation in guinea pig lungs (Vargaftig and Dao-Hai, 1971; Engineer et al., 1978). However, it should be noted that thus far this effect has only been reported in perfused lung preparations and may therefore involve an effect of SRS on vascular permeability that may or may not have relevance for asthmatic responses initiated in bronchi or nearby tissues outside the vascular system.

Since glutathione is required for SRS synthesis, agents which lower intracellular glutathione concentrations might also be of value in controlling SRS formation, at least on an emergency basis. We have recently demonstrated that SRS biosynthesis is inhibited almost completely when intracellular glutathione concentrations in RBL-1 cells are decreased to 10% or less of their original value by exposure of cells to unsaturated compounds which react enzymatically with glutathione. Moreover, some inhibition of SRS synthesis is observed even with much more modest reductions of glutathione levels (Parker et al., 1980b). While the sustained reduction of intracellular glutathione concentrations must be presumed to be undesirable, there is preliminary evidence to indicate that low glutathione levels are well tolerated for up to 2 weeks in rats treated with inhibitors of glutathione synthesis (Griffith and Meister, 1979), so perhaps this approach deserves further evaluation.

VII. Inhibition of SRS Action at the End Organ Level

The mechanism of action of SRS at the end organ level remains to be defined. SRS is extremely potent as a spasmogen in bronchial and ileal smooth muscle preparations, suggesting that specific receptors are involved in its actions, although this had not yet been directly demonstrated. This is preliminary evidence to indicate SRS may act by stimulating the formation of Ca^{2+} channels as with other spasmogenic agents. Nonspecific inhibition of SRS action on smooth muscle can be demonstrated with catecholamines and phosphodiesterase inhibitors, presumably through increases in intracellular cAMP. SRS responses on smooth muscle can be inhibited by high concentrations of indomethacin, although the basis for this effect is uncertain and it should be noted that indomethacin also inhibits responses to serotonin, histamine, and bradykinin (Aboulafia et al., 1976; Famaey et al., 1977). The only apparently selective SRS antagonist at the end organ level is the Fison product, FPL-55712 (and related chromone-2 carboxylic acids), but they appear to be too unstable for practical therapeutic use. These agents appear to act as competitive inhibitors of SRS binding although this has not yet been substantiated by direct binding studies.

VIII. Conclusion

Now that pure SRS has become available and its structure and mechanism of biosynthesis have been in large measure elucidated, it should be possible to develop quantitative immunochemical techniques for its measurment, learn more about both its formation and catabolism in vivo, and further define its physiological spectrum and mechanism of action (Parker, 1981). Out of this should emerge a better understanding of its role in human allergy. The possible development of selective inhibitors of SRS biosynthesis or action is now being extensively explored by the pharmaceutical industry, and the development of potentially useful SRS antogonists for evaluation on human asthma can be predicted. Hopefully these efforts will lead to better control of this common and medically important disease.

References

Aboulafia, J., Mendes, G. B., Miyamoto, M. E., Paiva, A. C. M., and Paiva, T. B. (1976). Effect of indomethacin and prostaglandin on the smooth muscle contracting activity of angiotensin and other agonists. *Br. J. Pharmacol., 58*:223-228.

Adkinson, N. F., Jr., Newball, H. H., Findlay, S., Adams, G. K., and Lichtenstein, L. M. (1980). Anaphylactic release of prostaglandins from human lung *in vitro. Am. Rev. Respir. Dis., 121*:911-920.

Anggard, E., Bergoqvist, U., Hoberg, B., Johansson, K., Thon, I. L., and Uvnäs, B. (1963). Biologically active principles occurring on histamine release from cat paw, guinea-pig lung and isolated rat mast cells. *Acta Physiol. Scand., 59*:97-110.

Bach, M. K., and Brashler, J. R. (1974). In vivo and in vitro production of a slow reacting substance in the rat upon treatment with calcium ionophores. *J. Immunol., 113*:2040-2044.

Bach, M. K., and Brashler, J. R. (1978). Stimulated production of slow reacting substance by mercaptans from ionophore A23187-induced mononuclear cells: Mercaptan structure-activity studies. *Life Sciences 23*:2119-2126.

Bach, M. K., Brashler, J. R., and Gorman, R. R. (1977). On the structure of slow reacting substance of anaphylaxis: Evidence of biosynthesis from arachidonic acid. *Prostaglandins, 14*:21-38.

Bach, M. K., Brachler, J. R., Brooks, C. D., and Neerken, A. J. (1979). Slow reacting substances: Comparison of some properties of human lung SRS-A and two distinct ractions from ionophore-induced rat mononuclear cells SRS. *J. Immunol., 122*:160-165.

Bach, M. K., Brashler, J. R., Hammarström, S., and Samuelsson, B. (1980a). Identification of a component of rat mononuclear cell SRS as leukotriene D. *Biochem Biophys. Res. Commun., 93*:1121-1126.

Bach, M. K., Brashler, J. R., Hammarström, S., and Samuelsson, B. (1980b). Identification of leukotriene C-1 as a major component of slow reacting substance from rat mononuclear cells. *J. Immunol., 125*:115-117.

Benveniste, J. (1980). Presentation at International Congress of Immunology, Paris, August, 1980.

Borgeat, P., Hamberg, M., and Samuelsson, B. (1976). Transformation of arachidonic acid and homo-γ-linolenic acid by rabbit polymorphonuclear leukocytes. Monohydroxy acids from novel lipoxygenase. *J. Biol. Chem., 251*:7816-7820.

Brocklehurst, W. E. (1960). The release of histamine and formation of a slow-reacting substance (SRS-A) during anaphylactic shock. *J. Physiol. 151*: 416-435.

Brocklehurst, W. E. (1962). Slow reacting substance and related compounds. In *Progress in Allergy.* Edited by P. Kallos. Basel, S. Karger AG, vol. 6, pp. 539-558.

Burka, J. F., and Eyre, P. (1974a). The immunological release of slow-reacting substance of anaphylaxis from bovine lung. *Can. J. Physiol. Pharm. 52*: 1201-1204.

Burka, J. F., and Eyre, P. (1974b): A study of prostaglandins and prostaglandin antagonists in relation to anaphylaxis in calves. *Can. J. Physiol. Pharmacol. 52*:942-951.

Burka, J. F., and Eyre, P. (1975). Modulation of the formation and release of bovine SRS-A in vitro by several anti-anaphylactic drugs. *Int. Arch. Allergy Appl. Immunol., 49*:774.

Clark, D. A., Goto, G., Marfat, A., and Corey, E. J. 1980). 11-*Trans* leukotriene C: A naturally occurring slow reacting substance. *Biochem. Biophys. Res. Commun., 94*:1133-1139.

Collier, H. O. J., and James, G. W. L. (1966). Bradykinin and slow reacting substance in anaphylactic bronchoconstriction in guinea pig in vivo. *J. Physiol., 185*:71P-72P.

Conroy, M. C., Orange, R. P., and Lichtenstein, L. M. (1976). Release of slow reacting substance of anaphylaxis (SRS-A) from human leukocytes by the calcium ionophore A23187. *J. Immunol., 116*:1677-1681.

Dawson, W., Lewis, R. L., McMahon, R. E., and Sweatman, W. J. F. (1974). Potent bronchoconstrictor activity of 15-keto prostaglandin $F_{2\alpha}$, *Nature, 250*:331-332.

Dessaint, J. P., Torpier, G., Capron, M., Brazin, H., and Cparon, A. (1979). Cytophilic binding of IgE to the macrophage I. Binding characteristics of IgE on the surface of macrophages in the rat. *Cell. Immunol., 46*:12-23.

Drazen, J. M., Lewis, R. A., Wasserman, S. I., Orange, R. P., and Austen, K. F. (1979). Differential effects of a partially purified preparation of slow-reacting substance of anaphylaxis on guinea pig tracheal spirals and parenchymal strips. *J. Clin. Invest., 63*:1-5.

Drazen, J. M., Austen, K. F., Lewis, R. A., Clark, D. A., Goto, G., Marfat, A., and Corey, E. J. (1980). Comparative airway and vascular activities of leukotrienes C-1 and D in vivo and in vitro. *Proc. Natl. Acad. Sci., 77*: 4354-4358.

Engineer, D. M., Niederhauser, U., Piper, P. J., and Sirois, P. (1978). Release mediators of anaphylaxis: Inhibition of prostaglandin synthesis and the modification of release of slow reacting substances of anaphylaxis and histamine. *Br. J. Pharmacol., 52*:61-66.

Falkenhein, S. C., MacDonald, H., Huber, M. M., Koch, D., and Parker, C. W. (1980). Effect of the 5-hydroperoxide of eicosatetraenoic acid and inhibitors of the lipoxygenase pathway on the formation of slow reacting substance by rat basophilic leukemia cells. Direct evidence that slow reacting substance is a product of the lipoxygenase pathway. *J. Immunol., 125*:163-168.

Famaey, J. P., Fontaine, J., Seaman, I., and Reuse, J. (1977). A possible role of prostaglandins in guinea-pig isolated ileum contractions to serotonin. *Prostaglandins, 14*:119-124.

Feldberg, W., and Kellaway, C. H. (1938). Liberation of histamine and formation of lysocithin-like substances by cobra venom. *J. Physiol., 94*:187-226.

Flower, R. J., and Blackwell, G. J. (1979). Anti-inflammatory steroids induce biosynthesis of a phospholipase A_2 inhibitor which prevents prostaglandin generation. *Nature, 278*:456-459.

Ford-Hutchinson, A. W., Bray, M. A., Doig, M. V., Shipley, M. E., and Smith, M. J. H. (1980). Leukotriene B: A potent chemokinetic and aggregating substance released from polymorphonuclear leukocytes. *Nature, 286*:264-276.

Gardner, H. W., Kleiman, R., Weisleder, D., and Inglett, G. E. (1977). Cysteine adds to lipid hydroperoxide. *Lipids, 12*:655-660.

Goetzl, E. J., Pickett, W. C. (1980). The human PMN leukocyte chemotactic activity of complex hydroxy-eicosatetraenoic acids (HETE's). *J. Immunol. 125*:1789-1791.

Grant, J. A., and Lichtenstein, L. M. (1974): Release of slow reacting substance of anaphylaxis from human leukocytes. *J. Immunol., 112*:897-904.

Griffith, O. W., and Meister, A. (1979). Glutathione: Interorgan translocation, turnover, and metabolism. *Proc. Natl. Acad. Sci. 65*:5606-5620.

Hammerström, S. (1980). Keukotriene C_5: A slow reacting substance derived from eicosapentaenoic acid. *J. Biol. Chem., 255*:7093-7094.

Hammerström, S., Murphy, R. C., Samuelsson, B., Clark, D. A., Mioskowski, C., and Corey, E. J. (1979). Structure of leukotriene C. Identification of the amino acid part. *Biochem. Biophys. Res. Commun., 91*:1266-1272.

Henderson, W. R., and Kaliner, M. (1979). Mast cell granule peroxidase: Location, secretion and SRS-A inactivation. *J. Immunol., 122*:1322-1328.

Herxheimer, H., and Stresemann, E. (1963). The effect of slow reacting substance (SRS-A) in guinea-pigs and in asthmatic patients. *J. Physiol., 165*: 78P-79P.

Hitchcock, M. (1978). Effect of inhibitors of prostaglandin synthesis and prostaglandins E_2 And $F_{2\alpha}$ on the immunologic release of mediators of inflammation from activity sensitized guinea pig lung. *J. Pharmacol. Exp. Ther., 207*:630-640.

Hyman, A. L., Spannhake, E. W., and Kadowitz, P. J. (1978): Prostaglandins and the lung. *Am. Rev. Respir. Dis., 117*:111-136.

Ishizaka, T., Ishizaka, K., Orange, R. P., and Austen, K. F. (1971). Pharmacologic inhibition of the antigen-induced release of histamine and slow reacting substance of anaphylaxis (SRS-A) from monkey lung tissues mediated by human IgE. *J. Immunol., 106*:1267-1273.

Jakschik, B. A., and Parker, C. W. (1976). (Abstract). Probable precursor role for arachidonic acid in slow reacting substance (SRS) biosynthesis. *Clin. Res., 24*:575A.

Jakschik, B. A., and Parker, C. W. (1977c). Presentation at the International Meeting on Prostaglandins, Vail, Colorado, March, 1977.

Jakschik, B. A., Falkenhein, S., and Parker, C. W. (1977a). Precursor role of arachidonic acid in slow reacting substance from rat basophilic leukemia cells. *Proc. Natl. Aurd. Sci., 74*:4577-4581.

Jakschik, B. A., Kulczycki, A., MacDonald, H. H., and Parker, C. W. (1977b). Release of slow reacting substance (SRS) from rat basophilic leukemia (RBL-1) cells. *J. Immunol., 119*:618-622.

Jakschik, B. A., Sun, F. F., Lee, L., and Steinhoff, M. M. (1980). Calcium stimulation of a novel lipoxygenase. *Biochem. Biophys. Res. Commun., 95*: 103-110.

Kellaway, C. H., and Trethewie, E. R. (1940). The liberation of a slow-reacting smooth muscle-stimulating substance in anaphylaxis. *Quart. J. Exp. Physiol., 30*:121-145.

Kennerly, D. A., Sullivan, T. J., Sylwester, P., and Parker, C. W. (1979). Diacylglycerol Metabolism in Mast Cells: A potential role in membrane fusion and arachidonic acid release. *J. Exp. Med., 150*:1039-1044.

Kulczycki, A., Jr., Isersky, C., and Metzger, H. (1974). The interaction of IgE with rat basophilic leukemia cells. I. Evidence for specific binding of IgE. *J. Exp. Med., 139*:600-616.

Lewis, R. A., Wasserman, S. I., Goetzl, E. J., and Austen, K. F. (1974). Formation of slow-reacting substance of anaphylaxis in human lung tissue and cells before release. *J. Exp. Med., 140*:1133-1146.

Lewis, R. A., Drazen, J. M., Austen, K. F., Clark, D. A., and Corey, E. J. (1980b). Identification of the C(6)-S-conjugate of leukotriene with a cysteine as a naturally occurring slow reacting substance of anaphylaxis (SRS-A). Importance of the 11-*cis*-geometry for biological activity. *Biochem. Biophys. Res. Commun., 96*:271-277.

Lewis, R. A., Austen, K. F., Drazen, J. M., Clark, D. A., Marfat, A., and Corey, E. J. (1980a). Slow reacting substances of anaphylaxis: Identification of leukotrienes C-1 and D from human and rat sources. *Proc. Natl. Acad. Sci., 77*:3710-3714.

Mathe, A. A. (1976). Studies on actions of prostaglandins in the lung. *Acta Physiol. Scand.* (Supp.), *441*:1-55.

Morris, H. R., Taylor, G. W., Piper, P. J., and Tippins, J. R. (1980). Structure of slow reacting substance of anaphylaxis from guinea-pig lung. *Nature, 285*: 104-105.

Morris, H. R., Taylor, G. W., Piper, P. J., Sirois, P., and Tippins, J. R. (1978). Slow reacting substance of anaphylaxis. Purification and characterization. *FEBS Lett., 87*:203-206.

Murphy, R. C., Hammarström, S., and Samuelsson, B. (1979). Leukotriene C: A slow-reacting substance from murine mastocytoma cells. *Proc. Natl. Acad. Sci., 76*:4275-4279.

Newball, H. H., and Lenfant, C. (1977). Influence of atropine and cromolyn on human bronchial hyperreactivity to aerosolized PGF-2α. *Respir. Physiol. 30*:125-136.

Newball, H. H., Keiser, H. R., and Lenfant, C. (1980). Prostaglandin F-2α functions as a local hormone on human airways. *Respir. Physiol. 41*:183-197.

Newball, H. H., Adkinson, N. F., Jr., Adams, G. K., Findlay, S. R., and Lichtenstein, L. M. (1978). Mechanism of anaphylactic release of prostaglandins (PG's) from human lung. *J. Allergy Clin. Immunol. 61*:148.

Ohnishi, H., Kosuzme, H., Kitamura, Y., Yamaguchi, K., Nobuhara, M., and Suzuki, Y. (1980). Structure of slow-reacting substance of anaphylaxis (SRS-A). *Prostaglandins, 20*:655-666.

Orange, R. P., and Austen, K. F. (1969). Slow reacting substance of anaphylaxis. *Adv. Immunol., 10*:105-144.

Orange, R. P., and Chang, P. L. (1975). The effect of thiols on immunologic release of slow reacting substance of anaphylaxis. *J. Immunol., 115*:1072-1077.

Orange, R. P., and Moore, E. G. (1976). The effect of thiols on the immunologic release of slow reacting substance of anaphylaxis. II. Other vitro and in vivo models. *J. Immunol., 116*:392-397.

Orange, R. P., Murphy, R. C., and Austen, K. F. (1974). Inactivation of slow reacting substance of anaphylaxis (SRS-A) by arylsulfatases. *J. Immunol., 113*:316-322.

Örning, L., Hammarström, S., and Samuelsson, B. (1980). Leukotriene D: A slow reacting substance from rat basophilic leukemia cells. *Proc. Natl. Acad. Sci., 77*:2014-2017.

Palmer, M. R., Mathews, R., Murphy, R. C., and Hoffer, B. (1980a). Leukotriene C elicits a prolonged excitation of cerebellar Purkinje neurons. *Neurosci. Lett., 18*:173-180.

Palmer, R. M. J., Stepney, R. J., Higgs, G. A., and Eakins, K. E. (1980b). Chemokinetic activity of arachidonic acid lipoxygenase products on leukocytes of different species. *Prostaglandins, 20*:411-418.

Parker, C. W. (1977). Aspirin sensitive asthma. In *Asthma: Physiology, Immunopharmacology and Treatment.* Edited by L. M. Lichtenstein, K. F. Austen, and A. S. Simon. New York, Academic Press, pp. 301-313.

Parker, C. W. (1979). Prostaglandins and slow reacting substance. *J. Allergy Clin. Immunol., 63*:1-14.

Parker, C. W. (1980a). Pulmonary effects of inhibitors. In *Prostaglandin in Synthetase Inhibitors in Clinical Medicine* New York, Alan R. Liss, Inc., vol. 1, pp. 30-43.

Parker, C. W. (1980b). SRS-A on rat leukemia and rat mast cells. Kroc Foundation Meeting in May 1980 at Santa Barbara, California. Fourth Symposium on Biochemistry of Allergic Reactions (In Press).

Parker, C. W., 1980c). *Asthma and Rhinitis in Clinical Immunology.* Philadelphia, W. B. Saunders, Vol. 2, pp. 1372-1438.

Parker, C. W. (1980d). Incorporation of ^{14}C-AA into SRS. In Proceedings of the Symposium on SRS-A and Leukotrienes. London, John Wiley & Sons Lit., (In Press).

Parker, C. W. (1981): Chemical nature of slow reacting substance in *Advances in Inflammation Research.* New York, Raven Press (In Press).

Parker, C. W., Falkenhein, S. F., and Huber, M. M. (1980a). Sequential conversion of the glutathionyl side chain of slow reacting substance (SRS) to cysteinyl-glycine and cysteine in rat basophilic leukemia cells stimulated with A-23187. *Prostaglandins, 20*:863-886.

Parker, C. W., Fischman, C. M., and Wedner, H. J. (1980b): Relationship of slow reacting substance biosynthesis to intracellular glutathione levels. *Proc. Natl. Acad. Sci., 77*:6876-6873.

Parker, C. W., Huber, M. M., Falkenhein, S. (1979a). (Abstract) Evidence that slow reacting substance (SRS) is a fatty acid thioether formed through a previously undefined pathway of arachidonate metabolism. *Clin. Res., 27*: 473A.

Parker, C. W., Huber, M. M., Falkenhein, S. (1979b). (Abstract) Incorporation of ^{35}S into slow reacting substance (SRS). *Fed. Proc., 38*:1167A.

Parker, C. W., Huber, M. M., Hoffman, M. K., and Falkenhein, S. F. (1979c). Characterization of the two major species of slow reacting substance from rat basophilic leukemia cells as glutathionyl thioethers of eicosatetraenoic acids oxygenated at the 5 position. Evidence that peroxy groups are present and important for spasmogenic activity. *Prostaglandins, 18*: 673-686.

Parker, C. W., Jakschik, B. A., Huber, M. M., and Falkenhein, S. F. (1979d). Characterization of slow reacting substance as a family of thiolipids derived from arachidonic acid. *Biochem. Biophys. Res. Commun., 89*:1186-1192.

Parker, C. W., Koch, D. A., Huber, M. M., and Falkenhein, S. F. (1980c). Arylsulfatase inactivation of slow reacting substance. Evidence for proteolysis as a major mechanism when ordinary commercial preparations of the enzyme are used. *Prostaglandins, 20*:887-908.

Parker, C. W., Koch, D. A., Huber, M. M., and Falkenhein, S. F. (1980d). Formation of the cysteinyl form of slow reacting substance (leukotriene E_4) in human plasma. *Biochem. Biophys. Res. Commun., 97*:1038-1046.

Parker, C. W., Koch, D. A., Huber, M. M., and Falkenhein, S. F. (1980e). Incorporation of radiolabel from [1-^{14}C] 5-hydroxy-eicosatetraenoic acid into slow reacting substances. *Biochem. Biophys. Res. Commun. 94*:1037-1043.

Paterson, N. A. M., and Craig, I. D. (1979). Inactivation by alveolar macrophages of a slow reacting substance released from pig lung cells. *Am. Rev. Respir. Dis., 119*:76A.

Patterson, R., and Suszko, I. M. (1971). Primate respiratory mast cells. Reactions with ascaris antigen and anti-heavy chain sera. *J. Immunol., 106*: 1274-1283.

Radmark, O., Malmstein, C., and Samuelsson, B. (1980). Leukotriene A: Stereochemistry and enzymatic conversion to leukotriene B. *Biochem. Biophys. Res. Commun., 92*:954-961.

Rokasch, J., Girard, Y., Guindon, Y., Atkinson, J. G., Larue, M., Young, R. N., Masson, P., and Holme, G. (1980). The synthesis of a leukotriene with SRS-like activity. *Tetrahedron Lett. 21*:1485-1488.

Rouzer, C. A., Scott, W. A., Cohn, Z. A., Blackburn, P., and Manning, J. M. (1980). Mouse peritoneal macrophages release leukortiene C in response to a phagocytic stimulus. *Proc. Natl. Acad. Sci., 77*:4928-4932.

Samuelsson, B., and Hammarström, S. (1980). Nomenclature for leukotrienes. *Prostaglandins, 19*:645-648.

Samuelsson, B., Borgeat, P., Hammarström, S., and Murphy, R. C. (1979). Introduction of a nomenclature: Leukotrienes. *Prostaglandins, 17*:785-787.

Schulman, E. S., Adkinson, N. F., Adams, G. K., Lichtenstein, L. M., and Newball, H. H. (1980a). Anaphylactic release of thromboxane A-2 from human bronchi and parenchyma. *J. Allergy Clin. Immunol., 65*:235.

Schulman, E. S., Adkinson, N. F., Demers, L. M., Fitzpatrick, F. A., Adams, G. K., Lichtenstein, L. M., and Newball, H. H. (1980b). Anaphylactic release of prostaglandins, thromboxane A-2 and prostacyclin from human lung. *Fed. Proc. 39*:931.

Schulman, E. S., Newball, H. H., Demers, L. M., Fitzpatrick, F. A., and Adkinson, N. F., Jr. (1981). Anaphylactic release of thromboxane A_2, prostaglandin D_2, and prostacyclin from human lung parenchyma. *Am. Rev. Respir. Dis., 124*:402-406.

Schulman, E. S., Adkinson, N. F., Jr., Newball, H. H. (1982). Cyclooxygenase metabolites in human lung anaphylaxis: Airway vs. parenchyma. *J. Appl. Physiol., 53*:589-595.

Siegel, M. I., McConnel, R. T., and Cuatrecasas, P. (1979). Aspirin-like drugs interfere with arachidonate metabolism by inhibition of the 12-hydroperoxy-5,8,10,14-eicosatetraenoic acid peroxidase activity of the lipoxygenase pathway. *Proc. Natl. Acad. Sci., 76*:3774-3778.

Siraganian, R. P., and Metzger, H. (1978). Evidence that the "mouse mastocytoma" cell line (MCT-1) is of rat origin. *J. Immunol., 121*:2584-2585.

Sirois, P. (1979). Inactivation of slow reacting substance of anaphylaxis (SRS-A) by lipoxygenase. *Prostaglandins, 17*:395-404.

Sok, D., Pai, J., Atrache, V., and Sih, C. J. (1980). Characterization of slow reacting substances (SRSs) of rat basophilic leukemia (RBL-1) cells: Effect of cysteine on SRS profile. *Proc. Natl. Acad. Sci., 77*:6481-6485.

Stenson, W. F., and Parker, C. W. (1979). Metabolism of arachidonic acid in ionophore stimulated neutrophils. Esterification of a hydroxylated metabolite into phospholipids. *J. Clin. Invest., 64*:1457-1465.

Stenson, W. F., and Parker, C. W. (1980). Monohydroxyeicosatetraenoic acids (HETEs) induced degranulation of human neutrophils. *J. Immunol., 124*: 210-214.

Stenson, W. F., Parker, C. W., and Sullivan, T. J. (1980b). Augmentation of IgE-mediated release of histamine by hydroxyeicosatetraenoic acid and 12-hydroxyeicosatetraenoic acid. *Biochem. Biophys. Res. Commun., 96*: 1045-1052.

Strandberg, K., and Uvnäs, B. (1971). Purification and properties of the slow reacting substance formed in the cat paw perfused with compound 48/80. *Acta Physiol. Scand., 82*:358-374.

Takahashi, H., Webster, M. E., and Newball, H. H. (1976). Separation of slow reacting substance of anaphylaxis (SRS-A) from human lung into four biologically active fractions. *J. Immunol., 117*:1039-1044.

van den Bosch, H. (1974). Phosphoglyceride metabolism. *Ann. Rev. Biochem., 43*:243-277.

Vargaftig, B. B., and Dao-Hai, N. (1971): Release of vasoactive substances from guinea pig lungs by slow reacting substance C and arachidonic acid. *Pharmacology 6*:99-108.

Walker, J. L. (1973). The regulatory function of prostaglandins in the release of histamine and SRS-A from passively sensitized human lung tissue. *Adv. Biosci., 9*:235-240.

Wasserman, S. I., Goetzl, E. J., and Austen, K. F. (1975). Inactivation of slow reacting substance of anaphylaxis in human eosinophil arylsulfatase. *J. Immunol., 114*:645-649.

Watanabe, S., and Koda, A. (1979). Purification and some physicochemical properties of slow reacting substance of anaphylaxis (SRS-A) from sensitized guinea pig lung. *Microbiol. Immunol., 23*:1009-1022.

Watanabe-Kohno, S., and Parker, C. W. (1980). Role of arachidonic acid in the biosynthesis of slow reacting substance of anaphylaxis (SRS-A) from sensitized guinea pig lung fragments. Evidence that SRS-A is a very similar or identical structurally to nonimmunologically induced forms of SRS. *J. Immunol., 125*:946-955.

Yecies, L. D., Watanabe, S., and Parker, C. W. (1979b). Slow reacting substance from ionophore A-23187-stimulated basophilic leukemia cells and peritoneal mast cells in the rat. I. Purification and comparison during sequential Sephadex LH-20 and thin layer chromatography. *Life Sciences, 25*:1909-1916.

Yecies, L. D., Wedner, H. J., and Parker, C. W. (1979d). Slow reacting substance (SRS) from ionophore A-23187 stimulated human leukemic basophils. I. Evidence for a precursor role of arachidonic acid and initial purification. *J. Immunol., 123*:2814-2816.

Yecies, L. D., Johnson, S. M., Wedner, H. J., and Parker, C. W. (1979a). Slow reacting substances (SRS) from ionophore A-23187 stimulated peritoneal mast cells of the normal rat. II. Evidence for a precursor role of arachidonic acid and further purification. *J. Immunol., 122*:2090-2095.

Yecies, L. D., Wedner, H. J., Johnson, S. M., Jakschik, B. A., and Parker, C. W. (1979c). Slow reacting substance (SRS) from ionophore A-23187 stimulated peritoneal mast cells of the normal rat. I. Conditions of generation and initial characterization. *J. Immunol., 122*:2083-2089.

3

Anaphylactic Release of Arachidonic Acid Metabolites from the Lung

N. FRANKLIN ADKINSON, JR., EDWARD S. SCHULMAN,*
and HAROLD H. NEWBALL†

The Johns Hopkins University School of Medicine
The Good Samaritan Hospital
Baltimore, Maryland

I. Introduction

Over the last decade, the important role of arachidonic acid metabolites in physiologic homeostasis and pathologic events in human lung has unfolded at an ever increasing rate. Cyclooxygenase products, including prostaglandins, thromboxanes, and prostacyclin, are produced by lung tissue in response to a variety of stimuli; these metabolites exert potent biologic effects on a number of cell functions. Both pulmonary vasculature and human airways appear to be influenced in a complex and as yet poorly understood manner by arachidonate metabolites. Reviews of the known effects of arachidonate metabolites on lung function have been published elsewhere (Mathe et al., 1977b; Hyman et al., 1978).

The scope of this chapter is limited to consideration of the origin and possible pathophysiologic effects of arachidonate metabolites released during IgE-

---

Present Affiliation
* Jefferson Medical College, Philadelphia, Pennsylvania
† Institute of Chemical Defense, Edgewood, Maryland
Supported in part by NIH Grants Nos. HL24938 and HL24210 and Grant No. 1392 from The Council For Tobacco Research U.S.A., Inc. Dr. Schulman was supported in part by a National Pulmonary Faculty Training Center Grant from the NHLBI (HL07159).

dependent anaphylaxis in human lung. This focus has potential relevance for bronchial asthma, where chronic mast cell activation appears to be a primary pathologic event (Austen and Orange, 1976). Lung anaphylaxis may also be a useful human model of systemic anaphylaxis. In man, unlike numerous experimental animals, the lung is one of the more important target organs during systemic anaphylaxis. Although this feature is common to the guinea pig (the most commonly employed experimental animal model for human bronchial asthma), it has now become clear that there are marked differences in arachidonate metabolism during anaphylaxis in human and guinea pig lung. For example, in guinea pig lung, thromboxane is clearly the predominant cyclooxygenase product during in vitro anaphylaxis (Dawson et al., 1976; Boot et al., 1978), in contrast to human lung where thromboxane is a minor metabolite (Schulman et al., 1981). Because of marked species differences, animal models are generally not suitable for study of the anaphylactic release of arachidonic acid metabolites from human lung.

II. Methods of Study

Experimental study of human lung anaphylaxis in vivo is limited to studies in which peripheral plasma and urine samples have been assayed for arachidonate metabolites following inhalation challenge using relevant antigens in allergic subjects. Following extraction and concentration of 30 ml peripheral venous plasma and analysis by gas-liquid chromatography/mass spectrometry, Green et al., (1974) were able to demonstrate a three- to eightfold rise in venous plasma levels of 15-keto-13,14-dihydro-$PGF_{2\alpha}$ following severe antigen-induced bronchospasm in four asthmatic subjects. No significant increase in this principal $PGF_{2\alpha}$ metabolite was observed in a fifth pateint who had a less than 10% fall in FEV_1. In similar studies in our laboratory (Fish et al., 1981), we were unable to confirm increases in this $PGF_{2\alpha}$ metabolite using radioimmunoassay of both extracted and unextracted peripheral plasma samples from asthmatics undergoing somewhat milder degrees of bronchospasm (unpublished observations, 1981). Thus, bronchial challenge of asthmatic subjects may release small quantities of cyclooxygenase metabolites into the peripheral circulation, but, for the metabolites that have been measured, the alterations are subtle and close to the threshold of sensitivity for radioimmunoassay. It would appear that large volumes of plasma must be extracted and/or concentrated to appreciate acute changes in venous plasma prostaglandin levels as a result of inhalational challenge with antigen. This requirement renders the method impractical for routine use in clinical studies.

Sherman et al. (1981) recently reported preliminary studies in which highly significant peripheral arterial-venous differences in $PGF_{2\alpha}$ and thromboxane B_2 concentrations were observed in normal subjects and in patients with pulmonary disease. However, the arterial concentrations observed were still quite low and not easily measured with precision. Further investigation of the spectrum and quantity of metabolites released in vivo is severely limited by the degree of mediator release that can be safely provoked in human subjects, as well as by the need for invasive techniques to sample lung output closer to its source.

Because of the difficulties of studying arachidonate metabolites in plasma, urinary metabolites have been examined. Morris et al. (1980, 1981a) recently observed that urine specimens obtained during status asthmaticus showed excretion rates for thromboxane B_2, $PGF_{2\alpha}$, and PGE_2 that were twice those observed in normal children or asymptomatic asthmatics. However, the same studies showed that only 8–32% of added prostaglandin standards were recoverable from urine in appropriate thin-layer chromatography (TLC) fractions after silica-gel chromatography of ether-extracted urine. Thus, radioimmunoassay of either unextracted or ether-extracted urine for arachidonate metabolites is fraught with difficulty due to a marked influence of unknown cross-reacting substances.

Another line of in vivo investigation of the role of arachidonate metabolites on antigen-induced lung disease has been the evaluation of cyclooxygenase inhibitors on antigen-induced bronchospasm in allergic individuals. Smith and Dunlop (1975) reported that 200 mg of indomethacin per day for 1 week had no effect on antigen-induced bronchospasm of nine atopic asthmatics challenged with a house dust mite extract. More recently, Fish et al. (1981) confirmed these results in asthmatic patients, but observed that indomethacin increased bronchial sensitivity to antigen inhalation in patients with ragweed rhinitis but having no history of asthma. This result suggests that arachidonate metabolism is somehow different in asthmatic patients compared with rhinitic, nonasthmatic controls. Whether the effect of indomethacin blockade of cyclooxygenase metabolism exerted its effect in nonasthmatic subjects by influencing mast cell secretion, secondary prostaglandin-producing cells, or smooth muscle function remains to be determined.

Because of the difficulties inherent in in vivo studies of human lung anaphylaxis, much interest has been focused on in vitro studies of surgically excised human lung fragments. The techniques employed by various investigators are similar (Mathe et al., 1977a; Platshon and Kaliner, 1978; Adkinson et al., 1980); that utilized in our laboratory will be briefly outlined. Macroscopically normal pieces of human lung removed at thoracotomy usually for lung cancer are dissected free of pleura and visible blood vessels. Subpleural parenchymal fragments and/or segmental and subsegmental bronchial fragments may be prepared. Bronchial fragments are dissected free of adhering parenchymal tissue. Passive sensitization with a potent reagenic serum is performed at 37°C for 3 hr or 22°C for 18 hr. After thorough washing, a suitable number of fragments of either bronchial or parenchymal tissue are suspended in Tyrode's buffer and challenged with antigen or pharmacologic agents. Mediator release is generally complete within 20-30 min; response to pharmacologic agents (methacholine, histamine, KCl) occurs more rapidly. After each challenge, supernatants are removed and assayed for arachidonate metabolites, as well as for the mast cell marker histamine. Residual tissue histamine may be extracted by boiling the lung tissues in 2% perchloric acid for 10 min so that total tissue histamine content may be determined.

Piper and Walker (1973) detected release of PGE_1, PGE_2, and $PGF_{2\alpha}$ during antigen challenge of human lung fragments previously passively sensitized in vitro. The quantity of these prostaglandins released was not related to antigen dose. RCS (rabbit aorta contracting substance; principally TxA_2) was not detectable during in vitro human lung anaphylaxis. Piper and Walker employed bioassay for quantitation of prostanoids. These early observations have been considerably extended in more recent work by a number of investigators employing radioimmunoassay, as reviewed below.

Although the sensitivity and specificity of bioassay for prostaglandins and thromboxane are well established (Piper and Vane, 1971; Palmer et al., 1973; Piper, 1977), recent advances in radioimmunoassay technology have led to this method being widely used for analysis of short-term in vitro tissue culture experiments, especially where large numbers of samples are involved (Adkinson, 1977; Platshon and Kaliner, 1978; Adkinson et al., 1980; Morris et al., 1981b). In recent years, agreement of radioimmunoassay with gas chromatography-mass spectroscopy has generally been quite good. In addition, we have found that prior organic extraction and lipid chromatography is not necessary to obtain accurate radioimmunoassay results in aqueous buffers which do not contain serum or large amounts of protein (Adkinson, 1977; Adkinson et al., 1980). Elimination of the need for tedious extraction and chromatography procedures prior to assay greatly expands the volume of samples that can be handled and has permitted detailed examination of kinetic courses and dose-response relationships.

III. Spectrum of Arachidonate Products Produced in Human Lung Anaphylaxis

Current knowledge of arachidonate metabolism indicates the involvement of at least two enzyme cascades. The cyclooxygenase pathway leads to the production via labile cyclic endoperoxides of the primary prostaglandins (PGE_2, $PGF_{2\alpha}$, and PGD_2), thromboxanes (TxA_2), as well as prostacyclin (PgI_2). The lipoxygenase enzymes produce hydroperoxy and hydroxy derivatives of arachidonate, among which are potent regulators of neutrophil and eosinophil function (reviewed in Goetzl, 1980). The lipoxygenase pathways also generate the biologically potent leukotriene series, and possibly other metabolites, some of which may facilitate biochemical events involved in secretory processes (Stenson and Parker, 1980; Peters et al., 1981). Except for the classical slow reacting substances of anaphylaxis (SRS-A), now identified as predominantly leukotrienes C and D in human lung (Lewis et al., 1980a), there have not yet been systematic studies of lipoxygenase pathway products released during human lung anaphylaxis. SRS-A is discussed in detail elsewhere in this volume (Chap. 2) and will not be addressed further here.

The lipoxygenase and cyclooxygenase enzymes are likely to be differentially distributed among the various cell types present in a complex tissue such as human lung. Recent evidence suggests that human mast cells preferentially produce PGD_2 through the cyclooxygenase pathway (Lewis et al., 1980a,b; Roberts et al., 1980). In contrast, human macrophages favor the production of PGE_2, with lesser quantities of thromboxane (Morley et al., 1979). Prostacyclin is the favored product from vascular endothelial cells (Moncada et al., 1977), while cultured human lung fibroblasts, but not skin fibroblasts, synthesize significant quantities of TxA_2 from exogenous arachidonate (Bryant et al., 1978). The predominant or favored arachidonate metabolites for other lung cell types are just now beginning to receive study.

Nijkamp et al. (1976) reported the appearance of an RCS (thromboxane)-releasing factor during guinea pig lung anaphylaxis. Preliminary characterization of the material suggested that it was a small molecular weight peptide. Steel and Kaliner (1981) have recently reported finding another factor released from antigen-challenged human lung fragments challenged with anti-IgE. They provide evidence that an oligopeptide of 13 amino acids is generated following lung mast cell activation. This peptide induces peripheral guinea pig lung fragments to produce both $PGF_{2\alpha}$ and TxB_2. No information is yet available as to whether this peptide prostaglandin-generating factor (PGF) is a primary mast cell mediator or is released secondarily from other cells following mast cell activation. Definitive study of this and perhaps other prostanoid releasing factors that may be produced during anaphylaxis has yet to be undertaken.

IV. Cyclooxygenase Products from Parenchymal versus Bronchial Tissue

Our studies of the relative quantities of cyclooxygenase products of arachidonic acid released during anaphylactic challenge of human bronchial and parenchymal lung tissue are summarized in Figure 1. The results shown represent the mean of four individual human lung experiments, among which there was considerable variability as indicated by the appreciable standard errors. Of the five cyclooxygenase products measured by radioimmunoassay, the prostacyclin metabolite 6-keto-$PGF_{1\alpha}$ and the primary prostaglandin PGD_2 predominated in parenchyma. Lesser quantities of PGE, $PGF_{2\alpha}$, and thromboxane B_2 were

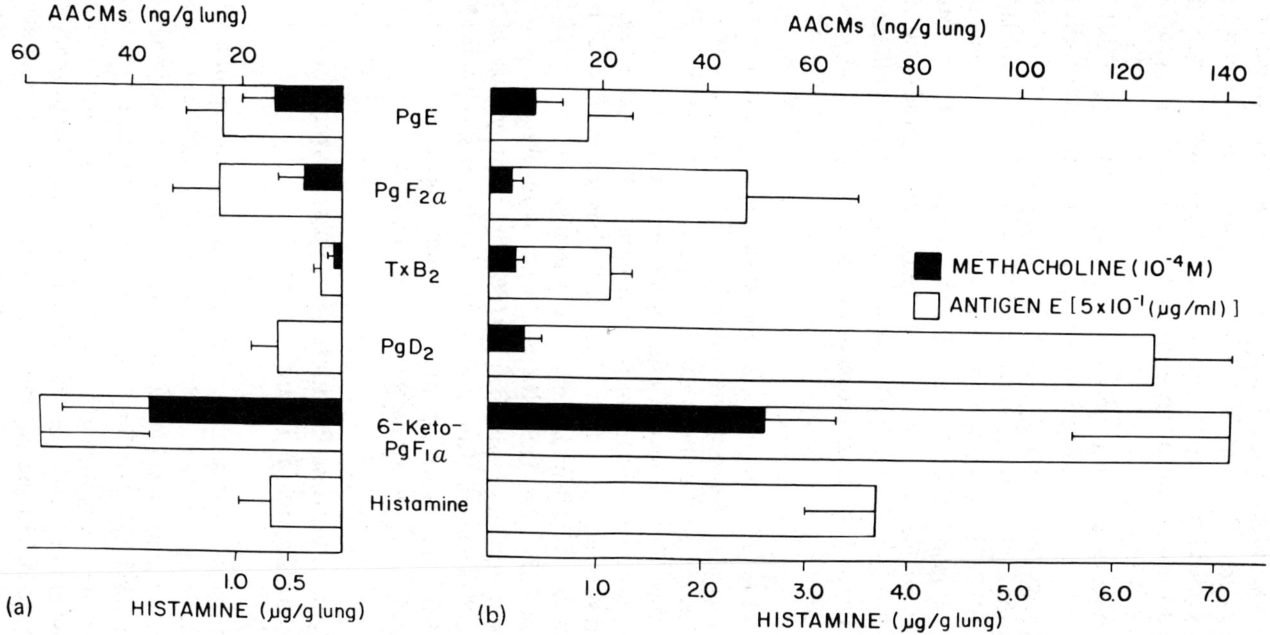

Figure 1 Anaphylactic production of arachidonic acid cyclooxygenase metabolites [(AACM) ng/g wet weight] in human lung tissue. Results shown are mean ± SEM of four individual lung studies. (*a*) Bronchial tissue; (*b*) parenchymal tissue.

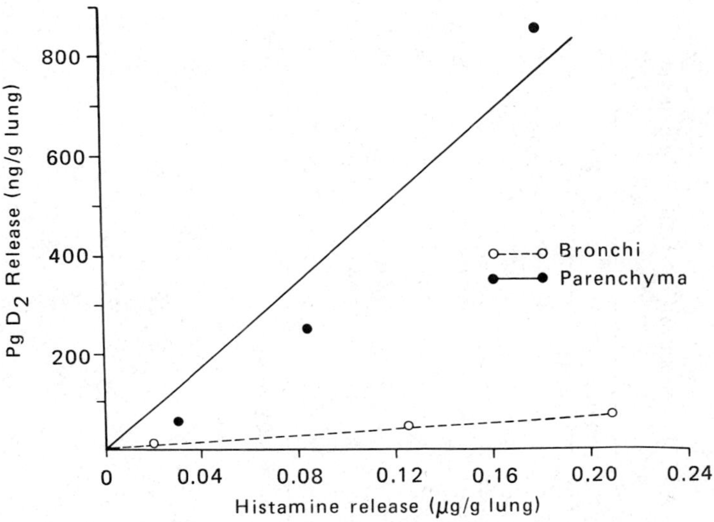

Figure 2 Illustration of typical linear relationship between antigen-induced histamine release and, in this case, PGD_2 generation.

detected. Submaximal methacholine concentrations (10^{-4} M) were used to evaluate the contribution of methacholine-sensitive tissues (especially smooth muscle) to the total cyclooxygenase output during lung anaphylaxis. Methacholine challenge produced an appreciable fraction of antigen-elicited synthesis only in the case of prostacyclin (37%) and PGE (42%). Thus, muscle contraction per se accounts for a significant portion of cyclooxygenase activity during in vitro anaphylaxis only for the two known bronchodilator metabolites. In these experiments histamine release averaged 3.7 ± 0.7 μg/g wet weight lung, which represents a mean of $22.9 \pm 4.5\%$ total histamine content.

With the exception of PGE_2, the cyclooxygenase production during anaphylactic challenge of human bronchial tissue is less than that observed with a comparable weight of parenchyma from the same lung (Fig. 1). In bronchial tissue, as in parenchyma, prostacyclin production predominates. PGD_2 release was only 10% of that seen in parenchyma, but this may be attributable to the much lower histamine release (0.67 ± 0.3 μg/g lung; $4.8 \pm 1.9\%$ total histamine) compared with parenchymal tissue (see above). As in parenchyma, submaximal methacholine challenge accounted for more than 50% of anaphylactic production only for PGE (58%) and prostacyclin (64%).

In order to normalize cyclooxygenase output for the disparate histamine release levels observed between bronchial and parenchymal tissue, the data from antigen dose-response experiments were subjected to linear regression analysis

Table 1 Comparison of Net Arachidonic Acid Cyclooxygenase Metabolite (AACM) Generation Per Unit of Histamine Release from Human Bronchi and Parenchyma

	Bronchi			Parenchyma				
AACM	AACM (ng)[a] / Histamine (μg)	r[b]	P[c]	AACM (ng)[a] / Histamine (μg)	r[b]	P[c]	F Ratio[d]	P[e]
PGE	26.5 ± 33.0	.494	.506	28.0 ± 9	.867	.057	1.1	.395
$PGF_{2\alpha}$	13.2 ± 6.6	.816	.184	50.0 ± 5.2	.984	.002	27.4	.002
TxB_2	3.3 ± 1.2	.890	.110	24.0 ± 6	.929	.023	20.5	.004
PGD_2	309.6 ± 26	.993	.007	5120.0 ± 580	.981	.003	51.0	.001
6-keto-$PgF_{1\alpha}$	56.9 ± 12	.957	.043	325 ± 66.8	.942	.017	21.6	.004

[a]Slope of the regression of Net AACM production ng/g lung vs. histamine release μg/g lung.
[b]Correlation coefficient for linear regression analysis.
[c]Probability of type-I error in rejecting hypothesis of nonlinearity.
[d]Test for differences in slopes of the regression lines for bronchi vs. parenchyma.
[e]Probability of type-I error in rejecting hypothesis that slopes are not different.

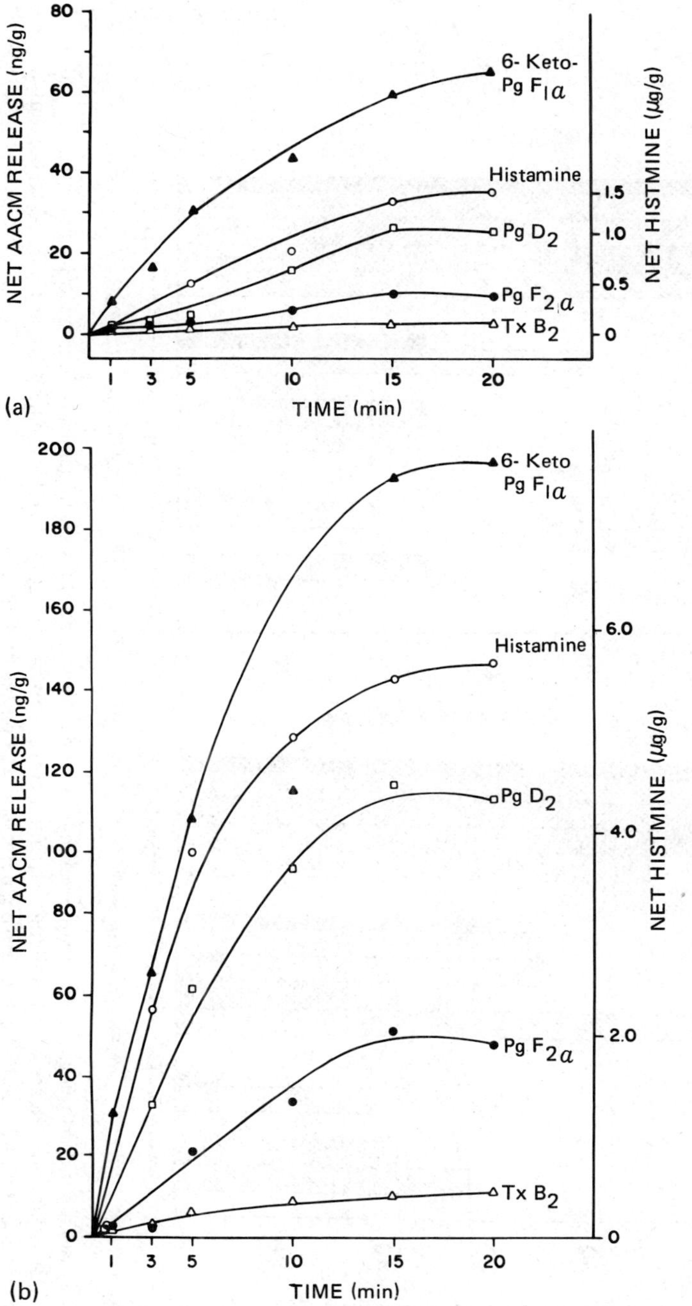

Figure 3 Kinetic release of histamine and arachidonic acid cyclooxygenase metabolites (AACM) after antigen challenge of passively sensitized human lung fragments. (*a*) Bronchial tissue; (*b*) parenchymal tissue.

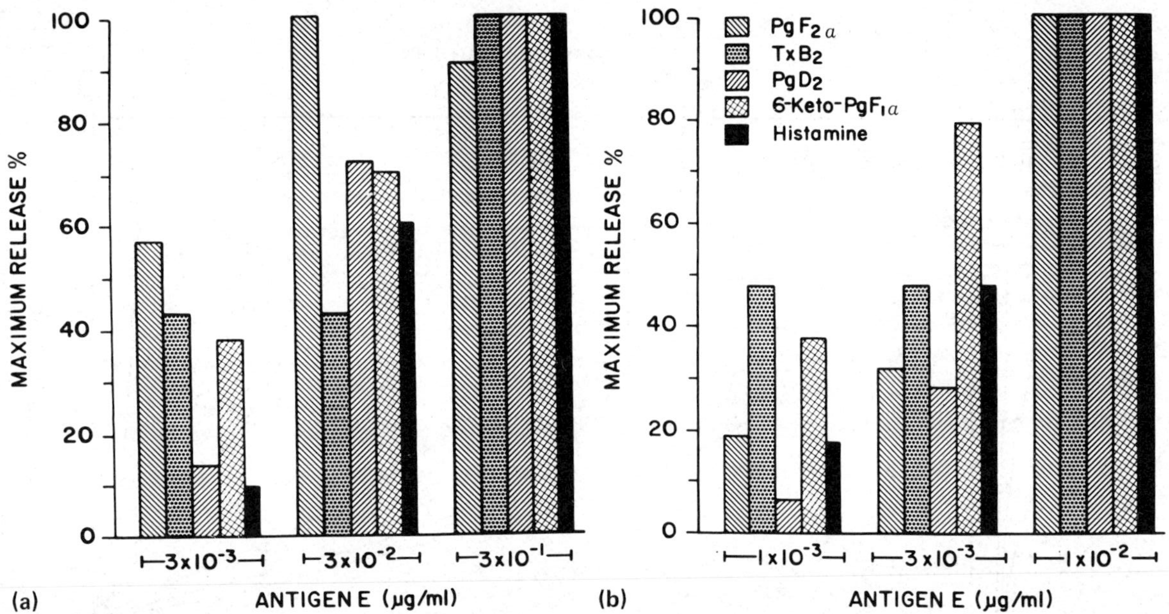

Figure 4 Dose-dependent release of histamine and cyclooxygenase metabolites from passively sensitized human lung fragments. Spontaneous release of unchallenged fragments was subtracted from all values, which are normalized to percent maximum release for each mediator. (*a*) Bronchial tissue; (*b*) parenchymal tissue.

to determine the best estimate of cyclooxygenase products per microgram of histamine release. Satisfactory correlation coefficients ($\geq 0.8; p < 0.1$) were found to support the general linearity of metabolite release as a function of histamine release for all metabolites except PGE in bronchial tissue. This linear relationship is illustrated for PGD_2 in Figure 2. Table 1 displays the normalized results. Normalization for histamine release amplifies the predominance of PGD_2 relative to the other cyclooxygenase metabolites. Except for PGE, parenchymal tissue produced more of each metabolite per microgram of histamine released than did bronchial tissue. Especially noteworthy is the sixteenfold greater release of PGD_2 per microgram of histamine release in parenchyma compared with bronchi. This observation is not easily reconciled with the concept that the activated mast cell is the sole source for PGD_2, unless one postulates biochemical differences between bronchial and parenchymal mast cells.

V. Relation of Mast Cell Activation to Arachidonate Metabolism

Figure 3 shows the kinetics of cyclooxygenase product formation compared with that for histamine release after antigen challenge of sensitized bronchial and parenchymal fragments. Release of both histamine and the assayed cyclooxygenase metabolites have a similar kinetic course which is complete by 15-20 min following antigen challenge. In contrast to the earlier findings of Piper and Walker (1973) using bioassay, our radioimmunoassay studies indicate an antigen dose-dependent increase in cyclooxygenase output in both bronchi and parenchyma (Fig. 4). It is clear from the results shown with four cyclooxygenase products, however, that the shape and position of the dose-response curves differ among the metabolites and most differ from that of histamine release as well.

VI. Source of Arachidonate Products Released During Anaphylaxis

Of great interest and relevance is the cellular source of the arachidonate products released during lung anaphylaxis. Available evidence suggests that contracting smooth muscle, or adjacent tissues which are physically distorted as a result of vascular or bronchial smooth muscle contraction, do not comprise a major source of bronchospastic cyclooxygenase products produced during anaphylaxis. Several investigators have observed that smooth muscle agonists, including maximally effective concentrations of histamine, methacholine, and the depolarizing agent potassium chloride, result in cyclooxygenase products accounting for relatively small fractions (usually $\leq 25\%$) of that produced during anaphylaxis (Platshon and Kaliner, 1978; Steel et al., 1979; Adkinson et al., 1980; Schulman et al., 1981).

The use of H_1 antihistamine only partially and variably inhibits anaphylactic prostaglandin production (Platshon and Kaliner, 1978; Adkinson et al., 1980). This finding, coupled with the low levels of $PgF_{2\alpha}$ and PgE_2 generated by exogenous histamine, suggests that histamine release from mast cells during anaphylaxis may not be a major secondary stimulus for anaphylactic prostaglandin production. While partially purified SRS-As have been shown to induce the release of prostaglandins from perfused guinea pig lungs and human lung fragments (Mathe et al., 1977a), the quantitative capacity of the leukotrienes to generate cyclooxygenase metabolites in human lung tissue remains to be examined. Preliminary studies in our laboratory indicate that leukotrienes C_4 and D_4 at micromolar concentrations can generate prostaglandins and thromboxanes from normal human lung tissue (unpublished observations 1981). Until the level of endogenous leukotrienes released during in vitro lung anaphylaxis is known, it will be difficult to assess the relative contribution of leukotriene-induced cyclooxygenase synthesis to total arachidonate metabolism during lung anaphylaxis.

Other than histamine and leukotrienes, the latter of which are themselves arachidonate metabolites, no other clearly defined human mast cell products have been reported to generate prostaglandin or thromboxane production secondarily from other lung cell types. The prostaglandin-generating factor described by Steel and Kaliner (1981) could be of mast cell origin, but this remains to be demonstrated. The capacity of chemotactic factors, heparin, mast cell enzymes, and other human mast cell constituents to induce arachidonate metabolism from adjacent tissue in the lung is currently unknown.

As discussed above, the major known source of prostacyclin in the lung appears to be from vascular endothelium. Pulmonary macrophages and alveolar type-II cells may be capable of limited prostacyclin production (Humes et al., 1977; Taylor et al., 1978). The principal source of the relatively large quantities of prostacyclin generated during human lung anaphylaxis remains to be determined.

The human lung mast cell produces predominantly PGD_2 when activated by immunologic or nonimmunologic stimuli (Schulman et al., 1981; Lewis et al., 1980a; Roberts et al., 1980). Lesser quantities of prostacyclin are also released. Our experimental observations discussed above leave open the possibility that there may be another major source(s) of PGD_2 production in human lung during anaphylaxis. An alternative explanation, which would leave the mast cell as the predominant if not exclusive source for PGD_2, is that biochemical differences exist between mast cells in bronchi and parenchyma, such that the more peripheral mast cells produce more PGD_2 per quantum of histamine released. Currently, however, there is little evidence to support the concept of biochemical heterogeneity among human lung mast cells.

The target tissues for prostaglandin- and thromboxane-releasing factor(s) are also unknown, since only intact guinea pig lung has thus far been used to

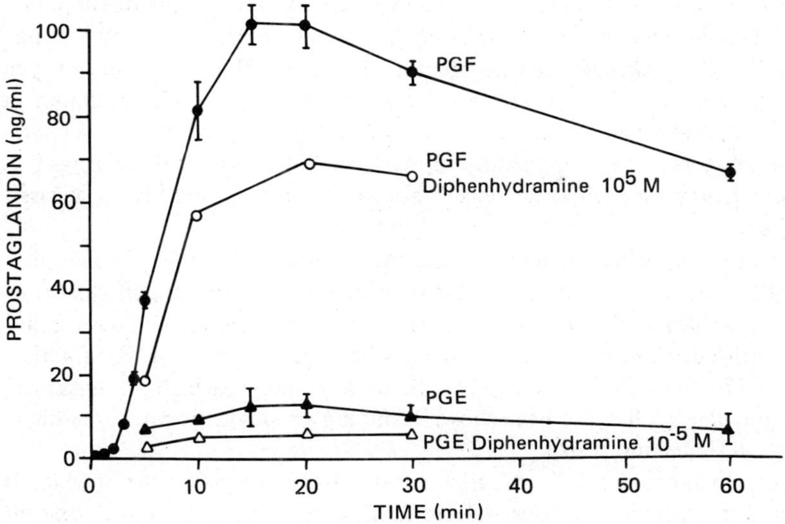

Figure 5 Incomplete inhibition of anaphylactic $PGF_{2\alpha}$ production by the H_1 antihistamine diphenhydramine (10^{-5} M) from human lung. Higher concentrations of this drug affected histamine release.

assay this factor(s). The guinea pig prostaglandin-releasing factor appears to favor production of thromboxane, which is the primary cyclooxygenase metabolite observed during guinea pig anaphylaxis (Nijkamp et al., 1976; Engineer et al., 1978). The human lung releasing factor reported by Steel and Kaliner (1981) generates more $PGF_{2\alpha}$ than TxB_2 from guinea pig lung fragments. There may well be, a spectrum of releasing factors with differing tissue specificities.

VII. Pharmacologic Modulation of the Production of Arachidonate Metabolites During Human Lung Anaphylaxis

Pharmacologic agents that antagonize known functions of mast cell mediators can also reduce the secondary activation of the arachidonate cyclooxygenase during antigen-induced anaphylaxis. For example, as mentioned above, H_1 antihistamines variably and only partially diminish cyclooxygenase production in human lung anaphylaxis in vitro (Platshon and Kaliner, 1978; Adkinson et al., 1980), as shown in Figure 5. In preliminary experiments, FPL-55712 (2 × 10^{-5} M), a pharmacologic antagonist of SRS-A (leukotrienes), completely blocks the ability of micromolar leukotrienes C_4 and D_4 to generate a variety of cyclooxygenase products from human and guinea pig lung fragments (unpublished observations). When the H_1 antagonist diphenhydramine (10^{-4} M) and FPL-55712 (2×10^{-5} M) are used together, inhibition of antigen-induced cyclooxygenase activity is incomplete. Failure to obtain complete inhibition may be due to the prostaglandin-generating activity of other mast cell mediators (e.g., releasing factors), or to the inability of pharmacologic doses of these drugs to antagonize fully the high local concentrations of histamine and SRS-A released into the microenvironment.

Since lung cyclooxygenase activity increases with increasing degrees of mast cell activation, it is not surprising that drugs which inhibit mast cell histamine release also inhibit production of arachidonate metabolites. These include cAMP-active drugs such as theophylline, β-adrenergic drugs, and PGE_2 (Mathe et al., 1977c; Strandberg et al., 1977). Sodium cromolyn, which prevents mast cell degranulation, has also been shown to inhibit anaphylactic prostaglandin generation (Piper and Walker, 1973).

Finally, nonsteroidal, anti-inflammatory drugs, the prototype of which is aspirin, directly inhibit in a dose-related fashion the generation of cyclooxygenase products, while increasing slightly antigen-induced histamine release from human lung fragments (Platshon and Kaliner, 1978). It is becoming increasingly clear that various cyclooxygenase enzymes have differential sensitivity to nonsteroidal anti-inflammatory drug inhibition. This has been best studied with regard to platelet thromboxane synthetase and the vascular endothelial prostacyclin synthetase enzymes (Moncada and Vane, 1979). Whether there are marked differential sensitivities to the aspirinlike drugs among the lung cell types responsible for cyclooxygenase production during lung anaphylaxis has yet to be determined.

VIII. Conclusions

IgE-dependent mast cell activation in human lung results in the production of biologically significant quantities of arachidonate metabolites. Of greatest potential interest for the pathogenesis of human allergic asthma are the SRSs, now identified as leukotrienes derived from the lipoxygenase pathway. Of the known biologically active products of the cyclooxygenase pathway, prostacyclin and PGD_2 predominate when sensitized human lung fragments are challenged with antigen in vitro. Thromboxane, the principle cyclooxygenase product in guinea pig lung anaphylaxis, is a relatively minor product during human lung anaphylaxis. With the exception of PGD_2, which may be largely derived from activated lung mast cells, little is known about either the primary stimuli or the target tissues for cyclooxygenase activation during human lung anaphylaxis. For all metabolites measured except PGE_2, the more peripheral parenchymal tissue appears to be a richer source of cyclooxygenase metabolites per unit of histamine release than the more central bronchial tissues. The possibility exists that drugs or metabolic circumstances may influence the ratio of bronchoconstrictor-to-bronchodilator cyclooxygenase products. This provides a possible opening for therapeutic intervention in bronchospastic states such as allergic bronchial asthma.

Acknowledgments

We appreciate the courtesy of the American Physiological Society in allowing us to reproduce portions of this manuscript (including Figs. 1-4), which have appeared previously in the *Journal of Applied Physiology* [Schulman et al. (1982)].

References

Adkinson, N. F., Jr. (1977). Prostaglandin production by human peripheral blood cells *in vitro*. *J. Lab. Clin. Med., 90*:1043-1053.

Adkinson, N. F., Jr., Newball, H. H., Findlay, S., Adams, G. K., and Lichtenstein, L. M. (1980). Anaphylactic release of prostaglandins from human lung *in vitro*. *Am. Rev. Respir. Dis., 121*:911-920.

Austen, K. F., and Orange, R. P. (1976). Bronchial asthma: The possible role of the chemical mediators of immediate hypersensitivity in the pathogenesis of subacute chronic disease. *Am. Rev. Respir. Dis., 112*:423-434.

Boot, J. R., Cockerill, A. F., Dawson, W., Mallen, D. N. B., and Osborne, D. J. (1978). Modification of prostaglandin and thromboxane release by immunological sensitisation and successive immunological challenges from guinea-pig lung. *Int. Arch. Allergy Appl. Immunol., 57*:159-164.

Bryant, R. W., Feinmark, S. J., Makheja, A. N., and Bailey, J. M. (1978). Lipid metabolism in cultured cells. *J. Biol. Chem., 253*:8134-8142.

Dawson, W., Boot, J., Cockerill, A., Mallen, D., and Osborne, D. (1976). Release of novel prostaglandins and thromboxanes after immunological challenge of guinea-pig lung. *Nature, 262*:699-702.

Engineer, D. M., Morris, H. R., Piper, P. J., and Sirois, P. (1978). The release of prostaglandins and thromboxanes from guinea pig lung by slow reacting substances of anaphylaxis, and its inhibition. *Br. J. Pharmacol., 64*:211-218.

Fish, J. E., Ankin, M. G., Adkinson, N. F., Jr., and Peterman, V. I. (1981). Indomethacin modification of immediate-type immunologic airway responses in allergic asthmatic and non-asthmatic subjects: Evidence for altered arachidonic acid metabolish in asthma. *Am. Rev. Respir. Dis., 123*:609-614.

Goetzl, E. J. (1980). Mediators of immediate hypersensitivity derived from arachidonic acid. *N. Engl. J. Med., 303*:822-825.

Green, K., Hedquist, H., and Svanborg, N. (1974). Increased plasma levels of 15-keto-13,14-dihydro-prostaglandin $F_{2\alpha}$ after allergen-provoked asthma in man. *Lancet, ii*:1419-1421.

Humes, J. L., Bonney, R. J., Pelus, L., Dahlgren, M. E., Sadowski, S. J., Kuehl, F. A., Jr., Davies, P. (1977). Macrophages synthesise and release prostaglandins in response to inflammatory stimuli. *Nature, 269*:149-151.

Hyman, A. L., Spannhake, E. W., and Kadowitz, P. J. (1978). Prostaglandins and the lung. *Am. Rev. Respir. Dis., 117*:111-136.

Lewis, R. A., Roberts, L. J., II, Holgate, S. T., Oates, J. A., and Austen, K. F. (1980b). Prostaglandin D_2 production by rat and human mast cells activated by reversed anaphylaxis. *Fed. Proc., 39*:905.

Lewis, R. A., Austen, K. F., Drazen, J. M., Clark, D. A., Marfat, A., and Corey, E. J. (1980a). Slow reacting substances of anaphylaxis: identification of leukotrienes C-1 and D from human and rat sources. *Proc. Natl. Acad. Sci., 77*:3710-3714.

Mathe, A. A., Strandberg, K., and Yen, S-S. (1977a). Prostaglandin release by slow reacting substance from guinea pig and human lung tissue. *Prostaglandins, 14*:1105-1115.

Mathe, A. A., Hedquist, P., Strandberg, K., and Leslie, C. A. (1977b). Aspects of prostaglandin function in the lung. *N. Eng. J. Med., 296*:850-855, 910-914.

Mathe, A. A., Yen, S-S., Sohn, R. J., and Hedquist, P. (1977c). Release of prostaglandins and histamine from sensitized and anaphylactic guinea pig lungs: Changes in cyclic AMP levels. *Biochem. Pharmacol., 26*:181-188.

Moncada, S., and Vane, J. R. (1979). Arachidonic acid metabolites and the interactions between platelets and blood-vessel walls. *N. Engl. J. Med., 300*: 1142-1147.

Moncada, S., Higgs, E. A., and Vane, J. R. (1977). Human arterial and venous tissues generate prostacyclin (prostaglandin x), a potent inhibitor of platelet aggregation. *Lancet, i*:18-20.

Morley, J., Bray, M. A., Jones, R. W., Nugteren, D. H., and van Dorp, D. A. (1979). Prostaglandin and thromboxane production by human and guinea-pig macrophages and leukocytes. *Prostaglandins, 17*:730-736.

Morris, H. G. and Sherman, N. A. (1980). Prostaglandin-like substances in urine of asthmatic patients. *Adv. Prostaglandin Thromboxane Res., 8*:1765-1770.

Morris, H. G., Sherman, N. A., and Shepperdson, F. T. (1981a). Effect of aspirin on plasma and urinary thromboxane in patients with EIB. Proceedings of The American Academy of Allergy, San Francisco, 37th Annual Meeting (Abstract #180).

Morris, H. G., Sherman, N. A., and Shepperdson, F. T. (1981b). Variables associated with radioimmunoassay of prostaglandins in plasma. *Prostaglandins, 21*:771-788.

Nijkamp, F. P., Flower, R. J., Moncada, S., and Vane, J. R. (1976). Partial purification of RCS-RF and inhibition of its activity by anti-inflammatory steroids. *Nature, 263*:479-480.

Palmer, M. A., Piper, P. J., and Vane, J. R. (1973). Release of rabbit aorta contracting substances (RCS) and prostaglandins induced by chemical or mechanical stimulation of guinea-pig lungs. *Br. J. Pharmacol., 49*:226-242.

Peters, S. P., Siegel, M. I., Kagey-Sobotka, A., and Lichtenstein, L. M. (1981). Lipoxygenase products modulate histamine release in human basophils. *Nature, 292*:455-457.

Piper, P. J. (1977). Anaphylaxis and the release of active substances in the lungs. *Pharmacol. Ther. B., 3*:75-98.

Piper, P. J., and Vane, J. R. (1971). The release of prostaglandins from lung and other tissues. *N.Y. Acad. Sci., 180*:363-385.

Piper, P. J., and Walker, J. C. (1973). The release of spasmogenic substances from human chopped lung tissue and its inhibition. *Br. J. Pharmacol., 47*:291-304.

Platshon, L. F., and Kaliner, M. (1978). The effects of the immunologic release of histamine upon human lung cyclic nucleotide levels and prostaglandin generation. *J. Clin. Invest., 62*:1113-1121.

Roberts, L. J., Sweetman, B. J., Lewis, R. A., Austen, K. F., and Oates, J. A. (1980). Increased production of prostaglandin D_2 in patients with systemic mastocytosis. *N. Engl. J. Med., 303*:1400-1404.

Schulman, E. S., Newball, H. H., Demers, L. M., Fitzpatrick, F. A., and Adkinson, N. F., Jr. (1981). Anaphylactic release of thromboxane A_2, prostaglandin D_2, and prostacyclin from human lung parenchyma. *Am. Rev. Respir. Dis., 124*:402-406.

Schulman, E. S., Adkinson, N. F., Jr., and Newball, H. H. (1982). Cyclooxygenase metabolites in human lung anaphylaxis: Airway vs. parenchyma. *J. Appl. Physiol., 53*:589-595.

Sherman, N. A., Morris, H. G., Silvers, W., and Shepperdson, F. T. (1981). Plasma and serum prostaglandins in patients with asthma. Proceedings of The American Academy of Allergy, San Francisco, 37th Annual Meeting (Abstract # 179).

Smith, A. P., and Dunlop, L. (1975). Prostaglandins and asthma. *Lancet i*:39.

Steel, L., and Kaliner, M. (1981). Prostaglandin-generating factor of anaphylaxis: identification and isolation. *J. Biol. Chem., 256*:12692-12698.

Steel, L., Platshon, L., and Kaliner, M. (1979). Prostaglandin generation by human and guinea pig lung tissue: comparison of parenchymal and airway responses. *J. Allergy Clin. Immunol., 64*:287-293.

Stenson, W. F., and Parker, C. W. (1980). Monohydroxyeicosatetraenoic Acids (Hetes) Induce Degranulation of Human Neutrophils. *J. Immunol., 124*:2100-2104.

Strandberg, K., Mathe, A. A., and Yen, S-S. (1977). Release of histamine and formation of prostaglandins in human lung tissue and rat mast cells. *Int. Arch. Allergy Appl. Immunol., 53*:520-529.

Taylor, L., Polgar, P., McAteer, J., and Doublas, W. H. J. (1978). Prostaglandin production by type II alveolar epithelial cells in culture. *Prostaglandins, 15*:699-700.

4

Immunopharmacology of Acetyl Glyceryl Ether Phosphorylcholine (AGEPC)

R. NEAL PINCKARD,
LINDA M. McMANUS,
and DONALD J. HANAHAN
The University of Texas
Health Science Center at San Antonio
San Antonio, Texas

MARILYN HALONEN
The University of Arizona
College of Medicine
Tucson, Arizona

I. Introduction

The lung is a principal and particularly sensitive target organ that is involved in a variety of acute allergic and inflammatory reactions. Several highly potent chemical mediators that are produced either endogenously in the lung or exogenously and then transported to the lung via the circulation have been implicated in modulating the physiologic and inflammatory sequelae of various pulmonary disease states (see Chap. 1). Some examples of these potent, chemically defined mediators include histamine, serotonin, bradykinin, arachidonic acid metabolites derived from the cyclooxygenase (PGE_2, $PGF_{2\alpha}$, PGD_2, PGI_2, and TxA_2) and the lipoxygenase (leukotrienes B, C, D, E and hydroperoxy-and hydroxy-eicosatetraenoic acids) pathways, and the C3a and C5a anaphylatoxins. Most of these highly potent chemical mediators possess a spectrum of pharmacologic activities and collectively may be classified into a group of compounds termed "autacoids" (Douglas, 1980). The term autacoid originally was derived (Schafer, 1916) from the Greek words *autos* ("self") and *akos* ("medicinal agent" or

Supported by NIH Grants HL-22555, HL-22582, HL-00463, and The American Heart Association, Texas Affiliate.

"remedy"). Douglas (1980) proposed that this generic term be used in place of the terms "local hormones" or "autopharmacologic agents" to distinguish this group of potent pharmacologic agents clearly from the more general classification of hormones.

Recently, the chemical structure of another chemical mediator, platelet-activating factor (PAF) has been characterized to be acetyl glyceryl ether phosphorylcholine (AGEPC; Hanahan et al., 1980) and the molecule synthesized (Demopoulos et al., 1979). These accomplishments have enabled the initiation of a series of studies to assess the biological activities of this molecule which clearly indicate that AGEPC unquestionably should be considered as a most potent autacoid. The following discussion will address this issue and the possible role of AGEPC in the immunopharmacology of the lung.

II. Identification and Structural Characterization of Platelet-Activating Factor

Historically, the development of this new, fascinating field of investigation occurred in two phases during the past 10 years. The first phase encompassed a period from 1970-1977 when PAF initially was defined and some of its biological properties were identified, including its involvement in IgE-acute allergic reactions. Table 1 lists some of the highlights that occurred during this first developmental phase. Initially, Henson (1970) reported an apparent leukocyte-platelet communication whereby antigen stimulation of buffy coat cells obtained from immunized rabbits resulted in the activation of platelets, i.e., the release of platelet vasoactive amines. Evidence was presented that indicated that platelet stimulation occurred either through direct leukocyte-platelet interaction or through the release of a soluble, fluid-phase factor(s) from sensitized leukocytes which then mediated platelet stimulation. Subsequently, two independent

Table 1 Platelet-Activating Factor: 1970–1979

Leukocyte-platelet communication	Henson (1970)
Fluid-phase platelet stimulator released from rabbit basophils	Siraganian and Osler (1971); Benveniste et al. (1972a)
Platelet-activating factor (PAF)	Benveniste et al. (1972b)
Lipid-like nature of PAF	Benveniste (1974)
1-Lyso-phosphatidylcholine proposed as PAF structure	Benveniste et al. (1977)
Implication of PAF in mediating IgE-induced systemic anaphylaxis	Henson and Pinckard (1977); Pinckard et al. (1977)

studies (Siraganian and Osler, 1971; Benveniste et al., 1972a) confirmed that a fluid-phase mediator was released and that the IgE-sensitized rabbit basophil most likely was the leukocyte that released this platelet stimulator. At this time, Benveniste et al. (1972b) named this newly described mediator "platelet-activating factor" or PAF to describe its biological activity, since the chemical nature of the material was not known. Subsequently, the lipidlike nature of PAF was suggested because the platelet-stimulating activity could be extracted into ethanol (Benveniste, 1974) and was soluble in chloroform (Benveniste et al., 1977); in the latter study, Benveniste and co-workers (1977) suggested that the structure of PAF likely was a 1-lyso-phospholipid that probably contained choline. This structure was postulated because of both the thin-layer chromatographic (TLC) behavior of PAF and the differential susceptibility of PAF to phospholipase attack.

While the above studies described a fascinating new mediator which was released by IgE-sensitized rabbit basophils and manifested potent platelet-stimulating activity in vitro, there was only circumstantial evidence for its possible role as a mediator of IgE-induced acute allergic reations in vivo. Two studies however, provided more convincing, although still indirect, evidence for the importance of PAF in allergic reactions. Pinckard et al. (1977) demonstrated the development of profound, but reversible, intravascular platelet aggregation and acute thrombocytopenia during the early phases of antigen-induced, IgE systemic anaphylaxis in the rabbit. These intravascular platelet alterations mimicked the biological actions of PAF as defined in vitro and suggested that PAF may have been operative in vivo. In addition, these studies indicated that the platelet was involved in some of the pathophysiologic sequelae of the anaphylactic syndrome. In a parallel series of experiments, Henson and Pinckard (1977) demonstrated that platelets obtained 60 min following the initiation of IgE-induced systemic anaphylaxis were specifically desensitized to PAF. These latter studies strongly suggested that PAF was produced and had interacted with circulating platelets. Thus, postanaphylaxis platelets were unresponsive to PAF stimulation; however, of importance, these PAF-desensitized platelets maintained normal responsiveness to other nonrelated platelet stimuli.

Following the first 7 years of PAF investigation, two very important pressing questions remained unanswered and were the focus of the next 3 years of investigation (Table 2): (a) unequivocal, direct evidence that PAF was produced in vivo during IgE-induced acute allergic reactions was lacking and (b) the chemical structure of PAF had not been elucidated. The answer to the first question derived from studies that further characterized the IgE-induced anaphylactic syndrome in the rabbit (Pinckard et al., 1979). In these investigations, the intravascular release of substantial amounts of PAF within 60 sec following intravenous antigen challenge of IgE-sensitized rabbits was documented. The PAF was methanol extracted from the plasmas of acidified (pH 3–4), citrated blood

Table 2 Platelet-Activating Factor: 1979–1980

Isolation and physicochemical characterization of PAF released during IgE anaphylaxis	Pinckard et al. (1979)
1-0-Alkyl-2-acetyl-*sn*-glyceryl-3-phosphorylcholine (AGEPC): Proposed structure for PAF and APRL	Demopoulos et al. (1979); Blank et al. (1979); Benveniste et al. (1979b)
AGEPC-induced anaphylactoid reactions: intravascular, cardiovascular, and pulmonary	McManus et al. (1980a); Halonen et al. (1980)
Direct structure-proof identification of rabbit basophil PAF as AGEPC	Hanahan et al. (1980)

samples followed by extraction into the chloroform-rich phase of a mixture of chloroform-methanol-water (1:1:0.9, v/v). Similar PAF activity could be extracted from the plasmas of antigen-challenged, normal rabbits that previously were transfused with IgE-sensitized rabbit basophils. In both of these studies, the temporal release of PAF into the plasma correlated with the development of basopenia, neutropenia, and thrombocytopenia. The TLC behavior (on silica gel G) of the PAF released during IgE anaphylaxis was identical to highly purified PAF obtained in vitro from antigen-stimulated rabbit buffy coat cells containing IgE-sensitized basophils.

Physicochemical studies provided evidence that PAF was indeed a lipid with properties that would be expected for a neutral phospholipid containing at least one carboxylic acid ester grouping required for its biological activity (Pinckard et al., 1979). In these studies, it was found that the biological activity of PAF (i.e., the stimulation of washed rabbit platelets) was exceedingly stable to a variety of physical and chemical treatments with the exception that PAF was rapidly and completely inactivated by exposure to NaOH, particularly in the presence of methanol. The loss of activity following base-catalyzed methanolysis suggested that a carboxylic acid ester grouping was essential for the biologic activity of the molecule. Subsequently, Demopoulos et al., (1979) demonstrated that the biological activity of PAF, previously destroyed by base-catalyzed methanolysis, could be completely restored by acylation of the PAF degradation product only with short-chain fatty acid anhydrides (i.e., acetic acid anhydride); in addition, it was shown that the PAF degradation product was completely soluble in chloroform. This latter observation indicated that the PAF molecule contained only one carboxylic acid ester grouping, a phosphate ester, and one other linkage to the glycerol backbone that was resistant to base treatment, e.g.,

(a)

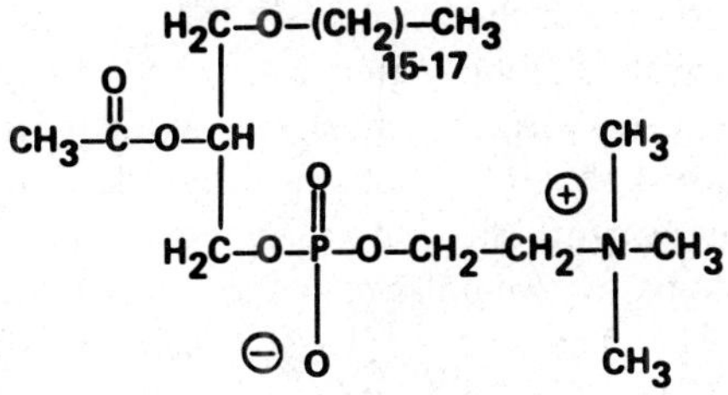

1-*O*-hexadecyl/octadecyl-2-acetyl-*sn*-glyceryl-3-phosphorylcholine (AGEPC)

(b)

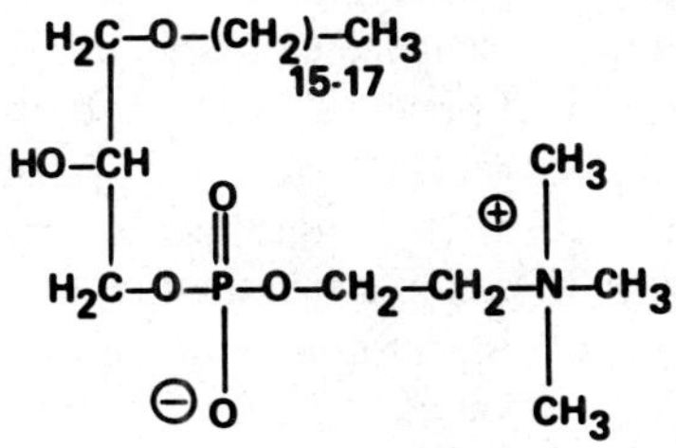

1-*O*-hexadecyl/octadecyl-*sn*-glyceryl-3-phosphorylcholine (Lyso-GEPC)

Figure 1 (*a*) Acetyl glyceryl ether phosphorylcholine (AGEPC); (*b*) lyso-glyceryl ether phosphorylcholine (lyso-GEPC).

an ether linkage. Since PAF was highly resistant to treatment with strong acid, this supported an alkyl grouping, rather than an alkenyl grouping (i.e., a plasmalogen), as the latter would be highly susceptible to acid cleavage. Thus, these findings were consistent for a PAF molecule with a structure similar to a 1-*O*-alkyl-2-acetyl-*sn*-glyceryl-3-phosphorylcholine (AGEPC, Fig. 1a).

In view of the above, the vinyl ether-containing phospholipids were isolated and purified from beef heart and were subjected to catalytic hydrogenation followed by base-catalyzed methanolysis to yield 1-*O*-hexadecyl/octadecyl-*sn*-glyceryl-3-phosphorylcholine (lyso-GEPC, Fig. 1b). The 2 position of lyso-GEPC then was acylated utilizing acetic, proprionic, or butyric acid anhydrides and the various derivatives were purified, structurally characterized, and tested for platelet-stimulating activity. While all three compounds manifested potent platelet-stimulating activity, the acetylated derivative (AGEPC) biologically was the most active and was the only derivative that shared all of the physicochemical properties with native PAF obtained from antigen-stimulated, IgE-sensitized basophils. These data, together with the observation that both native PAF and AGEPC cross-desensitized washed rabbit platelets to the same degree, led to the conclusion that AGEPC (Fig. 1a) was very similar, if not identical, to the native PAF molecule (Demopoulos et al., 1979). Subsequently, Blank and co-workers published results of a similarly synthesized molecule whose biological activity mimicked that of the antihypertensive polar renal medullary lipid (APRL) previously described by Prewitt and co-workers (1979). Thereafter, Benveniste and co-workers (1979b) also published a similar structure and proposed that it, too, likely was the same as PAF.

While the proceeding studies suggested that the native PAF released in vitro from IgE-sensitized rabbit basophils and AGEPC were one and the same molecule, direct structure-proof analysis of native PAF was mandatory to establish conclusively the answer to this most important question. To date, only one study has answered this question (Hanahan et al., 1980). These studies were made possible by a modification of previously published purification procedures involving sequential TLC on silica gel G using solvent systems differing in their relative polarities (Pinckard et al., 1979). Thus, highly purified PAF was obtained by utilizing two TLC purification steps; the first separation was performed using a solvent system of chloroform-methanol-water (65:35:6, v/v) followed by a second TLC separation using a solvent system of methanol-water (2:1, v/v) (Hanahan et al., 1980; see Fig. 2). Utilizing the highly purified PAF obtained from antigen-stimulated, IgE-sensitized rabbit basophils, the following studies were conducted and demonstrated that PAF and AGEPC were indeed one and the same molecule. First, the glyceryl ether component of PAF was established by gas-liquid chromatography and electron-impact mass spectrometry of its isopropylidene derivative. These studies not only documented the glyceryl ether composition of PAF, but also demonstrated that greater than 90% of the molecules were that of 1-*O*-octadecyl glyceryl ether (C-18) and less than 10% were 1-*O*-hexadecyl glyceryl ether (C-16). Other mass spectral studies of the trimethylsilylated residues of acid-hydrolyzed PAF samples documented the occurrence of glycerol and phosphate in the native PAF molecule. Choline as a component part of PAF was established by pyrolysis gas chromatography-mass spectrometry. Finally, the presence of the proposed fatty acid component of PAF as acetic acid was accomplished by gas-liquid chromatography where the level of acetic acid in native PAF was estimated to be in the range of 9–10%, a value similar to the calculated amount of 10.9% for 1-*O*-octadecyl-2-acetyl-*sn*-glyceryl-3-phosphorylcholine. Therefore, the preceding studies unequivocally demonstrated that native PAF was composed of at least two molecules of AGEPC, one containing a C-18 alkyl grouping ($>$ 90%) and the other containing a C-16 alkyl grouping ($<$ 10%) (Fig. 1a; Hanahan et al., 1980).

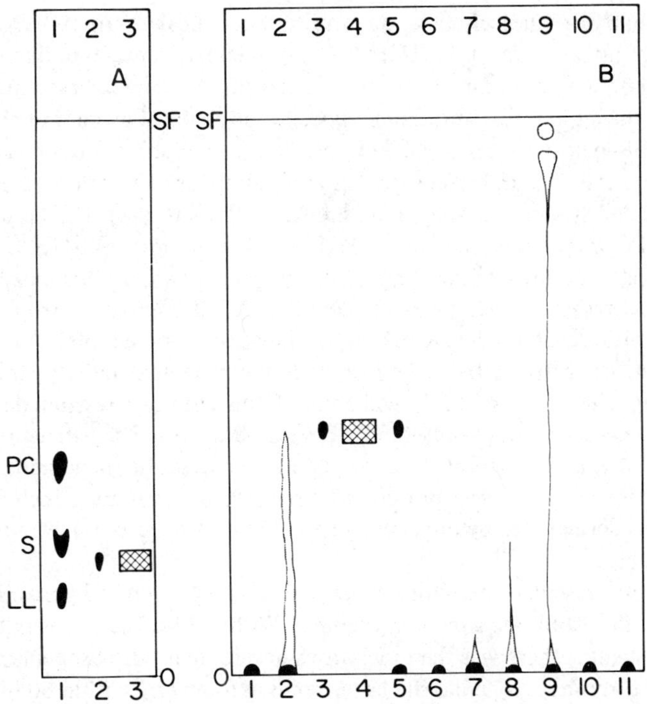

Figure 2 Thin-layer chromatography (TLC) of AGEPC, native rabbit PAF, and various other lipid standards. The plates were precoated silica gel G (250 μm), AnalTech). [hatched box], platelet-activating activity; SF, solvent front; and O, origin. (*a*) This TLC plate was developed in a solvent system of chloroform: methanol: water (65:35:6, v/v). Lane 1, phospholipid standards, lysolecithin (LL, $R_f = 0.15$), sphingomyelin (S, $R_f = 0.23$), and phosphatidylcholine (PC, $R_f = 0.40$); lane 2, AGEPC ($R_f = 0.21$); and lane 3, rabbit basophil-derived, antigen-induced, native PAF ($R_f = 0.21$). (*b*) This TLC plate was developed in a solvent system of methanol/water (2:1, v/v). Lane 1, phosphatidylcholine; lane 2, lysolecithin, lane 3, AGEPC ($R_f = 0.44$); lane 4, rabbit basophil-derived, antigen-induced, native PAF ($R_f = 0.44$); lane 5, mixture of AGEPC and sphingomyelin; lane 6, sphingomyelin; lane 7, neutral lipids; lane 8, phosphatidylethanolamine; lane 9 phosphoinositides; lane 10, phosphatidylserine; and lane 11, cardiolipin. (From McManus et al., 1980a. © 1980 The Williams & Wilkins Co., Baltimore.)

III. Biological Effects of AGEPC In Vivo—Intravascular Alterations

The availability of relatively large quantities of chemically pure AGEPC made possible definitive intravenous AGEPC infusion experiments to define those biological consequences that might occur if this mediator were released intravascularly (e.g., during IgE systemic anaphylaxis in the rabbit; Pinckard et al., 1979). Thus, the biological effects of AGEPC infusion in the rabbit could be compared with those intravascular, cardiovascular, and pulmonary alterations characteristic of IgE-induced systemic anaphylactic shock. At the outset of this discussion, the term AGEPC will be used in place of PAF for two reasons: (a) AGEPC describes the chemical structure of PAF, that is, acetyl glyceryl ether phosphorylcholine and (b) most recent studies have indicated that AGEPC has a spectrum of biological activities over and above platelet stimulation, for example, neutrophil stimulation, vasoactive activity, guinea pig ileal-contracting activity, and so forth (see below). The term "AGEPC" will be used, however, in a restricted sense, since presently it describes only the PAF released from IgE-sensitized rabbit basophils. At this time, AGEPC can not be used to describe the various platelet-activating factors that have reported to be released by a variety of cell types from several species (see below), since their chemical structures have not yet been elucidated.

The intravascular alterations characteristic of IgE-induced systemic anaphylaxis in the rabbit are shown in Figure 3. Within 30-60 sec after intravenous antigen challenge, there was the precipitous development of basopenia, neutropenia, and thrombocytopenia, the latter tending to reverse within 60 min after antigen challenge (Halonen and Pinckard, 1975; Pinckard et al., 1977). In concert with the development of thrombocytopenia, plasma levels of thromboxane B_2 (TxB_2) elevated within 60 sec after antigen challenge and reached maximum levels by 180 sec and then steadily declined (McManus et al., 1980b). The plasma levels of platelet factor 4 (PF4), a specific platelet α-granule protein, became elevated slightly after the elevations in TxB_2 and reached maximum values at between 4–5 min after antigen challenge; plasma PF4 levels then gradually returned toward preinfusion levels by 60 min. As would be expected, pretreatment of rabbits with aspirin (100 mg/kg, intraperitoneally) 18 hr prior to antigen challenge abrogated the elevations in plasma levels of TxB_2; in contrast, the intravascular release of PF4 still occurred, although the PF4 elevations were reduced and delayed when compared to nonaspirin-treated rabbits (McManus et al., 1980b). All of these intravascular alterations during IgE-induced systemic anaphylaxis correlated well with the intravascular release of PAF during this reaction (Pinckard et al., 1979); that is, plasma PAF activity increased within 60 sec after antigen challenge and reached a maximum within 2-3 min. Thus, the sequence of intravascular events (thrombocytopenia, basopenia, neutropenia,

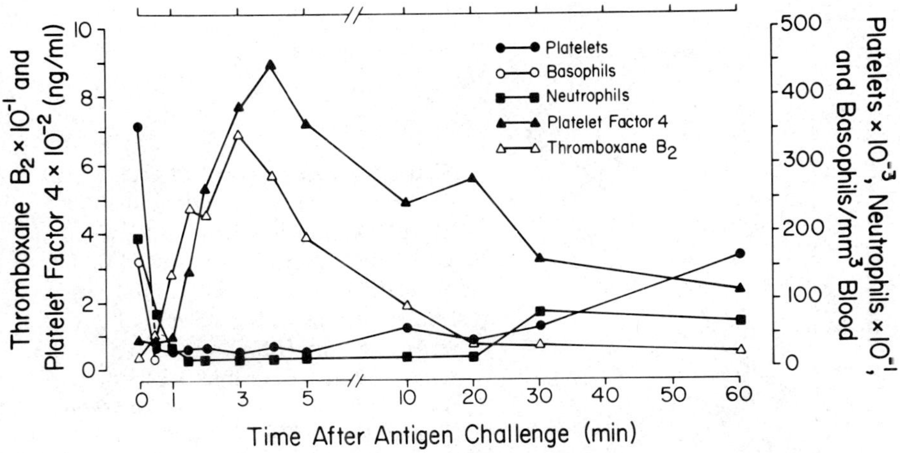

Figure 3 Temporal alterations in platelets, stainable basophils, neutrophils, and plasma PF4 and TxB_2 levels in an IgE-sensitized rabbit after intravenous antigen challenge with 5 mg horseradish peroxidase (HRP). The data are representative of all rabbits studied although the maximum TxB_2 and PF4 released varied between animals. (From McManus et al., 1980b. © 1980 The Williams & Wilkins Co., Baltimore.)

and intravascular PAF, TxB_2, and PF4 release) observed during anaphylaxis suggested a probable role for PAF in mediating these reactions.

Since the chemical structure of PAF had been elucidated and the molecule synthesized (i.e., AGEPC), the platelet-stimulating activity of PAF could be equated to the molar concentration of AGEPC (Fig. 4). Thus, retrospectively, we were in the position of estimating the actual amounts of PAF released intravascularly during IgE-induced systemic anaphylaxis in the rabbit (Pinckard et al., 1979). With this information at hand, it was apparent that the peak plasma concentrations of AGEPC during anaphylaxis approached 10^{-8} M, which would be equivalent to approximately 0.5 μg AGEPC released; it is likely however, that the total amount of AGEPC released during anaphylaxis greatly exceeded this value since functional PAF activity is rapidly degraded by an apparent plasma enzyme (Pinckard et al., 1979; Farr et al., 1980). In any event, rabbits were intravenously infused with concentrations of AGEPC to establish plasma AGEPC concentrations comparable with those estimated to occur during the IgE-induced anaphylactic syndrome (McManus et al., 1980a).

Figure 5 shows the characteristic intravascular alterations induced by a continuous 15-sec intravenous infusion of 1.27 μg AGEPC (total dose). The intravascular alterations induced by AGEPC infusion were virtually identical to

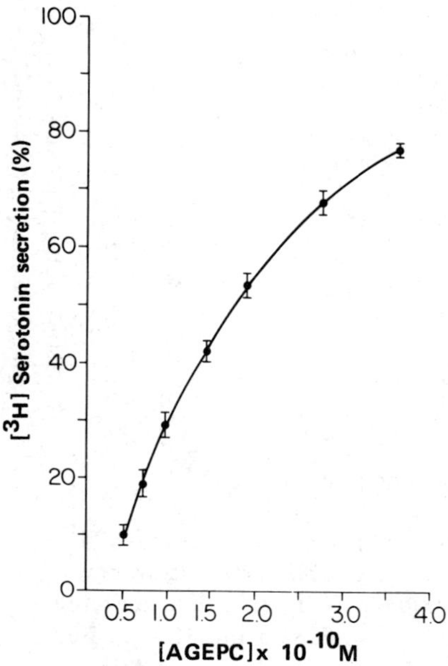

Figure 4 Dose-response of acetyl glyceryl ether phorphorylcholine (AGEPC)-induced release of [^{3}H]-serotonin from isolated, washed rabbit platelets. Purified AGEPC in pyrogen-free saline containing 2.5 mg/ml bovine serum albumin (BSA) was diluted in the same medium. Four microliters of various AGEPC-BSA saline dilutions were then added to 200 μl of platelets (250,000 platelets/μl) prewarmed to 37°C. After 60 sec, duplicate samples of the platelet suspension were removed to a 0°C ice bath and 20 μl of 1.5 M formalin was added. After centrifugation, specific [^{3}H] serotonin in the platelet-free supernatants was determined based on Triton X-100 controls. Each point represents the mean percent release derived utilizing six different platelet preparations. The bars indicate the standard error of the mean. (Adapted from Satouchi et al., 1981.)

those observed during IgE-induced systemic anaphylaxis with two noticeable differences. The first was that the development of basopenia, neutropenia, thrombocytopenia, and the release of TxB_2 and PF4 occurred at an earlier time in AGEPC-infused rabbits than during IgE-induced systemic anaphylaxis. The likely explanation for this small temporal difference can be explained by the observation that detectable plasma levels of PAF observed during anaphylaxis occurred between 30-60 sec after antigen challenge; this PAF then subsequently mediated the various intravascular alterations. The second difference was that in AGEPC-infused rabbits, the basopenia was reversible, whereas there was no return of basophils in anaphylactic rabbits 60 min after antigen challenge. The explanation for this difference likely is that during anaphylaxis, basophil degranulation would occur following interaction with antigen, thus preventing their identification using toluidine blue staining procedures. It is apparent that AGEPC does not induce basophil degranulation and therefore, following the development of leukopenia, the basophils returned to the peripheral circulation together with the neutrophils.

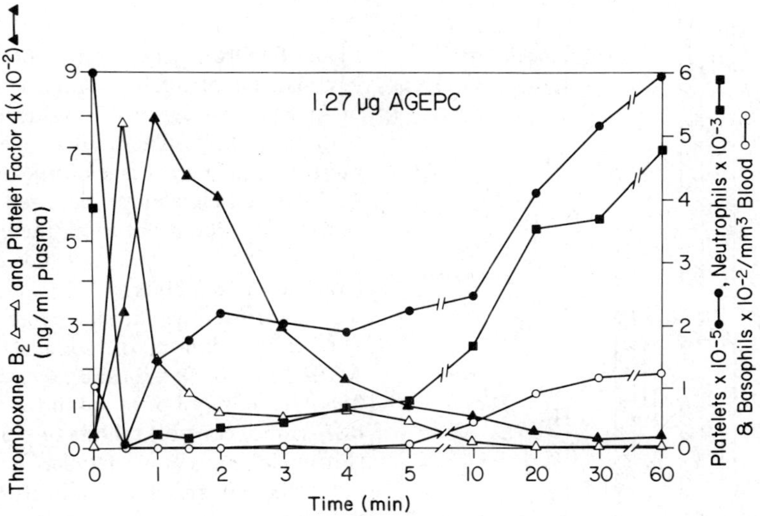

Figure 5 Intravascular effects of acetyl glyceryl ether phosphorylcholine (AGEPC) (1.27 μg) infusion on circulating levels of platelets, neutrophils, basophils, platelet factor 4, and thromboxane B_2 in the rabbit. (Modified from Mc Manus et al., 1980a. © 1980 The Williams & Wilkins Co., Baltimore.)

Other studies characterized the intravascular responses following infusion of several different amounts of AGEPC (McManus et al., 1980a). As little as 0.08 μg AGEPC induced the development of significant, but rapidly reversible thrombocytopenia, neutropenia, and basopenia; however, at this very low dose the platelet-release reaction was not initiated in view of no elevations in the plasma levels of PF4. Increasing the amounts of AGEPC infused resulted in an accentuation and a prolongation of the cellular changes with sequential increases in the elevations in plasma PF4 levels. Exceeding an AGEPC dose of 1.27 μg uniformly resulted in lethal reactions within 2-3 min after the initiation of AGEPC infusion. In these lethal reactions, the rabbits developed profound systemic hypotension and respiratory arrest (see below). In keeping with our in vitro observations that lyso-GEPC biologically was inactive with respect to stimulating washed rabbit platelets (Demopoulos et al., 1979), we assessed whether the intravenous infusion of relatively large quantities of lyso-GEPC (34.4 μg) would effect any intravascular alterations. The results demonstrated that removal of the acetyl group in the 2 position rendered the molecule (i.e., lyso-GEPC) biologically inactive when administered intravenously into rabbits.

Simultaneous estimation of ^{51}Cr-platelet distribution 30 sec after AGEPC infusion demonstrated that the platelets were preferentially sequestered in the

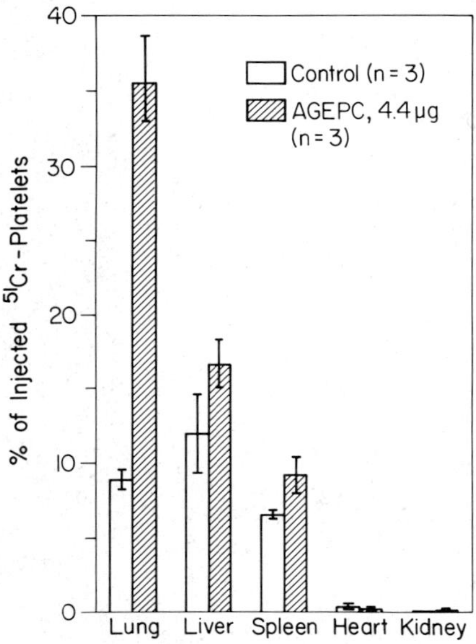

Figure 6 Organ sequestration of ^{51}Cr-labeled platelets after infusion of AGEPC (4.4 μg) or BSA-saline (control) into rabbits. The results are expressed as the percentage of injected ^{51}Cr-labeled platelets sequestered per organ ± SD. Before infusion, there were 6059 ± 1102 ^{51}Cr cpm/ml of blood in these rabbits (*n* = 6). Thirty seconds after infusion, there were 1446 ± ^{51}Cr cpm/ml of blood in the AGEPC rabbits (*n* = 3) and 5692 ± 858 ^{51}Cr cpm/ml of blood in the BSA-saline (control) rabbits (*n* = 3). (From McManus et al., 1980a. © 1980 The Williams and Wilkins Co., Baltimore.)

lung (Fig. 6). Similar patterns of specific pulmonary platelet sequestration had been previously demonstrated to occur during IgE-induced systemic anaphylaxis in the rabbit (Pinckard et al., 1977). Light microscopic examination of the lungs obtained from animals 30 sec after the infusion of 2.5 μg AGEPC (Fig. 7) confirmed that massive platelet aggregates were present in the pulmonary vasculature. In the same tissue samples, numerous neutrophils were also identified in association with the platelet aggregates. An additional striking feature in these tissue samples was significant muscular artery constriction (Fig. 8) where vascular lumina were virtually obliterated.

By electron microscopy, the platelets sequestered in the lung at 30 sec after the initiation of AGEPC infusion (2.5 μg) were aggregated; most of these aggregated platelets were not eliptical but were well-rounded with pseudopodia and apparently were in the process of undergoing granule extrusion (Fig. 9). In these aggregates, some platelet dense bodies were still observed, a not surprising observation since maximum platelet secretion of platelet factor 4 did not occur until 60 sec following AGEPC infusion (see above); therefore, these platelets were most likely in the process of undergoing granule extrusion. Of interest was that thromboxane release was maximal at 30 sec after AGEPC infusion (see above). Since the platelet is a likely source of thromboxane release following AGEPC infusion, these results indicate that thromboxane synthesis occurred at a time when platelets were sequestered in the pulmonary vasculature and thus the effects of thromboxanes and other prostaglandin intermediates directly onto vasculature surfaces in the lung would be expected.

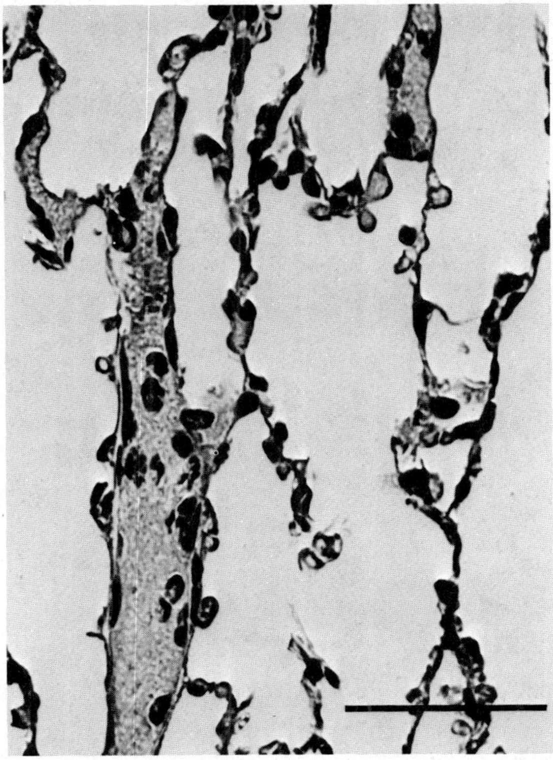

Figure 7 Light microscopic appearance of pulmonary platelet and neutrophil sequestration 30 sec after acetyl glyceryl ether phosphorylcholine (AGEPC) infusion (2.5 μg) in the rabbit. Six micrometer paraffin section. Hematoxylin and eosin stain. Bar represents 50 μm.

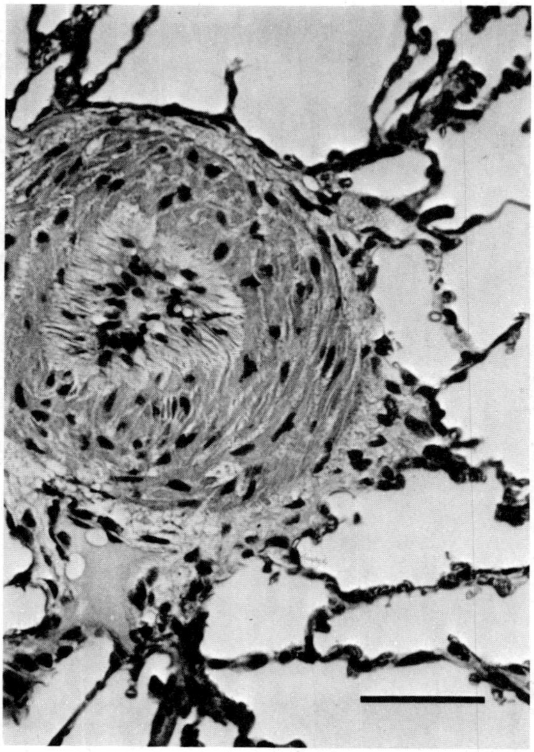

Figure 8 Light microscopic appearance of pulmonary vascular constriction 30 sec after acetyl glyceryl ether phosphorylcholine (AGEPC) infusion (2.5 μg) in the rabbit. Six micrometer paraffin section. Hematoxylin and eosin stain. Bar represents 50 μm.

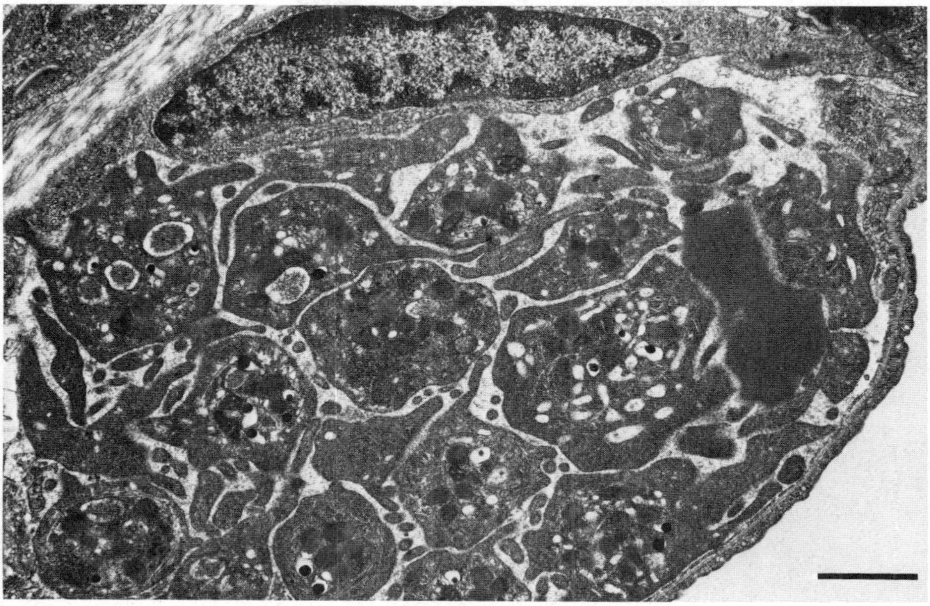

Figure 9 Electron microscopic appearance of platelets sequestered in the pulmonary vasculature after acetyl glyceryl ether phosphorylcholine (AGEPC) infusion in the rabbit. Thirty seconds after AGEPC infusion (2.5 μg), the lungs were fixed by transtracheal perfusion with glutaraldehyde. Blocks of tissue were postfixed with osmium tetroxide, dehydrated, and embedded in epon-araldite. Ultrathin sections were counterstained with uranyl acetate and lead citrate. Bar represents 1 μm.

IV. Biological Effects of AGEPC In Vivo— Respiratory and Cardiovascular Alterations

In addition to characterizing the intravascular effects induced by the intravenous administration of AGEPC, parallel studies were conducted to assess the development of respiratory and cardiovascular alterations (Halonen et al., 1980). As in the previous studies, any alterations then could be compared and contrasted to the respiratory and cardiovascular changes which occur during IgE-induced systemic anaphylactic shock in the rabbit (Halonen et al., 1976). Intravenous infusion of AGEPC (0.6 μg/kg) over a 15-sec period, resulted in abrupt and marked alterations in respiratory function (Fig. 10a; Table 3). Ventilatory alterations included an initial, brief cessation in breathing that occurred 10-15 sec after the infusion of AGEPC was begun; this was followed by a resumption of breathing in a rapid shallow pattern for approximately 15-30 sec. Apnea commonly devel-

Table 3 Mean Maximum Physiological Alterations Induced by Antigen and AGEPC

Group	HR[a]		P_{aorta}		P_{RV}	C_L	R_L	f (↓)		f (↓)	V_T
	1[b]	2[b]	1[b]	2[b]				1[b]	2[b]		
Antigen, platelet-intact											
$\overline{x}$	97.2[c]	61.0	41.0	20.7	196	46.5	479	98.7	37.7	138	68.5
SD	3.7	34.8	19.2	23.1	36.2	16.9	366	1.5	38.7	18.6	17.4
Antigen, platelet-depleted											
$\overline{x}$	89.0	66.8	62.9	47.4	167	51.9	315	93.9	59.5	137	72.0
SD	5.4	27.1	19.2	28.3	47.9	17.7	128	8.8	38.5	23.4	13.9
p[d]	<.02	>.2	=.05	>.05	>.2	>.5	>.3	>.2	>.2	>.7	>.6
Time to maximum[e] (min)	.25-1	2-8	1.5-3	6-8	1.5-3.5	.75-4	.75-5.5	.25-.75	1.5-3	.75-1	.75-1
AGEPC, platelet-intact											
$\overline{x}$	78.8	63.0	48.8	31.0	218	39.7	447	70.5	53.0	241	41.8
SD	17.7	26.8	17.6	24.9	59.3	17.5	221	31.4	49.6	69.4	4.6
p[d]	<.025	>.9	>.4	>.4	>.4	>.5	>.8	=.05	>.6	<.01	<.005

AGEPC, platelet-depleted											
$\overline{x}$	83.6	7.36	41.0	57.6	170	86.3	115	91.1	67.3	149	81.7
SD	5.3	18.8	19.1	22.8	34.9	9.8	13.9	23.4	44.9	34.6	16.8
p^f	>.4	>.3	>.4	<.05	>.05	<.001	<.005	>.05	>.8	<.02	<.001
Time to maximum[e] (min)	.17-.5	1.5-5	.25-2	3-9	.5-3	.25-3	.5-2	.17-.25	1.5-4	.25-.5	.25-.5

[a]Definitions of abbreviations: HR = heart rate; P_{aorta} = aortic systolic pressure; P_{RV} = right ventricular systolic pressure; C_L = dynamic compliance; R_L = total pulmonary resistance; f = breathing frequency; V_t = tidal volume; AGEPC = acetyl glyceryl ether phosphorylcholine (0.6 μg/kg); ANTIGEN = horseradish peroxidase (5 mg).

[b]HR, P_{aorta}, and f (↓) consistently exhibited bimodal responses in the AGEPC group; each response is assessed separately.

[c]All values are percent of prechallenge values.

[d]*p* value associated with Student's *t* test for difference between this group and Antigen, Platelet-Intact Group.

[e]Time (after antigen or AGEPC) range during which maximum values were achieved for all members of group.

[f]*p* value associated with Student's *t* test for difference between this group and AGEPC, Platelet-Intact Group.

Source: Modified from Halonen et al. (1981).

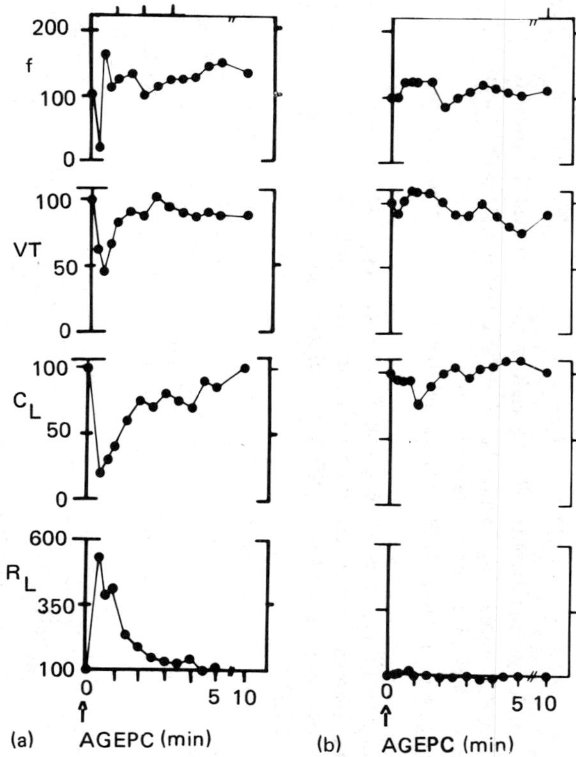

Figure 10 Typical respiratory alterations induced by acetyl glyceryl ether phosphorylcholine (AGEPC) in the rabbit. AGEPC (0.6 μg/kg) was administered intravenously over 15 sec in 2 ml. Variables are plotted as percent of prechallenge values. In *a*, platelets are intact; in *b*, platelets have been depleted prior to infusion by the administration of goat anti-platelet globulin. f = breathing frequency, V_T = tidal volume, C_L = dynamic compliance, and R_L = total pulmonary resistance. (Adapted from Halonen et al., 1981.)

oped beginning 1-4 min after AGEPC infusion and lasted from 36-72 sec; in the lethal reactions, respiratory arrest occurred at 90-120 sec after AGEPC infusion.

Lung mechanical changes included a significant increase in total pulmonary resistance and a decrease in dynamic lung compliance. The maximum change in both of these variables occurred within 15-60 sec after the initiation of intravenous AGEPC infusion. Total pulmonary resistance returned to preinfusion values between 3 and 5 min, while the alterations in the dynamic compliance returned to preinfusion values between 5 and 10 min. No differences with respect to the degree of the lung mechanical changes were observed between the lethal and nonlethal reactions.

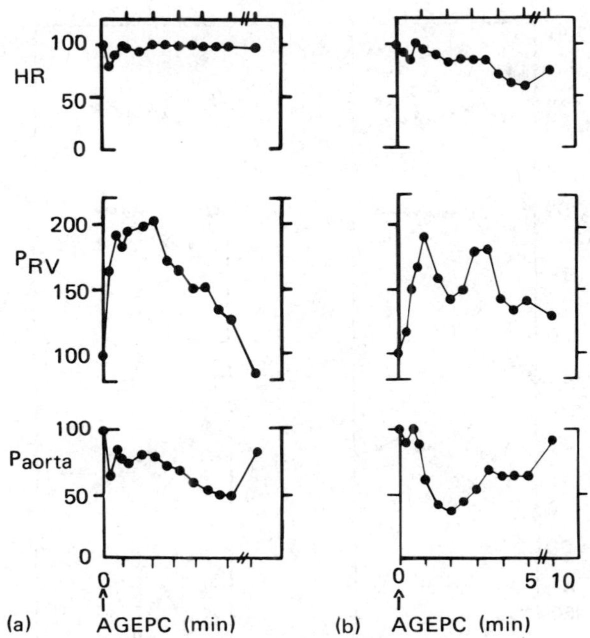

Figure 11 Typical cardiovascular alterations induced by acetyl glyceryl ether phosphorylcholine (AGEPC) in the rabbit. AGEPC (0.6 μg/kg) was administered intravenously over 15 sec in 2 ml. Variables are plotted as percent of prechallenge values. In *a*, platelets are intact; in *b*, platelets have been depleted prior to AGEPC infusion by the administration of goat anti-platelet globulin. HR = heart rate, P_{RV} = right ventricular systolic pressure, P_{aorta} = aortic systolic pressure. (Modified from Halonen et al., 1981.)

Severe cardiovascular alterations also were induced by AGEPC infusion and included episodes of transient bradycardia, a rise in right ventricular systolic pressure, and a fall in aortic systolic pressure, the latter occurring in two phases (Fig. 11a and Table 3). Bradycardia temporally corresponded with the periods of decreased breathing frequency and generally was more marked in those rabbits which exhibited more prolonged periods of apnea. Elevations in the right ventricular systolic pressure were maximal between 30-180 sec after AGEPC infusion and returned to preinfusion levels by 15 min. During the initial fall, aortic pressure reached a minimal value within 120 sec; this was followed either by a plateau or a rise with a subsequent secondary fall in aortic systolic pressure that reached their lowest values within 3-9 min after AGEPC infusion. In nonlethal reactions, aortic pressure did not return to within preinfusion levels until at least 15 min following AGEPC infusion.

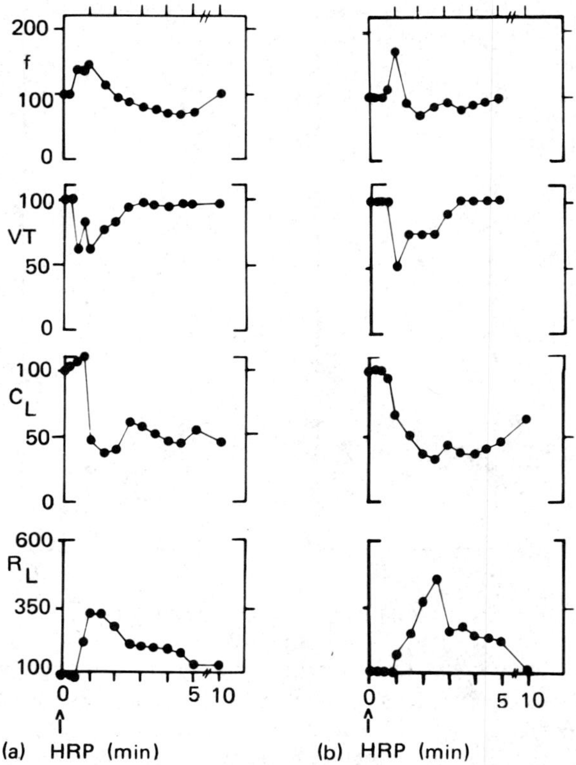

Figure 12 Typical respiratory alterations induced by antigen in the rabbit. Antigen [5 mg horseradish peroxidase (HRP)] was administered into the right ventricle in a bolus injection in 0.5 ml. (*a*) Platelet intact; (*b*) platelet depleted. VT = tidal volume; C_L = dynamic compliance; R_L = total pulmonary resistance. (Modified from Halonen et al., 1981.)

The physiologic responses induced by AGEPC infusion in the rabbit (Figs. 10a, 11a, and Table 3) were characteristic of the physiologic alterations that occurred during IgE-induced systemic anaphylaxis in the rabbit (Figs. 12a, 13a, and Table 3). The only differences observed were that the early bradycardia did not occur during IgE-induced systemic anaphylaxis, and during the episodes of rapid, shallow breathing, the AGEPC-induced increase in breathing frequency and decrease in tidal volume were of greater magnitude. The above data, together with the previous documentation for the intravascular release of PAF during systemic anaphylaxis (Pinckard et al., 1979), strongly suggest that AGEPC is an important mediator in the physiologic alterations observed in this syndrome.

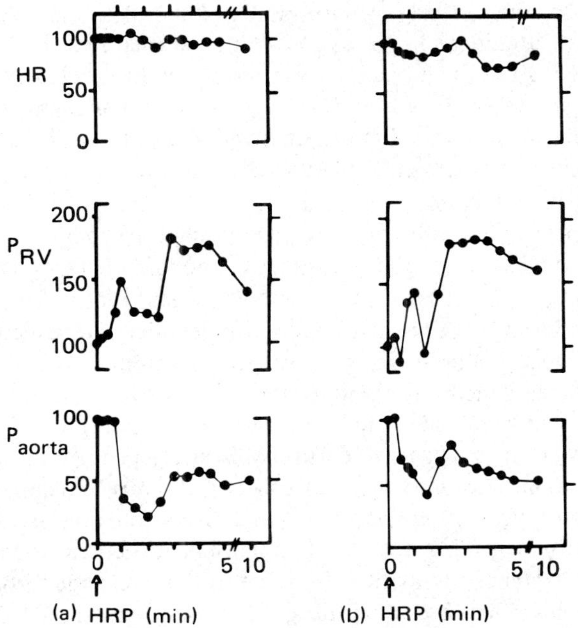

Figure 13 Typical cardiovascular alterations induced by acetyl glyceryl ether phosphorylcholine (AGEPC) in the rabbit. Antigen [5 mg horseradish peroxidase (HRP)] was administered into the right ventricle in a bolus injection in 0.5 ml. (*a*) Platelet intact; (*b*) platelet depleted. HR = heart rate; P_{RV} = right ventricular systolic pressure; P_{aorta} = aortic systolic pressure. (Modified from Halonen et al., 1981.)

Several other experiments have provided some additional insight into the nature of this physiologic activity of AGEPC. As with the intravascular alterations described earlier, the biological activity of AGEPC for initiating respiratory and cardiovascular alterations also was dependent upon the acetyl group in the 2 position; thus lyso-GEPC was completely inactive in inducing any alterations in respiratory and/or cardiovascular physiology and also did not antagonize these physiologic alterations induced by a subsequent infusion of AGEPC (Halonen et al., 1980).

Since AGEPC had been shown to be a potent platelet stimulator (Demopoulos et al., 1979), it was important to answer the obvious question as to whether the AGEPC-induced intravascular, respiratory, and cardiovascular alterations were platelet dependent. The answers to this question were derived from a series of studies utilizing rabbits depleted of circulating platelets by the administration of a specific anti-rabbit platelet antibody prior to intravenous AGEPC infusion (Halonen et al., 1981). As illustrated in Figure 10b and Table 3, the AGEPC-induced alterations in ventilation were somewhat reduced in platelet-depleted rabbits. Thus, the initial interruption in breathing did not occur and the episodes of rapid shallow breathing did not show as great an increase in frequency nor decrease in tidal volume as observed in platelet depletion. However, the lung mechanical changes induced by AGEPC infusion were completely abrogated by platelet depletion.

In contrast to the ventilatory and lung mechanical changes, the cardiovascular changed induced by AGEPC infusion were not affected by platelet depletion. Thus, the episodes of bradycardia, the rise in right ventricular pressure, and the aortic hypotension were not affected by platelet depletion, except for a slight but significant reduction in the second phase of aortic hypotension (Fig. 11b; Table 3). These data therefore demonstrated that AGEPC-induced cardiovascular alterations were platelet independent; however, the AGEPC-induced lung mechanical changes appear to occur by platelet-dependent mechanisms. Similar observations were made by Vargaftig et al. (1980) who demonstrated that in the guinea pig, partially purified PAF derived from hog leukocytes induced a platelet-independent systemic hypotension and a platelet-dependent rise in pulmonary resistance to inflation. It can be further concluded from the physiologic studies described above that the apneic episode was unrelated to bronchoconstriction. Thus, the apnea may reflect direct or indirect effects of AGEPC upon the breathing control center(s) that are not mediated through platelet stimulation. Finally, neither the AGEPC-induced alterations in ventilatory patterns that were only slightly diminished in platelet-depleted rabbits, nor the AGEPC-induced increase in right ventricular pressure can be ascribed to changes in the dynamic lung compliance and/or lung resistance that were observed in the platelet-intact rabbits.

As part of the platelet-depletion studies, we also determined the effects of platelet depletion upon IgE-induced systemic anaphylaxis in the rabbit for comparison. Platelet depletion had no effect upon any of the physiologic alterations of IgE-anaphylaxis except for a slight dimunition in the first fall in aortic pressure. (See Figs. 12b, 13b, and Table 3). Thus, whereas the lung mechanical changes induced by AGEPC were platelet dependent, the alterations occurring as a component part of the IgE anaphylactic response occurred independently of circulating platelets. Therefore, this phase of the anaphylactic response in platelet-depleted rabbits would not appear to be mediated by AGEPC; however, this does not rule out the participation of AGEPC and platelets in the lung mechanical changes in platelet-intact rabbits undergoing IgE anaphylaxis. It has been recently demonstrated that the administration of chlorpheniramine (an H_1 antagonist) partially inhibited the lung mechanical alterations of IgE-anaphylaxis (Halonen, unpublished observations). Thus, histamine appears to mediate these alterations partially and could arise either from the circulating platelet or alternatively, in platelet-depleted rabbits, from either the blood basophil or tissue mast cell. Other platelet-independent mediators released or activated during IgE-induced systemic anaphylaxis that might mediate the lung mechanical changes could include the leukotrienes C and D, bradykinin, and $PGF_{2\alpha}$. Nevertheless, our data to date are consistent with the likelihood that most of the ventilatory and cardiovascular alterations of IgE-induced anaphylaxis may be mediated at least in part by AGEPC through mechanisms independent of the circulating platelet.

V. Biological Activities of AGEPC In Vitro

Up until the time that the structure of PAF had been elucidated and AGEPC synthesized, the only biological activity for PAF or AGEPC that was unequivocally documented was its ability to act as a potent stimulator of washed rabbit platelets (Fig. 4). The results obtained with respect to the intravascular, cardiovascular, and pulmonary alterations following intravenous infusion of AGEPC in the rabbit (see above) and in the baboon (Pinckard et al., 1980b; McManus et al., 1981b) strongly suggested that AGEPC likely possessed other potent biological activities in addition to platelet stimulation. For instance, neutrophil-stimulating properties were suggested in view of the neutropenia induced by intravenous AGEPC infusion; similarly, vasoactive and smooth muscle-contracting properties were suggested by the profound AGEPC-induced cardiovascular and pulmonary alterations. Again, with the availability of chemically pure AGEPC, it was possible to initiate definitive studies to explore other possible biological activities intrinsic to the AGEPC molecule, as discussed below.

VI. Human Platelet Stimulation

Initial attempts to document AGEPC-induced aggregation of the secretion from washed human platelets met with little success and with a high degree of variability in the reproducibility of the experiments (McManus et al., 1981a); similar problems previously had been reported by Lotner and co-workers (1980) using partially purified PAF released from stimulated human neutrophils. Review of the literature indicated conflicting reports with respect to the ability of PAF to stimulate washed human platelets (c.f. McManus et al., 1981a). The variability in these various studies may have occurred due to the utilization of relatively crude PAF preparations or to the different procedures employed to prepare washed human platelets. An obvious solution to this problem, therefore, was to utilize AGEPC and to determine whether it could initiate platelet aggregation and secretion in human platelet-rich plasma (PRP).

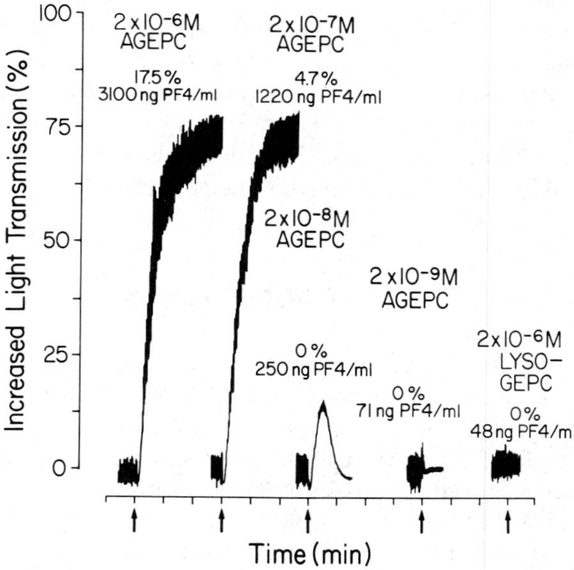

Figure 14 Acetyl glyceryl ether phosphorylcholine (AGEPC)-induced stimulation of citrated human platelet-rich plasma. The numbers above the aggregation curves indicate the final molar concentrations of AGEPC or lyso-GEPC added at the time indicated by the arrow, the percent [^{3}H] serotonin released (corrected for nonspecific release after the addition of human serum albumin-saline) and the amount of PF4 secreted (ng/ml). Secretion values were determined in separate assay tubes and the secretion reactions were terminated at 60 sec. (From McManus et al., 1981a.)

Figure 14 shows the results of a series of experiments that documented that AGEPC can initiate both platelet aggregation and secretion when added to human PRP. As was the case with rabbit PRP, AGEPC induced dose-dependent aggregation of human PRP with concomitant secretion of both [^{3}H] serotonin and PF4. A characteristic monophasic irreversible platelet aggregation response always was observed at high concentrations of AGEPC (2 μM); at lower AGEPC concentrations, biphasic platelet aggregation occurred (data not shown). Indomethacin (10 μM) or ADP scavengers prevented the second wave of platelet aggregation but had no effect on the platelet release of serotonin or PF4 at any AGEPC concentration. Chelation of extracellular calcium with either EDTA or EGTA (0.01 M) completely prevented AGEPC-induced platelet aggregation; however, these agents did not prevent AGEPC-induced platelet shape-change and, of interest, the platelet release reaction also was unaffected. These findings were different from those previously reported for washed rabbit platelets where chelation of extracellular calcium abrogated the platelet-release reaction induced by AGEPC (Demopoulos et al., 1979; Pinckard et al., 1979). The differences between these observations likely are due to an alteration in rabbit platelet responsiveness resulting from the washing procedures, since chelation of extracellular calcium in rabbit PRP also did not affect the release reaction following the addition of AGEPC (McManus et al., 1981a). As would be expected, prostacyclin (PGI_2 27nM) abrogated both AGEPC-induced platelet aggregation and secretion in both human and rabbit PRP (McManus et al., 1981a). It should be noted that the concentrations of AGEPC required to initiate platelet aggregation and secretion in PRP greatly exceeded those concentrations previously reported for washed rabbit platelets (Demopoulos et al., 1979). These observations could be due to the presence of an apparent enzyme in plasma that rapidly degrades AGEPC (Pinckard et al., 1979; Farr et al., 1980); or alternatively, high concentrations or plasma albumin or possibly other plasma proteins might competitively inhibit the association of AGEPC with the platelet membrane. Nevertheless, these studies clearly indicate that AGEPC is a potent stimulator of human platelets and therefore, platelet activation by AGEPC may play a role in various allergic and inflammatory reactions.

VII. Neutrophil Stimulation

The consistent observation of the development of profound and prolonged neutropenia after intravenous infusion of AGEPC into rabbits and baboons (McManus et al., 1980a, 1981b) suggested that AGEPC might be capable of interacting with and stimulating the neutrophil. In addition, AGEPC-induced neutropenia also occurred in platelet-depleted rabbits suggesting direct AGEPC effects (Halonen et al., 1981). Thus, studies were initiated to determine whether or not AGEPC could stimulate the human neutrophils in vitro (Shaw et al., 1981). In the presence of cytochalasin B (5 μg/ml), AGEPC induced a dose-dependent (10^{-10} to 10^{-5} M AGEPC) release of both specific (lysozyme, lactoferrin) and azurophilic (β-glucuronidase, myeloperoxidase) lysosomal enzymes. The secretion of lysosomal enzymes was rapid ($T_{1/2}$ = 20 sec), was dependent upon active glycolysis, and did not result in the release of lactate dehydrogenase. The threshold concentration for AGEPC-induced neutrophil stimulation of enzyme secretion occurred at 10^{-10} M with dose-related increases in enzyme release up to 10^{-6} M AGEPC. However, increasing concentration of AGEPC to greater than 10^{-6} M led to a subsequent reduction of granule enzyme secretion.

In addition to inducing human neutrophil enzyme secretion, AGEPC also induced the production of superoxide anion (Shaw et al., 1981). As would be expected for any potent neutrophil stimulator, AGEPC also induced a dose-dependent aggregation of human neutrophils. In addition, related studies documented that AGEPC was chemotactic for these cells. The specificity of the AGEPC-induced stimulation of human neutrophils was documented by experiments which demonstrated that desensitization of neutrophils to C5a did not subsequently desensitize the neutrophils to AGEPC and vice versa. As was shown to be the case for both human and rabbit platelet stimulation and the intravascular and cardiovascular alterations in rabbits induced by AGEPC, lyso-GEPC did not stimulate human neutrophils with respect to granule enzyme secretion, superoxide production, or aggregation (Shaw et al., 1981). Similar neutrophil stimulation by AGEPC and certain AGEPC analogs had been reported by Goetzl and co-workers (1980), although their dose-response characteristics did not show the same significant degree of lysosomal enzyme secretion as reported by Shaw et al. (1981) for reasons that are not as yet apparent. Nevertheless, these studies clearly demonstrate that AGEPC is a potent stimulator of human neutrophils and thus suggest that this acetylated alkyl phosphoglyceride may be of importance in acute inflammatory as well as allergic reactions.

VIII. Vasoactive Activity

Because of the emerging multiplicity of biological actions of AGEPC, studies were initiated to assess whether or not AGEPC possessed vasoactive properties as estimated by increased vascular permeability at intradermal injection sites. Following skin test studies in guinea pigs, rabbits, and baboons, an extensive examination of the vasoactive activity of AGEPC in the skin of human volunteers was conducted (Pinckard et al., 1980b). AGEPC, lyso-GEPC, and histamine were cotitrated in the skin of human volunteers who had not previously taken medication for 2 weeks prior to skin testing. Three important observations resulted from these studies. First, lyso-GEPC was skin-test negative at concentrations as high as 1000 pmol (i.e., 520 ng). In contrast, AGEPC manifested potent vasoactive properties eliciting wheal and flare reactions at AGEPC amounts as low as 0.1 pmol (52 pg). Following intradermal administration, AGEPC induced immediate skin blanching indicative of acute vasoconstriction which was often associated with burning pain and pruritis. Five minutes after AGEPC injection, intense erythema up to 30 mm in diameter developed. This reaction was accompanied by the subsequent development of central edema up to 12 mm in diameter. Both the erythema and edema generally were maximal within 10 min after AGEPC injection; thereafter, the wheal and flare reactions lessened in intensity, becoming negative within 60 min. No delayed cutaneous manifestations due to AGEPC administration were observed. Cotitration of histamine revealed that AGEPC (on a molar basis) was between 100 and 1000 times more vasoactive than histamine; thus, between 10 and 100 pmol (1 and 11 ng histamine base, respectively) were required to elicit comparable skin test end-points induced by 0.1 pmol of AGEPC. Initial drug intervention studies to assess possible mechanisms for the vasoactive properties of AGEPC in man have yielded equivocal findings. For example, administration of H_1 histamine antagonists did not effect significant blockage of either AGEPC or histamine-induced wheal and flare reactions.

In view of the above observations, additional studies were performed in both rabbits and guinea pigs to assess the relative potency of AGEPC and histamine in enhancing vascular permeability in the presence or absence of the H_1 blocker, chlorpheniramine (5-10 mg/kg). These studies (Humphrey et al., 1981, 1982) demonstrated that AGEPC was between 1000 and 10,000 times more vasoactive than histamine in both species. In the rabbit, between 1 and 10 pmol of AGEPC were required to initiate positive skin blueing, whereas in the guinea pig, only 0.1 pmol was required. In both species, prior administration of the H_1 antagonist, chlorpheniramine, had no effect upon AGEPC-induced skin blueing. In contrast, the vasoactive properties of histamine were reduced at least 100-fold by prior H_1 blockade. In related studies, histologic assessment of skin biopsies obtained from rabbits at various times after AGEPC adminstration were indicative of interstitial edema. In addition, within 15-30 min after intradermal AGEPC administration, neutrophil infiltrates developed and reached a maximum 3 hr later (Humphrey et al., 1981). These latter studies are consistent with the observations which have demonstrated that AGEPC serves as a chemotactic stimulus for neutrophils in vitro (see above).

IX. Smooth Muscle Contraction

In addition to the multiple biological activities of AGEPC described above, recent evidence has demonstrated that this acetylated alkyl phosphoglyceride is a potent agonist with respect to inducing smooth muscle contraction in the isolated guinea pig ileum (Findlay et al., 1981). In these studies, the isolated guinea pig ileum was evaluated since this tissue previously had been utilized to study other autacoids. At a final concentration of 10^{-7} M, AGEPC consistently induced comparable ileal contraction as was observed with 5×10^{-8} to 1×10^{-7} M histamine. As illustrated in Figure 15, the AGEPC-induced ileal contraction was slower in onset than histamine, but occurred more rapidly than the contraction induced by SRS. Following the development of maximum ileal contraction, removal of the fluid-phase agonists by washing with agonist-free Tyrode's buffer resulted in a rapid relaxation of the ileum in the case of histamine ($T_{1/2}$ = 10 sec) and SRS ($T_{1/2}$ = 10-90 sec); however, repeated ileal washing had lesser effect upon relaxation ($T_{1/2}$ = 30 sec to 7 min) after ileal contraction induced by AGEPC. The precise potency of AGEPC for inducing ileal contraction could not be determined since AGEPC induced complete desensitization of the guinea pig ileum to subsequent AGEPC-induced contraction. This desensitization was specific since prior exposure of the guinea pig ileum to AGEPC did not subsequently affect ileal contraction induced either by histamine or SRS. As would be anticipated, lyso-GEPC had no effect upon the guinea pig ileum and did not antagonize subsequent AGEPC-induced ileal contraction.

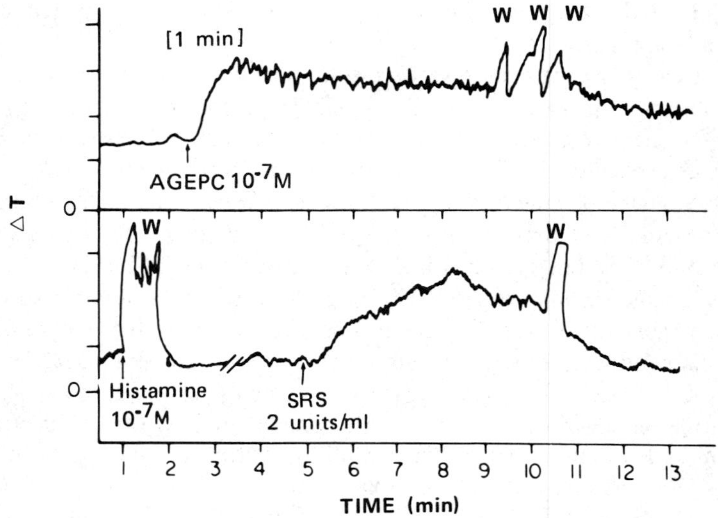

Figure 15 Acetyl glyceryl ether phosphorylcholine (AGEPC)-induced contraction of the isolated guinea pig ileum. This composite figure shows the responses of three separate guinea pig ileal preparations challenged with agonist (AGEPC, histamine, or SRS) at the times indicated by the arrows. After addition of each agonist, the change in ileal tension (ΔT) was continuously recorded. At various times after agonist addition, the tissue bath was washed (W) with Tyrode's buffer to remove fluid-phase agonist to allow muscle relaxation. (From Findlay et al., 1981.)

In the preceding investigations (Findley et al., 1981), AGEPC-induced ileal contraction was independent of the release of endogenous neurotransmitters, histamine, SRS, or products of the cyclooxygenase pathways of arachidonic acid metabolism. Thus, the presence of muscarinic (atropine, 10^{-6} M), H_1 (diphenhydramine, 10^{-6} M), and/or SRS (FPL-55712, 5×10^{-7} M) antagonists or indomethacin (10^{-5} M) had no effect upon AGEPC-induced ileal contraction. These studies, therefore, demonstrated that AGEPC is a relatively potent agonist for stimulating smooth muscle contraction in the guinea pig ileum through a mechanism that is independent from the stimulation of muscarinic, H_1, or SRS receptors. Whether or not AGEPC can induce smooth muscle contraction of tissues other than the guinea pig ileum remains to be studied. In this regard, it is likely that AGEPC can initiate vascular smooth muscle contraction in view of the apparent vasoconstricting effects observed immediately after intradermal administration in man and in experimental animals (Pinckard et al., 1980a; Humphrey et al., 1982) (see above). In addition, recent studies have indicated that AGEPC causes contraction of guinea pig lung parenchymal strips (O'Flaherty et al.,

1981). AGEPC may also contract coronary arteries since infusion of between 10-100 fmol of AGEPC into the isolated perfused guinea pig heart resulted in significant reductions in coronary artery flow; in this system, AGEPC also induced significant decreases in left ventricular myocardial contractility and the development of prolonged cardiac arrhythmias (Burke et al., 1982).

X. Summary

It is quite apparent from the preceding observations that AGEPC should be classified as an autacoid, in view of its multiple and extremely potent physiologic and inflammatory biological activities. However, as is the case with many other autacoids, it is premature to assess the possible pathophysiologic role of AGEPC in modulating various aspects of the acute allergic and inflammatory process in man for several reasons. First, although PAF has been shown to be produced by several inflammatory cell types obtained from various species including man (Table 4), a concerted effort must be made to identify those human cell types capable of releasing and/or synthesizing PAF and, of great importance, to determine whether the PAF is chemically identical to AGEPC. Second, at the present time, most of the biological activities of AGEPC have been assessed either in experimental animals or in in vitro experiments utilizing human cells. The intravascular alterations induced following AGEPC infusion have been conducted in the rabbit (McManus et al., 1980a) and in the nonhuman primate, the baboon (McManus et al., 1981b), the latter studies providing some possible insight to the human situation. Physiologically, AGEPC has been shown to have potent pharmacological properties in the rabbit (Halonen et al., 1980, 1981), rab (Blank et al., 1979), guinea pig (Vargaftig et al., 1980), and again, in the baboon (Pinckard et al., 1980b). To date, the only experiments that have indicated the biological activity of AGEPC in man have been the in vitro studies that have characterized AGEPC stimulation of isolated human neutrophils (Goetzl et al., 1980; Shaw et al., 1981), human platelets (McManus et al., 1981a), and the in vivo studies that have documented its potent vasoactive properties in human skin (Pinckard et al., 1980a). Due to ethical considerations, it is unlikely that it will be possible further to test directly the in vivo biological activities of AGEPC in man. Thus, as with most other autacoids, the role of AGEPC in normal as well as in various diseases in man likely may remain speculative for some time to come. One possible avenue to elucidate this important issue would be the development of highly specific drugs that would either specifically inhibit AGEPC synthesis or serve as a potent AGEPC antagonist, possibly an analog of AGEPC. Regarding the latter possibility, intensive investigations currently are being conducted in this area (Hanahan et al., 1981; Satouchi et al., 1981); however, to date, all of the AGEPC analogs synthesized have retained relatively potent biological activities and no specific antagonists have

Table 4 Cellular Sources of PAF or AGEPC

Rabbit	Basophil	Siraganian and Osler (1971); Benveniste et al. (1972a,b); Pinckard et al. (1979); Betz et al. (1980); Hanahan et al. (1980)
	Neutrophil	Lynch et al. (1979); Clark et al. (1980)
	Platelet	Chignard et al. (1979); Chignard et al. (1980); Namm and High (1980); Chap et al. (1981)
	Alveolar macrophage	Benveniste (1979); Benveniste et al. (1979a); Arnoux et al. (1980)
Rat	Peritoneal macrophage	Mencia-Huerta and Benveniste (1979); Benveniste (1979)
	Alveolar macrophage	Benveniste (1979); Arnoux et al. (1980)
Mouse	Peritoneal macrophage	Mencia-Huerta and Benveniste (1979)
Pig	Buffy coat cells	Benveniste et al. (1977); Tence et al. (1980)
Human	Basophil[a]	Benveniste (1974); Lewis et al. (1975); Clark et al. (1976); Camussi et al. (1981)
	Neutrophil	Clark et al. (1980); Lotner et al. (1980); Camussi et al. (1981)
	Monocyte	Clark et al. (1980); Camussi et al. (1981)
	Platelet	Chignard et al. (1979)
	Alveolar macrophage	Arnoux et al. (1980)

[a]Lack of PAF production by human basophils has also been reported (Betz et al., 1980; Sanchez Crespo et al., 1980).

been found. Alternatively, the process whereby AGEPC itself can initiate specific desensitization of various cells and tissues (Demopoulos et al., 1979; Findlay et al., 1981; Shaw et al., 1981) could be utilized as a probe, perhaps therapeutically, to modulate the biological effects of AGEPC. Nevertheless, this new field of basic and clinical investigation still is in its infancy and the coming years should present a wealth of fascinating information regarding the molecular pathophysiology of this unique and novel class of acetylated alkyl phosphoglycerides.

References

Arnoux, B., Duval, B., and Benveniste, J. (1980). Release of platelet-activating factor (PAF-acether) from alveolar macrophages by the calcium ionophore A23187 and phagocytosis. *Eur. J. Clin. Invest., 10*:437-441.

Benveniste, J. (1974). Platelet activating factor, a new mediator of anaphylaxis and immune complex deposition from rabbit and human basophils. *Nature, 249*:581-582.

Benveniste, J. (1979). Release of platelet-activating factor by peritoneal and alveolar macrophages. *Monogr. Allergy, 14*:138-141.

Benveniste, J., Henson, P. M., and Cochrane, C. G. (1972a). A possible role for IgE in immune complex disease. In *The Biological Role of the Immunoglobulin E System.* Edited by K. Ishizaka and D. H. Dayton, Jr. Proceedings of a Conference on the Biological Role of the Immunoglobulin E System. Vero Beach, Florida, Dept. Health, Education and Welfare, pp. 187-205.

Benveniste, J., Henson, P. M., and Cochrane, C. G. (1972b). Leukocyte-dependent histamine release from rabbit platelets. The role of IgE, basophils, and a platelet activating factor. *J. Exp. Med., 136*:1356-1377.

Benveniste, J., Le Couedic, J. P., Polonsky, J., and Tence, M. (1977). Structural analysis of purified platelet-activating factor by lipases. *Nature, 269*:170-171.

Benveniste, J., Duval, A., Arnoud, B., and Chretien, J. (1979a). Liberation du facteur activant les plaquettes (P.A.F.) par les macrophages alveolaires. *Nouv. Presse Med., 8*:2071-2072.

Benveniste, J., Tence, M., Varenne, P., Bidault, J., Boullet, C., and Polonsky, J. (1979b). Semi-synthese et structure proposee du facteur activant les plaquettes (P.A.F.): PAF-acether, un alkyl ether analogue de la lysophosphatidylcholine. *C. R. Acad. Sc. (Paris), 289*:1037-1040.

Betz, S. J., Lotner, G. Z., and Henson, P. M. (1980). Generation and release of platelet activating factor (PAF) from enriched preparations of rabbit basophils; failure of human basophils to release PAF. *J. Immunol., 125*:2749-2755.

Blank, M. L., Snyder, F., Byers, L. W., Brooks, B., and Muirhead, E. E. (1979). Antihypertensive activity of an alkyl ether analogue of phosphatidylcholine. *Biochem. Biophys. Res. Comm., 90*:1194-1200.

Burke, J. A., Levi, R., Hanahan, D. J., and Pinckard, R. N. (1982). Cardiac effects of acetyl glyceryl ether phosphorylcholine. *Fed. Proc., 41*:823.

Camussi, G., Aglietta, M., Coda, R., Bussolino, F., Piacibello, W., and Tetta, C. (1981). Release of platelet-activating factor (PAF) and histamine. II. The cellular origin of human PAF: monocytes, polymorphonuclear neutrophils and basophils. *Immunology, 42*:191-199.

Chap, H., Mauco, G., Simon, M. F., Benveniste, J., and Douste-Blazy, L. (1981). Biosynthetic labelling of platelet activating factor from radioactive acetate by stimulated platelets. *Nature 289*:312-314.

Chignard, M., Le Couedic, J. P., Tence, M., Vargaftig, B. B., and Benveniste, J. (1979). The role of platelet-activating factor in platelet aggregation. *Nature, 179*:799-800.

Chignard, M., Le Couedic, J. P., Vargaftig, B. B., and Benventiste, J. (1980). Platelet-activating factor (PAF-acether) secretion from platelets: Effect of aggregating agents. *Br. J. Haematol., 46*:455-464.

Clark, R. A. F., Gallin, J. I., and Kaplan, A. P. (1976). Mediator release from basophil granulocytes in chronic myelogenous leukemia. *J. Allergy Clin. Immunol., 58*:623-634.

Clark, P. O., Hanahan, D. J., and Pinckard, R. N. (1980). Physical and chemical properties of platelet-activating factor obtained from human neutrophils and monocytes and rabbit neutrophils and basophils. *Biochem. Biophys. Acta, 628*:69-75.

Demopoulos, C. A., Pinckard, R. N., and Hanahan, D. J. (1979). Platelet-activating factor. Evidence for 1-*O*-alkyl-2-acetyl-*sn*-glyceryl-3-phosphorylcholine as the active component (A new class of lipid chemical mediators). *J. Biol. Chem., 254*:9355-9358.

Douglas, W. W. (1980). Autacoids. In *The Pharmacological Basis of Therapeutics.* Edited by A. G. Gilman, L. S. Goodman, and A. Gilman. New York, Macmillan Publishing Co., Inc., pp. 608-646.

Farr, R. S., Cox, C. P., Wardlow, M. L., and Jorgensen, R. (1980). Preliminary studies of an acid-labile factor (ALF) in human sera that inactivates platelet activating factor (PAF). *Clin. Immunol. Immunopathol., 15*:318-330.

Findlay, S. R., Lichtenstein, L. M., Hanahan, D. J., and Pinckard, R. N. (1981). The contraction of guinea pig ileal smooth muscle by acetyl glyceryl ether phosphorylcholine. *Amer. J. Physiol., 241*:C130-134.

Goetzl, E. J., Derian, C. K., Tauber, A. I., and Valone, F. H. (1980). Novel effects of 1-*O*-hexadecyl-2-acyl-*sn*-glycero-3-phosphorylcholine mediators on human leukocyte function: Delineation of the specific roles of the acyl substituents. *Biochem. Biophys. Res. Commun., 94*:881-888.

Halonen, M., and Pinckard, R. N. (1975). Intravascular effects of IgE antibody upon basophils, neutrophils, platelets and blood coagulation in the rabbit. *J. Immunol., 115*:519-524.

Halonen, M., Fisher, H. K., Blair, C., Butler, C., and Pinckard, R. N. (1976). IgE-induced respiratory and circulatory changes during systemic anaphylaxis in the rabbit. *Am. Rev. Respir. Dis., 114*:961-969.

Halonen, M., Palmer, J. D., Lohman, I. C., McManus, L. M., and Pinckard, R. N. (1980). Respiratory and circulatory alterations induced by acetyl glyceryl ether phosphorylcholine (AGEPC), a mediator of IgE anaphylaxis in the rabbit. *Am. Rev. Respir. Dis., 122*:915-924.

Halonen, M., Palmer, J. D., Lohman, C., McManus, L. M., and Pinckard, R. N. (1981). Differential effects of platelet depletion on the physiologic alterations of IgE anaphylaxis and acetyl glyceryl ether phosphorylcholine infusion in the rabbit. *Am. Rev. Respir. Dis., 124*:416-421.

Hanahan, D. J., Demopoulos, C. A., Liehr, J., and Pinckard, R. N. (1980). Identification of platelet-activating factor isolated from rabbit basophils as acetyl glyceryl ether phosphorylcholine *J. Biol. Chem., 225*:5514-5516.

Hanahan, D. J., Munder, P. G., Satouchi, K., McManus, L. M., and Pinckard, R. N. (1981). Retention of potent platelet stimulating activity by the methoxy analogues and by the *sn*-1 stereochemical form of acetyl glyceryl ether phosphorylcholine. *Biochem. Biophys. Res. Commun., 99*:183-188.

Henson, P. M. (1970). Release of vasoactive amines from rabbit platelets induced by sensitized mononuclear leukocytes and antigen. *J. Exp. Med., 131*:287-306.

Henson, P. M., and Pinckard, R. N. (1977). Basophil derived platelet activating factor (PAF) as an *in vivo* mediator of acute allergic reactions. Demonstration of specific desensitization of platelets to PAF during IgE-induced anaphylaxis in the rabbit. *J. Immunol., 119*:2179-2184.

Humphrey, D. M., McManus, L. M., Hanahan, D. J., and Pinckard, R. N. (1982). Vasoactive properties of acetyl glyceryl ether phosphorylcholine (AGEPC) and AGEPC analogues. *Lab. Invest. 46*:422-427.

Humphrey, D. M., Pinckard, R. N., McManus, L. M., and Hanahan, D. J. (1981). Intradermal neutrophil infiltrates induced by 1-*O*-alkyl-2-acetyl-*sn*-glyceryl-3-phosphorylcholine (AGEPC). *Fed. Proc., 40*:1003.

Lewis, R. A., Goetzl, E. J., Wasserman, S. I., Valone, F. H., Rubin, R. H., and Austin, K. F. (1975). The release of four mediators of immediate hypersensitivity from human leukemic basophils. *J. Immunol., 114*:87-92.

Lotner, G. Z., Lynch, J. M., Betz, S. J., and Henson, P. M. (1980). Human neutrophil-derived platelet activating factor. *J. Immunol., 124*:676-684.

Lynch, J. M., Lotner, G. Z., Betz, S. J., and Henson, P. M. (1979). The release of a platelet-activating factor by stimulated rabbit neutrophils. *J. Immunol., 123*:1219-1226.

McManus, L. M., Shaw, J. O., and Pinckard, R. N. (1980b). Thromboxane B_2 (TxB_2) release during IgE anaphylaxis in the rabbit. *J. Immunol., 125*:1950-1954.

McManus, L. M., Hanahan, D. J., and Pinckard, R. N. (1981a). Human platelet stimulation by acetyl glyceryl ether phosphorylcholine (AGEPC). *J. Clin. Invest., 67*:903-906.

McManus, L. M., Hanahan, D. J., Demopoulos, C. A., and Pinckard, R. N. (1980a). Pathobiology of the intravenous infusion of acetyl glyceryl ether phosphorylcholine (AGEPC), a synthetic platelet-activating factor (PAF), in the rabbit. *J. Immunol., 124*:2919-2924.

McManus, L. M., Pinckard, R. N., Fitzpatrick, F. F., O'Rourke, R. A., Crawford, M. H., and Hanahan, D. J. (1981b). Acetyl glyceryl ether phosphorylcholine (AGPEC): Intravascular alterations following intravenous infusion in the baboon. *Lab. Invest., 45*:303-307.

Mencia-Huerta, J. M., and Benveniste, J. (1979). Platelet-activating factor in macrophages. I. Evidence for the release from rat and mouse peritoneal macrophages and not from mastocytes. *Eur. J. Immunol., 9*:409-415.

Namm, D. H., and High, J. A. (1980). Thrombin-induced formation of a polar lipid material within platelets that possesses platelet-activating activity. *Thromb. Res., 30*:285-292.

O'Flaherty, J. T., Lees, C. J., and Stimler, N. P. (1981). Anaphylatoxic and polymorphonuclear neutrophil (PMN)-stimulating actions of platelet activating factor (PAF). *Fed. Proc., 40*:1015.

Pinckard, R. N., Halonen, M., Palmer, J. D., Butler, C., Shaw, J. O., and Henson, P. M. (1977). Intravascular aggregation and pulmonary sequestration of platelets during IgE-induced systemic anaphylaxis in the rabbit. Abrogation of lethal anaphylactic shock by platelet depletion. *J. Immunol., 119*: 2185-2193.

Pinckard, R. N., Farr, R. S., and Hanahan, D. J. (1979). Physicochemical and functional identity of platelet-activating factor (PAF) released *in vivo* during IgE anaphylaxis with PAF released *in vitro* from IgE sensitized basophils. *J. Immunol., 123*:1847-1857.

Pinckard, R. N., Kniker, W. T., Lee, L., Hanahan, D. J., and McManus, L. M. (1980a). Vasoactive effects of 1-*O*-alkyl-2-acetyl-*sn*-glyceryl-3-phosphorylcholine (AcGEPC) in human skin. *J. Allergy Clin. Immunol., 65*: 196.

Pinckard, R. N., McManus, L. M., O'Rourke, R. A., Crawford, M. H., and Hanahan, D. J. (1980b). Intravascular and cardiovascular effects of acetyl glyceryl ether phosphorylcholine (AGEPC) infusion in the baboon. *Clin. Res., 28*:258A.

Prewitt, R. L., Leach, B. E., Byers, L. W., Brooks, B., Lands, W. E. M., and Muirhead, E. E. (1979). Antihypertensive polar renomedullary lipid, a semisynthetic vasocilator. *Hypertension 1*:299-308.

Sanchez Crespo, M., Alonso, F., and Egido, J. (1980). Platelet activating factor in anaphylaxis and phagocytosis. I. Release from human peripheral polymorphonuclear and monocytes during the stimulation by ionophore A23187 and phagocytosis and not from degranulating basophils. *Immunology, 40*:645-655.

Satouchi, K., Pinckard, R. N., McManus, L. M., and Hanahan, D. J. (1981). Modification of the polar head group of acetyl glyceryl ether phosphorylcholine and subsequent effects upon platelet activation. *J. Biol. Chem., 256*:4425-4432.

Schafer, E. A. (1916). *The Endocrine Organs: An Introduction to the Study of Internal Secretion.* New York, Longmans, Green and Co.

Shaw, J. O., Pinckard, R. N., Ferrigni, K. S., McManus, L. M., and Hanahan, D. J. (1981). Activation of human neutrophils with 1-*O*-hexadecyl/octadecyl-2-acetyl-*sn*-glyceryl-3-phosphorylcholine (platelet-activating factor). *J. Immunol., 127*:1250-1255.

Siraganian, R. P., and Osler, A. G. (1971). Destruction of rabbit platelets in the allergic response of sensitized leukocytes. I. Demonstration of a fluid phase intermediate. *J. Immunol., 106*:1244-1251.

Tence, M., Polonsky, J., Le Couedic, J. P., and Benveniste, J. (1980). Release, purification, and characterization of platelet-activating factor. *Biochemie, 62*:251-259.

Vargaftig, B. B., Lefort, J., Chignard, M., and Benveniste, J. (1980). Platelet-activating factor induces a platelet-dependent bronchoconstriction unrelated to the formation of prostaglandin derivatives. *Eur. J. Pharmacol., 65*:185-192.

5

Regulation of Bronchial Secretions

JAY A. NADEL
University of California
School of Medicine
San Francisco, California

I. Introduction

The role of abnormal secretion of fluid and mucus in the pathogenesis of disease is unknown. The symptomatology and pathology of various airway diseases suggests that abnormal secretion and/or ciliary transport play an important role in the pathogenesis of the diseases. In this chapter, I will review the present state of knowledge concerning the normal regulation of airway secretions, and I will suggest possible roles in disease. Ciliary action and secretions together produce normal mucociliary clearance; coughing also clears the airways of foreign materials and accumulated secretions. These integrated functions are reviewed elsewhere in this text. However, where relevant, I will indicate possible roles of the various secretory processes in clearance.

This study was supported in part by USPHS NIH Program Project Grant HL-24136, California Air Resources Board Contract A9-115-30, Grant #1311 from the Council for Tobacco Research-U.S.A., Inc., and a grant from the Vick Divisions Research and Development.

As a physiologic "subunit," the airway surface epithelium can be thought of as a "sheet," composed of cells that are attached by tight junctions. These surface cells appear to secrete (a) ions by active transport, and (b) mucins and other components of mucus by a form of cellular exocytosis. These two functions of the surface epithelium will be presented in separate sections. A second physiologic subunit is the airway submucosal gland, composed of acini and connected to the airway lumen via a short duct. Regulation of the glands will be reviewed separately.

Major advances have occurred in the understanding of the processes of secretion in airways during the last decade. This is due in no small part to the application of modern techniques of anatomy, cell biology, physiology, pharmacology, and biochemistry to these problems. Thus, use of morphometric methods of examining airway glands during secretion (Basbaum et al., 1982), use of autoradiography (Meyrick and Reid, 1975) and release (Gallagher et al., 1975) of specifically labeled radioactive precursors, application of the renal micropipette technique to airways (Nadel, 1977), and the application of the Ussing chamber technique to the study of airway ion transport (Olver et al., 1975) are examples of the exploitation of techniques to the problem of airway secretion. Knowledge of the regulation of airway secretion is advancing rapidly. The next step will be to begin to apply this knowledge to an understanding of the effects of modification of secretion on the effectiveness of mucociliary clearance and of cough. Ultimately, it is hoped that these insights can be applied to a better understanding of the pathogenesis of disease and to a rational basis for therapy.

II. Airway Submucosal Glands

Most (95%) of the airway secretions are composed of water. The remaining 5% are composed of proteins, carbohydrates, lipids, and inorganic materials. A substantial part of this material is incorporated into mucins by cells in the airway epithelium. Production of mucins is believed to occur in submucosal glands and in surface goblet cells. Because the submucosal glands occupy approximately 40 times more volume than surface goblet cells in the human large conducting airways (Reid, 1960), these structures are likely to be major contributors to the total secretion of mucus. Glands are rare in rabbits and guinea pigs (Mawdsley-Thomas et al., 1971), and nonexistent in chickens (Walsh and McLelland, 1974) and geese (Phipps et al., 1977); they are numerous in cats (Florey et al., 1932; Gallagher et al., 1975), pigs, and ferrets (Basbaum et al., 1982), and moderately numerous in dogs (B. Borson, personal communication). In healthy humans, they are also moderately numerous (one gland per square millimeter of trachea [Thurlbeck et al., 1961]). In chronic bronchitis and asthma, there is an increase in the size of the glands (Cardell and Pearson, 1959; Reid, 1960; Restrepo and Heard, 1963), and this hypertrophy is likely to play an important role in these diseases. Glands are made up of a short, funnel-shaped ciliated duct that leads into the surface epithelium, a nonciliated collecting duct, and mucous and serous tubules that are lined with mucous and serous cells, respectively (Meyrick et al., 1969). Mucous cells are characterized in the electron microscope by their electron-lucent and often confluent granules, while serous cells are characterized by their electron-dense discrete secretory granules and the presence of inter- and intracellular canaliculi (Meyrick and Reid, 1970). Myoepithelial cells are located at the base of each acinus, and their contraction may aid in the passage of secretions along the tubules (Basbaum et al., 1982). During stimulation, serous cells show loss of granules, diverticulation, and enlargement of their acinar lumens (Basbaum et al., 1982). Granule depletion can be assumed to be an index of protein secretion (Amsterdam et al., 1969; Jamieson and Palade, 1971). During stimulation, serous cells also show vacuolization (Basbaum et al., 1982), an effect considered by some to be indicative of secretion of ions and water (Garrett et al., 1978). Granule depletion and vacuolization may be independent, separately regulated processes (Batzri et al., 1971) implying that protein and water movement may be controlled separately. Morphometric studies of mucous cell depletion in airways are not available; in rectal goblet cells, membranes of adjacent mucous granules form contact areas that appear to be protein-poor membrane lipid bilayers which form the interaction sites. It is believed that these fused bilayers then break down to cause membrane fusion (Neutra and Schaeffer, 1977).

Understanding of the regulation of fluid requires a method for obtaining these secretions uncontaminated by other structures. Study of airway submucosal gland secretion has been hampered by the small size of the anatomic structures involved, the small volume of secretions normally produced, and the relative inaccessibility of the glands. Thus, control of the rate of flow and biochemical constituents of salivary gland secretion has been studied extensively, while even the rate of secretion of individual airway glands was unknown until relatively recently. Early methods of collecting airway secretions were contaminated with sputum or alveolar fluid (Wardell et al., 1970). Recently, Adams and coworkers developed a method for harvesting secretions in the airway lumen, but this method can not distinguish the source of the secretions (Adams et al., 1976).

The study of renal and salivary gland secretion have been made possible by the use of micropipettes which allow the removal of secretions from specific structures. With this in mind, we have developed a micropipette method for obtaining secretions from single airway submucosal gland ducts in cats (Ueki et al., 1980; German et al., 1980). Because the opening of the gland duct is funnel-shaped, it is relatively easy to seal the duct and harvest secretions without obstructing flow into the pipette. Originally, identification of the openings was made possible by topical application of neutral red dye (Nadel, 1977), but we can now identify the openings without dye by their elliptical shape and their proximity to blood vessels (Ueki et al., 1980). The individual gland secretory rate under basal conditions averaged 9 nl/min, and remained remarkably constant over several hours. Calculations suggested a total secretory rate from all the tracheal glands of approximately 24 ml/day. We have used the micropipette technique extensively to study the regulation of gland secretory rate and also to study the biochemical constituents of the secreted fluid. In dogs, secreted mucus is too viscous to harvest in pipettes. In this species, we expose the trachea and spray a fine layer of powdered tantalum on the exposed surface. During gland secretion, elevations occur in the tantalum layer at sites of gland duct openings which we call "hillocks" (Nadel, 1977). We visualize the hillocks through a dissecting microscope and use a television camera to record the images on tape. By measuring the rate of formation and growth of the hillocks, we obtain an estimation of the rate of gland secretion. Compared with the micropipette method, the major advantage of the hillock method is its ease of study, and its major disadvantage is its inability to obtain the secretions directly.

A third method used for studying airway submucosal gland secretion is the use of radioactively labeled precursors of mucin. Because it is relatively specific for mucins, [^{35}S] sodium sulfate labeling of large, nondialyzable materials is often used. [^{35}S] sodium sulfate is most avidly taken up by submucosal glands, less by epithelial ciliated cells and surface mucosubstance, and even less by surface goblet cells (Jeffery, 1978). Sulfate attachment occurs first in the Golgi area of the submucosal gland cells when examined autoradiographically; radioactivity is later seen within granules and moves from the base to the apex of the cell to be secreted (Meyrick and Reid, 1975).

Both parasympathetic and sympathetic nerves innervate airway submucosal glands, and stimulation of various sensory pathways increase secretory rate via autonomic reflex pathways. Recent evidence also indicates that α- and β-adrenergic stimultation produces selectively different effects on submucosal gland cells. Because abnormalities in the autonomic nervous system have been strongly implicated in the pathogenesis of asthma (Boushey et al., 1980) and because autonomic agonists and antagonists are used in the treatment of asthma, these systems will be reviewed in detail.

A. Modulation by the Parasympathetic System

The parasympathetic motor nerve supply to the glands is via the vagus nerves. One proof of vagal control of the glands is anatomic: the presence of acetylcholinesterase staining in fibers coursing among the tubules and ducts of the glands suggests the presence of parasympathetic nerve endings in glands (Wardell et al., 1970; Mann, 1971; El-Bermani and Grant, 1975; and Murlas et al., 1980), and this is confirmed by the electron microscopic demonstration of varicosities containing small agranular vesicles near gland tubules and ducts at all levels of the trachea (Murlas et al., 1980). Cholinergic and adrenergic varicosities were found near serous and mucous cells; no selectivity of axons to either type of gland cell was evident. There were approximately nine times as many cholinergic as adrenergic varicosities, and most of these varicosities were present in interstitial bundles located between the acini; only 4% of the cholinergic varicosities occurred in close contact with gland cells. The significance of these locations in relation to the regulation of specific gland cells is unclear. One might conclude from the predominance of cholinergic axons that cholinergic control of gland secretions might be more effective than adrenergic control. However, it is much more likely that the potency and specificity of neural control over effector cells in glands depends mainly on the distribution of adrenergic and cholinergic (muscarinic) receptors than on the distribution of axons. The second evidence of vagal control of airway submucosal glands derives from the effects of stimulation of the vagal motor pathway: early studies by Florey showed that electrical stimulation of the vagal motor nerves increased the volume of airway secretions, but the source of these secretions could not be determined (Florey et al., 1932). Electrical stimulation of the vagus nerves increased the rate of fluid secretion into micropipettes (Ueki et al., 1980) and the release of ^{35}S bound to mucins into the airway lumen (Gallagher et al., 1975) in cats, and increased the rate of hillock formation in dogs (Nadel, 1977; Nadel and Davis, 1980). The secretomotor fibers to the upper trachea travel in the superior laryngeal nerves, and the fibers to the lower trachea travel in the recurrent laryngeal nerves of the dog (Davis et al., 1976). The ^{35}S-labeled mucins released by vagal stimulation could have been derived from the surface epithelium (e.g., goblet cells) or from cells of the submucosal glands. However, the fact that prolonged electrical stimulation of the vagus nerves depleted the radioactively labeled ^{35}S-label from only submucosal glands indicates that the released radiolabeled materials were derived principally from gland cells (Gallagher et al., 1975). Further confirmatory evidence for the presence of parasympathetic nerves and muscarinic receptors was obtained in ferret trachea in vitro by electrical transmural stimulation of nerves in vitro (Borson et al., 1980).

There is evidence that responses in the motor pathway can be potentiated. Thus, the secretory response to stimulation of the vagus nerve was potentiated by serotonin, whereas the secretory response to infused acetylcholine was not (Popovac et al., 1979). This effect has also been described for airway smooth muscle (Hahn et al., 1978). Serotonin is reported to affect mucociliary clearance in cats (Dadaian et al., 1971). These effects could be due to stimulation of secretions via vagal motor pathways. The site of interaction of serotonin and parasympathetic nerves in airways is unknown. However, in the myenteric ganglion cells of the guinea pig small intestine, serotonin depolarized the somal membrane and augmented excitability when applied iontophoretically (Wood, 1978), and furthermore, stimulation of interganglionic fiber tracts released an excitatory substance that resembled serotonin (Wood and Mayer, 1979). This raises the question whether serotonin or other neurohumoral agents secreted by the body normally modulate the output of acetylcholine through prejunctional or ganglionic effects, and whether disease alters this modulation. Because the parasympathetic ganglia are located in the airway walls, their study has been neglected because of the inability to locate them in vivo and because of their inaccesibility. However, recently Grillo and Nadel (1980) have developed a vital staining technique to identify airway ganglia, and neurophysiologic studies have been initiated to study these structures.

Atropine prevented the responses to vagal stimulation, indicating that the effect was due to the release of acetylcholine acting on muscarinic receptors. The presence of muscarinic receptors on airway secretory cells is further shown by the fact that muscarinic agonists stimulated the secretion of fluid from submucosal glands (Ueki et al., 1980), the formation of hillocks (Davis et al., 1976), the output of radiolabeled mucins (Sturgess and Reid, 1972; Boat and Kleinerman, 1975), and the release of lysozyme (Tom-Moy et al., 1981), effects that were abolished by atropine. Morphometric studies of lung anatomy also confirm the stimulatory effects of muscarinic agonists: methacholine causes morphologic changes in airway submucosal gland cells of ferrets, effects that could be prevented by preincubation with atropine (Basbaum et al., 1982). Both serous (Basbaum et al., 1982) and mucous (C. B. Bausbaum, personal communication) cells were depleted by methacholine, suggesting that muscarinic receptors are plentiful on both serous and mucous cells and provide no evidence of selective regulation of either cell type by the parasympathetic system.

Cooling blockade of the cervical vagus nerves decreased the rate of secretion from gland ducts slightly in cats (Ueki et al., 1980) and decreased fluid collection rate in dogs (King et al., 1979), indicating that "tonic" vagal nervous activity plays a role in gland secretions in the resting state. This correlates well with the fact that vagal efferent nervous activity occurs spontaneously in fibers believed to innervate airway glands (Widdicombe, 1966). The fact that the muscarinic antagonist, atropine, reduced the basal secretory rate and that the acetylcholinesterase inhibitor, physostigmine increased the basal secretory rate in human airway submucosal glands in culture suggests that at least part of the resting muscarinic stimulus can occur in the absence of central nervous connections, at least under the special condition in vitro (Coles, 1977).

It has been suggested that cholinergic antagonists such as atropine are deleterious because they dry the airway mucosa. Atropine is a specific muscarinic antagonist. Therefore, it can be predicted to inhibit secretions only when the secretions are produced by the release of acetylcholine (e.g., from the vagus nerves). Thus, if excessive secretions are produced abnormally by reflex stimulation, atropine could have a beneficial effect on mucociliary clearance.

Similarly, in diseases where inadequate fluid and mucus production exist, stimulation of the glands by cholinergic agonists could improve clearance.

Many reflexes involving the vagus nerves are known to stimulate contraction of airway smooth muscle (Nadel, 1980). Although studies of reflex control of airway submucosal glands have only recently begun, several observations of possible important physiological and clinical significance have been made. Mechanical stimulation of the laryngeal epithelium in cats increases the rate of secretion of fluid from airway submucosal glands (German et al., 1982) and increases the rate of ^{35}S-labeled mucins into the tracheal lumen (Gallagher et al., 1975). Exercise is reported to increase mucociliary clearance rates (Wolff et al., 1977). Exercise increases the water loss in the large airways, and this could stimulate the production of mucus via a vagal reflex similar to the effect of mechanical irritation of the airway. Chemical stimulation of the tracheobronchial mucosa with ammonia stimulates secretion of mucins via a vagal reflex (Phipps and Richardson, 1976). The sensory pathway for this reflex is via the superior laryngeal nerves, and the efferent pathway is via the vagi. Various aromatic vapors are purported to stimulate the output of respiratory tract fluid (Boyd and Sheppard, 1970a,b,c, 1971; Richardson and Phipps, 1978), but their sites and mechanisms of action are presently unknown. They could act reflexly by stimulating reflex pathways in the nose, larynx, or airways. They could act locally on the airway epithelial cells, or they could act by releasing mediators which stimulate secretion.

Fluid secretion may be a part of the normal cough reflex. It is postulated that the volume and composition of secretions produced by this irritant reflex assists in the removal of foreign irritants during cough. It is probably not a coincidence that cough receptors are concentrated in the large airways. It is also interesting that airway submucosal glands are concentrated in these large airways where compression of the airways occurs during cough (Jones et al., 1975) and where cough is therefore most likely to be effective in clearance. While most authors concentrate on the effects of airway secretions on mucociliary clearance, it is likely that gland secretion also plays a major role in relation to cough. Chronic inflammatory changes in the airways in asthma and in bronchitis may be the cause of cough that may be a prominent symptom in these diseases. One could speculate that the epithelial inflammatory changes are primary and that secondary reflex stimulation causes the excessive production of airway secretions. Furthermore, chronic reflex gland stimulation could be the explanation of the gland hypertrophy and hyperplasia that occur in these diseases. Chronic treatment with muscarinic antagonists could possibly reverse this abnormal gland growth and thus provide a rationale for its therapeutic use.

Hypoxemia also stimulates submucosal gland secretion reflexly via stimulation of the carotid bodies and with efferent pathways in the vagi (Davis et al., 1980). Anatomic changes in the small airways are believed to be early manifestations of chronic bronchitis. Perhaps these changes cause hypoxemia and (presuming that the reflex exists in humans), the hypoxemia stimulates reflex production of mucus, further intensifying the disease. Chronic hypoxic reflex gland stimulation could also contribute to gland hypertrophy.

Stimulation of bronchial C fibers with bradykinin or capsaicin also accelerates the production of hillocks in dogs via a vagal reflex (Davis et al., 1982). Gastric distension also reflexly stimulates gland secretions with the afferent and efferent pathways located in the vagus nerves (German et al., 1980b). It is not known whether chemical stimulation of the stomach produces similar reflex secretion from airway submucosal glands, but such a reflex could explain purported effects of some drugs and foods. Thus far, all vagal reflexes described stimulate the production of secretions. Only one vagal reflex is known to inhibit the secretion from the airway submucosal glands: lung inflation diminishes the production of gland secretions via receptors in the lungs (presumably "Hering-Breuer" fibers), with afferent and efferent pathways in the vagi (Chinn et al., 1981).

Airway smooth muscle tone that normally exists in airways is due to the presence of vagal motor nerve activity. The degree of this tone is determined, at least in part, by a balance of two opposing stimuli: stimulation of rapidly adapting receptors produces bronchoconstriction, while stimulation of slowly adapting receptors inhibits vagal efferent activity and decreases bronchomotor tone. Lung inflation stimulates both types of receptors. We have suggested that the balance between the two determines the resting bronchomotor tone (Nadel et al., 1973). Similarly, the degree of vagally mediated secretions may depend on a balance of receptor inputs; abnormalities in these signals may affect secretion in disease.

B. Modulation by the Adrenergic System

The adrenergic system can influence airway submucosal glands both by the release of circulating catecholamines from chromaffin cells and by direct nervous innervation of the airways. The former plays a significant role in lower vertebrates, while the latter is better developed in higher vertebrates (Burnstock, 1969). The sympathetic nerve supply to the airways varies greatly among species, so information from one species cannot be extrapolated to another species (Richardson, 1979). Specific fluorescence studies indicated the presence of catecholamine-containing fibers among the tracheal gland tubules and ducts in cats (Murlas et al., 1980). Electron microscopic studies confirmed the presence of adrenergic nerve endings by demonstrating the existence of small dense-cored vesicles in nervous varicosities near gland cells in cats (Murlas et al., 1980) and in humans (Meyrick et al., 1969). Like cholinergic varicosities, very few adrenergic varicosities make close contact with gland cells; most were present in interstitial bundles between gland acini. Adrenergic varicosities were distributed in equal numbers near serous and mucous cells. Of all axon bundles containing adrenergic varicosities, 92% contained one or more cholinergic varicosities (Murlas et al., 1980). This close proximity provides the anatomic basis for possible postganglionic interaction between the cholinergic and adrenergic systems. Thus, release of a nervous mediator from one system could modulate the release of a mediator from the other system, as it does in canine and rabbit salivary glands (Emmelin and Gjorstrup, 1976; Gjorstrup, 1977). For example, it has been shown that endogenously released norepinephrine from nerves to airway smooth muscle can partially inhibit bronchoconstriction caused by stimulation of the cholinergic nerves (Vermeire and Vanhoutte, 1979). A similar inhibition of the release of norepinephrine from adrenergic nerves by stimulation of muscarinic receptors has been demonstrated for nerves supplying tracheal submucosal glands in ferrets (Borson and Nadel, 1981).

Electrical stimulation of the thoracic sympathetic nerves increased the release of ^{35}S-labeled mucins in cats (Gallagher et al., 1975; Peatfield and Richardson, 1980). In ferrets, field stimulation of tracheal segments in chambers after administration of atropine caused fluid secretion from submucosal glands, an effect that was abolished by tetrodotoxin (indicating that the effect was mediated by nerves) or by adrenergic antagonists. The absence of adrenergic effects in guinea pigs (Goco et al., 1963), rabbits (Korhonen et al., 1969), and geese (Breeze and Wheeldon, 1977) may be due to the fact that these species have poorly developed submucosal glands.

Weak effects of α-adrenergic agonists in some studies may be due to the fact that these agonists cause vascular constriction, thus limiting the amount of the agonist reaching the gland cells. Thus, Davis and associates showed that the stimulating effect of phenylephrine on submucosal gland secretion was increased by papaverine, a drug that dilated the tracheal blood vessels (Davis et al., 1979). Reflexes mediated via sympathetic nerves are only rarely studied, but present evidence indicates that irritation of the nose, pharynx, or larynx increases the release of ^{35}S-labeled mucins, partly via sympathetic pathways (Phipps and Richardson, 1976). Differential regulation of serous versus mucous cells is a relatively recently demonstrated phenomenon. Thus, when I raised the possibility of differential regulation of these two cell types at a Ciba Foundation meeting in 1977, existing evidence suggested that serous and mucous cells had the same response to drugs (Reid, 1977). We now know that muscarinic agonists deplete both serous and mucous cells of their granules nonselectively but that α- and β-adrenergic agonists are more selective. The fact that both α- and β adrenergic agonists stimulate the release of ^{35}S-labeled materials, effects that were abolished by α- and β-adrenergic antagonists respectively, suggested that both adrenergic receptors stimulation somehow cause airway submucosal gland secretion in cats (Phipps et al., 1980). However, in the same species, an α-adrenergic agonist increased fluid secretion markedly (Ueki et al., 1980), while

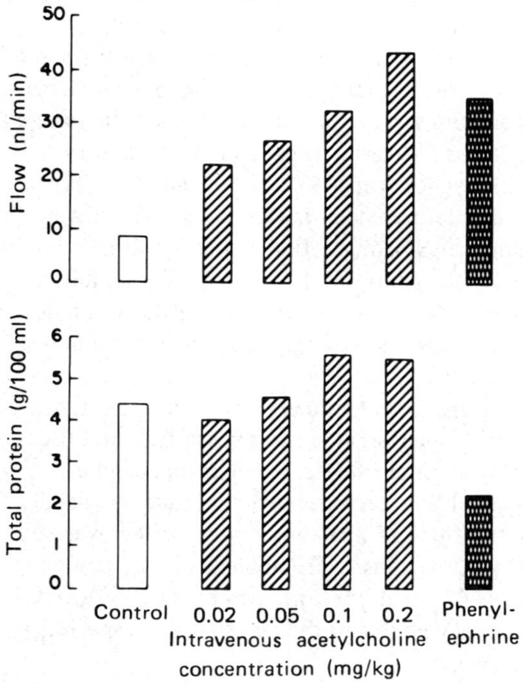

Figure 1 Effect of acetylcholine vs phenylephrine on fluid output (top) and total protein concentration (bottom) obtained in micropipettes in one cat. Increasing concentrations of acetylcholine caused progressive increases in fluid production and a modest increase in total protein concentration, while a comparable increase in fluid production by phenylephrine (5 μg/min iv, for 2 min) resulted in a striking decrease in the total protein concentration of the fluid produced.

a β-adrenergic agonist had little effect on fluid flow. (I. Ueki, personal communication). Similarly, Borson and coworkers demonstrated that sympathetic nerve stimulation produced fluid flow from ferret tracheal glands, an effect abolished by an α-adrenergic antagonist but not by a β-adrenergic antagonist (Borson et al., 1980). These studies suggest that α- and β-adrenergic stimulation affect airway submucosal glands differently. Morphometric studies performed in ferret tracheal epithelium indicate that α- and β-adrenergic agonists have markedly different morphologic effects on serous and mucous cells: α-adrenergic stimulation produced evidence of significant serous cell depletion, but β-adrenergic stimulation did not (Basbaum et al., 1982). Preliminary results suggest that mucous cells are depleted by β-adrenergic, but not by α-adrenergic stimulation. Thus, serous cells appear to contain predominantly α receptors, while mucous cells appear to contain β receptors. Of course, definitive studies to confirm this hypothesis will require autoradiographic localization of specific radioactive ligands. We have further evidence for selectivity of adrenergic receptors in ferret glands. Thus, Tom-Moy et al. used immunocytochemical methods to prove that lysozyme was localized within the secretory granules of the serous

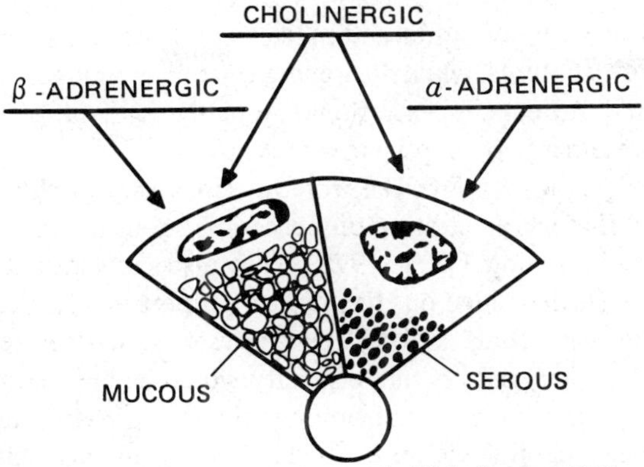

Figure 2 Diagrammatic representation of serous and mucous cells of airway submucosal gland and hypothesis of selective regulation. Cholinergic muscarinic agonists stimulate secretion from both cell types (indicated by arrows to serous and mucous cells). α-adrenergic stimulation selectively depletes serous cells (indicated by arrow to serous cell) producing high fluid output containing low sulfur (S) and total protein concentrations. β-Adrenergic stimulation selectively depletes mucous cells (indicated by arrow to mucous cell), producing low fluid output containing high sulfur and protein concentrations.

cells; mucous cells and surface cells did not contain lysozyme (Tom-Moy et al., 1980). They also showed that an α-adrenergic agonist stimulated the release of large amounts of lysozyme compared to a β-adrenergic agonist; this α-adrenergic effect was abolished by an α-adrenergic antagonist (Tom-Moy et al., 1981). Micropipette studies in cats also indicate striking differences. Thus, α-adrenergic stimulation increases fluid output markedly (Ueki et al., 1980), while β-adrenergic agonists stimulate only little fluid production (I. Ueki, personal communication). Similarly, Ueki and Nadel (1981) showed that α-adrenergic stimulation decreases the total protein concentration in fluid harvested from gland ducts in micropipettes (Fig. 1), while β-adrenergic agonists increase the protein concentration (I. Ueki, personal communication). Presumably, the proteins derived from serous cells come predominantly from the electron-dense granules, and the proteins derived from mucous cells come from electron-lucent granules. Other studies show that α-adrenergic agonists produce fluid with lower concentrations of sulfur than β-adrenergic agonists do (Quinton, 1979). The effects of autonomic agonists are summarized diagrammatically in Figure 2: α-adrenergic agonists stimulate the production of copious secretions containing high concentrations of lysozyme with low sulfur and protein concentrations, presumably by depleting serous cell contents, while β-adrenergic agonists produce scanty fluid with high sulfur and protein concentrations (probably containing highly concentrated mucins), presumably by depleting serous cells.

The physiologic properties of the secretions may vary markedly. King and coworkers showed that administration of muscarinic agonists decreased mucus viscosity and elasticity in dogs (King, 1979). They also showed that the effect of muscarinic antagonists depended on the physical properties of the mucus present in the control state (King et al., 1979). They suggested that when resting cholinergic vagal "tone" is low, viscosity and elasticity would be high; stimulation of muscarinic receptors under these conditions would decrease viscosity and elasticity. However, when cholinergic tone is high, viscosity and elasticity of control secretions would be low, and further stimulation of muscarinic receptors would not affect viscoelastic properties. The viscoelastic properties of secretions selectively produced by serous or mucous cells might have markedly different viscoelastic and other properties. Further, effects of these differences might have important implications about the effectiveness of mucociliary clearance and about the effectiveness of cough in producing clearance. Imbalance between α- and β-adrenergic systems in disease or during drug therapy could markedly affect the secretory process. The mechanism underlying the decrease in mucociliary clearance rate that occurs during sleep is unknown (Bateman et al., 1978); it could be due to changes in the autonomic nervous system during sleep.

III. Surface Epithelial Cells

Goblet cells and serous cells are the two surface cell types believed to be sources of glycoproteins. Airway goblet cells resemble goblet cells of the intestine and mucous cells of the airway submucosal glands. Like submucosal glands, they are found mainly in the trachea and bronchi and decrease toward the periphery of the lungs. Their number varies among species, being numerous in humans, cats, pigs, and geese (Nadel et al., 1979). Serous cells in the epithelium and in submucosal glands appear similar; their distribution is the same as epithelial goblet cells. Clara cells are found in the peripheral airways in some species (Breeze and Wheeldon, 1977). They may secrete lipids or proteins. Airway irritation with smoke or SO_2 is believed to induce transition of Clara cells to goblet cells (Jeffrey and Reid, 1977).

The luminal surface of the ciliated airway cells is lined with sulfated glycoprotein (Spicer et al., 1971), a material believed to be secreted by the epithelial cells (Gallagher et al., 1977, 1978). Motor innervation of the airway epithelium is not clearly defined. It probably varies with species, being functional only in species which do not have submucosal glands (e.g., geese) (Phipps and Richardson, 1976; Nadel et al., 1979).

Only a few studies have been performed to examine secretory effects of surface cells; these studies utilize autoradiographic, morphologic, and radioactive counting methods.

Muscarinic agonists did not deplete surface goblet cells in cats, suggesting that muscarinic receptors are not present in these cells, although they appear plentiful in morphologically similar mucous cells of the airway submucosal glands (Jeffery, 1978). This difference between morphologically similar cells is similar to the large intestinal mucosa, where the goblet cells in the crypts are stimulated to secrete in response to muscarinic agonists, while the goblet cells on the mucosal surface are unaffected (Specian and Neutra, 1980).

Direct airway irritation and a few drugs appear to be effective in stimulating secretion from surface epithelial cells. Administration of tobacco smoke or ammonia directly into the lumen of the airways of cats resulted in a marked decrease in goblet cell number. In cats, ammonia caused the release of [^{3}H] glucose into the lumen from both goblet cells and from the surface mucosubstance. Thus, irritants may cause secretion from both of these sources. Ammonia also increased the output of radiolabeled mucins in geese but not in cats, evidently by a local effect on the cells (Richardson et al., 1978). Effects on the epithelial surface may be due to active release of materials or to damage to the cells. The exact stimulus and mechanism of these local irritant responses is unknown. It has been suggested that the irritants may release prostaglandins which then act as secretagogues (Richardson et al., 1978).

IV. Effects of Drugs and Other Substances

Various drugs affect secretion from airways. In some cases, the source of the secretion (e.g., glands vs surface cells) is clear; in many cases, the evidence is circumstantial; in still other cases, no attempt was made to determine the source of the secretion (Widdicombe, 1978).

Lidocaine applied locally to the tracheas of cats or geese stimulated mucin production (Phipps, 1977; Phipps et al., 1977); this effect may involve the displacement of calcium ions from extra- and intracellular binding sites (Phipps, 1977). A common secretory mechanism appears to regulate cells whose secretory product is contained in membrane-limited secretory granules (Douglas, 1978). Stimuli on the plasma membrane lead to a rise in the concentration of free calcium ions at specific loci inside the cell (e.g., the inner aspect of the plasma membrane) which cause an energy-dependent step, resulting in the merging of membranes of the secretory granules and subsequent rupture and expulsion of the granules to the exterior (a process called exocytosis). The role of calcium in airway secretion is not well understood, but calcium appears to play a ubiquitous role in stimulus-secretion coupling. Thus, calcium ionophore increased the release of [^{3}H] glucose-labeled mucins, presumably from mucus-secreting cells of chicken tracheas in vitro (Balfre, 1977).

A. Serotonin and Vasoactive Intestinal Peptide

Serotonin potentiated the effect of vagal stimulation on secretion from airway submucosal glands in dogs, possibly by an effect on parasympathetic ganglia in the airways (Popovac et al., 1979), but serotonin had no effect on mucin secretion locally when delivered into a tracheal segment in cats (Richardson et al., 1978). Vasoactive intestinal peptide (VIP) has not been studied in the airway secretory system, but there are several reasons to suspect that it may play a role. Vasoactive intestinal peptide was first identified on the basis of its vasodilator activity and considered to be a hormone (Said and Mutt, 1969), More recently, immunohistochemical studies have revealed that VIP occurs in neurons, including those in airways of cats and rabbits (Uddman et al., 1978; Uddman and Sundler, 1979). Vasoactive intestinal peptide nerves were found around seromucous glands, as well as blood vessels and smooth muscle; ganglia also stained for VIP. Because of their location in the cholinergic nerves of the exocrine glands in cats, it was suggested that they might be a neurotransmitter. Lundberg and associates (1980) showed that preganglionic stimulation of cholinergic nerves to the cat submandibular gland caused nonmuscarinic vasodilation and secretion, associated with the release of VIP, effects that were reduced by infusion of VIP antiserum. The results suggested that VIP and acetylcholine might coexist and, together, might modulate effector responses (Lundberg et al., 1980). Perhaps VIP is a mediator for the nonadrenergic inhibitory nervous system in airways (Richardson, 1975; Richardson and Beland, 1976). Evidence for this is based on the studies of airway smooth muscle in guinea pigs (Matsuzaki et al., 1980).

VIP relaxes airway smooth muscle independent of adrenergic or cholinergic receptors (Piper et al., 1970). Further, VIP was released during electrical field stimulation of guinea pig trachea, an effect blocked by tetrodotoxin. Modulation of secretion from airway submucosal glands by VIP is also likely, but not yet studied.

B. Bradykinin

Bradykinin reflexly stimulated fluid secretion from airway submucosal glands in vivo (Davis et al., 1982), but did not influence the rate of release of tagged mucins from explants (Sturgess and Reid, 1972). Bradykinin is released endogenously under various conditions such as acidosis (O'Brodovich et al., 1981) and bradykinin may play a role in the inflammatory response (Regoli and Barabe, 1980). Thus, the endogenous release of bradykinins could cause epithelial inflammation and thereby modify other (e.g., autonomic) responses. Basic polypeptides (e.g., kallidin and substance P) increased mucin production in dogs in vitro, while hexadimethrine, a kalladin antagonist, decreased it (Baker et al., 1977).

C. Histamine

Histamine aerosol delivered to the lungs in cats failed to stimulate secretions in the trachea; tracheal instillation of histamine stimulated mucin production in cats and geese, but the cells of origin were not determined (Richardson et al., 1978). Histamine had no effect on secretion in dogs in vitro (Chakrin et al., 1973) or in humans (Sturgess and Reid, 1972). Clearly, the role of histamine (a putative mediator in asthma) in airway secretion requires more investigation.

D. Prostaglandins and Leukotreines

Two metabolic pathways of arachidonic acid metabolism have been described. The cyclooxygenase pathway includes prostaglandins and prostaglandin intermediates. The other, lipoxygenase, pathway produces the leukotriene derivatives, including the major functional components of slow-reacting substance of anaphylaxis (SRS-A) (Hammarstrom et al., 1979; Murphy et al., 1979; Lewis et al., 1980; Orning et al., 1980).

Prostaglandin effects are not well worked out. Local application of PGE_1 stimulated mucin production in cats (Richardson et al., 1978), and several prostaglandins PGA_2, PGD_2, and $PGF_{2\alpha}$) caused release of tagged mucins in human bronchi in vitro; PGE_2 was the only prostaglandin which significantly reduced secretion significantly (Marom et al., 1981). Various prostaglandins (A_1, E_1, E_2, $F_{1\alpha}$, and $F_{2\alpha}$) appear to stimulate fluid secretion when applied directly to cat tracheas (Iravani and Melville, 1975). $PGF_{2\alpha}$ stimulates irritant receptors, producing reflex increases in airway smooth muscle tone mediated via vagal nervous pathways (Wasserman, 1975); a similar reflex could be present in the secretomotor system. Reflex stimulation of C-fiber, afferent nerves in the lungs by capsaicin or bradykinin has been shown to stimulate the production of hillocks reflexly in dogs (Davis et al., 1980), and stimulation of irritant receptors by prostaglandins might cause similar vagal reflex responses. Local prostaglandin release secondary to tissue inflammation could account for the increase in mucous production found in association with inflammatory diseases of the airways.

Lung inflation causes the release of prostaglandins and prostacyclin (Berry et al., 1971; Utsunomiya et al., 1982) and experimental pulmonary embolism causes the release of thromboxane A_2 (Utsunomiya et al., 1982). These released prostaglandins could in turn stimulate or inhibit the release of secretions and provide part of a "feedback" system of regulation.

Progress in the study of the structure and functions of SRS-A has accelerated during the past decade, but very little is known of its effect on airway secretions. Leukotriene (LTC_4) appears to stimulate the secretion of fluid from airway submucosal glands in dogs, an effect that appears to involve the vagal motor pathway, with no residual local effect (Johnson, personal communication).

Leukotrienes contract airway smooth muscle (Drazen et al., 1979); their effects on airway secretions need further study.

Autologous serum promoted tracheal secretion in cats by an unknown mechanism (Hall et al., 1978). Preliminary studies suggest that a similar effect occurs in humans (Peatfield, 1980). $C5_a$, a peptide derived from the fifth component of complement, contracts guinea pig tracheal muscle, an effect apparently due to a product of arachidonate metabolism, at least in part by SRS-A (Regal and Pickering, 1981). This and other components of blood could stimulate secretions in airways.

V. Active Ion Transport

A thin aqueous solution lines the airways. The secretion is a complex mixture, containing approximately 95% water. The top layer is believed to consist of a gel of hydrated mucus, while underneath lies a more watery sol layer (Yoneda, 1976). The cilia beat freely in the gel; the tips of the cilia make contact with the viscoelastic gel of mucus and sweep it up the airway, along with trapped deposited particles. Such a system requires a finely tuned regulation of the volume of liquid, because a small decrease in the thickness of the sol layer will prevent effective motion of the cilia, while an increase in the thickness of the sol layer will not allow the tips of the cilia to make proper contact with the gel. In other epithelia, fluid movement is brought about by active transport of ions across the epithelium, and water moves as a result of the local osmotic gradients produced by the movement of ions. In 1975, using Ussing's short-circuit current technique, we described active transport of ions across the posterior membranous portion of the canine trachea (Olver et al., 1975). We showed that there was a net movement of Cl^- toward the lumen and a smaller net movement of Na^+ toward the submucosa. When net Cl^- movement toward the lumen predominates, net secretion of fluid occurs toward the lumen; when net Na^+ movement toward the submucosa predominates, water reabsorption should occur. Multiple studies have confirmed the original observations in the trachea. The exact ratio of net Cl^- and Na^+ movements has varied, but generally net Cl^- movement accounts for about 75% of the short-circuit current generated. Studies have been performed in dogs (Al-Bazzaz and Al-Awqati, 1977) and cats (Phipps et al., 1980). Although demonstration of net ion movement suggests that changes in the volume of respiratory tract fluid occur, measurement of fluid movement must be made directly in order to validate this impression. Therefore, we developed a sensitive method for measuring volume flow across the canine tracheal epithelium (Welsh et al., 1980), and we showed that the baseline volume flow from the submucosa to the mucosa was usually not measurable in the resting state. However, stimulation with aminophylline (2 ×

10^{-3} M), a drug which stimulates C1 secretion, increased the flow to 137 ± 29 $nl \cdot min^{-1} \cdot cm^{-2}$. Thus, measurement of small amounts of fluid movement is now possible and should be useful in the study of airway fluid secretion. Recent studies suggest that while net $C1^-$ movement toward the lumen predominates in the trachea, net Na^+ movement toward the submucosa may predominate in bronchi (Knowles et al., 1980).

The canine trachea normally produces a net movement of fluid into the airways because the net flux of $C1^-$ toward the lumen exceeds the net flux of Na^+ toward the submucosa. This tissue can be transformed into an absorbing surface by adding a drug (MK-196) that inhibits $C1^-$ transport (Nathanson et al., 1981). Thus, not only the degree, but also the direction, of fluid movement can be modified by drugs and perhaps by disease. Sampling of fluid obtained in canine trachea and bronchi also suggests that regional differences exist (Boucher et al., 1981). Surface epithelial cells and airway submucosal glands may both contribute to active ion transport. However, the fact that the posterior segment of the trachea contains very few glands but is an actively transporting epithelium suggests that surface cells may predominate in the active transport demonstrated. The secretion of $C1^-$ that occurs in tracheal epithelium may be a ubiquitous property of epithelial tissues derived from the primitive foregut (Nadel et al., 1979). This epithelium consists of columnar cells which extend across the epithelial surface. Basal and intermediate cells lie between the columnar cells and have no contact with the airway lumen. Most columnar cells are ciliated, but others (e.g., goblet cells) are also present. The epithelium exists as a sheet, and it is not possible to determine which cell typ͏e in the sheet actively transports ions. In order to study individual types of cells, Widdicombe and co-workers have developed a preparation of isolated cells from canine tracheal mucosa (Widdicombe et al., 1982). These cells show excellent viability; separation of the three cell types should allow their separate study.

If net movement of Na^+ in tracheal epithelium follows the basic model proposed for Na^+-transporting epithelia (Koefoed-Johnsen and Ussing, 1958), it would be predicted that the apical membrane of the tracheal epithelium is permeable to Na^+ and that Na^+, K^+-ATPase should be located on the basolateral membrane (Widdicombe and Welsh, 1980). Widdicombe has recently shown that Na^+ K^+-ATPase is localized on the basolateral membranes in the airway epithelium (Widdicombe et al., 1979). Widdicombe also found that the uptake of [^{3}H] ouabain was greatly inhibited by removal of Na^+, by low temperature, by addition of K^+, and by anoxia (Widdicombe et al., 1979), further evidence that the uptake of ouabain occurred onto tissue Na^+ K^+-ATPase. Ouabain in the serosal medium decreased net Na^+ movement to zero by decreasing net Na^+ flux toward the submucosa; this is further evidence for the basolateral location of Na^+ K^+-ATPase (Widdicombe et al., 1979). Amiloride inhibited the passive Na^+ entry step across the apical cell membranes in other Na^+-transporting tissues, and Widdicombe showed that it did so in canine tracheal epiethlium (Widdicombe and Welsh, 1980). Details of a model to explain the Na^+ and Cl^- transport properties of tracheal epitheliums is given by Widdicombe and Welsh (1980).

Many drugs and mediators affect active ion transport in the airways (Marin et al., 1976). Acetylcholine increased net transport toward the lumen, an effect that was abolished by atropine, indicating that the effect was due to stimulation of muscarinic receptors. The adrenergic agonists, terbutaline (Davis et al., 1975), epinephrine (Al-Bazzaz et al., 1977), and theophylline (Al-Bazzaz and Al-Awqati, 1979) all increased net flux toward the lumen, presumably via a β-adrenerigc effect, probably via cAMP (Al-Bazzaz, 1981). Other putative mediators also stimulate active transport. Thus, histamine increased net fluxes toward the lumen, an effect prevented by an H_1 blocker (Marin et al., 1977). $PGF_{2\alpha}$ also affects tracheal ion transport (Al-Bazzaz and Yadava, 1978).

The control system for secretion and removal of fluid may be markedly altered by disease. Thus, the abnormally viscid mucus in cystic fibrosis may be due to an abnormality in active transport. Similarly, status asthmaticus could be due to the release of mediators that affect active transport of ions into the airway, thus preventing the normal movement of water and causing inspissation of mucus.

VI. Evidence of Mucociliary Abnormalities in Asthma and in Experimental Anaphylaxis

Pathologic findings at postmortem provide strong evidence of mucociliary abnormalities in asthma: mucous glands are hypertrophic, goblet cells are increased in number, and excessive secretions are present in the airway lumen (Huber and Koessler, 1922). Ciliated epithelium is often denuded (Hilding, 1943), and mucous plugs are conspicuous in patients who die in status asthmaticus (Dunnill, 1960; Alexander, 1963). Studies of patients during life provides some evidence concerning possible causes of the postmortem findings. Studies of mucociliary clearance suggest that abnormal clearance occurs in at least some asymptomatic asthmatic subjects (Santa Cruz et al., 1974; Mezey et al., 1978); other studies show normal clearance (Mossberg et al., 1976). This variability could reflect the disease process itself, selection of patients, or the relative insensitivity of the methods for examining focal effects. Sputum from asthmatic patients has been reported to be more viscous than from other patients (Charman and Reid, 1972), and the sputum showed a marked decrease in viscosity at low shear rates (Keal and Reid, 1975).

Two mechanisms appear likely to explain effects on airway secretion in asthma: (a) antigen-mediated effects and (b) inflammatory effects.

Studies in animals provide some evidence of mucociliary changes following antigen administration: in sensitive dogs, inhalation of *Ascaris suum* aerosols produces a reagin-mediated, immediate-type hypersensitivity reaction (Chiesa et al., 1975). Using this model, Wanner and associates showed that inhalation of *Ascaris* antigen decreased tracheal mucous velocity (Wanner et al., 1975). Compound FPL-55712, a selective antagonist of slow-reacting substance of anaphylaxis (SRS-A) prevented this decrease in tracheal mucous veolicty, suggesting that SRS-A release was responsible for the slowing of mucus velocity caused by antigen inhalation. The delayed clearance could be due to effects either on cilia or on the secretory process. Studies have been performed to examine the role of antigen-antibody reactions on the secretory process. In cats sensitized to horseradish peroxidase, delivery of the antigen intravenously, by aerosol, or into a bypassed tracheal segment had no significant effect on mucin production (Richardson et al., 1978).

Studies in humans showed that tracheal mucus velocity decreased after bronchial challenge with ragweed extract (Wanner, 1979). Sodium cromolyn prevented this slowing, suggesting that mediator release from mast cells was responsible for the effect. The fact that changes in mucus velocity were clearly separable from bronchoconstriction in the animal and human studies suggests that different mechanisms might be involved. Anaphylaxis of human airways in vitro is reported to stimulate mucin secretion, at least partially by stimulating histamine H_2 receptors (Shelhamer et al., 1980); abnormal secretions could be the cause of the reported decreases in mucus velocity found after bronchial challenge in patients in vivo.

Products of arachidonic acid metabolism may play an important role in immediate-type hypersensitivity reactions. Products of the cyclooxygenase pathway of arachidonate metabolism, including prostaglandin intermediates, are released during immediate hypersensitivity reactions (Piper and Walker, 1973; Schulman et al., 1980, 1981, 1982). Studies indicate that some of these products could participate in airway smooth muscle contractions (Sweatman and Collier, 1968; Hedqvist et al., 1978; Hyman et al., 1978), but the fact that the specific cyclooxygenase inhibitor, indomethacin, had no effect on the bronchomotor responses to inhaled antigen in allergic asthmatic humans (Hammarstrom et al., 1979) suggests that products of the cyclooxygenase pathways are not major mediators of the bronchomotor response to inhaled antigen in human asthma.

Exciting new work indicates that products of the lipoxygenation of arachidonic acid may play an even more important role as mediators of immediate hypersensitivity reactions. Several leukotrienes, derivatives of the lipoxygenase pathway, probably constitute the major functional components of slow-reacting substance of anaphylaxis (Hammarstrom et al., 1979; Murphy et al., 1979; Lewis et al., 1980; Orning et al., 1980). Leukotrienes C_4 and D_4 are very potent constrictors of airway smooth muscle in some species (Drazen et al., 1980).

In experimental canine asthma, the decrease in mucus velocity produced by inhalation of *Ascaris suum* antigen was prevented by FPL-55712 (Wanner et al., 1975), a compound that selectively antagonizes SRS-A (Augstein et al., 1973). The fact that histamine and acetylcholine increased mucus velocity in their preparation indicates that these agonists could not explain the slowing of mucus velocity that occurred after antigen. Similarly, they found that antigen challenge decreased mucus velocity in asthmatic subjects, an effect also prevented by the SRS-A antagonist (Ahmed et al., 1980). They concluded that the effect of antigen was due to the effects of SRS-A released by the antigen-antibody reaction. Studies of the effects of SRS-A antagonists on the impaired clearance of stable asthmatic subjects without antigen challenge might have further therapeutic implications. Effects of SRS-A on airway secretions need to be performed to assess the mechanism of impaired clearance following antigen.

Inflammation could also result in changes that might produce abnormal airway secretion. First, damage to the airway epithelium exaggerates reflex bronchomotor responses (Nadel, 1977). Thus, viral infections (Empey et al., 1976) and ozone (Lee et al., 1979; Golden et al., 1978) damage the airway epithelium and cause temporary airway hyperreactivity. The mechanism of these effects is unknown, but it could be secondary to the release of inflammatory mediators. Similar effects on the airway secretomotor system might occur. A second mechanism by which inflammation might affect airway secretions is by a direct effect of released mediators on the target secretory cells. Third, inflammatory mediators, by increasing vascular permeability, may allow the escape into the airway lumen of plasma components that are capable of affecting airway secretion. The fact that abnormally high concentrations of plasma proteins have been found in airway secretions of asthmatic patients (Brogan et al., 1971; Brogan et al., 1975) may be due to "leakage" from the blood into the airway, due to increased vascular permeability.

Asthma is a disease which produces symptoms (e.g., cough, bronchospasm, mucous production) which vary in degree and character. Perhaps the release of different mediators under varying conditions determines the target cells affected and thus the symptomatology.

References

Adams, G. K., Aharonson, E. F., Reasor, M. J., and Proctor, D. F. (1976). Collection of normal canine tracheobronchial secretions. *J. Appl. Physiol., 40*:247-249.

Ahmed, T., Greenblatt, D. W., Birch, S., Marchette, B., and Wanner, A. (1980). Mucociliary transport in allergic patients with antigen-induced bronchospasm: role of slow reacting substance of anaphylaxis (SRS-A). *Am. Rev. Respir. Dis., 121*:106.

Al-Bazzaz, F. J. (1981). Role of cyclic AMP in regulation of chloride secretion by canine tracheal mucosa. *Am. Rev. Respir. Dis., 123*:295-298.

Al-Bazzaz, F., and Al-Awqati, Q. (1977). Characteristics of ion transport in canine tracheal epithelia. *Fed. Proc. 36*:479.

Al-Bazzaz, F., and Al-Awqati, Q. (1979). Interaction between sodium and chloride transport in canine tracheal mucosa. *J. Appl. Physiol., 46*:111-119.

Al-Bazzaz, F., and Yadava, V. P. (1978). Ion transport across tracheal epithelium: effect of prostaglandins. *Clin. Res. 26*:687A.

Al-Bazzaz, F., Khan, A., and Cheng, E. (1977). Stimulation of chloride secretion across canine tracheal epithelia by theophylline and epinephrine. *Clin. Rs. 25*:414A.

Alexander, H. L. (1963). A historical account of death from asthma. *J. Allergy, 34*:305-322.

Amsterdam, A., Chad, I., and Schramm, M. (1969). Dynamic changes in the ultrastructure of the acinar cell of the rat parotid gland during the secretory cycle. *J. Cell Biol., 41*:753-773.

Augstein, J., Farmer, J. B., Lee, T. B., Sheard, P., and Tattersall, M. L. (1973). Selective inhibitor of slow reacting substance of anaphylaxis. *Nature, 245*: 215-217.

Baker, A. P., Hillegass, L. M., Holden, D. A., and Smith, W. J. (1977). Effect of kallidin, substance P, and other basic polypeptides on the production of respiratory macromolecules. *Am. Rev. Respir. Dis., 115*:811-817.

Balfre, K. (1977). The effects of calcium and calcium ionophore A23187 on mucin secretion and potential difference in the isolated chicken trachea. *J. Physiol.* (Lond.), *275*:80-81P.

Basbaum, C. B., Ueki, I., Brezina, L., and Nadel, J. A. (1981). Tracheal submucosal gland serous cells stimulated in vitro with adrenergic and cholinergic agonists: A morphometric study. *Cell Tissue Res., 220*:481-498.

Bateman, J. R. M., Pavia, D., and Clarke, S. W. (1978). The retention of lung secretions during the night in normal subjects. *Clin. Sci. Mol. Med., 55*: 523-527.

Batzri, S., Amsterdam, A., Selinger, Z., Ohad, I., and Schramm, M. (1971). Epinephrine-induced vacuole formation in parotid gland cells and its independence of the secretory process. *Proc. Natl. Acad. Sci., 68*:121-123.

Berry, E. M., Edmonds, J. F., and Wyllie, J. H. (1971). Release of prostaglandin E_2 an unidentified factors from ventilated lungs. *Br. J. Surg. 58*:189-193.

Boat, T. F., and Kleinerman, J. I. (1975). Human respiratory tract secretions. 2. Effect of cholinergic and adrenergic agents on in vitro release of protein and mucous glycoprotein. *Chest 67*:32S-34S.

Borson, D. B., Chinn, R. A., Davis, B., and Nadel, J. A. (1980). Adrenergic and cholinergic nerves mediate fluid secretion from tracheal glands of ferrets. *J. Appl. Physiol., 49*:1027-1031.

Borson, D. B., and Nadel, J. A. (1981). Cholinergic nerves inhibit adrenergic neurotransmisstion to tracheal submucosal glands of ferrets. *Fed. Proc. 40*: 254.

Boucher, R. C., Stutts, M. J., Bromberg, P. A., and Gatzy, J. T. (1981). Regional differences in airway surface liquid composition. *J. Appl. Physiol., 50*: 613-620.

Boushey, H. A., Holtzman, M. J., Sheller, J. R., and Nadel, J. A. (1980). State of the Art. Bronchial hyperreactivity. *Am. Rev. Respir. Dis., 121*:389-413.

Boyd, E. M., and Sheppard, E. P. (1970a). Inhaled anisaldehyde and respiratory tract fluid. *Pharmacology, 3*:345-352.

Boyd, E. M., and Sheppard, E. P. (1970b). Nutmeg oil and camphene as inhaled expectorants. *Arch. Otolaryngol., 92*:372-378.

Boyd, E. M., and Sheppard, E. P. (1970c). The effect of inhalation of citral and geraniol on the output and composition of respiratory tract fluid. *Arch. Int. Pharmacodyn. Ther., 188*:5-13.

Boyd, E. M., and Sheppard, E. P. (1971). An autumn-enhanced mucotropic action of inhaled terpenes and related volatile agents. *Pharmacology, 6*:65-80.

Breeze, R. G., and Wheeldon, E. B. (1977). The cells of the pulmonary airways. *Am. Rev. Respir. Dis., 116*:705-777.

Brogan, T. D., Ryley, H. C., Allen, L., and Hutt, H. (1971). Relation between sputum sol phase composition and diagnosis in chronic chest diseases. *Thorax, 26*:418-423.

Brogan, T. D., Ryley, H. C., Neale, L., and Yassa, J. (1975). Soluble proteins of bronchopulmonary secretions from patients with cystic fibrosis. *Thorax, 30*:72-79.

Burnstock, G. (1969). Evolution of the autonomic innervation of visceral and cardiovascular systems in vertebrates. *Pharmacol. Rev., 21*:247-324.

Cardell, B. S., and Pearson, R. S. B. (1959). Death in asthmatics. *Thorax, 14*: 341-352.

Chakrin, L. W., Baker, A. P., Christian, P., and Wardell, J. R. Jr. (1973). Effect of cholinergic stimulation on the release of macromolecules by canine trachea in vitro. *Am. Rev. Respir. Dis., 108*:69-76.

Charman, J., and Reid, L. (1972). Sputum viscosity in chronic bronchitis, bronchiectasis, asthma and cystic fibrosis. *Biorheology, 9*:185-199.

Chiesa, A., Dain, D., Meyers, G. L., Kessler, G. F., and Gold, W. M. (1975). Histamine release during antigen inhalation in experimental asthma in dogs. *Am. Rev. Respir. Dis., 111*:148-156.

Chinn, R. A., Johnson, H. G., Davis, B., and Nadel, J. A. (1981). Reflex effects of lung inflation on submucosal gland secretion in canine trachea. *Cystic Fibrosis Club Abstracts 22*:102.

Coles, S. (1977). Regulation of the secretory cycles of mucous and serous cells in the human bronchial gland. In *Mucus in Health and Disease.* Edited by M. Elstein and D. V. Parke. London, Plenum Press, pp. 155-168.

Dadaian, J. H., Yin, S., and Laurenzi, G. A. (1971). Studies of mucus flow in the mammalian respiratory tract. II. The effects of serotonin and related compounds on respiratory tract mucus flow. *Am. Rev. Respir. Dis., 103*: 808-815.

Davis, B., Marin, M. G., and Nadel, J. A. (1975). Adrenergic receptor in canine tracheal epithelium. *Am. Rev. Respir. Dis. 111*:947.

Davis, B., Roberts, A. M., Coleridge, H. M., and Coleridge, J. C. G. (1981). Reflex increase of canine tracheal gland secretion caused by stimulating bronchial C-fibers. Physiologist, *24*:105.

Davis, B., Chinn, R., Graf, P., Popovac, D., and Nadel, J. (1979). Papaverine enhances alpha-adrenergic stimulation of mucus glands in canine trachea in vivo. *Physiologist 22*:26A.

Davis, B., Chinn, R., Popovac, D., Widdicombe, J. G., and Nadel, J. (1980). Hypoxia stimulates mucus gland secretion via a carotid body reflex in dogs. *Am. Rev. Respir. Dis. 121*:332.

Davis, B., Marin, M., Fischer, S., Graf, P., Widdicombe, J., and J. Nadel. (1976). New method for study of canine mucous gland secretion in vivo: cholinergic regulation. *Am. Rev. Respir. Dis. 113*:257.

Douglas, W. W. (1978). Stimulus-secretion coupling: variations on the theme of calcium-activated exocytosis involving cellular and extracellular sources of calcium. In *Respiratory Tract Mucus.* Ciba Foundation Symposium 54 (new series). Amsterdam, Elsevier/Excerpta Medica/North-Holland, pp. 61-87.

Drazen, J. M., Austen, K. F., and Lewis, R. A. (1980). Comparative airway and vascular activities of leukotrienes C-1 and D in vivo and in vitro. *Proc. Natl. Acad. Sci. 77*:4354-4358.

Drazen, J. M., Lewis, R. A., Wasserman, S. I., Orange, R. P., and Austen, K. F. (1979). Differential effects of a partially purified preparation of slow reacting substance of anaphylaxis on guinea pig tracheal spirals and parenchymal strips. *J. Clin. Invest., 63*:1-5.

Dunnill, M. S. (1960). The pathology of asthma, with special reference to changes in the bronchial mucosa. *J. Clin. Pathol., 13*:27-33.

El-Bermani, A.-W., and Grant, M. (1975). Acetylcholinesterase-positive nerves of the rhesus monkey bronchial tree. *Thorax, 30*:162-170.

Emmelin, N., and Gjorstrup, P. (1976). Interaction between sympathetic and parasympathetic salivary nerves in anaesthetized dogs. *Arch. Oral Biol., 21*:27-32.

Empey, D. W., Laitinen, L. A., Jacobs, L., Gold, W. M., and Nadel, J. A. (1976). Mechanisms of bronchial hyperreactivity in normal subjects following respiratory tract infection. *Am. Rev. Respir. Dis., 113*:131-139.

Florey, H., Carleton, H. M., and Wells, A. Q. (1932). Mucus secretion in the trachea. *Br. J. Exp. Pathol., 13*:269-284.

Gallagher, J. T., Kent, P. W., Phipps, R. J., and Richardson, P. S. (1977). Influence of pilocarpine and ammonia vapor on the secretion and structure of cat tracheal mucins: differentiation of goblet and submucosal gland cell secretions. In *Mucus in Health Disease.*

Gallagher, J. T., Hall, R. L., Jeffery, P. K., Phipps, R. J., and Richardson, P. S. (1978). The nature and origin of tracheal secretions released in response to pilocarpine and ammonia. *J. Physiol.* (Lond.), *275*:36-37P.

Gallagher, J. T., Kent, P. W., Passatore, M., Phipps, R. J., and Richardson, P. S. (1975). The composition of tracheal mucus and the nervous control of its secretion in the cat. *Proc. R. Soc. Lond. B., 192*:49-76.

Garrett, J. R., Thulin, A., and Kidd, A. (1978). Variations in parasympathetic secretory and structural responses resulting from differences in the prestimulation of parotid acini in rats. Some factors affecting watery vacuolation. *Cell Tissue Res., 188*:235-250.

German, V. F., Ueki, I. F., and Nadel, J. A. (1980). Micropipette measurement of airway submucosal gland secretion: Laryngeal reflex. *Am. Rev. Respir. Dis., 122*:413-416.

German, V. F., Corrales, R., Ueki, I. F., and Nadel, J. A. (1982). Relax stimulation of tracheal submucosal gland secretion by gastric irritation in cats. *J. Appl. Physiol., 52*:1153-1155.

Gjorstrup, P. (1977). Effects of sympathetic nerve stimulation in the presence of a slow parasympathetic secretion in the parotid and submaxillary glands of the rabbit. *Acta Physiol. Scand., 101*:211-218.

Goco, R. V., Kress, M. B., and Brantigan, O. C. (1963). Comparison of mucus glands in the tracheobronchial tree of man and animals. *Ann. N.Y. Acad. Sci., 106*:555-571.

Golden, J. A., Nadel, J. A., and Boushey, H. A. (1978). Bronchial hyperirritability in healthy subjects after exposure to ozone. *Am. Rev. Respir. Dis., 118*:287-294.

Grillo, M. A., and Nadel, J. A. (1980). Vital staining of tracheal ganglia. *Physiologist, 178*:77.

Hahn, H. L., Wilson, A. G., Graf, P. D., Fischer, S. P., and Nadel, J. A. (1978). Interaction between serotonin and efferent vagus nerves in dog lungs. *J. Appl. Physiol., 44*:144-149.

Hall, R. L., Peatfield, A. C., and Richardson, P. S. (1978). The effect of serum on mucus secretion in the trachea of the cat. *J. Physiol.* (Lond.), *282*:47-48P.

Hammarstrom, S., Murphy, R. C., Samuelsson, B., Clark, D. A., Mioskowski, C., and Corey, E. J. (1979). Structure of leukotriene C: identification of the amino acid part. *Biochem. Biophys. Res. Commun., 91*:1266-1272.

Hedqvist, P., Stradberg, K., and Hamberg, M. (1978). Bronchial and cardiovascular actions of prostaglandin endoperoxides and an endoperoxide analogue. *Acta Physiol. Scand., 103*:299-307.

Hilding, A. C. (1943). The relation of ciliary insufficiency to death from asthma and other respiratory diseases. *Ann. Otol. Rhinol. Laryngol., 52*:5-19.

Huber, H. L., and Koessler, K. K. (1922). Pathology of bronchial asthma. *Arch. Intern. Med., 30*:689-760.

Hyman, A. L., Spannhake, E. W., and Kadowitz, P. J. (1978). Prostaglandins and the lung. *Am. Rev. Respir. Dis., 117*:111-136.

Iravani, J., and Melville, G. N. (1975). Mucociliary activity in the respiratory tract as influenced by prostaglandin E_1. *Respiration, 32*:305-315.

Jamieson, J. D., and Palade, G. E. (1971). Synthesis, intracellular transport, and discharge of secretory proteins in stimulated pancreatic exocrine cells. *J. Cell Biol., 50*:135-158.

Jeffery, P. K. (1978). Structure and function of mucus-secreting cells of cat and goose airway epithelium. In *Respiratory Tract Mucus.* Ciba Foundation Symposium 54 (new series). Amsterdam, Elsevier/Excerpta Medica/North-Holland, pp. 5-20.

Jeffery, P. K., and Reid, L. (1977). The respiratory mucous membrane. In *Respiratory Defense Mechanisms.* Edited by J. D. Brain, D. F. Proctor, and L. Reid, New York, Marcel Dekker, Inc. pp. 193-245.

Jones, J. G., Fraser, R. B., and Nadel, J. A. (1975). Prediction of maximum expiratory flow rate from the compliance of the compressed airway. *J. Appl. Physiol., 38*:1002-1011.

Keal, E. E., and Reid, L. (1975). Pathologic alterations in mucous in asthma within and without the cell. In *New Directions in Asthma.* Edited by M. Stein. Park Ridge, Il., American College of Chest Physicians, pp. 223-239.

King, M., Cohen, C., and Viires, N. (1979). Influence of vagal tone on rheology and transportability of canine tracheal mucus. *Am. Rev. Respir. Dis., 120*: 1215-1219.

Knowles, M. R., Murray, G. F., Shallal, J. A., Gatzy, J. T., and Boucher, R. C. (1980). Bioelectrical properties (BEP) and ion transport (IT) in excised human bronchi. *Physiologist, 23*:100.

Koefoed-Johnsen, V., and Ussing, H. H. (1958). The nature of the frog skin potential. *Acta Physiol. Scand., 42*:298-308.

Korhonen, L. K., Holopainen, E., and Paavolainen, M. (1969). Some histochemical characteristics of tracheobronchial tree and pulmonary neoplasms. *Acta Histochem.* (Jena), *32*: 57-73.

Lee, L.-Y., Dumont, C., Djokic, T. D., Menzel, T. E., and Nadel, J. A. (1979). Mechanism of rapid, shallow breathing after ozone exposure in conscious dogs. *J. Appl. Physiol., 46*:1108-1114.

Lewis, R. A., Austen, K. F., Drazen, J. M., Clark, D. A., Marfat, A., and Corey, E. J. (1980). Slow reacting substances of anaphylaxis: identification of leukotrienes C-1 and D from human and rat sources. *proc. Natl. Acad. Sci., 77*:3710-3714.

Lundberg, J. M., Anders, A., Fahrenkrug, J., Hokfelt, T., and Mutt, V. (1980). Vasoactive intestinal polypeptide in cholinergic neurons of exocrine glands: Functional significance of coexisting transmitters for vasodilation and secretion. *Proc. Natl. Acad. Sci., 77*:1651-1655.

Mann, S. P. (1971). The innervation of mammalian bronchial smooth muscle: the localization of catecholamines and cholinesterases. *Histochem. J., 3*: 319-331.

Marin, M. G., Davis, B., and Nadel, J. A. (1976). Effect of acetylcholine on Cl^- and Na^+ fluxes across dog tracheal epithelium in vitro. *Am. J. Physiol., 231*:1546-1549.

Marin, M. G., Davis, B., and Nadel, J. A. (1977). Effects of histamine on electrical and ion transport properties of tracheal epithelium. *J. Appl. Physiol., 42*:735-738.

Marom, Z., Shelhamer, J. H., and Kaliner, M. (1981). Effects of arachidonic acid, monohydroxyeicosatetraenoic acid and prostaglandins on the release of mucous glycoproteins from human airways in vitro. *J. Clin. Invest., 67*: 1695-1702.

Matsuzaki, Y., Hamasaki, Y., and Said, S. I. (1980). Vasoactive intestinal peptide: A possible transmitter of nonadrenergic relaxation of guinea pig airways. *Science, 210*:1252-1253.

Mawdsley-Thomas, L. E., Healey, P., and Barry, D. H. (1971). Experimental bronchitis in animals due to sulphur dioxide and cigarette smoke. An automated quantitative study. In *Inhaled Particles III.* Edited by W. H. Walton, London, Unwin, pp. 509-526.

Meyrick, B., and Reid, L. (1970). Ultrastructure of cells in the human bronchial submucosal glands. *J. Anat., 107*:281-299.

Meyrick, B., and Reid, L. (1975). In vitro incorporation of H^3-threonine and H^3-glucose by the mucous and serous cells of the human bronchial submucosal gland; a quantitative electron microscopic study. *J. Cell Biol., 67*: 320-344.

Meyrick, B., Sturgess, J. M., and Reid, L. (1969). A reconstruction of the duct system and secretory tubules of the human bronchial submucosal gland. *Thorax, 24*:729-736.

Mezey, R. J., Cohn, M. A., Fernandez, R. J., Januszkiewicz, A. J., and Wanner, A. (1978). Mucociliary transport in allergic patients with antigen-induced bronchospasm. *Am. Rev. Respir. Dis., 118*:677-684.

Mossberg, B., Strandberg, L., and Philipson, K. (1976). Tracheobronchial clearance in bronchial asthma. Response to beta-adrenoreceptor stimulation. *Scand. J. Respir. Dis.*, *57*:119-128.

Murlas, C., Nadel, J. A., and Basbaum, C. B. (1980). A morphometric analysis of the autonomic innervation of cat tracheal glands. *J. Auton. Nerv. Syst.*, *2*:23-37.

Murphy, R. C., Hammarstrom, S., and Samuelsson, B. (1979). Leukotriene C: a slow reacting substance from murine mastocytoma cells. *Proc. Natl. Acad. Sci.*, *76*:4275-4279.

Nadel, J. A. (1977). Autonomic control of airway smooth muscle and airway secretions. *Am. Rev. Respir. Dis.*, *115*:117-126.

Nadel, J. A. (1980). Autonomic regulation of airway smooth muscle. In *Physiology and Pharmacology of the Airways.* Edited by J. A. Nadel. New York, Marcel Dekker, Inc., pp. 217-257.

Nadel, J. A., and Davis, B. (1980). Parasympathetic and sympathetic regulation of secretion from submucosal glands in airways. *Fed. Proc.*, *39*:3075-3079.

Nadel, J. A., Davis, B., and Phipps, R. J. (1979). Control of mucus secretion and ion transport in airways. *Ann. Rev. Physiol.*, *41*:369-381.

Nadel, J. A., Phillipson, E. A., Fishman, N. H., and Hickey, R. F. (1973). Regulation of respiration by bronchopulmonary receptors in conscious dogs. *Acta Neurobiol. Exp.*, *33*:33-50.

Nathanson, I. T., Widdicombe, J. H., and Highland, E. (1981). Effect of MK-196 on ion transport by dog tracheal epithelium. *Fed. Proc.*, *40*:373.

Neutra, M. R., and Schaeffer, S. F. (1977). Membrane interactions between adjacent mucous secretion granules. *J. Cell. Biol.*, *74*:983-991.

O'Brodovich, H. M., Stalcup, S. A., Pang, L. M., Lipset, J. S., and Mellins, R. B. (1981). Bradykinin production and increased pulmonary endothelial permeability during acute respiratory failure in unanesthetized sheep. *J. Clin. Invest.*, *67*:514-522.

Olver, R. E., Davis, B., Marin, M. G., and Nadel, J. A. (1975). Active transport of Na^+ and $C1^-$ across the canine tracheal epithelium in vitro. *Am. Rev. Respir. Dis.*, *112*:811-815.

Orning, L., Hammarstrom, S., and Samuelson, B. (1980). Leukotriene D: a slow reacting substance from rat basophilic leukemia cells. *Proc. Natl. Acad. Sci.*, *77*:2014-2017.

Peatfield, A. C. (1980). The control of mucus secretion into the lumen of the trachea. Ph.D. Thesis, London University, England.

Peatfield, A. C., and Richardson, P. S. (1980). Sympathetic nerve activity stimulates cat tracheal mucin secretion via beta-adrenorecptors. *J. Physiol.* (Lond.), *305*:78P-79P.

Phipps, R. J. (1977). The control of tracheal mucin secretion. Ph.D. Thesis, London University, England.

Phipps, R. J., and Richardson, P. S. (1976). The effects of irritation at various levels of the airway upon tracheal mucus secretion in the cat. *J. Physiol.* (Lond.), *261*:563-581.

Phipps, R. J., Nadel, J. A., and Davis, B. (1980). Effect of alpha-adrenergic stimulation on mucus secretion and on ion transport in cat trachea in vitro. *Am. Rev. Respir. Dis.*, *121*:359-365.

Phipps, R. J., Richardson, P. S., Corfield, A., Gallagher, J. T., Jeffery, P. K., Kent, P. W., and Passatore. M. (1977). A physiological, biochemical and histological study of goose tracheal mucin and its secretion. *Philos. Trans. R. Soc. Lond.*, *279*:513-540.

Piper, P. J., and Walker, J. L. (1973). The release of spasmogenic substances from chopped human lung tissue and its inhibition. *Br. J. Pharmacol.*, *47*:291-304.

Piper, P. J., Said, S. I., and Vane, J. R. (1970). Effects on smooth muscle preparations of unidentified vasoactive peptides from intestine and lung. *Nature*, *225*:1144-1146.

Popovac, D., Chinn, R., Graf, P., Nadel, J., and Davis, B. (1979). Serotonin potentiates nervous stimulation of mucus gland secretion in canine trachea in vivo. *Physiologist*, *22*:102.

Quinton, P. M. (1979). Composition and control of secretions from tracheal bronchial submucosal glands. *Nature*, *279*:551-552.

Regal, J. F., and Pickering, R. J. (1981). C5a-induced tracheal contraction: effect of an SRS-A antagonist and inhibitors of arachidonate metabolism. *J. Immunol.*, *126*:313-316.

Regoli, D., and Barabe, J. (1980). Pharmacology of bradykinin and related kinins. *Pharmacol. Rev.*, *32*:1-46.

Reid, L. (1960). Measurement of the bronchial mucous gland layer: a diagnostic yardstick in chronic bronchitis. *Thorax*, *15*:132-141.

Reid, L. M. (1977). Secretory cells. *Fed. Proc.*, *36*:2703-2707.

Restrepo, G. L., and Heard, B. E. (1963). Mucous gland enlargement in chronic bronchitis: extent of enlargement in the tracheo-bronchial tree. *Thorax*, *18*:334-339.

Richardson, J., and Beland, J. (1976). Nonadrenergic inhibitory nervous system in human airways. *J. Appl. Physiol.*, *41*:764-771.

Richardson, J. B. (1975). Demonstration of a nonadrenergic inhibitory nervous system in the trachea of the guinea pig. *J. Allergy Clin. Immunol.*, *56*: 473-480.

Richardson, J. B. (1979). Nerve supply to the lung. *Am. Rev. Respir. Dis.*, *119*: 785-802.

Richardson, P. S., and Phipps, R. J. (1978). The anatomy, physiology, pharmacology and pathology of tracheobronchial mucus secretion and the use of expectorant drugs in human disease. *Pharmacol. Ther.*, *3*:441-479.

Richardson, P. S., Phipps, R. J., Balfre, K., and Hall, R. L. (1978). The roles of mediators, irritants and allergens in causing mucin secretion from the trachea. In *Respiratory Tract Mucus.* Ciba Foundation Symposium 54 (new series). Amsterdam, Elsevier/Excerpta Medica/North-Haolland, pp. 111-131.

Said, S. I., and Mutt, V. (1969). Polypeptide with broad biological activity: Isolation from small intestine. *Science, 169*:1217-1218.

Santa Cruz, R., Landa, J., Hirsch, J., and Sackner, M. A. (1974). Tracheal mucous velocity in normal man and patients with obstructive lung disease; effects of terbutaline. *Am. Rev. Respir. Dis., 109*:458-463.

Schulman, E. S., Adkinson, N. F., Demers, L. M., Fitzpatrick, F. A., Adams, G. K., Lichtenstein, L. M., and Newball, H. H. (1980). Anaphylactic release of prostaglandins, thromboxane A_2 and prostacyclin from human lung. *Fed. Proc., 39*:444.

Schulman, E. S., Newball, H. H., Demers, L. M., Fitzpatrick, F. A., and Adkinson, N. F., Jr. (1981). Anaphylactic release of thromboxane A_2, prostaglandin D_2, and prostacyclin from human lung parenchyma. *Am. Rev. Respir. Dis., 124*:402-406.

Schulman, E. S., Adkinson, N. F., Jr., Newball, H. H. (1982). Cyclooxygenase metabolites in human lung anaphylaxis: Airway vs. parenchyma. *J. Appl. Physiol., 53*:589-595.

Shelhamer, J. H., Marom, Z., and Kaliner, M. (1980). Immunologic and neuropharmacologic stimulation of mucous glycoprotein release from human airways in vitro. *J. Clin. Invest., 66*:1400-1408.

Specian, R. D., and Neutra, M. R. (1980). Mechanism of rapid mucus secretion in goblet cells stimulated by acetylcholine *J. Cell Biol., 85*:626-640.

Spicer, S. S., Chakrin, L. W., Wardell, J. R., Jr., and Kendrick, W. (1971). Histochemistry of mucosubstances in the canine and human respiratory tract. *Lab. Invest., 25*:483-490.

Sturgess, J., and Reid, L. (1972). An organ culture study of the effect of drugs on the secretory activity of the human bronchial submucosal gland. *Clin. Sci., 43*:533-543.

Sweatman, W. J., and Collier, H. O. J. (1968). Effects of prostaglandins on human bronchial muscle. *Nature, 217*:69-71.

Thurlbeck, W. M., Benjamin, B., and Reid, L. (1961). Development and distribution of mucous glands in the foetal human trachea. *Br. J. Dis. Chest, 55*: 54-64.

Tom-Moy, M., Basbaum, C., and Nadel, J. A. (1981). Effects of cholinergic and adrenergic stimulation on lysozyme secretion in ferret trachea. *Fed. Proc., 40*:622.

Tom-Moy, M., Basbaum, C. B., and Nadel, J. A. (1980). Immunocytochemical localization of lysozyme in the ferret trachea. *Physiologist, 178*:99.

Uddman, R., and Sundler, F. (1979). Vasoactive intestinal polypeptide nerves in human upper respiratory tract. *ORL, 41*:221-226.

Uddman, R., Alumets, J., Densert, O., Hakanson, R., and Sundler, F. (1978). Occurrence and distribution of VIP nerves in the nasal mucosa and tracheobronchial wall. *Acta Otolaryngol., 86*:443-448.

Ueki, I., and Nadel, J. A. (1981). Differences in total protein concentration in submucosal gland fluid: alpha-adrenergic vs cholinergic. *Fed. Proc., 40*: 622.

Ueki, I., German, V. F., and Nadel, J. A. (1980). Micropipette measurement of airway submucosal gland secretion. Autonomic effects. *Am. Rev. Respir. Dis., 121*:351-357.

Utsunomiya, T., Krausz, M. M., Valeri, C. R., Levine, L., Shepro, D., and Hechtman, H. B. (1982). Treatment of pulmonary embolism with positive end-expiratory pressure and prostaglandin E_1. Surg. Gynecol. Obstet., (In Press).

Vermeire, P. A., and Vanhoutte, P. M. (1979). Inhibitory effects of catecholamines in isolated canine bronchial smooth muscle. *J. Appl. Physiol., 46*: 787-791.

Walsh, C., and McLelland, J. (1974). The ultrastructure of the avian extrapulmonary respiratory epithelium. *Acta Anat., 89*:412-422.

Wanner, A. (1979). The role of mucociliary dysfunction in bronchial asthma. *Am. J. Med., 67*:477-485.

Wanner, A., Zarzecki, S., Hirsch, J., and Epstein, S. (1975). Tracheal mucous transport in experimental canine asthma. *J. Appl. Physiol., 39*:950-957.

Wardell, J. R., Jr., Chakrin, L. W., and Payne, B. J. (1970). The canine tracheal pouch. A model for use in respiratory mucus research. *Am. Rev. Respir. Dis., 101*:741-754.

Wasserman, M. A. (1975). Bronchopulmonary responses to prostaglandin F_{2alpha}, histamine and acetylcholine in the dog. *Eur. J. Pharmacol., 32*: 146-155.

Welsh, M. J., Widdicombe, J. H., and Nadel, J. A. (1980). Fluid transport across the canine tracheal epithelium. *J. Appl. Physiol., 49*:905-909.

Widdicombe, J. G. (1966). Action potentials in parasympathetic and sympathetic efferent fibres to the trachea and lungs of dogs and cats. *J. Physiol.* (Lond.), *186*:56-88.

Widdicombe, J. G. (1978). Control of secretion of tracheobronchial mucus. *Br. Med. Bull., 34*:57-61.

Widdicombe, J. H., and Welsh, M. J. (1980). Ion transport by dog tracheal epithelium. *Fed. Proc., 39*:3062-3066.

Widdicombe, J. H., Basbaum, C. B., and Highland, E. (1981). Ion contents and other properties of isolated cells from dog tracheal epithelium. *Am. J. Physiol., 241*:C184-C192.

Widdicombe, J. H., Basbaum, C. B., and Yee, J. Y. (1979). Localization of Na pumps in the tracheal epithelium of the dog. *J. Cell Biol.*, *82*:380-390.

Widdicombe, J. H., Ueki, I. F., Bruderman, I., and Nadel, J. A. (1979). The effects of sodium substitution and ouabain on ion transport by dog tracheal epithelium. *Am. Rev. Respir. Dis.*, *120*:385-392.

Wolff, R. K., Dolovich, M. B., Obminski, G., and Newhouse, M. T. (1977). Effects of exercise and eucapnic hyperventilation on bronchial clearance in man. *J. Appl. Physiol.*, *43*:46-50.

Wood, J. D. (1978). Slow synaptic excitation mediated by serotonin in Auerbach's plexus. *Nature*, *276*:836-837.

Wood, J. D., and Mayer, C. J. (1979). Serotonergic activation of tonic-type enteric neurons in guinea pig small bowel. *J. Neurophysiol.*, *42*:582-593.

Yoneda, K. (1976). Mucous blanket of rat bronchus: ultrastructural study. *Am. Rev. Respir. Dis.*, *114*:837-842.

6

Immune Release from Human Lung of Activators of the Hageman Factor-Dependent Pathways

HAROLD H. NEWBALL* and HENRY L. MEIER*

The Johns Hopkins University School of Medicine
The Good Samaritan Hospital
Baltimore, Maryland

I. Introduction

When challenged with the appropriate antigens, passively sensitized human lung fragments and human peripheral leukocyte preparations from allergic donors release several chemical mediators, including histamine, the slow-reacting substances of anaphylaxis (leukotrienes), and eosinophil chemotactic factors (Webster et al., 1974; Lichtenstein, 1977). The release processes that are involved have been described extensively. In each instance, the mediators are actively secreted by a process that is temperature- and calcium-dependent, requires metabolic energy, and is controlled by hormone-receptor interactions which influence the intracellular level of cyclic nucleotides (Lichtenstein and Margolis, 1968; Newball et al., 1980; Newball and Lichtenstein, 1981). While much attention has been given to the possible role of low molecular weight mediators in inflammatory or allergic reactions, little data has been available pertaining to the possible role of high molecular weight mediators, which are also actively secreted

Present Affiliation
*Institute of Chemical Defense, Edgewood, Maryland
Supported in part by NIH Grant No. HL24210, and Grant No. 1392 from The Council for Tobacco Research–U.S.A., Inc.

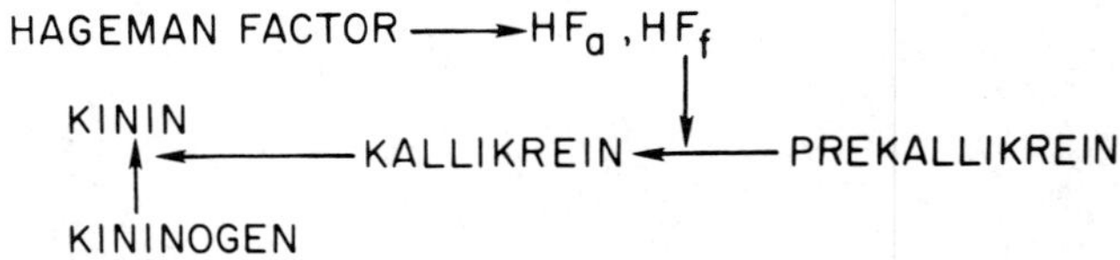

Figure 1 Hageman factor, prekallikrein, and kininogen were three of the initial proteins discovered in the Hageman factor-dependent pathways. Activated Hageman factor (HF_a) and Hageman factor fragment (HF_f) are the activated form of human Hageman factor.

during the IgE-mediated response. Recent studies of mast cell systems have revealed that large molecular weight complexes containing biologically active molecules may be secreted during secretory events. Thus, heparin bound to a large molecular weight proteoglycan is secreted and is biologically active (Metcalf et al., 1979).

Our work in mast cell and basophil systems also suggests that biologically active molecules are secreted in association with large molecular weight complexes (possibly fragments of granular matrices). We have described the IgE-mediated release of a high molecular weight complex from human peripheral leukocytes that has at least three activities associated with it: (a) a tosyl arginine methyl ester (TAMe) esterase activity, (b) a kinin-generating activity, and (c) a Hageman factor cleaving activity (Newball et al., 1975, 1978, 1979a,b,c). We have also demonstrated that proteases in supernatants from passively sensitized, antigen-challenged human lung directly cleave three proteins (Hageman factor, prekallikrein, and kininogen) of the human Hageman factor-dependent pathways (Newball and Lichtenstein, 1981; Newball et al., 1981a,b). Human Hageman factor plays a critical role in the activation of a number of pathways that participate in inflammatory events. Hageman factor (HF) circulates in plasma as a proenzyme and is activated through proteolytic cleavage to its active forms, HF_a and HF_f. Activated Hageman factor can activate the coagulation system and the complement system. Activated Hageman factor can also activate the proenzyme prekallikrein to kallikrein which, in turn, may activate the fibrinolytic system, or cleave kininogen to generate kinins, or reciprocally activate Hageman factor (Figs. 1 and 2). The activation of the complement, the coagulation, the fibrinolytic, and the kallikrein-kinin systems results in the generation of biologically active molecules. The mechanism by which these pathways become activated in vivo during inflammatory events is unknown; however, our studies of IgE-mediated human anaphylaxis indicate that these pathways do become activated in vivo. We suggest that the lung proteases, described below, may function as a triggering mechanism in the activation of the Hageman factor-dependent pathways.

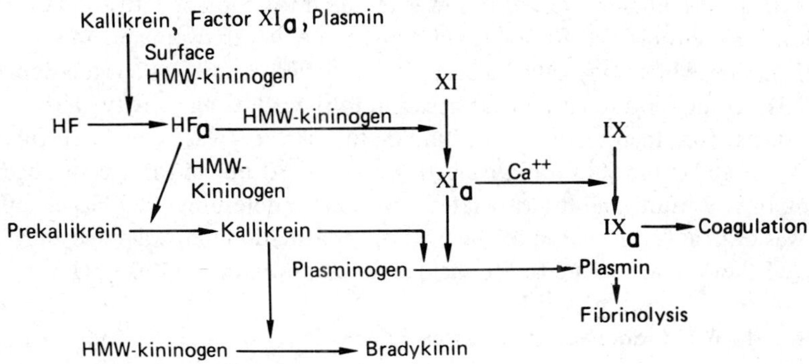

Figure 2 Interactions of the Hageman factor-dependent pathways of coagulation, fibrinolysis, and kinin generation. High molecular weight kininogen (HMW kininogen) serves as a cofactor in the activation of HF to HF_a, the activation of coagulation factor XI to XIa, and the activation of prekallikrein to kallikrein. Kallikrein may reciprocally activate Hageman factor to HF_a and HF_f.

In this chapter, we will address ourselves primarily to the newly described high molecular weight mediators that are derived from the lung and interact with the Hageman factor-dependent pathways, and then only briefly review data on the high molecular weight mediators that are derived from basophils. We will discuss two models of anaphylaxis: (a) the chopped human lung model, and (b) the human peripheral leukocyte model. These two models complement each other and data derived from the two models are generally similar.

II. Hageman Factor-Dependent Pathways

A. The Discovery of Hageman Factor

The observation that coagulation was initiated when blood came in contact with glass was made by Bordet and Genou (1901). However, it was not until the 1950s that the mechanism which initiates the intrinsic coagulation cascade was studied in any detail. Ratnoff and Conley (1951), in their study of the role of factor XI (PTA, plasma thromboplastin antecedent) in the coagulation cascade, predicted that there was a substance in plasma that preceded factor XI and was required for its activation. Soon thereafter, a patient named John Hageman entered Crile Veterans Administration Hospital with a liver disorder and upon routine evaluation exhibited a markedly prolonged partial thromboplastin time (PTT). The plasma of patients deficient in each of the coagulation factors known at that time could correct his PTT, indicating that this represented a deficiency of a then unknown clotting factor. Ratnoff and Colopy (1955) determined that

Mr. Hageman was missing a factor that was required for contact activation of coagulation, and Ratnoff and Rosenblum (1958) subsequently were able to show that this factor, which they called Hageman factor (also known as coagulation factor XII), could bind to certain surfaces and initiate clotting activity. They proposed that Hageman factor, by its binding to a surface, was being freed from an inhibitor, and could thus initiate clotting activity. Although this has not been substantiated, Ratnoff and his associates were able to determine that Hageman factor was critical for initiation of the intrinsic coagulation pathway, and they concluded that it had to bind to the surface for this initiation to take place.

B. Physical Properties of Hageman Factor

Since Ratnoff's discovery of Hageman factor, its structure and mechanism of action has been extensively studied in many laboratories. Hageman factor has been shown to be a glycoprotein that circulates in plasma in a concentration of 25-45 μg/ml and represents the zymogen of a proteolytic enzyme (Revak et al., 1974). The unactivated Hageman factor molecule has been reported to have a molecular weight of 115,000 (Kaplan and Austen, 1971) by molecular sieving techniques, and 80,000 (Cochrane and Wuepper, 1971) by SDS electrophoresis. It has been shown to be a single-chain glycoprotein with β-globulin mobility (Cochrane and Wuepper, 1971). Schoenmakers et al. (1965) studied the carbohydrate composition of bovine Hageman factor and found that it contained 5.9% neutral carbohydrate, 4.8% amino sugars, and 4.4% sialic acid residues. The amino acid composition of human Hageman factor has been determined by many groups (Speer et al., 1965; Cochrane and Wuepper, 1971; McMillin et al., 1974).

The secondary and tertiary structures of the molecule have been studied with the objective of determining whether it changes during activation. McMillin et al. (1974) reported shifts in the circular dichroism spectrum of factor XII during its activation by ellagic acid. They explained this shift as a change in the environment of some basic amino acids and tyrosine residues. However, since it has been shown that surfaces alone do not activate Hageman factor (Griffin, 1977, Meier et al., 1977), these results may be due to conformational changes that occur upon binding, but do not represent activation.

The activated forms of Hageman factor (many forms have been reported; see Kaplan and Austen, 1970, 1971) have not been characterized to the same extent as the unactivated form, because of their instability. At least four molecular species of activated Hageman factor (mol wt 115,000, 90,000, 60,000, and 40,000) have been shown to exist when serum was fractionated by gel filtration (Kaplan et al., 1971). However, upon further fractionation, all forms appeared to be transformed to the 40,000 molecular weight Hageman factor fragment (HF_f) form. Hageman factor fragment is reported to be heterogeneous, as demonstrated by the prealbumin doublet observed when it is electrophoresed on alkaline disc gels (Kaplan et al., 1971).

C. Activation of the Hageman-Factor Dependent Pathways

The interrelationship between the forms of Hageman factor and other proteins in plasma has been approached from different perspectives, depending on which of the three Hageman factor-dependent pathways (intrinsic coagulation, fibrinolysis, kinin generation) the investigator was persuing.

The Role of Hageman Factor in the Kinin-Generating Pathway

Margolis (1957, 1958, 1959, 1963) in his study of pain-producing substance (kinin), which was first described by Armstrong et al. (1957), demonstrated the interrelationship between glass activation of the intrinsic coagulation pathway and glass initiated production of pain-producing substance (PPS). He concluded that the production of PPS was a two-step process in which the first step required glass activation of Hageman factor. He demonstrated that this activity (HF_f) was not labile at 56°C. The second step involved the formation of PPS. Margolis also showed that, although both the intrinsic coagulation pathway and PPS production involved glass activation of Hageman factor, the second step in each of these processes appeared to be different. He demonstrated divergence of these two pathways by generating PPS in plasma that was known to be deficient in factor XI.

During the 1960s, Webster and co-workers (Webster and Pierce, 1961, 1963; Moriya et al., 1963; Webster et al., 1963) investigated a group of proteins known as kallikreins. Kallikreins were defined as proteins that were responsible for liberating potent pharmacological peptides, kinins, from plasma proteins termed kininogens. Bradykinin (Rocha e Silva et al., 1949) in turn caused vasodilation, smooth muscle contraction, increased capillary permeability, the production of pain, and influenced the migration of leukocytes. These workers demonstrated that there was a plasma kallikrein that was distinct from the kallikrein found in urine and other tissues (tissue kallikreins), and they were able to purify partially this plasma kallikrein. They, along with Sherry and his co-workers (Sherry et al., 1964) demonstrated that kallikrein was responsible for most of the lysine and arginine esterase activity in plasma. Sherry and colleagues (Colman et al., 1969a,b) were also able to demonstrate, using partially pure reagents, that this esterase activity was Hageman factor dependent. Therefore, by the early 1970s, the Hageman factor-dependent kinin-generating pathway had been partially defined and related to the PPS system of Margolis (Webster, 1968; Kaplan and Austen, 1970, 1971; Wuepper and Cochrane, 1971; Wuepper, 1972, 1973). Soon thereafter, a second form of Hageman factor known as Hageman factor fragment (HF_f) was shown by Kaplan and Austen (1970, 1971) to be capable of directly activating prekallikrein to its active form, kallikrein. The Hageman factor-dependent kinin-generating pathway in plasma at this time was reported to be composed of three proteins (Fig. 1): (a) Hageman factor, (b) prekallikrein, and (c) a kininogen (a source of kinin).

The Role of Hageman Factor in the Fibrinolytic Pathway

Although Ratnoff (1953) was the first to suggest that Hageman factor may play a role in fibrinolysis, it was the work of Niewiarowski and Prow-Wartelle (1959) that demonstrated that kaolin could initiate the generation of clot lysis activity and that this activity required the presence of Hageman factor. Iatridis and Ferguson (1961, 1962) elaborated on this observation by demonstrating that Hageman factor was not an activator of plasminogen, but acted as a "lysokinase" in plasma. They defined a lysokinase as an enzyme that activates a substrate (a proenzyme to an enzyme) which, in turn, converts plasminogen to the fibrinolytic enzyme plasmin. Thus, they postulated a multistep reaction that takes place in plasma when it is exposed to kaolin. This multistep pathway to fibrinolysis did not occur when Hageman factor-deficient plasma instead of normal plasma was used. The lysokinase was later shown to be HF_a or HF_f, which activates prekallikrein to its active form, kallikrein (Fig. 2).

The Role of Hageman Factor in the Intrinsic Coagulation Pathway

In the early 1960s, investigation of the initial step in coagulation progressed to a point where partially purified proteins were used to study individual enzymatic interactions. The method of purification of Hageman factor progressed from adsorption onto glass (Haanen et al., 1961), to the use of the charge properties of the molecule and the employment of newly developed ion-exchange techniques (Ratnoff et al., 1961; Ratnoff and Davie, 1962). It had been established by this time that factor XII, factor XI, factor VIII (anti-hemophilic factor), and factor IX (PTC, plasma thromboplastin component or Christmas factor) were all involved in the early stages of intrinsic coagulation. Ratnoff and Davie (1962) were able to purify Hageman factor free of the other early components of coagulation by using factor XI-deficient plasma and absorbing the plasma with dilute aluminum hydroxide. Although this preparation of Hageman factor was crude and active, it enabled them to demonstrate that Hageman factor did directly activate factor XI to XIa (Fig. 2).

Hageman Factor-Dependent Activation of Complement

Hageman factor has been reported to be indirectly (Donaldson, 1967) and directly (Ghebrehimet et al., 1981) involved in the activation of the complement cascade. However, it is generally agreed that Hageman factor is directly involved in the activation of the intrinsic blood coagulation, and of the kinin-generating and fibrinolytic pathways (Fig. 2). Much is known regarding the interaction of the activated forms of Hageman factor with the proenzymes of the latter pathways; however, our present knowledge of the interaction of the activated forms of Hageman factor with the complement cascade is very limited.

Feedback Activation of Hageman Factor by Kallikrein

In 1963, an 11-year-old girl, B. Fletcher, was hospitalized in Kentucky after her family's cabin was destroyed by fire. When a PTT was performed in a routine preoperative evaluation for an adenoidectomy, it was discovered that she had a prolonged clotting time. She was referred to Hathaway et al. (1965) at the University of Kentucky Medical Center, where a defect in her coagulation cascade was found; it was also shown to be present in three of her siblings. A similar defect was later reported in three unrelated patients by Hattersley and Hayse (1970). The factor missing in these patients (Fletcher factor) was shown to result in a prolonged PTT which could be corrected by increasing the time that the plasma was in contact with the activating surface prior to recalcification (Hathaway and Alsever, 1970). Using the procedure of Schiffman et al. (1960) for separating Hageman factor and factor XI, Hathaway was also able to demonstrate that the missing factor in Fletcher-trait plasma was distinct from Hageman factor and factor XI. Hathaway was also able to determine that activated Hageman factor corrected the coagulation defect in Fletcher-trait plasma. At that time, Davie and Ratnoff (1964) concluded that Fletcher factor was a coagulation factor that preceded Hageman factor in the coagulation cascade.

Wuepper and Cochrane (1971) then established a link between the investigations of the kinin-generating system and the studies of the autocorrecting coagulation abnormality present in Fletcher-trait plasma. They demonstrated that incubation of Fletcher-trait plasma with kaolin failed to generate any bradykinin but, when prekallikrein was added back to Fletcher-trait plasma, it was not only capable of generating bradykinin but it also corrected the coagulation defect (Fig. 2). Other studies (Webster, 1968; Wuepper, 1973; Saito et al., 1974; Weiss et al., 1974) demonstrated that Fletcher-trait plasma also exhibited a slower rate of Hageman factor-dependent fibrinolysis which autocorrected as the time of incubation with the surface was increased. Weiss et al. (1974) demonstrated that the addition of activated Hageman factor to Fletcher-trait plasma corrected the defect in both Hageman factor-dependent fibrinolysis and the intrinsic coagulation pathway, but had no effect upon the ability of Fletcher-trait plasma to generate bradykinin. From these observations, it was concluded that prekallikrein affected both coagulation and fibrinolysis by accelerating the rate of formation of activated Hageman factor (Fig. 2). However, the autocorrective nature of the abnormality suggested that there must be an alternate but slower mechanism by which Hageman factor can be activated upon contact with surfaces.

Other Activators of the Hageman Factor-Dependent Pathways

In order to explain the autocorrective nature of the prekallikrein-deficient plasma, other possible activators of Hageman factor had to be found. It was determined that both factor XIa (Cochrane et al., 1973) and plasmin (Kaplan and Austen, 1971) were capable of activating Hageman factor in both the fluid and solid phases; however, in both phases these enzymes are at least 10-fold less efficient as activators of Hageman factor, than is kallikrein (Griffin and Cochrane, 1976). Either factor XIa or plasmin might explain the ability of prekallikrein-deficient plasma to activate its Hageman factor slowly. Figure 2 illustrates the amplification loops that are involved in the activation of the Hageman factor-dependent pathways.

The Role of High Molecular Weight Kininogen as a Cofactor in the Activation of the Hageman Factor-Dependent Pathways

The next development in the identification of the factors required for the activation and/or function of Hageman factor came when Webster and Pierce (1973) and Schiffman and Lee (1974) reported that they could not maximally activate Hageman factor with a surface and "purified" preparations of each of the known constituents. Webster and Pierce (1973), studying the generation of arginine esterase activity (kallikrein formation), and Schiffman and Lee (1974), investigating the activation of factor XI, were not able to generate the same amount of activity using purified components at physiological concentrations, as they observed upon surface activation of whole plasma. Both groups postulated that there existed an additional cofactor that was required for optimal activation of Hageman factor in plasma. While the problem of maximizing Hageman factor activity was studied, the question concerning the nature of the last protein in the kinin-generating sequence was being debated. Jacobsen (1967) and Jacobsen and Kriz (1967) reported that two kininogens existed in plasma. A high molecular weight form of kininogen appeared to be the primary substrate for plasma kallikrein, while high and low molecular weight forms of kininogen were equally active as substrates for glandular kallikreins. This view was supported by Pierce and co-workers (Pierce and Webster, 1966; Pierce and Giumaraes, 1976; Giumaraes et al. 1974) who were able to purify high and low molecular weight kininogens and demonstrated that high molecular weight kininogen (HMW kininogen) was much more susceptible to cleavage and release of bradykinin by plasma kallikrein than was the low molecular weight kininogen (LMW kininogen). However, other investigators such as Spragg and Austen (1971) presented evidence that HMW kininogen was an aggregated form of LMW kininogen. Again, a new plasma deficiency was discovered with a prolonged clotting time, which helped resolve the question of the missing factor required for optimal Hageman factor activation and of the molecular nature of kininogen.

Almost simultaneously, three patients were observed (Colman, Bagdasarian, Talamo, et al., 1974; Lacombe, 1974; Saito and Ratnoff, 1974) in whom asymptomatic coagulation abnormalities were observed. The clotting time of these patients, named Fitzgerald, Flaujeac, and Williams, was greatly prolonged, and their PTTs did not autocorrect with increased incubation time as was the case in prekallikrein deficiency. It was shown independently that both Flaujeac and Williams lacked normal quantities of kininogen (Colman et al., 1975a; Wuepper et al., 1975a) and that, upon addition of a protein fraction containing HMW kininogen (Wuepper et al., 1975b) or purified HMW kininogen (Colman et al., 1975b) the abnormal PTT was corrected to normal values. The analysis of Fitzgerald's plasma showed that although he possessed half normal amounts of LMW kininogen, he was totally deficient in HMW kininogen (Saito et al., 1975; Waldman and Abraham, 1975). The existence of Fitzgerald's plasma, which contained only LMW kininogen, reinforced the argument that there are at least two genetically and functionally distinct kininogens in plasma. These findings were confirmed by Donaldson et al. (1976) in a fourth patient. Schiffman et al. (1975) were then able to show that Fitzgerald plasma was deficient in a "contact activation co-factor" which enables plasma to activate factor XI maximally. Subsequently, she demonstrated that HMW kininogen was identical to the contact activation cofactor (Schiffman and Lee, 1975; Schiffman et al., 1977). Meier et al. (1976) examined the model used by Webster and Pierce (1973) and found that there was a large augmentation in esterase activity when HMW kininogen was added to a mixture of purified Hageman factor and prekallikrein. Thus, HMW kininogen appeared to be the missing cofactor for optimal activation of Hageman factor (Fig. 2).

In order to ascertain whether HMW kininogen increased the amount of active Hageman factor generated by the same mechanism as kallikrein, activated factor XII in the presence of a surface was added to HMW kininogen-deficient plasma (Liu et al., 1976; Meier et al., 1976). The addition of active Hageman factor did not appreciably shorten the clotting time of HMW kininogen-deficient plasma as it would shorten the clotting time of Fletcher plasma. Thus, HMW kininogen appeared to be required for the expression of Hageman factor activity. HMW kininogen has actually been shown to have a multifaceted level of action in that it seems to be involved in the activation of Hageman factor as well as the expression of the activity of activated Hageman factor. The task of ascertaining HMW kininogen's role was difficult since the only assay (Ulevitch and Cochrane, 1974), until recently, by which active Hageman factor could be directly measured was not sensitive enough to detect physiological concentrations. Therefore, most studies of Hageman factor activation have utilized [^{3}H] DFP uptake (Meier et al., 1977a,b) and proteolytic digestion of Hageman factor (Griffin and Cochrane, 1976; Griffin, 1977a), neither of which is a direct measure of enzyme activity. The activity of Hageman factor has been followed by the ability of kallikrein to digest arginine esterases after activated Hageman factor converts prekallikrein to kallikrein. Liu and co-workers (Liu et al., 1976, 1977) were able to utilize acetyl-glycyl-lysyl-methyl ester in a study of the effect of HMW kininogen upon the activity of the Hageman factor fragments. They showed that HMW kininogen was able to increase the amount of methanol liberated by Hageman factor fragments, thereby demonstrating a direct effect of HMW kininogen upon the activity of Hageman factor. Shown in Figure 2 are mechanisms that can explain the data gathered from studies of the interaction between Hageman factor, kallikrein, and HMW kininogen.

Though the mechanism of activation of Hageman factor and its interactions with other plasma proteins have been extensively studied, the initial step in the activation of the Hageman factor-dependent pathways has not been determined. At least three plasma proteins (kallikrein, plasmin, factor XIa) have been shown to be capable of activating Hageman factor; however, all of these enzymes circulate as zymogens in plasma and require prior activation before they can activate Hageman factor. Though the initial mechanism for activating these pathways has not been determined, as a result of the feedback amplification loops in the Hageman factor-dependent pathways (Fig. 2) only a small number of active molecules may be sufficient to activate these pathways. Below is a discussion of the immune release of certain lung tissue proteases which may well function as a triggering event in the activation of the Hageman factor-dependent pathways of inflammation.

III. IgE-Mediated Release of Activators of the Hageman Factor-Dependent Pathways

A. Models Used for Studying the Release of High Molecular Weight Mediators

Experimental Studies with the Chopped Human Lung Model

Specimens of macroscopically normal human lung that were recovered from lungs usually excised for carcinoma were dissected free of pleura, cartilage, and large vessels, cut into fragments ($\simeq$100 mg), washed with tyrodes buffer, then passively sensitized with serum from a ragweed sensitive donor (Schulman et al., 1981). Challenge of the sensitized lung fragments with ragweed antigen E (AgE) resulted in a dose-dependent release of histamine (Fig. 3). Also released were other low molecular weight mediators such as prostaglandin $F_{2\alpha}$ ($PGF_{2\alpha}$) (Fig.

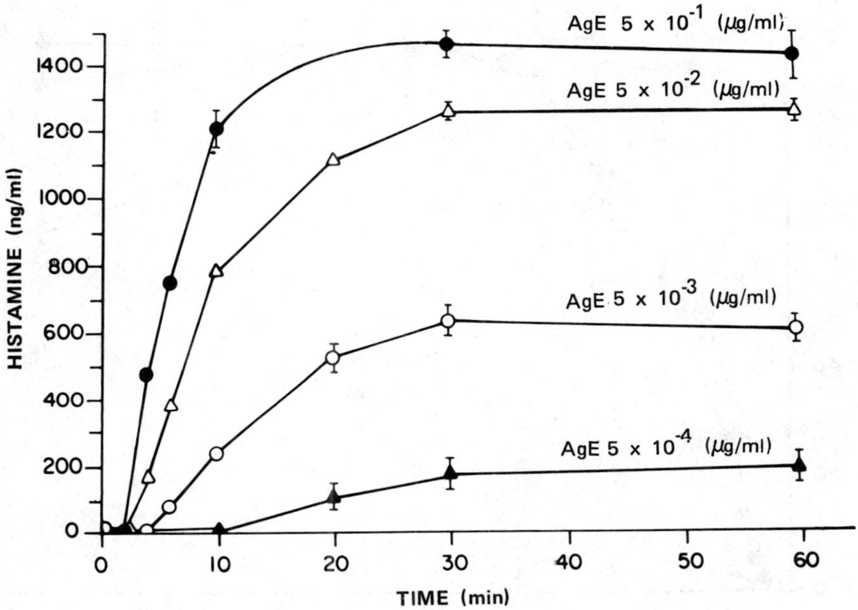

Figure 3 Kinetic and dose-response studies on human lung fragments. Challenge of passively sensitized human lung fragments with ragweed antigen E (AgE) resulted in a dose-dependent release of histamine. Triplicate beakers, each with 20 lung fragments, were challenged with antigen E at the concentrations noted in the figure. At the time intervals indicated, aliquots were removed and assayed for histamine.

4; Adkinson et al., 1979, 1980), a prostaglandin with potent agonist effects on human airways (Newball and Lenfant, 1977; Newball et al., 1980). Antigen challenge of the lung fragments also led to the release of a lung kallikrein-like activity (LK-A) that has TAMe esterase activity (Fig. 4), a lung Hageman factor activator (LHFA), and a lung prekallikrein activator (LPKA) (vide infra).

Experimental Studies with the Basophil Model

Human peripheral leukocyte preparations, challenged with either purified protein antigens, such as ragweed antigen E (AgE), or with highly specific anti-IgE, release a TAMe esterase activity. Our studies on the mechanism of release of a basophil kallikrein-like activity (BK-A) have primarily concentrated on this esterase activity, since its measurement is relatively easy and precise. As will be indicated below, however, it cannot be assumed that TAMe esterase activity parallels each of the biological activities of BK-A.

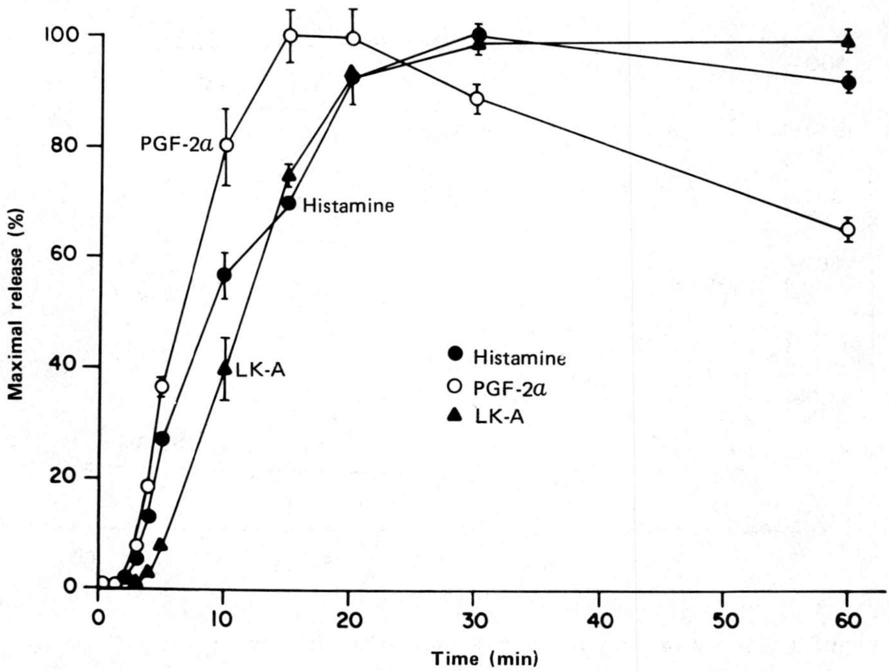

Figure 4 Antigen challenge of passively sensitized human lung fragments released low molecular weight mediators (histamine, PGF-2_α) and a high molecular weight mediator, a lung kallikrein-like activity (LK-A), all of which had similar release kinetics. The lung kallikrein-like activity (LK-A) generates a kinin from both high molecular weight kininogen and low molecular weight kininogen. The kinin contracts both the estrous rat uterus and the guinea pig ileum.

A typical dose-response curve for the release of TAMe esterase is shown in Fig. 5. In general, the pattern of histamine and TAMe esterase release is similar, whether the release is initiated by antigen or anti-IgE. The maximal percentage of histamine or TAMe esterase release has, however, no fixed relationship. This differential release of histamine and TAMe esterase is similar to the observations of others relating to differential release of enzymes from the neutrophil (Wright et al., 1977). In this cell type, which shares a common cell of origin with the basophil, the release of β-glucuronidase from the azurophil granule and lysozyme from the specific granule are often quite different. There have also been reports showing differential release of histamine and SRS-A from mast cells (Orange and Langer, 1973).

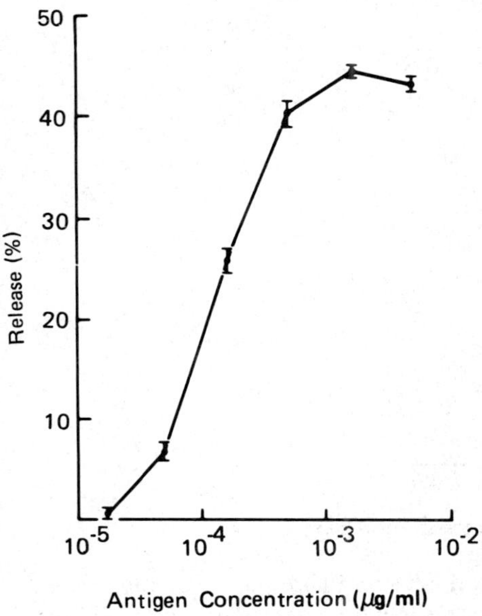

Figure 5 Dose-response of ragweed antigen E-induced release of a basophil kallikrein-like activity (BK-A). The basophil kallikrein-like activity (BK-A) generates a kinin from high molecular weight kininogen. The precision of the [^{3}H]TAMe arginine esterase assay is indicated by the standard deviations. (From Newball et al., 1979.)

While the quantity of histamine and TAMe esterase release may differ, the rate of release of the two mediators shows no significant difference. Similarly, release of both histamine and TAMe esterase is temperature and calcium dependent. Not only is the initiation of release of TAMe esterase temperature sensitive, but decreasing the temperature at any time during the release process stops the reaction abruptly. The release is also absolutely dependent upon the extracellular calcium concentration and the addition of EDTA at any time during the process causes a similar rapid cessation of release (Newball et al., 1979a).

Modulation of TAMe esterase release has been studied using the same series of agonists utilized to explore the control of histamine release. Agonists that act on specific receptors to activate adenylate cyclase inhibit the two processes similarly. For example, Fig. 6 shows that prostaglandin E_1 (PGE_1) inhibits both processes in a dose-dependent fashion. Similar experiments have been carried out with β-adrenergic agonists, histamine, and cholera enterotoxin. In each case, the inhibition dose-response curves were essentially identical. Agents, such as theophylline, which act by inhibiting the cAMP phosphodiesterase, inhibit the release of histamine and of TAMe esterase with similar dose-response relationships. Colchicine, which causes disaggregation of microtubules, is a potent inhibitor of histamine release while heavy water (D_2O), which favors microtubular aggregation, is a potent enhancer of this process; together, the two agents are

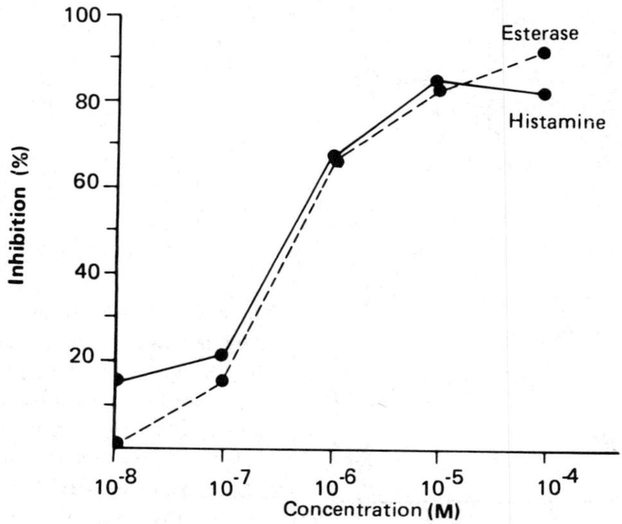

Figure 6 Inhibitory effect of prostaglandin E_1 on BK-A and histamine release. PGE-1 inhibits the release of both mediators in a dose-dependent fashion (From Newball et al., 1979a).

antagonistic, so that their effects cancel. Similar studies with respect to esterase release showed that colchicine inhibited the process while D_2O caused a potentiation of release (Newball et al., 1979a). The need for metabolic processes in the release of TAMe esterase was studied with 2-deoxyglucose, an inhibitor of glucose phosphorylation. These studies indicate that the TAMe esterase release is entirely energy dependent. The concentration of 2-deoxyglucose required for 50% inhibition of release is similar for the TAMe esterase (0.4 mM) and histamine release (0.3 mM) (Newball et al., 1979a).

After demonstrating that the release process and the pharmacologic control of TAMe esterase release was similar to that of the previously described mediators, we next attempted to purify the esterase and to ascertain its relationship to the biological activities (cleavage of kininogen) which had been observed in the crude supernatants. For this purpose, large quantities of the basophil supernatant were obtained by challenge of leukocyte preparations with anti-IgE or antigen E, and then chromatographed on Sepharose 6B, as shown in Figure 7. A major peak of TAMe esterase activity was observed that coincided with the first absorption peak and eluted with an estimated molecular weight of 1.2 million. A second esterase peak was present but was quantitatively of smaller magnitude and smaller molecular weight ($\simeq$ 400,000). A third arginine esterase peak was variably present and was quantitatively of even smaller magnitude than the other two forms.

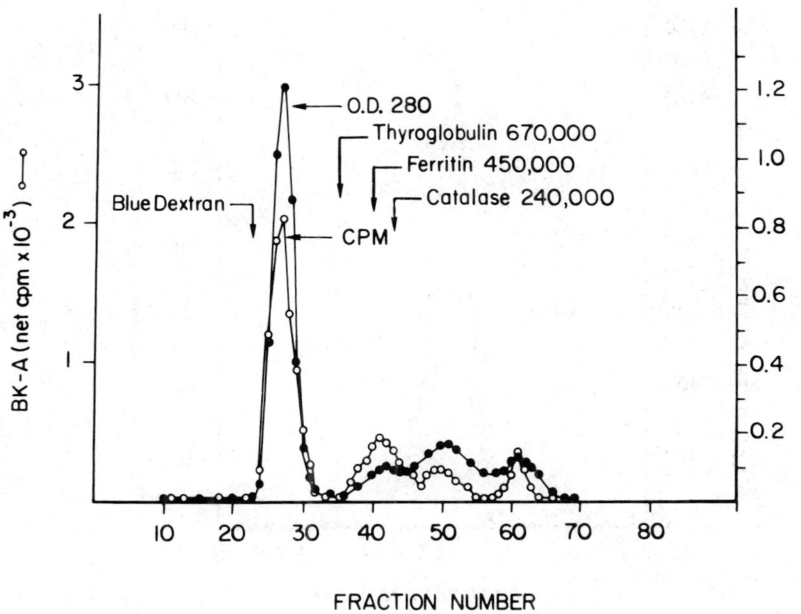

Figure 7 Sepharose 6B chromatography of a basophil kallikrein-like activity (BK-A). The TAMe esterase active fractions from DEAE-Sephacel were applied to Sepharose 6B. (From Newball et al., 1980. © 1980 The Williams & Wilkins Co., Baltimore.)

These fractions were then examined for their ability to generate immunoreactive kinin and to cleave Hageman factor. Figure 8 shows the relationship between TAMe esterase activity and the generation of immunoreactive kinin kinin from the first, high molecular weight peak of the Sepharose 6B column eluate. It is evident that the two activities cochromatagraph. This assay was carried out with acid-treated, heat-inactivated plasma as the source of kininogen. More recently, it has been shown that the same protease can cleave purified, high molecular weight kininogen to yield immunoreactive kinin (Newball et al., 1979a,b). Similar studies have not been completed with respect to the mediator that cleaves Hageman factor. It is clear, however, that while there is TAMe esterase activity associated with the first two peaks (Fig. 7), there is little present in the last, low molecular weight peak; fractions from the last peak were, however, most potent in cleaving Hageman factor.

The activity of the basophil Hageman factor (HF) protease is shown in Figure 9. Radiolabeled Hageman factor was adsorbed to a glass surface after which it was cleaved by either purified human plasma kallikrein or the basophil Hage-

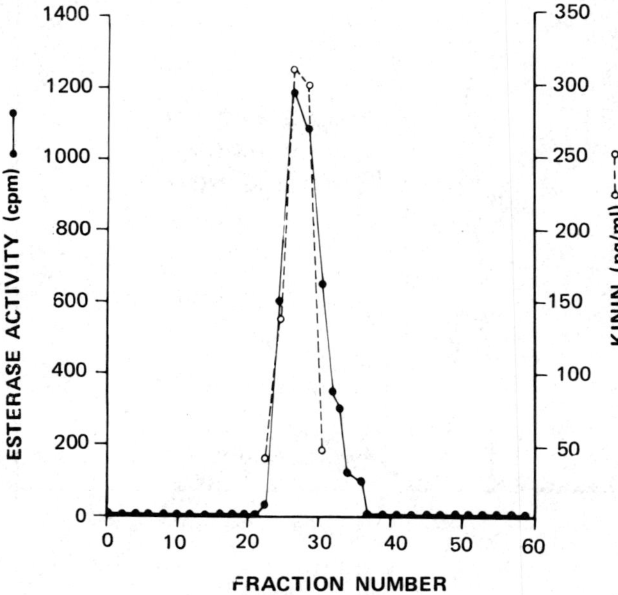

Figure 8 TAMe esterase activity (BK-A) and kinin generation by anti-IgE-generated supernatant chromatographed on Sepharose 6B (cpm X 10^{-1}). (From Newball et al., 1979a.)

man factor protease. After cleavage, samples were analyzed by electrophoresis on SDS-PAGE, as previously described (Revak et al., 1978; Newball et al., 1979c). In Figure 9, the top panel shows intact Hageman factor, with a molecular weight of 80,000. The middle panel shows the cleavage of Hageman factor by purified human plasma kallikrein. Part of the radiolabeled Hageman factor remains intact while the rest is cleaved into fragments of approximately 28,000 and 52,000 daltons. The lower panel shows cleavage of the Hageman factor by the basophil protease. As with plasma kallikrein, part of the radiolabeled Hageman factor remains uncleaved while the rest is cleaved into fragments of 28,000 and 52,000 daltons. Additional studies have suggested that the 28,000-molecular-weight fragment produced by the basophil enzyme has functional activity as assessed by its ability to activate prekallikrein to kallikrein (Newball et al., 1979).

B. A Human Lung Hageman Factor Activator

Mast cells and basophils are effector cells of IgE-mediated reactions in the human lung. We had earlier described the IgE-mediated release of a basophil kalli-

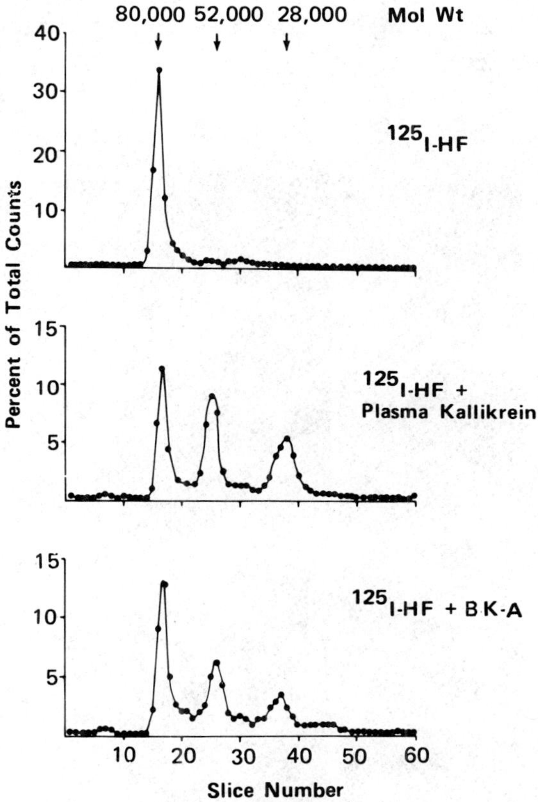

Figure 9 Cleavage of purified human Hageman factor by the basophil Hageman factor protease (BK-A). (From Newball, et al., 1980. © 1980 The Williams & Wilkins Co., Baltimore.)

krein-like activity (BK-A) from basophils of peripheral blood, which had Hageman factor cleaving activity. It seemed reasonable to challenge human lung fragments and dispersed human lung mast cells to determine whether we could, likewise, observe the IgE-mediated release of a lung Hageman factor activator (LHFA). The lung Hageman factor activator was isolated from supernatants of antigen-challenged, passively sensitized human lung fragments and partially purified human lung mast cells. In the example shown in Figure 10, supernatants were obtained from anti-IgE-challenged lung mast cells. Purified ^{125}I-radiolabeled human Hageman factor was exposed to the supernatant and the mixture was analyzed by electrophoresis on SDS slab gels, as earlier described (Newball et al., 1979c). The gels were dried and applied to x-ray films which resulted

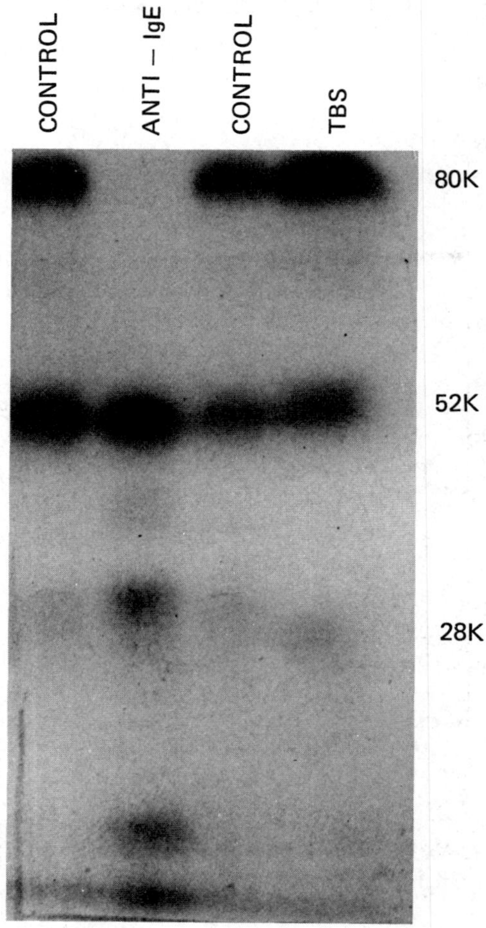

Figure 10 Autoradiogram of the cleavage of ^{125}I-Hageman factor by the lung Hageman factor activator (LHFA). Supernatant from anti-IgE-challenged human lung completely cleaved the 80K ^{125}I-Hageman factor while the control supernatants caused only minimal cleavage, that was no greater than Tris-buffered saline (TBS). (From Newball et al., 1981b.)

in the autoradiogram shown in Figure 10. The first track of the autoradiogram (labeled control) demonstrates minimal cleavage of the 80,000 molecular-weight Hageman factor that was exposed to supernatants from buffer-challenged lung. Depletion of the 80,000-molecular-weight Hageman factor is no greater for the

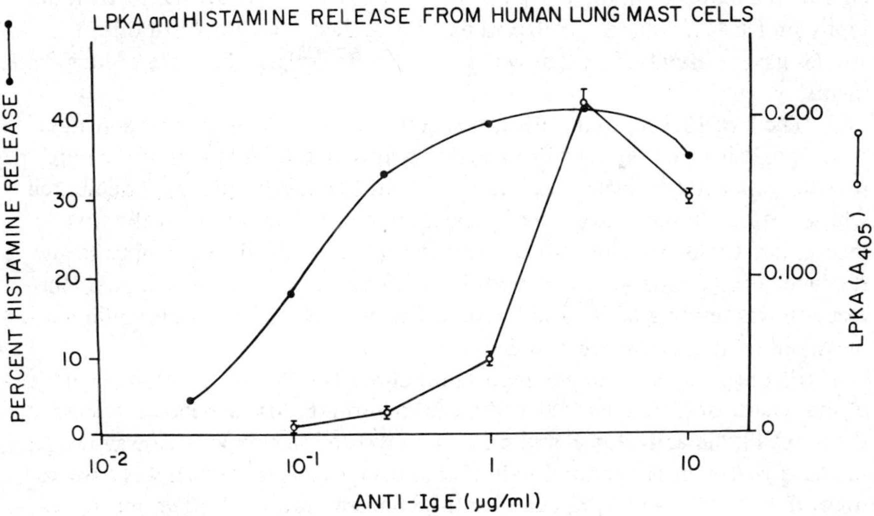

Figure 11 Anti-IgE-induced release of a lung prekallikrein activator (LPKA) and histamine from partially purified human lung mast cells. Both LPKA and histamine demonstrate antigen excess inhibition. (From Newball et al., 1981b.)

control supernatant than it is for the Tris-buffered saline (TBS). In contrast, as shown in the second track, there is complete cleavage of the Hageman factor that was exposed to the anti-IgE-challenged lung cell supernatant. These data indicate that the lung Hageman factor activator is generated by an IgE-mediated mechanism. Preliminary experiments with preparations of human lung mast cells of 98% purity show that they secrete a protease that cleaves human Hageman factor in a fashion similar to that obtained with the LHFA. It should be noted that, like human plasma kallikrein, the human lung Hageman factor activator cleaves zymogen Hageman factor in a fashion which yields a 52,000-molecular-weight heavy chain and a 28,000-molecular-weight light chain. Unlike plasma kallikrein, however, only a small portion of the 28,000-molecular-weight light chains that are generated by the LHFA appear to be functional in the activation of prekallikrein to kallikrein. The latter suggests that Hageman factor may not be the natural substrate of LHFA.

C. A Human Lung Prekallikrein Activator

Supernatants from antigen challenge of passively sensitized lung fragments were used for the purification of the lung prekallikrein activator (LPKA). The techniques used during purification included affinity chromatography on aminocaproyl-*p*-aminobenzamidine Sepharose 4B, followed by sequential chromatography on DEAE-Sephacel, SP-Sephadex, and Sephadex G-200. Most of our studies have utilized LPKA that was purified from antigen challenge of lung fragments.

The lung prekallikrein activator is detected by the action of its activated substrate, kallikrein, on Benz-Pro-Phe-Arg-*p*-nitroanilide. Aliquots of the lung prekallikrein activator were incubated with purified human plasma prekallikrein which resulted in the activation of prekallikrein to kallikrein. After the first incubation, the Benz-Pro-Phe-Arg-pNA substrate was added to the mixture and the incubation continued for an additional 30 min at 37°C, at which point the reaction was terminated by acidification. The amount of free *p*-nitroaniline was measured by its absorbance at 405 nm.

Figure 11 illustrates two important points. The first is the IgE-dependence of the release of LPKA. Note that there is an anti-IgE dose-dependent release of the prekallikrein activator. Simultaneous analysis of histamine release showed a similar dose-response relationship in that antigen excess inhibition was observed for both histamine and LPKA at an anti-IgE concentration of 10 μg/ml. A second point relates to the fact that, in this experiment, the prekallikrein activator was released from a suspension of partially purified mast cells. Preliminary experiments show that prekallikrein activator activity can be obtained from human mast cells that have been purified to 98%, suggesting that mast cells are the source of LPKA. It was important, however, that we exclude the possible contamination of our enzyme with serum components, specifically, the activated forms of Hageman factor (HF_a and HF_f), which were, heretofore, the only known physiological activator of prekallikrein. This was accomplished in the experiment illustrated in Figure 12, which demonstrated that LPKA is not one of the forms of activated Hageman factor. We utilized a monospecific sheep antibody to Hageman factor and an inhibitor of Hageman factor derived from corn (Swartz et al., 1977; Hojima et al., 1980). The antibody to Hageman factor and the corn inhibitor were interacted with Hageman factor fragment (HF_f), activated Hageman factor (HF_a, not shown in Fig. 12), and LPKA. The effects of the antibody and the corn inhibitor on HF_f, HF_a, and LPKA were evaluated utilizing the amidolytic assay as described above. The upper panel of Figure 12 shows that normal sheep IgG had no effect on the activity of HF_f, while the anti-Hageman factor antibody and the corn inhibitor completely inhibited its activity. Similar data were obtained for HF_a. The lower panel shows that neither the anti-Hageman factor antibody nor the corn inhibitor had any effect on the activity of the purified LPKA.

The data clearly show that anti-IgE or antigen challenge of human lung fragments and partially purified human lung mast cells lead to the active secretion of a tissue protease-a lung prekallikrein activator. The release of LPKA is antigen dose-dependent. The activated forms of Hageman factor (HF_a, HF_f)

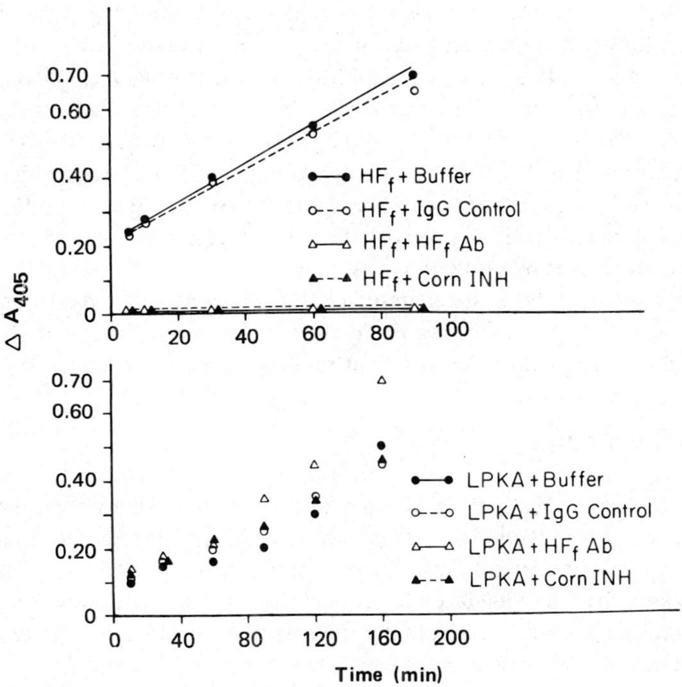

Figure 12 Effects of an anti-Hageman factor antibody and a corn inhibitor on the prekallikrein activator activity of HF_f and the lung prekallikrein activator (LPKA). The antibody to Hageman factor and the corn inhibitor completely inhibited the activity of HF_f. In contrast, neither the antibody to Hageman factor nor the corn inhibitor had any effect on the activity of the LPKA. (From Newball et al., 1981b.)

have, therefore, represented the only known physiological activators of prekallikrein. The data in Figure 12, utilizing monospecific antibody to Hageman factor, clearly show that the lung prekallikrein activator is a molecule that is distinct from the activated forms of Hageman factor.

D. A Human Lung Kininogenase

We earlier showed that antigen challenge of human peripheral basophils resulted in the generation of a kininogenase (Newball et al., 1979a,b). We have, likewise, shown that antigen challenge of human lung fragments and partially purified human mast cell preparations secrete a kininogenase. The lung kininogenase, or lung kinin-generating activity (LK-A), generates biologically active kinin from purified high and low molecular weight kininogen. The kinin that is generated is assayed on the estrous rat uterus and on the guinea pig ileum.

We have also studied the cleavage of high molecular weight kininogen by the kininogenase, utilizing SDS-slab gels. The kininogenase produced limited cleavage of the high molecular weight kininogen (three distinct fragments) which was similar, but not identical, to the cleavage of high molecular weight kininogen that is produced by plasma kallikrein. Much remains to be learned regarding the lung kininogenase. However, it is clear that the kininogenase is secreted from dispersed human lung cells by an IgE-mediated mechanism, that its release is antigen dose-dependent, and that it generates a kinin that contracts the estrous rat uterus and the guinea pig ileum, suggesting that the kinin that is generated is either bradykinin, lysbradykinin, or one of the larger kinins (unpublished data).

IV. Conclusions

We have tried to point out that, in addition to the low molecular weight mediators of inflammatory reactions, there is a group of high molecular weight mediators which are released from human lung (presumably mast cells) and human peripheral basophils following interaction of antigen and IgE antibody. These mediators have the ability to activate the Hageman factor-dependent pathways. The importance of these mediators is illustrated in Figure 13. Thus, LHFA, by acting on Hageman factor, proteolytically cleaves zymogen Hageman factor and appears to generate an active 28,000-molecular-weight fragment, which is capable of activating prekallikrein to kallikrein; kallikrein can either cleave plasminogen to produce plasmin, or act on kininogen to generate kinin. LPKA is a second tissue protease which can directly activate the zymogen prekallikrein to its active form, kallikrein. Each of these activation steps is subject to control by inhibitors, so that the additional ability of LK-A to generate a kinin from kininogen is an important "feed forward" aspect of these reactions. These are the first mediators from mast cells and basophils that are capable of interacting with the Hageman factor-dependent pathways to generate biologically relevant peptides. In fact, this represents the only known IgE-mediated pathway into the Hageman factor-dependent systems.

We have previously suggested that certain of the chemical mediators, such as histamine, participate not only in immediate-type inflammatory reactions, but also function in important aspects of the entire inflammatory process. While the role of LHFA, LPKA, and LK-A in immediate hypersensitivity reactions and in other inflammatory processes is not clear, they do represent a first and important interface between IgE-mediated reactions and the Hageman factor-dependent pathways of the inflammatory response. By virtue of these activities, LHFA, LPKA, and LK-A may influence mechanisms which are involved in both subacute and chronic cell-mediated inflammatory processes.

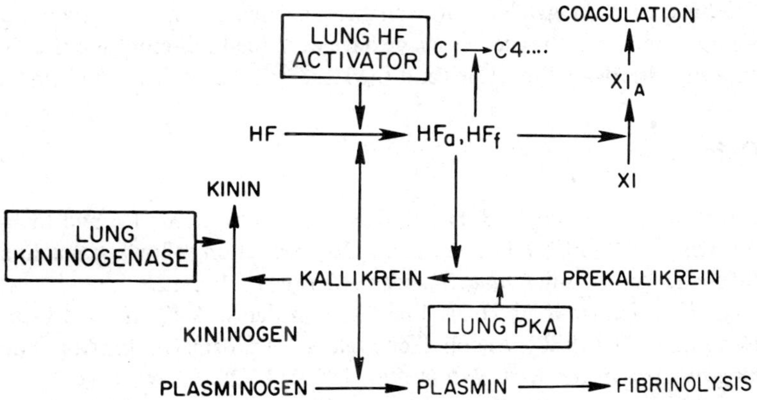

Figure 13 Partial outline of the Hageman factor-dependent pathways showing how activation of the pathways could occur by the lung Hageman factor activator (LHFA) or the lung prekallikrein activator (LPKA). The lung kininogenase represents a third protease that can directly generate kinins from kininogen.

There has been recent interest in the involvement of IgE-mediated mechanisms in delayed cutaneous reactions and in cutaneous basophil hypersensitivity, both of which represent subacute or chronic phases of inflammation. It has been shown that, in these types of reactions, there is activation of the coagulation system (DeShazo et al., 1979). Perhaps, during an IgE-mediated lung reaction, mast cells and basophils secrete the above described proteases which activate the Hageman factor-dependent pathways, thus resulting in inflammatory processes similar to those observed during delayed skin reactions. Further studies have also shown the deposition of fibrin in and around inflammatory lesions associated with cutaneous basophil hypersensitivity (Dvorak and Dvorak, 1974; Askenase, 1977). It is possible that mast cells and basophils, through the mechanisms described above, activate the coagulation system and are responsible for the fibrin deposition. In addition to being involved in subacute and chronic inflammatory reactions, the mediators described here may be involved in more acute reactions. Thus, we have reported the consumption of coagulation factors during human anaphylaxis (Kaplan et al., 1977), and other investigators have observed the same phenomenon in systemic anaphylaxis in rabbits (Pinckard et al., 1975). There has been clinical evidence that there are coagulation abnormalities in anaphylactic reactions, and the above described proteases may well provide the mechanism by which this occurs.

The basic biochemistry of the Hageman factor-dependent systems has been appreciated for a considerable period of time. The triggering event for the activation of these systems in vivo has not been clear, particularly from an immunologic point of view, and the mediators we have described represent the first link between antigen-activated reactions and the Hageman factor-dependent systems.

References

Adkinson, N. F., Jr., Newball, H. H., Findlay, S., Adams, G. K., III, and Lichtenstein, L. M. (1979). Origin of PGF-2α production following anaphylactic challenge of human lung. *Monogr. Allergy, 14*:122-125.

Adkinson, N. F., Jr., Newball, H. H., Findlay, S., Adams, G. K., III, and Lichtenstein, L. M. (1980). Anaphylactic release of prostaglandins from human lung *in vitro. Amer. Rev. Respir. Dis., 121*:911-920.

Armstrong, D., Jepson, J. B., Keele, C. A., and Stewart, J. W. (1957). Pain producing substance in human inflammatory exudates and plasma. *J. Physiol., 135*:350-370.

Askenase, P. S. (1977). The role of basophils, mast cells and vasomines in hypersensitivity reactions with a delayed time course. *Prog. Allergy,* 199-320.

Bordet, J., and Genou, O. (1901). Recherches sur la coagulation du sang et les serums anticoagulants. *Ann. Inst. Pasteur 14*:129-144.

Cochrane, C. G., and Wuepper, K. D. (1971). The first component of the kinin-forming system in human and rabbit plasma. Its relationship to clotting factor XII (Hageman factor). *J. Exp. Med. 134*:986-1004.

Cochrane, C. G., Revak, S. D., and Wuepper, K. D. (1973). Activation of Hageman factor in solid and fluid phases. A critical role of kallikrein. *J. Exp. Med., 138*:1564-1583.

Colman, R. W., Mattler, L., and Sherry, S. (1969a). Studies on the prekallikrein (kallikreinogen)–kallikrein enzyme system or human plasma. I. Evidence relating the kaolin activated arginine esterase to plasma kallikrein. *J. Clin. Invest., 48*:11-21.

Colman, R. W., Mattler, L., and Sherry, S. (1969b). Studies on the prekallikrein (kallikreinogen)–kallikrein enzyme system of human plasma. II. Evicence relating the kaolin activated arginine esterase to plasma kallikrein. *J. Clin. Invest., 48*:23-32.

Colman, R. W., Bagdasarian, A., Talamo, R. C., and Kaplan, A. P. (1976). Williams trait: A new deficiency with abnormal levels of prekallikrein, plasminogen proactivator, and kininogen. In *The Chemistry and Biology of the Kallikrein-Kinin System in Health and Disease.* Edited by J. J. Pisano and K. F. Austen. Washington, D.C., U.S. Government Printing Office, Fogarty International Proceedings, No. 27, pp. 65-72.

Colman, R. W., Bagdasarian, A., Talamo, R. C., Scott, C. F., Seavey, M., Guimaraes, J. A., Pierce, J. V., and Kaplan, A. P. (1975a). Williams trait:

Human kininogen deficiency with diminished levels of plasminogen, proactivator and prekallikrein associated with abnormalities of the Hageman factor-dependent pathways. *J. Clin. Invest., 56*:1650-1662.

Colman, R. W., Bagdasarian, A., Talamo, R. C., Seavey, M., Scott, C. F., and Kaplan, A. P. (1975b). Williams trait: Combined deficiency of plasma plasminogen proactivator, kininogen, and a new procoagulant factor. *Fed. Proc., 34*:859.

Davie, E. W., and Ratnoff, O. D. (1964). Waterfall sequence for intrinsic blood clotting. *Science, 145*:1310-1311.

DeShazo, R. D., Levinson, A. I., Dvorak, H. F., and Davis, R. W. (1979). The late skin reaction: Evidence for activation of the coagulation system in an IgE-dependent reaction in man. *J. Immunol., 122*:692-698.

Donaldson, V. H. (1967). Mechanisms of activation of C1 esterase in hereditary angioneurotic edema plasma in vitro. *J. Exp. Med. 127*:411-429.

Donaldson, V. H., Glueck, H. I., Miller, M. A., Movat, H. Z., and Habal, F. (1976). Kininogen deficiency in Fitzgerald trait: Role of high molecular weight kininogen in clotting and fibrinolysis. *J. Lab. Clin. Med., 87*:327-337.

Dvorak, H. F., and Dvorak, A. M. (1974). Cutaneous basophil hypersensitivity. In *Progress in Immunology II,* Vol. 3. Edited by L. Brent and J. Holborow. Amsterdam, North Holland Publishing Company, pp. 171-181.

Ghebrehiwet, B., Silverberg, M., and Kaplan, A. P. (1981). Activation of the classical pathway of complement by Hageman factor fragment. *J. Exp. Med. 153*:665-676.

Griffin, J. H. (1977a). Molecular mechanism of surface-dependent activation of Hageman factor (HF) (coagulation factor XII). *Fed. Proc., 36*:129.

Griffin, J. H. (1977b). New hypoehesis for the molecular mechanism of surface dependent activation of Hageman factor. *Thromb. Haemostasis, 38*:50.

Griffin, J. H., and Cochrane, C. G. (1976). Mechanism for the involvement of high molecular weight kininogen in surface-dependent reactions of Hageman factor. *Proc. Natl. Acad. Sci. USA, 73*:2559-2563.

Guimaraes, J. A., Liu, C. Y., Webster, M. E., and Pierce, J. V. (1974). Multiple forms of human plasma kininogen. *Fed. Proc., 33*:641.

Haanen, C., Hommes, F., and Morselt, G. (1961). Some observations on the role of Hageman factor in blood coagulation. *Thromb. Diath. Haemorrhag., 6*: 261-269.

Hathaway, W. E., and Alsever, J. (1970). The relation of "Fletcher factor" to factors XI and XII. *Brit. J. Haemat., 18*:161-169.

Hathaway, W. E., Belhausen, L. P., and Hathaway, H. S. (1965). Evidence of a new plasma coagulation factor I. Case report, coagulation studies and physiochemical properties. *Br. J. Haemat., 26*:521-532.

Hattersley, P. G., and Hayse, D. (1970). Fletcher factor deficiency. A report of three unrelated cases. *Br. J. Haemat., 18*:411-416.

Hojima, Y., Pierce, J. V., and Pisano, J. J. (1980). Hageman factor fragment inhibitor in corn seeds: Purification and characterization. *Thromb. Res., 20*: 149-154.

Iatridis, S. G., and Ferguson, J. H. (1961). Effect of surface and Hageman factor on the endogenous or spontaneous activation of the fibrinolytic system. *Thromb. Diath. Haemorrhag., 61*:411-423.

Iatridis, S. G., and Ferguson, J. H. (1962). Active Hageman factor. A plasma lysokinase of the human fibrinolytic system. *J. Clin. Invest., 41*:1277-1287.

Jacobsen, S. (1967). Substrates for plasma kinin-forming enzymes in human, dog and rabbit plasma. *Brit. J. Pharmacol., 26*:403-411.

Jacobsen, S., and Kriz, M. (1967). Some data on two purified kininogens from human plasma. *Brit. J. Pharmacol., 29*:25-36.

Kaplan, A. P., and Austen, K. F. (1970). A prealbumin activator of prekallikrein. *J. Immunol., 105*:802-811.

Kaplan, A. P., and Austen, K. F. (1971). A prealbumin activator of prekallikrein. II. Derivation of activators of prekallikrein from active Hageman factor by digestion with plasmin. *J. Exp. Med., 133*:696-712.

Kaplan, A. P., Spragg, J., and Austen, K. F. (1971). The bradykinin-forming system of man. In *Biochemistry of the Acute Allergic Reaction.* Edited by K. F. Austen and E. L. Becker. Oxford, Blackwell Scientific Publication Ltd., pp. 279-298.

Kaplan, A. P., Hunt, K. J., Sobotka, A. K., Smith, P., Horakova, Z., Gralnick, H., and Lichtenstein, L. M. (1977). Human anaphylaxis: A study of mediator systems. *Clin. Res., 25*:361A.

Lacombe, M. J. (1974). Deficit constitutionnel en un nouveau facteur de la coagulation intervenant au niveau de contact: Le facteur "Flaujeac". C. R. Hebd. *Seances Acad. Sc. Ser. D. Sci. Nat., 380*:1039-1041.

Lichtenstein, L. M. (1971). The immediate allergic response: in vitro separation of antigen activation, decay and histamine release. *J. Immunol. 107*:1122-1130.

Lichtenstein, L. M. (1977). Mechanisms of allergic inflammation. In *Progress in Immunology III.* Edited by T. E. Mandel. Amsterdam, North Holland Publishing, pp. 430-438.

Lichtenstein, L. M., and Margolis, S. (1968). Histamine release in vitro: inhibition by cathecholamines and methylxanthines. *Science 161*:902-903.

Lichtenstein, L. M., Foreman, J. C., Conroy, M. C., Marone, G., and Newball, H. H. (1979). Differences between histamine release from rat mast cells and human basophils and mast cells. In *The Mast Cell: Its Role in Health and Disease.* Edited by J. Pepys and A. M. Edwards, Kent, England, Pitman Medical Publishing Co., Ltd., pp. 83-96.

Liu, C. Y., Bagdasarian, A., Meier, H., Scott, C. F., Pierce, J., Kaplan, A. P., and Colman, R. W. (1976). Potentiation of the action of Hageman factor fragments (HF_f) by high molecular weight kininogen (HMW kng.). *Fed. Proc., 35*:692.

Liu, C. Y., Scott, C. F., Bagdasarian, A., Pierce, J. V., Kaplan, A. P., and Colman, R. W. (1977). Potentiation of the function of Hageman factor fragments by high molecular weight kininogen. *J. Clin. Invest., 60*:7-17.

Margolis, J. (1957). Plasma pain-producing substance and blood clotting. *Nature, 180*:1464-1465.

Margolis, J. (1958). Activation of a permeability factor in plasma by contact with glass. *Nature, 180*:635-636.

Margolis, J. (1959). Activation of plasma by contact with glass. Evidence of a common reaction which releases plasma kinin and initiates coagulation. *J. Physiol., 144*:1-22.

Margolis, J. (1963). The interrelationship of coagulation of plasma and release of peptides. *Ann. N.Y. Acad. Sci., 104*:133-145.

McMillin, C. R., Saito, H., Ratnoff, O. D., and Walton, A. G. (1974). The secondary structure of human Hageman factor (factor XII). *J. Clin. Invest. 54*: 1312-1322.

Meier, H. L., Webster, M., Liu, C. Y., Colman, R. W., and Kaplan, A. P. (1976). Enhancement of surface dependent Hageman factor activation of high molecular weight kininogen. *Fed. Proc., 35*:692.

Meier, H. L., Pierce, J. V., Colman, R. W., and Kaplan, A. P. (1977a). Activation and function of human Hageman factor. The role of high molecular weight kininogen and prekallikrein. *J. Clin. Invest., 60*:18-31.

Meier, H. L., Scott, C. F., Mandle, R., Jr., Webster, M. E., Pierce, J. V., Colman, R. W., and Kaplan, A. P. (1977b). Requirements for contact activation of human Hageman factor. *Ann. N.Y. Acad. Sci., 283*:93-103.

Metcalf, D. D., Lewis, R. A., Silbert, J. E., Rosenberg, R. D., Wasserman, S. I., and Austen, K. F. (1979). Isolation, identification, and characterization of heparin from human lungs. *J. Allergy Clin. Immunol., 63*:191.

Moriya, H., Pierce, J. V., and Webster, M. E. (1963). Purification and some properties of three kallikreins. *Ann. N.Y. Acad. Sci., 104*:172-176.

Newball, H. H., and Lenfant, C. (1977). Influence of atropine and cromolyn on human bronchial hyperreactivity to aerosolized PGF-2α. *Resp. Physiol., 30*:125-136.

Newball, H. H. and Lichtenstein, L. M. (1980). Lung hypersensitivity. In *Proceedings of the 10th Conference on Environmental Toxicology.* Washington, D.C. U.S. Government Printing Office (AFAMRL-TR-79-121), pp. 141-153.

Newball, H. H., and Lichtenstein, L. M. (1981). Mast cells and basophils-effector cells of inflammatory disorders in the lung. *Thorax 36*:721-725.

Newball, H. H., Keiser, H. R., and Lenfant, C. (1980a). Prostaglandin F-2α functions as a local hormone on human airways. *Resp. Physiol., 41*:183-197.

Newball, H. H., Meier, H. L., and Lichtenstein, L. M. (1980b). Basophil mediators and their release, with emphasis on BK-A. *J. Invest. Derm. 74*:344-348.

Newball, H. H., Talamo, R. C., and Lichtenstein, L. M. (1975). Release of leukocyte kallikrein mediated by IgE. *Nature, 254*(No. 5501):635-636.

Newball, H. H., Talamo, R. C., and Lichtenstein, L. M. (1979a). Anaphylactic release of a basophil kallikrein-like activity. II. A mediator of immediate hypersensitivity reactions. *J. Clin. Invest., 64*:466-475.

Newball, H. H., Berninger, R. W., Talamo, R. C., and Lichtenstein, L. M. (1979b). Anaphylactic release of a basophil kallikrein-like activity. I. Purification and characterization. *J. Clin. Invest., 64*:457-465.

Newball, H. H., Revak, S. D., Cochrane, C. G., Griffin, J. H., and Lichtenstein, L. M. (1978). Cleavage of Hageman factor (HF) by a basophil kallikrein of anaphylaxis (BK-A). *Clin. Res., 26*:519A.

Newball, H. H., Revak, S. D., Cochrane, C. G., Griffin, J. H., and Lichtenstein, L. M. (1979c). Activation of human Hageman factor by a leukocytic protease. In *Kinins II, Systemic Proteases and Cellular Function,* Part B. New York, Plenum Publishing Co., pp. 139-151.

Newball, H. H., Meier, H. L., Kaplan, A. P., Revak, S., Cochrane, C. G., and Lichtenstein, L. M. (1981a). Activation of the Hageman factor dependent systems during IgE-mediated reactions of the human lung. *Int. Arch. Allergy Appl. Immunol., 66*:165-167.

Newball, H. H., Meier, H. L., Kaplan, A. P., Revak, S. D., Cochrane, C. G., and Lichtenstein, L. M. (1981b). Activation of Hageman Factor by proteases released during antigen challenge of human lung. *Transactions of the Association of American Physicians,* pp. 429-432.

Orange, R. P., and Langer, H. (1973). Bronchial asthma: hyperreactivity of airways and target cells. In *Proceedings of 8th International Congress of Allergology, Tokyo.* Amsterdam, Excerpta Medica, p. 325.

Pierce, J. V., and Guimaraes, J. A. (1976). Further characterization of highly purified human plasma kininogens. In *The Kallikrein System in Health and Disease.* Edited by J. J. Pisano and K. F. Austen. Fogarty International Center Proceedings, No. 27. Washington, D.C., U.S. Government Printing Office, pp. 121-126.

Pierce, J. V., and Webster, M. E. (1966). The purification and some properties of two different kallidinogens from human plasma. In *Hypotensive Peptides.* Edited by E. G. Erdos, N. Back, and F. Sicriteri. New York, Springer-Verlag, pp. 130-193.

Pinckard, R. N., Tanigawa, C., and Halonen, M. (1975). IgE-induced blood coagulation alterations in the rabbit: consumption of coagulation factors XII, XI, and IX in vivo. *J. Immunol., 115*:525-532.

Ratnoff, O. D. (1953). Fibrinogen and fibrin as substrates for the proteolytic enzyme of plasma. *J. Clin. Invest. 32*:473-479.

Ratnoff, O. D., and Colopy, J. E. (1955). A familial hemorrhagic trait associated with a deficiency of clot-promoting fraction of plasma. *J. Clin. Invest. 34*: 602-613.

Ratnoff, O. D., and Conley, C. L. (1951). The role of surface and of calcium in the coagulation of a globulin fraction of platelet-dependent plasma. *Bull. J. Hopkins Hospital, 89*:245-254.

Ratnoff, O. D., and Davie, E. W. (1962). The purification of activated Hageman factor (activated XII). *Biochemistry 1*:964-967.

Ratnoff, O. D., and Rosenblum, J. M. (1958). Role of Hageman factor in the initiation of clotting by glass: evidence that glass frees Hageman factor from inhibition. *Am.J. Med. 25*:160-168.

Ratnoff, O. D., Davie, E. W. and Mallett, D. L. (1961). Studies on the action of Hageman factor: Evidence that activated Hageman factor in turn activates plasma thromboplastin antecedent. *J. Clin. Invest., 40*:803-819.

Revak, S. D., Cochrane, C. G., Bouma, B. N., and Griffin, J. H. (1978). Surface and fluid phase activities of two forms of activated Hageman factor produced during contact activation of plasma. *J. Exp. Med., 147*:719-729.

Revak, S. D., Cochrane, C. G., Johnston, A., and Hugli, T. (1974). Structural changes accompanying enzymatic activation of human Hageman factor. *J. Clin. Invest., 54*:619-627.

Rocha e Silva, M., Beraldo, W. T., and Rosenfeld, G. (1949). Bradykinin a hypotensive and smooth muscle stimulating factor released from plasma globulins by snake venom and by trypsin. *Am. J. Physiol., 1567*:261-273.

Saito, H., and Ratnoff, O. D. (1974). Fitzgerald trait: An asymptomatic disorder with impaired blood coagulation, fibrinolysis, kinin generation, and generation of permeability factor of dilution. In *The Chemistry and Biology of the Kallikrein-kinin System in Health and Disease.* Edited by J. J. Pisano and K. F. Austen. Fogarty International Proceedings, No. 27. Washington, D.C., U.S. Government Printing Office, pp. 73-74.

Saito, H., Ratnoff, O. D., and Donaldson, V. H. (1968). Defective activation of clotting, fibrinolytic and permeability enhancing systems in human Fletcher trait plasma. *Circ. Res., 34*:641-651.

Saito, H., Ratnoff, O. D., Waldmann, R., and Abraham, J. P. (1975). Fitzgerald trait. Deficiency of a hitherto unrecognized agent, Fitzgerald factor, participating in surface-mediated reactions of clotting, fibrinolysis, generation of kinins and the property of diluted plasma enhancing vascular permeability (PF-dil). *J. Clin. Invest., 55*:1082-1089.

Schiffman, S., and Lee, P. (1974). Preparation, characterization, activation of a highly purified factor XI. Evidence that a hitherto unrecognized plasma activity participates in interaction of factor XI and XII. *Brit. J. Haematol., 27*:101-114.

Schiffman, S., and Lee, P. (1975). Partial purification and characterization of contact activation cofactor. *J. Clin. Invest., 56*:1082-1092.

Schiffman, S., Lee, P., and Waldmann, R. (1975). Identity of contact activation cofactor and Fitzgerald factor. *Thromb. Res., 6*:451-454.

Schiffman, S., Lee, P., Feinstein, D. I., and Pecci, R. (1977). Relationship of contact activation cofactor (CAC) procoagulant activity to kininogen. *Blood, 49*:935-945.

Schiffman, S., Rapaport, S. I., Ware, A. G., and Mehl, J. W. (1960). Separation of plasma thromboplastin antecedent (PTA) and Hageman factor (HF) from human plasma. *Proc. Soc. Exp. Biol. Med., 105*:453-454.

Schoenmakers, J. G. G., Matze, R., Haanen, C., and Zilliken, F. (1965). Hageman factor a novel sialoglycoprotein with esterase activity. *Biochem. Biophys. Acta., 101*:166-176.

Schulman, E. S., Newball, H. H., Demers, L. M., Fitzpatrick, F. A., and Adkinson, N. F., Jr. (1981). Anaphylactic release of thromboxane A_2, and prostaglandin D_2, and prostacyclin from human lung parenchyma. *Am. Rev. Respir. Dis., 124*:402-406.

Sherry, S., Alkjaersig, N., and Fletcher, A. P. (1964). Assay of urokinase preparations with synthetic substrate acetyl-l-lysine methyl ester. *J. Lab. Clin. Med., 64*:145-153.

Speer, R. J., Ridgeway, H., and Hill, J. M. (1965). Activation of human Hageman factor (XII). *Thromb. Diath. Haemorrhag., 14*:1-11.

Spragg, J., and Austen, K. F. (1971). The preparation of human kininogen. II. Further characterization of purified human kininogen. *J. Immunol., 107*: 1512-1519.

Swartz, M. J., Mitchell, H. W., Cox, D. J., and Reeck, G. R. (1977). Isolation and characterization of trypsin inhibitor from opaque-2 corn seeds. *J. Biol. Chem., 255*:7281-7284.

Ulevitch, R., and Cochrane, C. G. (1974). A direct enzymatic assay for the esterolytic activity of activated Hageman factor. *Thromb. Diath. Haemorrh., 31*:30-39.

Waldman, R., and Abraham, J. (1975). Fitzgerald factor: A heretofore unrecognized coagulation factor. *Blood, 46*:761-768.

Webster, M. E. (1968). Human plasma kallikrein, its activation and pathological role. *Fed. Proc., 27*:84-89.

Webster, M. E., and Pierce, J. W. (1961). Action of kallikreins on synthetic ester substrates. *Proc. Soc. Exp. Biol. Med., 107*:186-191.

Webster, M. E., and Pierce, J. V. (1963). The nature of the kallidins released from human plasma by kallikreins and other enzymes. *Ann. N.Y. Acad. Sci., 104*:91-105.

Webster, M. E., and Pierce, J. V. (1973). Activators of Hageman factor (Factor XII): Identification and relationship to kallikrein-kinin system. *Fed. Proc., 32*:845.

Webster, M. E., Emmart, E. W., Turner, W. A., Moriya, H., and Pierce, J. (1963). Immunological properties of the kallikreins. *Biochem. Pharmacol., 12*:511-519.

Webster, M. E., Newball, H. H., Oh-Ishi, S., Takahashi, H., Horakova, Z., Atkins, F. L., and Beaven, M. A. (1974). Release of histamine and argining esterase activity from passively sensitized human lung by ragweed antigen. *Ciencia E Cultura, 26*:372-376.

Weiss, A. S., Gallin, J. I., and Kaplan, A. P. (1974). Fletcher factor deficiency. Abnormalities of coagulation, fibrinolysis chemotactic activity and kinin generation attributable to absence of prekallikrein. *J. Clin. Invest., 53*: 622-633.

Wright, D. G., Bralove, D. A., and Gallin, J. I. (1977). The differential mobilization of human neutrophil granules: Effects of phorbol myristate acetate and ionophore A23187. *Amer. J. Pathol., 87*:273-283.

Wuepper, K. D., and Cochrane, C. G. (1971). Plasma prekallikrein: isolation, characterization, and mechanism of activation. *J. Exp. Med., 135*:1-20.

Wuepper, K. D. (1972). Biochemistry and biology of components of the plasma kinin-forming system. In *Inflammation: Mechanism and Control.* Edited by I. H. Lepow and P. A. Ward. New York, Academic Press, pp. 93-117.

Wuepper, K. D. (1973). Prekallikrein deficiency in man. *J. Exp. Med., 138*:1345-1355.

Wuepper, K. D., Miller, D. R., and Lacombe, M. J. (1975a). Flaujeac trait: Deficiency of human plasma kininogen. *J. Clin. Invest., 56*:1663-1672.

Wuepper, K. D., Miller, D. R., and Lacombe, M. J. (1975b). Flaujeac trait: Deficiency of kininogen in man. *Fed. Proc., 34*:859.

7

Proteases and Antiproteases in the Lung

AARON JANOFF and HARVEY CARP*

State University of New York
Stony Brook, New York

I. Introduction: Protease-Antiprotease Balance in the Lung

Proteases and antiproteases in the lung have received increasing attention over the past 15 years, because of growing evidence that an imbalance between proteolytic enzymes and their inhibitors may give rise to certain features of chronic obstructive lung diseases (COLD) in man. For example, many investigators have suggested that unrestrained elastolytic activity in the lung may be responsible for the alveolar deformation seen in pulmonary emphysema (for a recent review, see Kuhn and Senior, 1978). Other workers have shown that elastolytic attack

---

Present Affiliation

*University of Miami School of Medicine, Miami, Florida.

This work was supported, in part, by USPHS grant 14262 from The National Heart, Lung and Blood Institute and by grant 1143 from The Council for Tobacco Research–U.S.A., Inc. H. Carp is a Postdoctoral Fellow of The National Institute of Environment Health Sciences (grant 5-T32-07088).

also causes alterations in the conducting airways similar to those associated with chronic bronchitis (Christensen et al., 1977; Hayes and Christensen, 1978). Much of the earlier evidence favoring protease mediation of pulmonary emphysema was reviewed by Mittman (1972) and, more recently, Eriksson (1978) has reexamined the role of protease-antiprotease imbalance in COLD.

The so-called protease-pathogenesis model of COLD received its original impetus from two major and almost simultaneous discoveries. The first was the induction of experimental pulmonary emphysema by treatment of animals with elastolytic proteases. This work has recently been summarized by Karlinsky and Snider (1978). The second was the observation of a frequent association between early-onset, panacinar emphysema and genetically determined deficiencies in alpha-1 antitrypsin (Laurell and Eriksson, 1963). The latter antiprotease is the predominant endogenous regulator of leukocyte elastase activity (Ohlsson, 1978). The majority of individuals affected by COLD, however, have normal concentrations of alpha-1 antitrypsin in their circulation. The major risk factor associated with development of emphysema in this group appears to be cigarette smoking (Auerbach et al., 1972). Therefore, recent research has focussed on possible mechanisms whereby inhaled tobacco smoke may disrupt the lung's protease-antiprotease balance.

In the present chapter, we will first discuss some of the elastolytic proteases in the lung and some of the major lung antiproteases that regulate the activity of these enzymes. We will then propose potential mechanisms by which cigarette smoking could elevate the elastase "burden" of the lung and/or depress the lung's elastase-inhibitor "screen." Finally, the protease-pathogenesis model of COLD will be reexamined to show how cigarette smoking and other environmental and genetic factors might influence the balance between proteases and antiproteases in the lung.

II. Proteases in the Lung

A. Proteases of the Alveolar Macrophage

Recently, a considerably body of evidence has accumulated showing that stimulated macrophages secrete a variety of neutral proteases in cell culture systems. Protease secretion can be induced by a phagocytic challenge (Gordon et al., 1974), by nonspecific inflammatory stimuli such as intraperitoneal injection of thioglycollate (Werb and Gordon, 1975a,b), or by lymphokines secreted from thymus-derived lymphocytes after exposure to specific antigens (Wahl et al., 1975; Klimetzek and Sorg, 1977; Noguiera et al., 1977; Vassali and Reich, 1977; Gordon et al., 1978). Most of this evidence derives from studies of peritoneal exudative macrophages of mice, but secretion of elastase by mouse alveolar macrophages has also been recently demonstrated (White et al., 1977). The enzymes produced by mouse peritoneal exudative macrophages include a serine-dependent plasminogen activator with trypsin-like specificity (Unkeless et al., 1974) and a metalloenzyme with specific collagenolytic activity (Werb and Gordon, 1975a), which is secreted in proenzyme form and can be activated by trypsin or plasmin (Werb et al., 1977). Perhaps of greater interest, in the context of the present discussion, is the fact that mouse macrophages also secrete an elastolytic protease that appears to be quite different from other known mammalian elastases.

The demonstration of elastase secretion by mouse alveolar macrophages (White et al., 1977) led to the suggestion that a similar enzyme might play a role in the degradation of lung elastin in pulmonary emphysema in man. This suggestion was supported by the fact that increased numbers of macrophages occur in the centroacinar zones of asymptomatic cigarette smokers prior to the onset of significant destructive changes in their lungs (Niewoehner et al., 1974). Because of the possible role of macrophage elastase in emphysema, several studies have been undertaken recently to search for a similar enzyme in human macrophages, to isolate the enzyme, to characterize its properties and mechanism of action on elastin, and to explore the interactions of macrophage elastase with endogenous antiproteases. Progress has been made in some areas but, in others, major questions remain to be solved.

In the first place, secretion of an elastase by human macrophages is not yet clearly established. De Cremoux and his colleagues (1978) reported secretion of an elastase-like enzyme by human and monkey alveolar macrophages, and Green et al. (1979) observed elastolytic activity produced by alveolar macrophages of dogs and man. Rodriguez et al. (1977) also detected elastase secretion from cultured alveolar macrophages of human smokers, but not from those of nonsmokers. However, Hinman and co-workers (1980) showed that the hydrolysis of insoluble elastin by human alveolar macrophages is probably due to polymorphonuclear neutrophil (PMN) elastase previously sequestered in the macrophages. (These workers also detected a second enzyme in human macrophages that hydrolyzed a synthetic amide substrate of elastase and was clearly different from the PMN enzyme. However, this second enzyme was secreted in very small amounts and it failed to hydrolyze insoluble elastin. Thus, its biological significance remains to be determined.) In support of Hinman's findings, the elastolytic enzyme of human alveolar macrophages described by Green et al. (1979) closely resembles human PMN elastase (a serine protease) and differs markedly from mouse macrophage elastase (a metalloenzyme). Furthermore, there is direct evidence that human alveolar macrophages can endocytose human PMN elastase (Campbell et al., 1979). For these reasons, it is still too early to say with certainty that a true elastase is synthesized and secreted by human alveolar macrophages.

In the meantime, good progress has been made in characterizing the elastase that is synthesized and secreted by mouse macrophages. Murine macrophage elastase is a calcium-dependent metalloenzyme (Werb and Gordon, 1975b; Banda and Werb, 1979; White et al., 1980b) with a molecular weight of 21,000 to 28,000 (White et al., 1980b). Mouse macrophage elastase appears to be resistant to inhibition by human alpha-1 antitrypsin* (White et al., 1980b). Using the oxidized B chain of insulin as substrate, Kettner et al. (1981) showed that the enzyme preferentially hydrolyzed peptide bonds to which leucine contributes the amino group (the major cleavage sites being Ala-Leu and Tyr-Leu). On the basis of this latter observation, highly specific and sensitive substrates may soon become available for the murine macrophage elastase. Such agents should prove highly useful in determining if a similar enzyme is produced by human alveolar macrophages.

B. Proteases of the Polymorphonuclear Neutrophil

Unlike the macrophage, which synthesizes and secretes proteolytic enzymes upon exposure to appropriate stimuli (see above), the polymorphonuclear neutrophil (PMN) contains preformed proteases in its cytoplasmic lysosomal granules. These enzymes are discharged when the cell encounters objects to be phagocytosed or undergoes postmortem autolysis. [For a recent review on the mechanisms of lysosomal enzyme discharge by PMN, see Weissmann et al. (1980).]

Interest in the neutral proteases of the PMN was heightened among investigators of lung disease when it was observed that homogenates of human or dog PMNs could reproduce the effect of papain or purified elastolytic proteases in the production of experimental emphysema (Mass et al., 1972). A short while earlier, an elastolytic protease had in fact been demonstrated in the cytoplasmic granule fraction of these cells (Janoff, 1970; Janoff and Scherer, 1968).

The protease content of the cytoplasmic granules of human PMNs has recently been reviewed by Baggiolini and co-workers (1978). The azurophil granules of these cells contain elastase (see above), cathepsin G (which is responsible for the chymotrypsin-like activity first described in PMNs by Mounter and Atiyeh in 1960 and characterized by Rindler et al. in 1973), and a third enzyme, which (like the aforementioned two) is also a serine protease (Baggiolini et al., 1978). In addition, azurophil granules of human PMNs contain small amounts of the carboxyl protease cathepsin D (active at acid pH) as well as the thiol protease cathepsin B. Two metalloproteases are contained in the specific granules of human PMNs, of which one is the specific collagenase originally described by Lazarus et al. (1968). Thus, all four families of proteolytic enzymes (aspartic acid,

---

*See addendum (5) on p. 207.

cysteine, serine, and metallo) are represented in the two granule classes of the human PMN.

Of the various PMN proteases mentioned above, the elastase has attracted greatest attention on the part of those interested in the pathogenesis of pulmonary emphysema. Intratracheal instillations of purified preparations of human PMN elastase were shown to produce lesions in dogs (Janoff et al., 1977) and hamsters (Senior et al., 1977) resembling those of human pulmonary emphysema. Recently, a completely uniform animal model of this disease has been described, in which pure dog PMN elastase was used to induce alveolar deformation in the homologous species (Sloan et al., 1980).

Human PMN elastase is a well-characterized enzyme and it has been purified and described by many investigators (Janoff, 1973; Ohlsson and Olsson, 1974a; Schmidt and Havemann, 1974; Taylor and Crawford, 1975; Feinstein and Janoff, 1975; Baugh and Travis, 1976; Twumasi and Liener, 1977). The enzyme has a molecular weight of about 33,000 and is a glycoprotein with variably reported carbohydrate content. PMN elastase is a serine protease that is inhibited by diisopropyl fluorophosphate and by active-site-directed chloromethyl ketone inactivators of pancreatic elastase. PMN elastase hydrolyzes most synthetic substrates of pancreatic elastase, including those with high specificity for the latter enzyme, but the two proteases can be distinguished by immunologic and other criteria, as well as on the basis of their different molecular weights. Studies by Blow (1977) showed preferential cleavage of the oxidized insulin B chain at peptide bonds to which valine contributes the carboxyl group.

Unlike the alveolar macrophage, which is a normal resident of the pulmonary air spaces, the bulk of lung PMNs are normally found in the pulmonary circulation and are rarely seen invading lung interstitium or alveolar air spaces (Damiano et al., 1980; Jamuar and Cronkite, 1980). It may therefore be of interest to summarize briefly some current ideas regarding possible routes of access of PMN elastase to lung connective tissues, in the absence of overt inflammation. Cohen et al. (1979) have shown the existence of a constant, small pool of alveolar PMNs in the lungs of normal rabbits. Cohen and Batra (1980) detected increases in this pool after mild chronic irritation, as occurs with repeated sterile saline lavage. Hunninghake et al. (1980) have shown that cigarette smoking can also increase the size of the alveolar PMN pool. Although PMNs only constitute a small percent of the lavage cell population in cigarette smokers, death of these cells in the air spaces may still constitute a major source of the lung's elastase "burden," if one considers the very short life-span of PMNs in the tissues (in comparison with macrophages) and the relatively enormous elastase content of the PMN. (A single PMN contains 4-5 pg elastase, which is about three orders of magnitude greater than the total amount of elastase secreted by a murine alveolar macrophage during 48-hr in culture). Thus, a steady, albeit low, level of PMN emigration into the alveolar airspaces and subsequent release of PMN enzymes could represent a significant challenge to susceptible lung connective tissue components. Some of these components will be described in the immediately following section. Further study of PMN turnover in healthy and diseased lungs is obviously needed. Such studies may be facilitated in the future by a recently described novel method for the detection of PMN constituents in tissues (Fagerhol et al., 1980).

C. Potential Targets of Macrophage and PMN Elastases in Lung Connective Tissue

The elastase secreted by murine macrophages slowly hydrolyzes insoluble elastin, and the rate of solubilization can be markedly enhanced if the particulate substrate is first complexed with anionic detergents like sodium dodecyl sulfate (SDS) (Werb and Gordon, 1975b; White et al., 1977). Kagan and Lerch (1976) have suggested that the increased susceptibility of SDS-elastin to elastolytic attack may be due to enhancement of charge complementarity between enzyme and substrate when the latter bears negatively charged SDS ligands. Galdston (1978) has conjectured that fatty acids and other anionic lipids may similarly affect lung elastin and render it more susceptible to elastolysis by macrophage and PMN enzymes. This worker has also pointed out that serum fatty acids are elevated in some smokers. Macrophage elastase can also hydrolyze proteoglycan molecules (White and McDevitt, unpublished observations) and immunoglobulins (Banda and Werb, 1980).

Whereas little is presently known regarding the natural substrate(s) of the macrophage elastase, it is well established that a wide variety of proteins can be readily hydrolyzed by PMN elastase. In addition to solubilizing lung elastin (Janoff et al., 1972, 1977), this enzyme can attack cartilage proteoglycan (Janoff et al., 1976; Keiser et al., 1976; Barrett, 1978) and several types of collagen molecules (Starkey et al., 1977; Gadek et al., 1980a; Mainardi et al., 1980a). Types-I and -II collagen are apparently cleaved by elastase at the nonhelical, telopeptide regions of the molecules, which contain the intermolecular cross-links. Resultant depolymerization and denaturation facilitates further nonspecific proteolytic attack. By contrast, types-III and-IV collagen (the latter is present primarily in basement membranes) are cleaved by PMN elastase across the helical portion of the tropocollagen molecules, randomly in the case of type-IV collagen but at a single cleavage-site in type-III collagen. This site has been localized to a peptide bond that is only four amino acid residues away from the specific cleavage site of true mammalian collagenases (Mainardi et al., 1980b).

In addition to the foregoing structural components, a variety of functionally important molecules in the lung can be degraded by PMN elastase. These include surfactant apoprotein (King and Janoff, unpublished observations, 1977), immunoglobulins (Folds et al., 1978; Prince et al., 1979), and intermediates of the kinin, complement, fibrinolytic, and clotting cascades (for a review, see Havemann and Janoff, 1978).

In the normal lung, the foregoing targets of PMN elastase are largely protected against attack through the action of powerful endogenous inhibitors of the enzyme. Some of these inhibitors are locally produced in the lung, while others are transported into lung fluids from the circulation.

III. Antiproteases in the Lung*

A. Bronchial Mucous Proteinase Inhibitor

Human mucous secretions, including bronchial mucus, contain locally produced inhibitors of leukocyte proteases (Fritz et al., 1978). The inhibitors present in seminal plasma, cervical mucus, and bronchial secretions have been purified and appear identical in their immunological and antiprotease activities, although some differences may exist in their primary amino acid sequences (Hochstrasser, 1980). In contrast to the circulating inhibitors, the local mucous proteinase inhibitors are low molecular weight and acid stable and they are found in only trace amounts in the circulation (micrograms per decaliter).

The low molecular weight, acid-stable proteinase inhibitor present in human bronchial mucus (BMPi) was first described by Hochstrasser et al. (1972) and, later, was isolated and partly characterized by Ohlsson et al. (1977). This substance is a cationic polypeptide with a molecular weight of 10,322. It is thought to represent the major antiprotease (on a molar basis) protecting the upper, mucous-lined airways against the destructive effects of inflammatory cell proteases (Tegner, 1978). Both PMN elastase and cathepsin G are well inhibited by this agent; by contrast, macrophage elastase appears to resist inhibition by BMPi (Carp and White, unpublished observations).

The precise secretory source of BMPi in the lung is presently uncertain, although immunoperoxidase staining techniques have demonstrated its presence in the seromucous glands of tracheal and maxillary-sinus mucosa (Tegner and Ohlsson, 1977). The serous cells of bronchial mucous glands as well as goblet cells and Clara cells have been suggested as possible sources of BMPi (Franken et al., 1980). Gadek and colleagues (1980b) reported undetectable levels of BMPi in bronchioalveolar lavage fluids of humans, obtained by washing below the major airways. They suggested that BMPi is present in only small amounts in peripheral airways and that its primary function is to protect the upper airways (bronchi, trachea, and nasopharynx) against proteolytically mediated injury.

---

*See Table 1.

Table 1 Some Important Lung Antiproteases in Humans

Name	Source(s) in lung	Molecular ratio $\times 10^{-3}$	PMN protease(s) inhibited[a]	References
Bronchial mucous proteinase inhibitor	Local production by mucous epithelium	~ 10	PMN elastase and cathepsin G[b]	Hochstrasser et al., 1972; Ohlsson et al., 1977; Tegner and Ohlsson, 1977; Tegner, 1978; Fritz et al., 1978; Hochstrasser, 1980
Alpha-1 proteinase inhibitor	Plasma, lymph, alveolar macrophage	52	PMN elastase[c]	Tuttle and Westerberg, 1974; Ohlsson, 1978; Johnson and Travis, 1978; Gadek et al., 1980b
Alpha-1 antichymotrypsin	Plasma, lymph	68	PMN cathepsin G[c]	Aronson et al., 1972; Ohlsson and Akesson, 1976; Travis et al., 1978a,b; Beatty et al., 1980
Alpha-2 macroglobulin[d]	Plasma, lymph, alveolar macrophage?	725	PMN elastase and cathepsin G	Ohlsson and Olsson, 1974b; Starkey and Barret, 1977; White et al., 1980a

[a]The physiological inhibitor(s) of macrophage elastase is presently unknown.
[b]Proximal airways.
[c]Peripheral airways and alveoli.
[d]Normally present in trace amount in pulmonary secretions; concentration increases with inflammation.

B. Alpha-1 Proteinase Inhibitor (Alpha-1 Antitrypsin)

In their assessment of the relative contribution of different inhibitors to the "anti-elastase" screen of the lower respiratory tract, Gadek et al. (1980b) concluded that "alpha-1-antitrypsin is the primary anti-elastase present at the level of the alveolar structures in the normal lung." [In view of its broad inhibitory spectrum and the fact that it is the predominant endogenous regulator of leukocyte elastase activity (Ohlsson, 1978), alpha-1 antitrypsin will be referred to hereafter as alpha-1 proteinase inhibitor (α1Pi), a name originally suggested by Johnson and Travis (1976).]

Lung α1Pi is primarily derived from the circulation and is present in the alveolar lining fluids as a component of transudated interstitial lymph (Tuttle and Westerberg, 1974). Alveolar macrophages also contain the inhibitor in their cytoplasm (Cohen, 1973; Olsen et al., 1975), probably as a result of endocytosis of free α1Pi or α1Pi-protease complexes from surrounding tissue fluids. However, some recent evidence suggests that these cells may also synthesize and secrete small amounts of α1Pi (White et al., 1981).

In man, α1Pi is a glycoprotein with a molecular weight of 52,000 and it is synthesized primarily in hepatocytes. α1Pi is a relatively broad-spectrum proteinase inhibitor, but its principal physiologic role is probably the inhibition of elastase released from phagocytically active or dying PMNs throughout the body. Macrophage elastase, by contrast, resists inhibition by α1Pi (White et al., 1980b). The active-site structure of this inhibitor has recently been determined by Johnson and Travis (1978), who showed that it contains a methionine-serine peptide bond. It is apparently this bond that is attacked by elastase early in a series of reactions that rapidly leads to formation of highly stable complexes between one mole of protease and one mole of antiprotease. The high stability of this complex (which allows α1Pi to act as a "pseudo-irreversible" inhibitor) may be based on either a very low dissociation constant or on covalent bonding or tetrahedral complex formation between the enzyme's active center serine residue and a carbonyl group at the active site of the inhibitor (Moroi and Yamasaki, 1974; Cohen et al., 1977). In any event, the inhibition of elastase by α1Pi depends on the state of the methionyl residue in the inhibitor's active site, and this dependence will figure prominently in our discussion of the effects of cigarette smoking on α1Pi activity in the lung (see Sec. V.A, below).

C. Alpha-1 Antichymotrypsin

Alpha-1 antichymotrypsin (Heimburger and Haupt, 1965) is also synthesized in the liver and reaches the lung via the circulation. Like α1Pi, alpha-1 antichymotrypsin (α1AChy) is an acute phase-reactant protein, but plasma concentrations of α1AChy increase more rapidly and to higher levels following injury than do those of α1Pi. Although the normal plasma molar concentration of α1AChy is only about one-fifth that of α1Pi, the concentration of the former inhibitor may double within 8 hr after injury, whereas α1Pi elevation requires 24-48 hr to reach peak values and, even then, seldom reaches 150% of its baseline concentration (Aronsen et al., 1972). The rapid and large acute phase response of α1AChy suggests an important protective function for this agent in inflammatory reactions, and this function may be to inhibit PMN cathepsin G (the chymotrypsin-like enzyme of the azurophil granules in human PMNs) (Ohlsson and Akesson, 1976; Ohlsson, 1978; Beatty et al., 1980). In addition, other chymotrypsin-like enzymes in the lungs, for example mast cell "chymase," may be regulated by α1AChy. Further details of the properties and reactions of this inhibitor can be found in recent articles by Travis and his co-workers (Travis et al., 1978a,b).

D. Alpha-2 Macroglobulin

In contrast to the inhibitors discussed above, alpha-2 macroglobulin (α2M) posesses several highly unusual properties. This liver-synthesized molecule has the broadest enzyme inhibitory spectrum of all the circulating anti-proteases, being active against many enzymes of bacterial, plant, and animal origin (Starkey and Barrett, 1977). In addition, α2M has two combining sites for many mammalian enzymes, including PMN elastase, so that one mole of α2M can inhibit 2 mol of the PMN enzyme (Ohlsson and Olsson, 1974b). Third, α2M does not form a rigid structural complex with proteases involving covalent bonding or tetrahedral complex formation between active centers of enzyme and inhibitor. Instead, following cleavage by the enzyme of susceptible peptide bonds in the inhibitor, the latter undergoes a conformational change which "traps the protease within its confines, sterically hindering further interaction of the enzyme and its substrates" (Starkey and Barrett, 1977).* The degree of inhibition, however, is dependent on substrate size; small synthetic substrates are readily hydrolyzed and even some high molecular weight substrates can be degraded by α2M:protease complexes under certain circumstances. It may be worth noting, in the context of the present discussion, that tropoelastin, soluble elastin, and even insoluble elastin have been reported to undergo attack by α2M:elastase complexes (Galdston, 1978; Galdston and Levytska, 1978). Finally, as would be expected in view of an "endopeptidase-trapping" mechanism of inhibition, α2M is a very large molecule (725,000 in molecular weight). This last feature probably accounts for the very low molar concentrations of α2M in plasma transudates in comparison with α1Pi and α1AChy, except when inflammation with attendant increased

*Recently, however, some evidence has been obtained suggesting that α2M: protease complexes may be partly stabilized by covalent bonds. Nevertheless, these bonds do not involve the active center of the enzyme (Salvesen and Barrett, 1980). Also see addendum (2) on p. 207.

vascular permeability is present. The concentration of α2M in normal bronchoalveolar lavage fluid is often below detection limits using standard assay techniques (Warr et al., 1977; Gadek et al., 1980b). However, using more sensitive methods, White et al. (1980a) detected the synthesis and secretion of α2M by human alveolar macrophages in vitro. In addition, others have reported synthesis by embryonic lung cells (Mosher et al., 1977). Thus, α2M may still perform some alveolar defense function in the normal lung.

IV. Elevation of Lung Proteases in Smokers

Cigarette smoking has two independent but mutually reinforcing actions that could lead to protease:anti-protease imbalance in the lung. One of these, an elevation of the lung's protease "burden" will now be discussed.

Cigarette smoke appears able to recruit PMNs to the airways (Kilburn and McKenzie, 1975; Hunninghake et al., 1981). Recruitment of PMNs in smoke-exposed hamsters is dependent on both particle and gas-phase components (Kilburn and McKenzie, 1975) and can be reproduced by aerosols of formaldehyde or acrolein absorbed onto carbon grains (Kilburn and McKenzie, 1978). Human smokers have been reported to have increased numbers of circulating PMN, and the cell counts correlate with number of cigarettes smoked rather than with the severity of chronic bronchitis (Corre et al., 1971; Galdston et al., 1977). In addition to recruitment of leukocytes, smoke components also cause elastase to be released from PMNs, both by cytotoxic reactions (Janoff and Blue, 1978) and by stimulating secretion from viable cells (Eliraz et al., 1977). Finally, PMNs from emphysema patients show greater secretion of lysosomal enzymes during phagocytosis than do PMNs from normal subjects, provided that particle-free, filtered smoke solution is added to the incubation medium of the cells (Desai et al., 1978).

Recruitment of PMNs into the lungs of smokers may also be amplified by chemoattractants derived from stimulated alveolar macrophages (Hunninghake et al., 1978; Gadek et al., 1979b). Two different chemotactic factors for PMNs have been demonstrated in the culture medium of alveolar macrophages. One of these has a molecular weight of 10,000, is inactivated by trypsin, and is distinct from formylmethionyl-peptide and C_{5a} (Merril et al., 1980). The second factor has a molecular weight below 1400 and may be a product of the lipoxygenase pathway of the macrophage (Valone et al., 1979; Merril et al., 1980). Cigarette smoke appears capable of stimulating alveolar macrophages to release both of these attractants for PMNs (Hunninghake et al., 1981).

Besides attracting PMNs into the lungs (with resultant potential for PMN elastase and other proteases to induce pulmonary damage), increases in the numbers of pulmonary macrophages themselves also occur in the cigarette smoker and can add to the lung's protease "burden." In this regard, it is important to remember that murine macrophage elastase appears resistant to endogenous antiproteases (see Sec. II.A, above). Bone marrow-derived monocytes are the apparent source of the increased numbers of alveolar macrophages in smokers rather than increased mitotic activity of resident macrophages (Matulionis, 1979a,b). The effects of tobacco smoke on numbers, morphology, enzyme content, metabolic responses, and bactericidal function of alveolar macrophages have been extensively described [for a recent review see Hocking and Golde (1979)]. In addition to increased numbers of macrophages in the lungs of smokers, several laboratories have recently reported increased elastase secretion per cell by macrophages exposed to cigarette smoke, both in vivo (Rodriguez et al., 1977; White et al., 1979; Hinman et al., 1980) and in vitro (Eliraz et al., 1977; White et al., 1979). It may be interesting to consider possible mechanisms by which cigarette smoking could activate macrophages and augment their elastase secretion. One possibility is that this occurs in smokers who develop hypersensitivity to tobacco antigens and that the process is mediated via lymphokines secreted from sensitized pulmonary lymphocytes. The presence of tobacco antigens in cigarette smoke is well established (Lehrer et al., 1978; Becker et al., 1979), and immune responses to tobacco antigens have been demonstrated in some smokers (Romanski and Broda, 1977). Other macrophage products, including the proteases plasminogen activator and collagenase, can be regulated by lymphocyte products (Wahl et al., 1975; Pantalone and Page, 1975; Gordon and Cohn, 1978). Thus, variation in hypersensitivity to tobacco antigens could be one factor affecting development of emphysema among smokers.

Taken together, the foregoing results suggest that significant elevations in the "protease-burden" of the lung may occur in cigarette smokers. Increased numbers of metabolically activated alveolar macrophages may be present. There may be augmented secretion per cell of an elastase which is resistant to endogenous proteinase inhibitors. Also, smokers' macrophages may elaborate chemotactic factors for PMN and these cells, in turn, may release large amounts of preformed elastase.

A second mechanism has also been suggested, however, to account for disturbed protease:antiprotease balance in the lungs of smokers. According to this view, the "anti-elastase screen" of the respiratory tract may be functionally impaired as a result of tobacco smoke inhalation. Obviously, both elevated lung proteases and depressed antiproteases can occur simultaneously in smokers. In the following section, the effects of cigarette smoking on the activity of lung proteinase inhibitors will be covered in some detail.

V. Depression of Lung Antiproteases in Smokers

According to this view, lung antiproteases may be inactivated by oxidizing agents, present either in cigarette smoke (exogenous oxidants) and/or generated by lung cells of smokers (endogenous oxidants).

A. Oxidation Hypothesis

In an earlier part of this chapter (Sec. III.B), we briefly discussed the molecular mechanism of elastase inhibition by α1Pi and pointed out that an important early step in the process involves attack upon a methionyl-seryl bond in the active site of the inhibitor (Johnson and Travis, 1978). All subsequent steps leading to the formation of stable complexes between the protease and the antiprotease depend on recognition of this peptide bond. In their more recent work, Johnson and Travis (1979) showed that oxidation of the active-site methionine thioether side chain to methionine sulfoxide prevented attack upon the adjacent peptide bond by elastase (a prerequisite for inhibition of the enzyme). Oxidized α1Pi interacts with PMN elastase at only 1/2000th of the rate given by the native inhibitor (Beatty et al., 1980). Similar findings have been obtained with synthetic elastase substrates containing methionine in the P_1 position. Oxidation of the methionine side chain in these synthetic peptides also prevents hydrolysis of adjacent amide or ester bonds by PMN elastase (Nakajima et al., 1979).

The active site structure of BMPi is not presently known, however, oxidizable residues also appear to be present close to the reactive center of this inhibitor (Fritz, personal communication, 1979). [A closely related, low molecular weight, acid-stable inhibitor in dog submandibularis glands contains a methionyl-aspartyl bond in its elastase and chymotrypsin-directed reactive center (Hochstrasser et al., 1975)]. As might be expected, BMPi can also be inactivated by chemical oxidants in vitro (Carp and Janoff, 1980a).

Thus, oxidants in tobacco smoke and/or oxidants generated in the lungs of tobacco smokers could theoretically cause functional deficiencies in two important components of the lung's anti-elastase "screen"; namely the anti-elastase of the conducting airways (BMPi) and the anti-elastase of the lower respiratory tract (α1Pi). In the succeeding two sections, we will review some experiments that were designed to test this possibility.

B. Inactivation of Antiproteases by Oxidants in Tobacco Smoke

Demonstration of Oxidants in Tobacco Smoke

Cigarette smoke displays a wide range of free-radical-mediated activities, including peroxidation and alkylation reactions both in vitro and in vivo (Stedman,

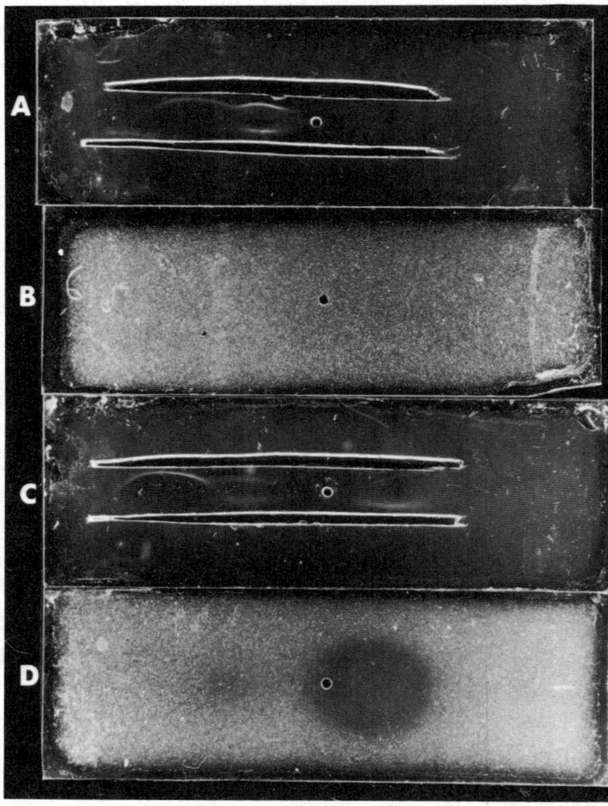

Figure 1 Electrophoretic analysis of mixtures of serum and elastase with and without cigarette smoke. (*A* and *C*) Immunoelectrophoresis in agarose gels at a pH of 8.6. Upper trough, rabbit antiserum to human α1Pi. Lower trough, rabbit antiserum to porcine elastase. (*B* and *D*) Electrophoresis in agarose gels at a pH of 8.6 containing finely divided ligament elastin. Anode to left, cathode to right. In *A* and *B*, untreated serum was incubated with elastase. Note presence of free alpha-1 proteinase inhibitor (α1Pi) migrating anodally, followed by complexes of α1Pi/elastase. No free elastase was detectable immunologically (*A*) or enzymatically (*B*). In *C* and *D*, smoke-treated serum was incubated with elastase. Note increased free α1Pi, decreased complexes of α1Pi/elastase, and cathodally migrating active uncomplexed elastase detected immunologically (*C*) and enzymatically (*D*). Note also that weak elastolytic activity was present in the region of the gel containing enzyme/inhibitor complexes (*D*). Thus, inhibition of elastase was incomplete, even in the case of complexes formed in the presence of smoke. (From Carp and Janoff, 1978.)

1968). Aqueous solutions of cigarette smoke can oxidize cysteine sulfhydryl groups, a reaction which is blocked by the free-radical scavenger, thymol (Tonge, 1962). Cigarette smoke contains approximately 2×10^{15} free radicals per puff (Pryor, 1980). Half of these appear to be polymeric phenoxy radicals related to melanin-like tobacco leaf pigments and are present in the particle fraction of cigarette smoke. They have a half-life of 10 hr on cigarette filters or in organic solvents following extraction of filters. An equal number of free radicals are found in the gas phase of cigarette smoke. These, however, are mainly oxygen-centered radicals with half-lives of 10 min in the gas phase and 1 min in aqueous solution.

In Vitro Inactivation of Antiproteases by Smoke Solutions

Freshly prepared aqueous solutions of unfractionated cigarette smoke, partly clarified by low-speed centrifugation, can suppress the elastase-inhibitory capacity of human serum (Carp and Janoff, 1978). Immunoelectrophoresis of mixtures of aqueous smoke solution, human serum, and elastase show decreased elastase:α1Pi complexes and increased free, active protease. Smoke-treated α1Pi and control α1Pi are indistinguishable with respect to total quantity, electrophoretic mobility, and antigenic behavior of the inhibitors. Figure 1 shows a typical experiment of the type just described. An important finding is that free-radical scavengers such as thymol or hydroquinone prevent the suppression of serum elastase inhibition by cigarette smoke. In the presence of such agents, elastase:α1Pi complexes can again be detected following immunoelectrophoretic analysis of enzyme-smoke-serum reaction mixtures, and free enzyme is not seen. Also, treatment of serum with model oxidants under conditions that favor selective oxidation of methionine groups leads to a similar suppression of serum elastase inhibition (Carp and Janoff, 1978; Cohen, 1979; Abrams et al., 1980). All of these observations suggest that oxidation reactions, perhaps mediated by smoke radicals, may be responsible for the observed results.

Similar findings have recently been obtained using ozone in place of cigarette smoke, as a source of oxidizing activity. "Ozone decreased the trypsin, chymotrypsin and elastase inhibitory activities of human α1Pi both in plasma and in solutions of the pure inhibitor. Total loss of pancreatic elastase inhibitory activity required 18 moles of ozone per mole of pure α1Pi. A corresponding loss of the ability to inhibit human leukocyte elastase was observed. The inactivated α1Pi contained four residues of methionine sulfoxide, in addition to oxidized tyrosine and tryptophan. Ozone inactivated α1Pi did not form normal complexes with serine proteases" (Johnson, 1980).

Inactivation of BMPi in vitro by aqueous cigarette smoke solutions has also been demonstrated (Carp and Janoff, 1980a). Thin-layer gel-immunofiltration analysis of mixtures of smoke-treated BMPi and human leukocyte elastase showed decreased elastase:BMPi complexes, increased uncomplexed BMPi, and increased free elastase (Fig. 2). Phenolic antioxidants prevented the suppression

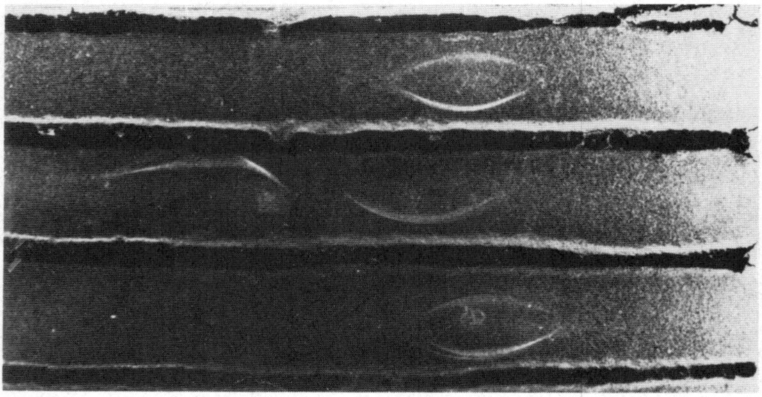

Figure 2 Analysis of mixtures of human leukocyte elastase and BMPi, under different experimental conditions, by thin-layer gel immunofiltration. Troughs 1 and 3 contain rabbit antiserum directed against human leukocyte elastase. Troughs 2 and 4 contain rabbit antibodies directed against bronchial mucous proteinase inhibitor (BMPi). The direction of filtration is from left to right. (*A*) Elastase added to untreated BMPi (control). Note the presence of BMPi: elastase complexes. Free BMPi and free elastase are not detected. (*B*) Elastase added to BMPi in the presence of aqueous smoke components. Proceeding from left to right, note free BMPi, free elastase, and absent BMPi:elastase complexes (some complexes were present, although not visible in the photograph). (*C*) Conditions identical to *B*, except that thymol was added to aqueous smoke solutions before the addition of BMPi. Note that BMPi:elastase complexes are once again present, whereas free BMPi and free elastase are not. (From Carp and Janoff, 1980a.)

of the elastase-inhibiting capacity of BMPi by cigarette smoke. In addition, treatment of BMPi with chemical oxidants caused a similar suppression of elastase-inhibition.

In Vivo Inactivation of Antiproteases by Inhaled Cigarette Smoke

Functional activity of BMPi was found to be significantly reduced in tracheal aspirates of human smokers compared with those of nonsmokers (Carp and Janoff, 1980a). The differences were unrelated to age or sex of the patients. In these studies, BMPi was partly purified from tracheal aspirates of patients undergoing elective surgery for nonpulmonary disorders (only nonpurulent aspirates were analyzed). Total BMPi content of the samples was determined immunochemically, using specific antibody, while BMPi activity was determined biochemically against trypsin or human leukocyte elastase.

Table 2 Elastase-Inhibiting Capacity (EIC) of Lung α1Pi in Rats Exposed to Cigarette Smoke Inhalation

Number of animals	Exposure (number of puffs)	EIC[a]	Decrease from control value (%)
16	0	0.59 ± 0.06	
9	3	0.42 ± 0.05	29[b]
14	6	0.36 ± 0.06	39[b]

[a]Mg pancreatic elastase inhibited/mg total α1Pi (measured immunologically) ±1 SDM in lung lavage fluid obtained 1 hr after smoke inhalation.
[b]Significantly different from control value at $P \leq 0.01$ (t test).
Source: Data from Janoff et al. (1979). Copyright 1979 by the American Association for the Advancement of Science.

Using similar techniques, it was also shown that cigarette smoke inhalation decreased α1Pi activity in the lungs of rats (Janoff et al., 1979) and in the lower respiratory tract of humans (Gadek et al., 1979a). In the former study, unadapted animals were subjected to brief exposures to inhaled, unfractionated cigarette smoke and, immediately thereafter, analysis of bronchopulmonary lavage fluids showed a significant decrease in the elastase-inhibiting capacity of immunologically measurable α1Pi. Results of one such experiment are shown in Table 2. It was also found that α1Pi activity in lavage fluids of smoke-exposed animals could be largely restored by dialyzing the fluids against reducing agents. Moreover, loss of a α1Pi activity following cigarette smoking was prevented if the test animals were first rendered tolerant to ozone. These experiments suggested that oxidation of α1Pi in the lungs of smoking animals was responsible for the loss of inhibitory activity. In the second of the two studies mentioned above, the authors determined elastase-inhibitory activity of immunologically measurable α1Pi in lavage fluids obtained from the lower respiratory tract of human smokers and nonsmokers. Both asymptomatic volunteers and patients with idiopathic pulmonary fibrosis were tested. There was about a 50% decrease in α1Pi activity of smokers' lavage fluids in both the volunteers and patients.

Thus, major anti-elastases of both the upper and lower respiratory tract appear to be inactivated by inhalation of cigarette smoke in vivo. Indirect evidence supports an oxidative pathway to account for the inactivation, however, direct proof of this is still lacking.* Oxidative mechanisms would be consistent with the demonstrated mechanism of α1Pi inactivation by chemical oxidants, as well as the established presence of oxidizing free-radical species in tobacco smoke (Pryor, 1980).

*However, see addendum (6) on p. 207.

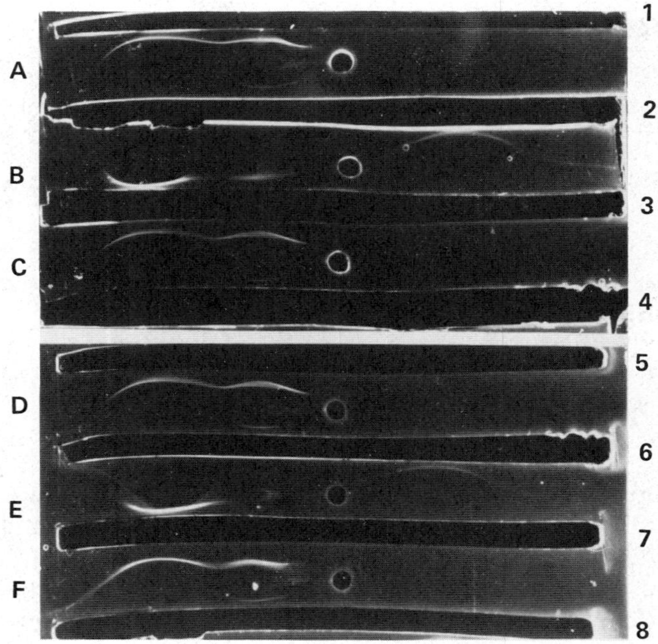

Figure 3 Immunoelectrophoretic analysis of mixtures of elastase and serum under various experimental conditions. Troughs 1, 3, 5, and 7 contain rabbit antiserum to human alpha-1 proteinase inhibitor (α1Pi). Troughs 2, 4, 6, and 8 contain rabbit antiserum to porcine pancreatic elastase. Anode to the left, cathode to the right. (*A*) Elastase added to control serum that had been incubated with unstimulated polymorphonuclear neutrophils (PMN). Note the presence of free α1Pi migrating toward the anode, followed by complexes of α1Pi and elastase. No free elastase was detected. (*B*) Elastase added to serum that had been incubated with phorbol ester-stimulated PMN. Note increased free α1Pi, decreased α1Pi:elastase complexes and uncomplexed elastase migrating toward the cathode. (*C*) Elastase added to serum that had been previously treated as in *B*, followed by treatment with dithiothreitol (a reducing agent). In contrast to *B*, no free elastase was detected and increased α1Pi:elastase complexes were present. (*D*) Elastase added to control serum that had been previously incubated with glucose oxidase as a source of hydrogen peroxide + Cl^-. Note the presence of α1Pi:elastase complexes. No free elastase was detected. (*E*) Elastase added to serum that had been previously incubated with myeloperoxidase + glucose oxidase + Cl^-. Note decreased α1Pi:elastase complexes and uncomplexed elastase migrating toward the cathode. (*F*) Elastase added to serum that had been previously treated as in *E*, followed by treatment with dithiothreitol. In contrast to *E*, no free elastase was detected and increased α1Pi:elastase complexes were present. (From Carp and Janoff, 1980b.)

Table 3 Effects of Cell-Generated Oxidants on Elastase Inhibition by Human Serum

Cell type	Phorbol myristate acetate (ng/ml)	Protective agent	Superoxide anion production (nM/1.6 × 10^6 cells)	Serum elastase-inhibition (% of control)
PMN	0	0	0	97 ± 9
PMN	1.5	0	37 ± 7	45 ± 6
PMN	1.5	SOD[a]	0	64 ± 7
PMN	1.5	HISOD[b]	36 ± 8	42 ± 6
PMN	1.5	CAT[c]	35 ± 6	89 ± 5
PMN	1.5	HICAT	36 ± 7	47 ± 5
PMN	1.5	NaN_3[d]	35 ± 7	75 ± 6
PMN (CGD)[e]	1.5	0	0	97 ± 9
Monocyte	0	0	2 ± 1	95 ± 5
Monocyte	1.5	0	22 ± 5	52 ± 8
Monocyte	1.5	SOD	0	70 ± 6
Monocyte	1.5	CAT	21 ± 5	95 ± 7
Monocyte	1.5	NaN_3	22 ± 4	77 ± 6
Monocyte (CGD)	1.5	0	0	96 ± 8
Alveolar macrophage	0	0	4 ± 2	90 ± 11
Alveolar macrophage	100	0	18 ± 4	55 ± 5

[a]Superoxide dismutase, 400 U/ml.
[b]Heat-inactivated superoxide dismutase.
[c]Catalase, 1500 U/ml.
[d]Sodium azide, 0.3 mM.
[e]Chronic granulomatous disease.
Source: Data from Carp and Janoff (1980b).

C. Inactivation of Antiproteases by Cell-Generated Oxidants

Chronic cigarette smoking not only increases the numbers of PMN leukocytes and macrophages in the alveoli, but it also activates these cells (Hocking and Golde, 1979). Among the metabolic pathways that are stimulated in smokers' macrophages are those which generate oxygen-free radicals and other activated species of oxygen (Holian and Daniele, 1979; Hoidal et al., 1980). It would therefore be of interest to know if such agents as superoxide anion, hydrogen peroxide, and products of the interaction of these two substances, as well as the myeloperoxidase-peroxide-halide oxidizing system of PMN and monocytes can inactivate lung antiproteases through oxidative reactions.

Carp and Janoff (1979) showed that human PMN, phagocytosing opsonized antigen-antibody complexes adsorbed to the outer surface of dialysis membranes, produce diffusable substances that are capable of suppressing the elastase-inhibiting capacity of whole serum or purified α1Pi present within the membrane-bounded compartment. Superoxide dismutase (which catalyzes the dismutation of superoxide anion to hydrogen peroxide), catalase (which breaks down hydrogen peroxide to water and oxygen), and mannitol (a scavenger of hydroxyl radical) partly protected α1Pi against inactivation, suggesting that "respiratory burst" oxidants derived from stimulated PMN were responsible for the observed effects. An artificial superoxide radical-generating system, involving xanthine and xanthine oxidase, could be substituted for phagocytosing PMN with similar results. More recently, the same authors (Carp and Janoff, 1980b) extended their observations to human mononuclear phagocytes (blood monocytes and alveolar macrophages) in addition to PMN, and they activated the cells with a nonphagocytic stimulus (cell membrane excitation with phorbol myristate acetate). Such stimulated cells also released reactive oxygen species able to suppress elastase-inhibition by human serum. Immunoelectrophoretic analysis of the enzyme-serum reaction mixtures showed decreased α1Pi:elastase complexes and free elastase. Treatment of phagocyte-inactivated serum with dithiothreitol (a reducing agent) resulted in significant recovery of inhibitory activity, suggesting that α1Pi had been oxidatively inactivated. (Typical results are shown in Fig. 3). Again, superoxide dismutase and catalase were partly protective. PMN and monocytes from a patient with chronic granulomatous disease, as expected, failed to produce detectable levels of superoxide anion following stimulation with phorbol ester and these cells also failed to suppress serum elastase inhibition. Some of the foregoing results are summarized in Table 3.

Matheson et al. (1979) demonstrated the inactivation of α1Pi by purified PMN myeloperoxidase. [This enzyme, along with hydrogen peroxide as cofactor, forms powerful oxidants from chloride or iodide anions. The halides (converted to hypochlorous acid and iodine, respectively) appear to serve as the ultimate oxidants in myeloperoxidase-catalyzed reactions.] Carp and Janoff (1980b) confirmed Matheson's finding with purified enzyme (see Fig. 3) and they also implicated myeloperoxidase secretion in the inactivation of α1Pi by phagocytosing PMN (Carp and Janoff, 1979) and by PMN and monocytes stimulated with phorbol ester (Carp and Janoff, 1980b). They showed that azide (an inhibitor of myeloperoxidase and other heme enzymes) partly protected serum elastase-inhibition against inactivation by the phagocytes (Table 3). Carp and Janoff (1980a) also demonstrated inactivation of BMPi by myeloperoxidase acting together with hydrogen peroxide and chloride anion.

Thus, endogenous oxidants generated by metabolically stimulated PMN and macrophages in the lungs of cigarette smokers and oxidants present in cigarette smoke itself may cause functional decreases in the activity of elastase-inhibitors such as BMPi and α1Pi. These effects of smoking on antiproteases may further strain the maintenance of protease:antiprotease balance in the lung. In the next and final section of this chapter we will reassess the protease-pathogenesis model of chronic obstructive lung disease in light of the foregoing observations.

VI. Conclusions and Speculations

A. The Protease-Pathogenesis Model Revisited.

The major hypotheses put forward in this chapter can now be integrated and summarized. Pulmonary emphysema in smokers may result from an *acquired* imbalance in protease:antiprotease levels in the lung. The disease in smokers would thus be distinct in its etiology from emphysema associated with α1Pi deficiency, in which the protease:antiprotease imbalance is *genetic* in origin. Still, both forms of the disease would share a common pathogenetic mechanism, namely, destruction of alveolar septa by unrestrained proteases released from pulmonary neutrophils and macrophages. The acquired imbalance in lung protease:antiprotease levels in cigarette smokers could result from two simultaneous actions of inhaled tobacco smoke. First, free radicals in smoke may decrease the activity of lung antiproteases directly, by oxidation of susceptible methionyl residues in or near the enzyme-combining sites of the inhibitors, and/or smoking may act indirectly by stimulating production of oxidants by lung cells. Second, smoking could cause a simultaneous increase in the activity of lung proteases by stimulating the migration of neutrophils and monocytes into this organ and activating their protease-secreting functions. Since a chymotrypsin-like serine protease in the cell membrane is thought to activate formation of oxygen-derived free radicals by neutrophils and macrophages (Kitagawa et al., 1980), small decreases in local antiprotease function or increases in protease activity could stimulate oxidant generation by these cells and lead to further inactivation of lung antiproteases. In effect, this would constitute an amplification loop in the anti-

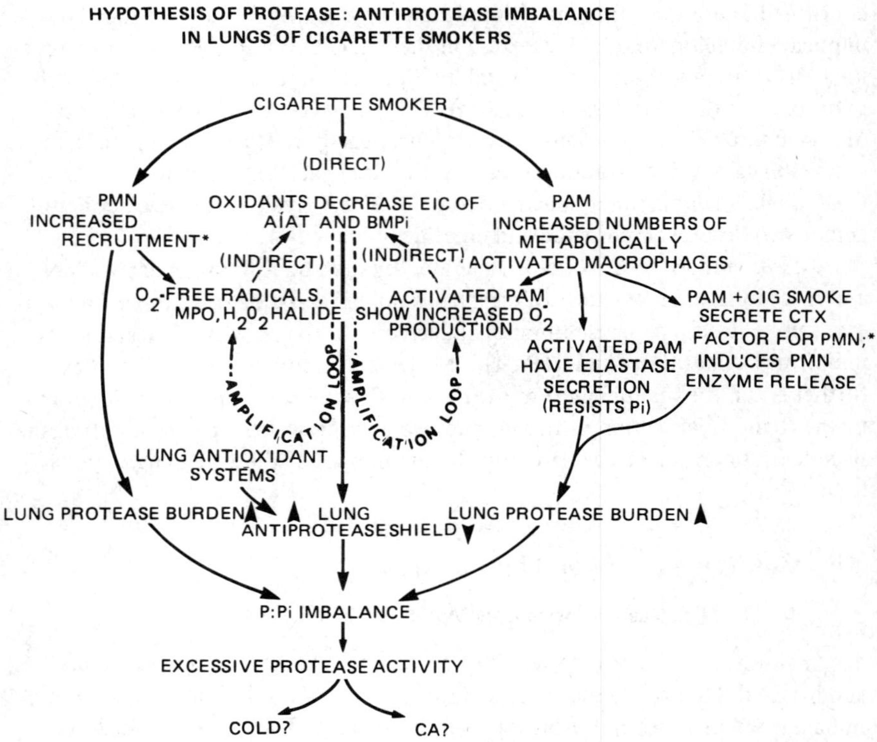

Figure 4 The protease-pathogenesis model revisited. Figure symbols: PMN, polymorphonuclear neutrophil; PAM, pulmonary alveolar macrophage: EIC, elastase inhibitory capacity; A1AT, alpha-1 antitrypsin (alpha-1 proteinase inhibitor); BMPi, bronchial mucous proteinase inhibitor; MPO, myeloperoxidase; O_2^- superoxide radical; CTX, chemotactic; P, protease; Pi, proteinase inhibitor; ▲, increase; ▼ , decrease; COLD, chronic obstructive lung disease; CA, cancer. See text for fuller description. (From Janoff et al., 1980.)

protease inactivating system. Lung antioxidants (catalase, superoxide dismutase, the glutathione peroxidase-glutathione reductase-glucose-6-phosphate dehydrogenase system) may also have important effects on protease:antiprotease balance. The foregoing pathways are schematically depicted in Figure 4.

One feature of chronic obstructive lung disease that this hypothesis may help to account for is the difference in lung pathology observed in smokers as opposed to α1Pi-deficient patients. Subjects in the latter category may develop pulmonary emphysema with little chronic bronchitis, whereas chronic obstructive lung disease in smokers is usually a mixture of destructive changes in respiratory units (emphysema) and airway inflammation plus mucous gland hyperplasia (bronchitis). One explanation for this difference may be that nonsmoking, α1Pi-deficient individuals suffer diminished antiprotease levels primarily in respiratory units which depend almost entirely on α1Pi for antiprotease defense. By contrast, chronic smokers may suffer acquired decreases in antiprotease activity in both major lung compartments (conducting airways and respiratory units) as a result of oxidant-inactivation of both BMPi and α1Pi. Another important anatomical difference is that in patients with α1Pi deficiency the emphysema is usually panacinar in form, whereas emphysema in smokers is typically centroacinar. This may occur because, in α1Pi deficiency, the entire respiratory unit is deprived of inhibitor and is therefore subject to destruction by enzymes present throughout the lung parenchyma (hence a panacinar lesion). By contrast, in the smoker "noxious gases would tend to concentrate and indeed have their first impact on the alveoli adjacent to respiratory bronchioles" (Dunnil, 1979). Thus, antiprotease inactivation and neutrophil or macrophage activation would be localized to this zone, leading to a centroacinar lesion.

B. The Alveolar Macrophage: On Which Side?

At present, the effects of alveolar macrophages on the equilibrium between lung proteases and antiproteases are not well understood. It may therefore be worthwhile to restate some of the points raised earlier, regarding functions of this cell, and to indicate which functions might promote an imbalance between lung proteases and antiproteases and which might favor the opposite. Thus, on the one hand, mouse macrophages secrete an elastase which is unusual in its ability to withstand endogenous antiproteases important to lung defense, such as α1Pi and BMPi. Stimulated macrophages also secrete chemotactic factors for PMNs. Furthermore, activated macrophages generate increased amounts of oxygen free-radicals capable of inactivating proteinase inhibitors. The numbers of alveolar macrophages in the lungs of smokers are greater than in nonsmokers, and the earliest concentration of these cells occurs in the centroacinar zone where septal destruction often begins. These, then, are some of the factors that cast the macrophage in the role of a "disruptor" of protease:antiprotease balance in the lung.

On the other hand, it is not yet proven with certainty that human alveolar macrophages (like their counterparts in murine species) secrete a true elastase* (see Sec. II.A, above). Some evidence favors the view that the elastolytic activity of the human alveolar macrophage is due, in reality, to PMN elastase previously sequestered within the cytoplasm of these cells (reviewed in Sec. II.A). Moreover, whatever the source of the macrophage activity, it is trivial in amount by comparison with PMN elastase content. The fact that macrophages have specific receptors for uptake of PMN elastase as well as elastase:inhibitor complexes

---

*However, see addendum (5) on p. 207 (Gadek et al., 1981).

(Campbell et al., 1979) suggests that these cells may exert a positive effect on lung protease:antiprotease balance by removing enzyme liberated from neutrophils. The increased numbers and centroacinar accumulation of macrophages in smokers' lungs may therefore, in reality, reflect their defensive function. Finally, recent demonstrations of α2M secretion (White et al., 1980a) and α1Pi secretion (White et al., 1981) by alveolar macrophages lend further support to a defensive role for these cells. It will be important to resolve this question if we are to identify the pathogenetic determinants operating in chronic obstructive lung disease.

C. Other Genetic and Environmental Factors That May Affect Protease: Antiprotease Balance

Not all smokers develop COLD, and those that do develop the disease at different rates. Depression of lung antiproteases by oxidants in inhaled smoke may be necessary for development of COLD but, by itself, this appears not to be sufficient. Thus, if the hypothesis is correct that disturbance of lung protease: antiprotease balance caused by smoking underlies the development of COLD in smokers, other factors (genetic and/or environmental) must also influence the risk of disease and its rate of progression. This can be surmised from the fact that although lung α1Pi is markedly decreased in activity in smokers (in comparison with nonsmoking controls), a correlation cannot be demonstrated between the amount of α1Pi inactivated and the severity of airflow obstruction (Carp, Hoidal, and Janoff, unpublished observations).

What other factors, then, may influence the eventual risk of COLD in the smoker? We can speculate on some of the possibilities. First, genetic factors could play a role and might include genetically induced variations in the activity of lung antioxidant enzymes or genetically determined differences in the immunologic response to smoke antigens. Additional variables might involve differences within the M genotype of α1Pi, affecting its susceptibility to oxidation, or variations in the efficiency of connective tissue repair mechanisms in the lung. In addition to genetic factors, a number of environmental agents may affect lung protease:antiprotease balance in the smoker. For example, inhalation of other oxidants such as ozone (Johnson, 1980), photolytically activated automobile emissions, the oxides of sulfur and nitrogen, and other urban or industrial air pollutants could play an exacerbating role, as could inadequate dietary intake of antioxidants (Chow, 1979). Additional aspects of the complex and multifactorial epidemiology of COLD have been discussed recently by Cohen (1980).

D. Future Perspectives in Prevention of COLD

Future discoveries may make it possible to reduce the source of oxidizing free radicals in cigarette smoke. Failing that, it may be possible to manipulate lung antioxidant defenses in order to diminish risks associated with cigarette smoking, or to develop safe, synthetic antiproteases to reinforce elastase inhibition in heavy smokers. Such agents should not contain methionine or other readily oxidized residues in their enzyme-combining sites. Finally, the same mechanism involved in disturbance of protease: antiprotease balance in subjects with chronic obstructive lung disease could also play a role in the pathogenesis of lung cancer in the smoker (see Fig. 4). This possibility is supported by the observation that antiproteases suppress initiation, promotion, and spread of tumors (Rossman and Troll, 1980). These questions represent some additional goals for future research in this area.

References

Abrams, W. R., Eliraz, A., Kimbel, P., and Weinbaum, G. (1980). The effect of the oxidizing agents chloramine-T and cigarette smoke on dog serum proteinase inhibitor(s). *Exp. Lung Res., 1*:211-223.

Aronsen, K. F., Ekelund, G., Kindmark, C. O., and Laurell, C. B. (1972). Sequential changes of plasma proteins after surgical trauma. *Scand. J. Clin. Lab. Invest., 29* (Suppl. 124):127-136.

Auerbach, O., Hammond, E. C., Garfinkel, L., and Benante, C. (1972). Relation of smoking and age to emphysema. Whole lung section study. *New Engl. J. Med., 286*:853-860.

Baggiolini, M., Bretz, U., Dewald, B., and Feigensen, M. E. (1978). The polymorphonuclear leukocyte. *Agents Actions, 8*:3-10.

Banda, M. J., and Werb, Z. (1979). Purification and characterization of macrophage elastase. *Fed. Proc., 38*1339 (Abstract).

Banda, M. J., and Werb, Z. (1980). Macrophage elastase degradation of immunoglobulins regulates binding to macrophage Fc receptors. *Fed. Proc., 39*: 799 (Abstract).

Barrett, A. J. (1978). The possible role of neutrophil proteinases in damage to articular cartilage. *Agents Actions, 8*:11-18.

Baugh, R. J., and Travis, J. (1976). Human leukocyte granule elastase: Rapid isolation and characterization. *Biochemistry, 15*:836-841.

Beatty, K., Bieth, J., and Travis, J. (1980). Kinetics of association of serine proteinases with native and oxidized α-1 proteinase inhibitor and α-1-antichymotrypsin. *J. Biol. Chem., 255*:3931-3934.

Becker, C. G., Levi, R., and Zavecz, J. (1979). Induction of IgE antibodies to antigen isolated from tobacco leaves and from cigarette smoke condensate. *Am. J. Pathol., 96*:249-255.

Blow, A. M. J. (1977). Action of human lysosomal elastase on the oxidized B chain of insulin. *Biochem. J., 161*:13-16.

Campbell, E. J., White, R. R., Senior, R. M., Rodriguez, R. J., and Kuhn, C.

(1979). Receptor-mediated binding and internalization of leukocyte elastase by alveolar macrophages *in vitro. J. Clin. Invest., 64*:824-833.

Carp, H., and Janoff, A. (1978). Possible mechanisms of emphysema in smokers. In vitro suppression of serum elastase inhibitory capacity by fresh cigarette smoke and its prevention by antioxidants. *Am. Rev. Respir. Dis., 118*: 617-621.

Carp, H., and Janoff, A. (1979). In vitro suppression of serum elastase-inhibitory capacity by reactive oxygen species generated by phagocytosing polymorphonuclear leukocytes. *J. Clin. Invest., 63*:793-797.

Carp, H., and Janoff, A. (1980a). Inactivation of bronchial mucous proteinase inhibitor by cigarette smoke and phagocyte-derived oxidants. *Exp. Lung Res., 1*:225-237.

Carp, H., and Janoff, A. (1980b). Potential mediator of inflammation. Phagocyte-derived oxidants suppress the elastase-inhibitory capacity of alpha 1-proteinase inhibitor *in vitro. J. Clin. Invest., 66*:987-995.

Chow, C. K. (1979). Nutritional influence on cellular antioxidant defense system. *Am. J. Clin. Nutr., 32*:1066-1081.

Christensen, T. G., Korthy, A. L., Snider, G. L., and Hayes, J. A. (1977). Irreversible bronchial goblet cell metaplasia in hamsters with elastase-induced panacinar emphysema. *J. Clin. Invest., 59*:397-404.

Cohen, A. B. (1973). Interrelationships between the human alveolar macrophage and alpha 1-antitrypsin. *J. Clin. Invest., 52*:2793-2799.

Cohen, A. B. (1979). The effects in vivo and in vitro of oxidative damage to purified alpha 1-antitrypsin and to the enzyme-inhibiting activity of plasma. *Am. Rev. Respir. Dis., 119*:953-960.

Cohen, B. H. (1980). Chronic obstructive pulmonary disease-a challenge in genetic epidemiology. *Am. J. Epidemiol., 112*:274-288.

Cohen, A. B., and Batra, G. K. (1980). Bronchoscopy and lung lavage induced bilateral pulmonary neutrophil influx and blood leukocytosis in dogs and monkeys. *Am. Rev. Respir. Dis., 122*:239-247.

Cohen, A. B., Gruenke, L. D., Craig, J. C., Geczy, D. (1977). Specific lysine labeling by $^{18}OH^-$ during alkaline cleavage of the α-1-antitrypisn-trypsin complex. *Proc. Natl. Acad. Sci. U.S.A., 74*:4311-4314.

Cohen, A. B., Batra, G., Petersen, R., Podany, J., and Nguyen, D. (1979). The size of the pool of alveolar neutrophils in normal rabbit lungs. *J. Appl. Physiol., 47*:440-444.

Corre, F., Lellouch, J., and Schwarz, D. (1971). Smoking and leukocyte counts. *Lancet, 2*:632-634.

Damiano, V. V., Cohen, A., Tsang, A. L., Batra, G., and Petersen, R. (1980). A morphologic study of the influx of neutrophils into dog lung alveoli after lavage with sterile saline. *Am. J. Pathol., 100*:349-354.

DeCremoux, H., Hornebeck, W., Jaurand, M., Bignon, J., and Robert, L. (1978). Partial characterization of an elastase-like enzyme secreted by human and monkey alveolar macrophages. *J. Pathol., 125*:171-177.

Desai, R., Baum, H., Bellamy, D., and Hutchison, D. C. S. (1978). The induction of lysosomal enzyme release from leukocytes of normal and emphysematous subjects and the effects of cigarette smoke. *Clin. Sci. Mol. Pathol., 54*:15p (Abstract).

Dunnill, M. S. (1979). Aetiology of emphysema. *Bull. Eur. Physiopathol., Respir., 15*:1015-1029.

Eliraz, A., Kimbel, P., and Weinbaum, G. (1977). Canine alveolar macrophage and neutrophil exposure to cigarette smoke: Regulation of elastase secretion. *Chest, 72*:239 (Abstract).

Eriksson, S. (1978). Proteases and protease inhibitors in chronic obstructive lung disease. *Acta Med. Scand., 203*:449-455.

Fagerhol, M. K., Dale, I., and Andersson, T. (1980). Release and quantitation of a leukocyte derived protein (L1). *Scand. J. Haematol., 24*:393-398.

Feinstein, G., and Janoff, A. (1975). A rapid method of purification of human granulocyte cationic neutral proteases: Purification and further characterization of human granulocyte elastase. *Biochim. Biophys. Acta., 403*: 493-505.

Folds, J. D., Prince, H. E., and Spitznagel, J. K. (1978). Limited cleavage of human immunoglobulins by elastase of human neutrophil polymorphonuclear granulocytes: possible modulator of immune complex disease. *Lab. Invest., 39*:313-321.

Franken, C., Kramps, J. A., Meyer, C. J. C. M., and Dijkman, J. H. (1980). Localization of the low molecular weight proteinase inhibitor in the respiratory tract. In *Biochemistry, Pathology and Genetics of Pulmonary Emphysema.* Edited by P. Sadoul and J. Bignon. Paris, Pergamon Press, 16 (Suppl):231-236.

Fritz, H., Schiessler, H., and Geiger, R. (1978). Naturally occurring low molecular weight inhibitors of neutral proteinases from PMN-granulocytes and of kallikreins. *Agents Actions, 8*:57-64.

Gadek, J. E., Fells, G. A., Crystal, R. G. (1979a). Cigarette smoking induces functional antiprotease deficiency in the lower respiratory tract of humans *Science, 206*:1315-1316.

Gadek, J. E., Fells, G. A., Wright, D. G., and Crystal, R. G. (1980a). Human neutrophil elastase functions as a type III collagen collagenase. *Biochem. Biophys. Res. Commun., 95*:1815-1822.

Gadek, J., Fells, G., Zimmerman, R., and Crystal, R. (1980b). The antielastase screen of the human lower respiratory tract: An assessment of the alpha 1-antitrypsin hypothesis. *Am. Rev. Respir. Dis., 121*:341 (Abstract).

Gadek, J., Fells, G., Hunninghake, G., Zimmerman, R., and Crystal, R. (1979b). Alveolar macrophage-neutrophil interaction: A role for inflammatory cell cooperation in the disruption of lung connective tissue. *Clin. Res., 27*: 397a (Abstract).

Galdston, M. (1978). Enhanced activity of human neutrophil elastase complexed to alpha 2-macroglobulin in serum of alpha 1-antitrypsin deficient individuals. In *Neutral Proteases of Human Polymorphonuclear Leukocytes.* Edited by K. Havemann and A. Janoff, Baltimore, Urban and Schwarzenberg, pp. 191-194.

Galdston, M., and Levytska, V. (1978). Enhanced proteolysis of ^{3}H-labeled insoluble elastin by human neutrophil elastase bound to alpha 2-macroglobulin in MM and ZZ (Pi) phenotype sera for alpha 1-antitrypsin. *Am. Rev. Respir. Dis., 117*:117 (Abstract).

Galdston, M., Melnick, E. L., Goldring, R. M., Levytska, V., Curasi, C. A., and Davis, A. L. (1977). Interactions of neutrophil elastase, serum trypsin inhibitory activity and smoking history as risk factors for chronic obstructive pulmonary disease in patients with MM, MZ and ZZ phenotype for alpha 1-antitrypsin. *Am. Rev. Respir. Dis., 116*:837-846.

Gordon, S., and Cohn, Z. (1978). Bacile Calmette-Guerin infections in the mouse. Regulation of macrophage plasminogen activator by T lymphocytes and specific antigens. *J. Exp. Med., 147*:1175-1188.

Gordon, S., Newman, W., and Bloom, B. (1978). Macrophage proteases and rheumatic diseases: Regulation of plasminogen activator by thymus-derived lymphocytes. *Agents Actions, 8*:19-26.

Gordon, S., Unkeless, J. C., and Cohn, Z. A. (1974). Induction of macrophage plasminogen activator by endotoxin stimulation and phagocytosis. Evidence for a two-stage process. *J. Exp. Med., 140*:995-1010.

Green, M. R., Lin, J. S., Berman, L. B., Osman, M. M., Cerreta, J. M., Mandl, I., and Turino, G. M. (1979). Elastolytic activity of alveolar macrophages in normal dogs and human subjects. *J. Lab. Clin. Med., 94*:549-562.

Havemann, K., and Janoff, A. (Editors) (1978). *Neutral Proteases of Human Polymorphonuclear Leukocytes.* Baltimore, Urban and Schwarzenberg, 468 pp.

Hayes, J. A., and Christensen, T. G. (1978). Bronchial mucous hypersecretion induced by elastase in hamsters: Ultrastructural appearances. *J. Pathol., 125*:25-31.

Heimburger, M., and Haupt, H. (1965). Karacterisierung von Alpha 1-x-Glycoprotein als Chymotrypsininhibitor des Human-plasma. *Clin. Chim. Acta., 12*:116-118.

Hinman, L. M., Stevens, C. A., Matthay, R. A., and Gee, J. B. L. (1980). Elastase and lysozyme activities in human alveolar macrophages. Effects of cigarette smoking. *Am. Rev. Respir. Dis., 121*:263-271.

Hochstrasser, K. (1980). Low molecular weight proteinase inhibitors in the respiratory tract. Biochemistry and function. In *Biochemistry, Pathology and Genetics of Pulmonary Emphysema.* Edited by P. Sadoul and J. Bignon. Paris, Pergamon Press, 16 (Suppl.):223-230.

Hochstrasser, K., Bretzel, G., Wachter, E., and Heindl, S. (1975). The amino acid sequence of the double-headed proteinase inhibitor from canine submandibularis glands. *Hoppe-Seyler's Z. Physiol. Chem., 356*:1865-1877.

Hochstrasser, K., Reichert, R., Schwarz, S., and Werle, E. (1972). Isolierung und Characterisierung eines Proteaseninhibitors aus menschlichem Bronchialsekret. *Hoppe Seyler's Z. Physiol. Chem., 353*:221-226.

Hocking, W. G., and Golde, D. W. (1979). The pulmonary alveolar macrophage. *New Engl. J. Med., 301*:639-645.

Hoidal, J. R., Fox, R. B., LeMarbe, P. A., Takiff, H. E., and Repine, J. E. (1980). Oxidative metabolism of alveolar macrophages from young asymptomatic cigarette smokers. Increased superoxide anion release and its potential consequences. *Chest, 77*:270S.

Holian, A., and Daniele, R. (1979). Stimulation of oxygen consumption and superoxide anion production in pulmonary macrophages by N-formyl methionyl peptides. *FEBS Letters, 108*:47-50.

Hunninghake, G., Gadek, J., and Crystal, R. (1980). Mechanism by which smoke attracts polymorphonuclear leukocytes to lung. *Chest, 77*:273-276.

Hunninghake, J. W., Gallin, J. I., and Fauci, A. S. (1978). Immunological reactivity in the lung: The *in vivo* and *in vitro* generation of a neutrophil chemotactic factor by alveolar macrophages. *Am. Rev. Respir. Dis., 117*:15-23.

Hunninghake, G. W., Szapiel, S. V., and Crystal, R. G. (1981). Cigarette smoking and lung destruction: Accumulation of neutrophils in the lungs of smokers. Ms. submitted for publication.

Jamuar, M. P., and Cronkite, E. P. (1980). The fate of blood granulocytes. *Exp. Hematol., 8*:884-894.

Janoff, A. (1970). Mediators of tissue damage in leukocyte lysosomes: X. Further studies on human granulocyte elastase. *Lab. Invest., 22*:228-236.

Janoff, A. (1973). Purification of human granulocyte elastase by affinity chromatography. *Lab. Invest., 29*:458-464.

Janoff, A., and Blue, M. L. (1978). Possible mechanisms of emphysema in cigarette smokers. Release of elastase from human polymorphonuclear leukocytes by cigarette smoke condensate in vitro. *Am. Rev. Respir. Dis., 117*: 317-325.

Janoff, A., and Scherer, J. (1968). Mediators of inflammation in leukocyte lysosomes: IX. Elastinolytic activity in granules of human polymorphonuclear leukocytes. *J. Exp. Med., 128*:1137-1155.

Janoff, A., Carp, H., and Lee, D. K. (1980). Inactivation of alpha 1-proteinase inhibitor by cigarette smoke *in vitro* and *in vivo. Bull. Europ. Pathophysiol. Respir., 16* (Suppl.):321-338.

Janoff, A., Carp, H., Lee, D. K., and Drew, R. T. (1979). Cigarette smoke inhalation decreases α 1-antitrypsin activity in rat lung. *Science, 206*:1313-1314.

Janoff, A., Feinstein, G., Malemud, C. J., and Elias, J. M. (1976). Degradation of cartilage proteoglycan by human leukocyte granule neutral proteases—a model of joint injury. I. Penetration of enzyme into rabbit articular cartilage and release of $^{35}SO_4$-labelled material from the tissue. *J. Clin. Invest., 57*:615-624.

Janoff, A., Sandhaus, R. A., Hospelhorn, V. D., and Rosenberg, R. (1972). Digestion of lung proteins by human leukocyte granules *in vitro. Proc. Soc. Exp. Biol. Med., 140*:516-519.

Janoff, A., Sloan, B., Weinbaum, G., Damiano, V., Sandhaus, R. A., Elias, J., and Kimbel, P. (1977). Experimental emphysema induced with purified human neutrophil elastase: Tissue localization of the instilled protease. *Am. Rev. Respir. Dis. 115*:461-478.

Johnson, D. A. (1980). Ozone inactivation of human α 1-proteinase inhibitor. *Am. Rev. Respir. Dis., 121*:1031-1038.

Johnson, D., and Travis, J. (1976). Human alpha 1-proteinase inhibitor mechanism of action: evidence for activation by limited proteolysis. *Biochem. Biophys. Res. Commun., 72*:33-39.

Johnson, D., and Travis, J. (1978). Structural evidence for methionine at the reactive site of human alpha 1-proteinase inhibitor. *J. Biol. Chem., 253*:7142-7144.

Johnson, D., and Travis, J. (1979). The oxidative inactivation of human alpha-1-proteinase inhibitor. Further evidence for methionine at the reactive center. *J. Biol. Chem., 254*:4022-4026.

Kagan, H. M., and Lerch, R. M. (1976). Amidated carboxyl groups in elastin. *Biochim. Biophys. Acta., 434*:223-232.

Karlinsky, J. B., and Snider, G. L. (1978). Animal models of emphysema. *Am. Rev. Respir. Dis., 117*:1109-1133.

Keiser, H., Greenwald, R. A., Feinstein, G., and Janoff, A. (1976). Degradation of cartilage proteoglycan by human leukocyte granule neutral proteases—a model of joint injury. II. Degradation of isolated bovine nasal cartilage proteoglycan. *J. Clin. Invest., 57*:625-632.

Kettner, C., Shaw, E., White, R., and Janoff, A. (1981). The specificity of macrophage elastase on the insulin B-chain. *Biochem. J.* (In Press).

Kilburn, K. H., and McKenzie, W. (1975). Leukocyte recruitment to airways by cigarette smoke and particle phase in contrast to cytotoxicity of vapor. *Science, 189*:634-637.

Kilburn, K. H., and McKenzie, W. (1978). Leukocyte recruitment to airways by aldehyde-carbon combinations that mimic cigarette smoke. *Lab. Invest., 38*:134-142.

Kitagawa, S., Takaku, F., and Sakamoto, S. (1980). Evidence that proteases are involved in superoxide production by human PMN leukocytes and monocytes. *J. Clin. Invest., 65*:74-81.

Klimetzek, V., and Sorg, C. (1977). Lymphokine-induced secretion of plasminogen activator by murine macrophages. *Eur. J. Immunol., 7*:185-187.

Kuhn, C., and Senior, R. M. (1978). The role of elastase in the development of emphysema. *Lung, 155*:185-197.

Laurell, C. B., and Eriksson, S. (1963). The electrophoretic alpha 1-globulin pattern of serum in alpha-1-antitrypsin deficiency. *Scand. J. Clin. Invest., 15*:132-140.

Lazarus, G. S., Daniels, J. R., Brown, R. S., Bladen, H. A., and Fullmer, H. M. (1968). Degradation of collagen by human granulocyte collagenolytic system. *J. Clin. Invest., 47*:2622-2629.

Lehrer, S. B., Wilson, M. R., and Salvaggio, J. E. (1978). Immunogenic properties of tobacco smoke. *J. Allergy Clin. Immunol., 62*:368-370.

Mainardi, C. L., Dixit, S. N., and Kang, A. H. (1980a). Degradation of type IV (basement membrane) collagen by a proteinase isolated from human polymorphonuclear leukocyte granules. *J. Biol. Chem., 255*:5435-5441.

Mainardi, C. L., Hasty, D. L., Sayer, J. M., and Kang, A. H. (1980b). Specific cleavage of human type III collagen by human polymorphonuclear leukocyte elastase. *J. Biol. Chem., 255*:12006-12010.

Mass, B., Ikeda, T., Meranze, D., Weinbaum, G., and Kimbel, P. (1972). Induction of experimental emphysema: Cellular and species specificity. *Am. Rev. Respir. Dis., 106*:384-391.

Matheson, N. R., Wong, P. S., and Travis, J. (1979). Enzymatic inactivation of human alpha 1-proteinase inhibitor by neutrophil myeloperoxidase. *Biochem. Biophys. Res. Commun., 88*:402-409.

Matulionis, D. H. (1979a). Reaction of macrophages to cigarette smoke. 1. Recruitment of pulmonary macrophages. *Arch. Environ. Health, 34*:293-298.

Matulionis, D. H. (1979b). Reaction of macrophages to cigarette smoke. 2. Immigration of macrophages to the lungs. *Arch. Environ. Health, 34*:298-301.

Merril, W. W., Naegel, G. P., Matthay, R. A., and Reynolds, H. Y. (1980). Alveolar macrophage-derived chemotactic factor. Kinetics of in vitro production and potential characterization. *J. Clin. Invest., 65*:268-276.

Mittman, C. (Editor) (1972). *Pulmonary Emphysema and Proteolysis.* New York, Academic Press, 539 pp.

Moroi, M., and Yamasaki, M. (1974). Mechanism of interaction of bovine trypsin with human alpha 1-antitrypsin. *Biochim. Biophys. Acta, 359*:130-141.

Mosher, D. F., Saksela, O., and Vaheri, A. (1977). Synthesis of alpha-2-macroglobulin by cultured adherant lung cells. *J. Clin. Invest., 60*:1036-1045.

Mounter, L. A., and Atiyeh, W. (1960). Proteases of human leukocytes. *Blood, 15*:52-59.

Nakajima, K., Powers, J. C., Ashe, B. M., and Zimmerman, M. (1979). Mapping the extended substrate binding site of cathepsin G and human leukocyte elastase. Studies with peptide substrates related to the α 1-protease inhibitor reactive site. *J. Biol. Chem., 254*:4027-4032.

Niewoehner, D. R., Kleinerman, J., and Rice, D. B. (1974). Pathologic changes in the peripheral airways of young cigarette smokers. *N. Engl. J. Med., 291*:755-758.

Noguiera, N., Gordon, S., and Cohn, Z. (1977). Trypanosoma cruzi: The immunological induction of macrophage plasminogen activator requires thymus-derived lymphocytes. *J. Exp. Med., 146*:172-183.

Ohlsson, K. (1978). Interaction of granulocyte neutral proteases with alpha 1-antitrypsin, alpha 2-macroglobulin and alpha 1-antichymotrypsin. In *Neutral Proteases of Human Polymorphonuclear Leukocytes.* Edited by K. Havemann and A. Janoff. Baltimore, Urban and Schwarzenberg, pp. 167-178.

Ohlsson, K., and Akesson, U. (1976). Alpha 1-antichymotrypsin interaction with cationic proteins from granulocytes. *Clin. Chim. Acta, 73*:285-291.

Ohlsson, K., and Olsson, I. (1974a). The neutral proteases of human granulocytes. Isolation and partial characterization of granulocyte elastases. *Europ. J. Biochem., 42*:519-527.

Ohlsson, K., and Olsson, I. (1974b). Neutral proteases of human granulocytes. III. Interaction between human granulocyte elastase and plasma protease inhibitors. *Scand. J. Clin. Lab. Invest., 34*:349-355.

Ohlsson, K., Tegner, T., and Akesson, U. (1977). Isolation and partial characterization of a low molecular weight acid stable protease inhibitor from human bronchial secretion. *Hoppe-Seyler's Z. Physiol. Chem., 358*:583-589.

Olsen, G. N., Harris, J. O., Castle, J. R., Waldman, R. H., and Karmgard, H. J. (1975). Alpha 1-antitrypsin content in serum, alveolar macrophages, and alveolar lavage fluid of smoking and non-smoking normal subjects. *J. Clin. Invest., 55*:427-430.

Pantalone, R. M., and Page, R. C. (1975). Lymphokine-induced production and release of lysosomal enzymes by macrophages. *Proc. Natl. Acad. Sci. U.S.A., 72*:2091-2094.

Prince, H. E., Folds, J. D., and Spitznagel, J. K. (1979). Interaction of human polymorphonuclear leukocyte elastase with human IgM. In vitro production of an Fabμ-like fragment. *Molec. Immunol., 16*:301-306.

Pryor, W. A. (1980). Methods of detecting free radicals and free radical-mediated pathology in environmental toxicology. In *Molecular Basis of Environmental Toxicity.* Edited by R. S. Bhatnagar. Ann Arbor, Ann Arbor Science Publishers, pp. 3-36.

Rindler, R., Hortnagl, H., Schmaltz, F., and Braunsteiner, H. (1973). Hydrolysis of a chymotrypsin substrate and of naphthol AS-D chloroacetate by human leukocyte granules. *Blut, 26*:239-249.

Rodriguez, R. J., White, R. R., Senior, R. M., and Levine, E. A. (1977). Elastase release from human alveolar macrophages: Comparison between smokers and non-smokers. *Science, 198*:313-314.

Romanski, B., and Broda, S. (1977). The immunological response to tobacco antigens in the smoker. 1. Specific precipitins against tobacco antigens in the serum of healthy cigarette smokers. *Allergol. Immunopathol., 5*:659-662.

Rossmann, T. G., and Troll, W. (1980). Protease inhibitors in carcinogenesis: possible sites of action. In *Carcinogenesis,* Vol. 5: Modifiers of Chemical Carcinogenesis. Edited by T. J. Slaga. New York, Raven Press, pp. 127-143.

Salvesen, G. S., and Barrett, A. J. (1980). Covalent binding of proteinases in their reaction with α2-macroglobulin. *Biochem. J., 187*:695-701.

Schmidt, W., and Havemann, K. (1974). Isolation of elastase-like and chymotrypsin-like neutral proteases from human granulocytes. *Hoppe-Seyler's Z. Physiol. Chem., 355*:1077-1082.

Senior, R. M., Tegner, H., Kuhn, C., Ohlsson, K., Starcher, B. C., and Pierce, J. A. (1977). The induction of pulmonary emphysema with human leukocyte elastase. *Am. Rev. Respir. Dis., 116*:469-475.

Sloan, B., Abrams, W. R., and Meranze, D. R. (1980). Emphysema induced *in vitro* and *in vivo* in dogs by a purified elastase from homologous leukocytes. *Am. Rev. Respir. Dis.* (In Press).

Starkey, P. M., and Barrett, A. J. (1977). α-2 Macroglobulin, a physiological regulator of proteinase activity. In *Proteinases in Mammalian Cells and Tissues.* Edited by A. J. Barrett. New York, North-Holland, pp. 663-696.

Starkey, P. M., Barrett, A. J., and Burleigh, M. C. (1977). The degradation of articular collagen by neutrophil proteinases. *Biochim. Biophys. Acta, 483*:386-397.

Stedman, R. L. (1968). The chemical composition of tobacco and tobacco smoke. *Chem. Rev., 68*:153-207.

Taylor, J. C., and Crawford, I. P. (1975). Purification and preliminary characterization of human leukocyte elastase. *Arch. Biochem. Biophys., 169*:91-101.

Tegner, H. (1978). Quantitation of human granulocyte protease inhibitors in non-purulent bronchial lavage fluids. *Acta Otolaryngol., 85*:282-289.

Tegner, H., and Ohlsson, K. (1977). Localization of a low molecular weight protease inhibitor to tracheal and maxillary sinus mucosa. *Hoppe-Seyler's Z. Physiol. Chem., 358*:425-429.

Tonge, B. L. (1962). Effect of tobacco smoke condensate on the aerial oxidation of cysteine. *Nature, 194*:284-285.

Travis, J., Bowen, J., and Baugh, R. (1978a). Human α-1-antichymotrypsin: Interaction with chymotrypsin-like proteinases. *Biochemistry, 17*:5651-5656.

Travis, J., Garner, D., and Bowen, J. (1978b). Human α-1-antichymotrypsin: Purification and properties. *Biochemistry, 17*:5647-5651.

Tuttle, W. C., and Westerberg, S. C. (1974). Alpha-1 globulin trypsin inhibitor in canine surfactant protein. *Proc. Soc. Exp. Biol. Med., 146*:232-235.

Twumasi, D. Y., and Liener, I. E. (1977). Proteases from purulent sputum: Purificaction and properties of the elastase and chymotrypsin-like enzymes. *J. Biol. Chem., 252*:1917-1926.

Unkeless, J. C., Gordon, S., and Reich, E. (1974). Secretion of plasminogen activator by stimulated macrophages. *J. Exp. Med., 139*:834-850.

Valone, F. H., Franklin, M. F., and Goetzl, E. J. (1979). Generation of a human polymorphonuclear leukocyte chemotactic factor by the lipoxygenase pathway of alveolar macrophages. *Clin. Res., 27*:476a (Abstract).

Vassali, J. D., and Reich, E. (1977). Macrophage plasminogen activator: Induction by products of activated lymphoid cells. *J. Exp. Med., 145*:429-437.

Wahl, L. M., Wahl, S. M., Mergenhagen, S. E., and Martin, G. R. (1975). Collagenase production by lymphokine-activated macrophages. *Science, 187*: 261-263.

Warr, G. A., Martin, R., Sharp, P. W., and Rossen, R. O. (1977). Normal human bronchial immunoglobulins and proteins. Effects of cigarette smoking. *Am. Rev. Respir. Dis., 116*:25-30.

Weissmann, G., Smolen, J. E., and Korchak, H. M. (1980). Release of inflammatory mediators from stimulated neutrophils. *New Engl. J. Med., 303*: 27-34.

Werb, Z., and Gordon, S. (1975a). Secretion of a specific collagenase by stimulated macrophages. *J. Exp. Med., 142*:346-360.

Werb, Z., and Gordon, S. (1975b). Elastase secretion by stimulated macrophages. *J. Exp. Med., 142*:361-377.

Werb, Z., Mainardi, C. L., Vater, C. A., and Harris, E. D., Jr. (1977). Endogenous activation of latent collagenase by rheumatoid synovial cells: Evidence for a role of plasminogen-activator. *N. Engl. J. Med., 296*:1017-1023.

White, R., Lee, D., Habicht, G., and Janoff, A. (1981). Secretion of alpha 1-proteinase inhibitor by cultured rat alveolar macrophages. *Am. Rev. Respir. Dis., 123*:447-449.

White, R., Janoff, A., and Godfrey, H. P. (1980a). Secretion of alpha-2-macroglobulin by human alveolar macrophages. *Lung, 158*:9-14.

White, R. R., Lin, H. S., and Kuhn, C. (1977). Elastase secretion by peritoneal exudative and alveolar macrophages. *J. Exp. Med., 146*:802-808.

White, R., White, J., and Janoff, A. (1979). Effects of cigarette smoke on elastase secretion by murine macrophages. *J. Lab. Clin. Med.*, *94*:489-499.

White, R. R., Norby, D., Janoff, A., and Dearing, R. (1980b). Partial purification and characterization of mouse peritoneal exudative macrophage elastase. *Biochim. Biophys. Acta*, *612*:233-244.

Since this article was submitted, several significant publications have appeared which provide important new information of the subject of this chapter. Some of these are listed here.

1. On the mechanism of action of α1Pi, see: Martodam, R. R., and Liener, I. E. (1981). The interaction of antitrypsin with trypsin, chymotrypsin and human leukocyte elastase as revealed by end group analysis. *Biochim. Biophys. Acta*, *667*:328-340.
2. On the mechanism of action of α2 macroglobulin, see: Sottrup-Jensen, L., Petersen, T. E., and Magnusson, S. (1980). A thiol-ester in α2 macroglobulin cleaved during proteinase complex formation. *FEBS Lett.*, *121*:275-279.
3. On the inactivation of α1Pi by cell-derived oxidizing agents, see: Clark, R. A., Stone, P. J., Hag, A. E., Calore, J. D., and Franzblau, C. (1981). Myeloperoxidase-catalyzed inactivation of α1-protease inhibitor by human neutrophils. *J. Biol. Chem.*, *256*:3348-3353.
4. On increased numbers of macrophages in asymptomatic cigarette smokers, see: Senior, R. M., Griffin, G. L., and Mecham, R. P. (1980). Chemotactic activity of elastin-derived peptides. *J. Clin. Invest.*, *66*:859-862.
5. On the elastolytic protease of macrophages, see: Banda, M. J., Clark, E. J., and Werb, Z. (1980). Limited proteolysis by macrophage elastase inactivates human α1-proteinase inhibitor. *J. Exp. Med.*, *152*:1563-1570; and Gadek, J., Hunninghake, G., Fells, G., Zimmerman, R., and Crystal, R. (1981). Production of connective tissue-specific proteases by human alveolar macrophages is constitutive (nonregulatable). *Am. Rev. Respir. Dis.*, *123*:55 (Abstract).
6. On direct evidence of oxidized α1Pi in smokers' lungs, see: Carp, H., Miller, F., Hoidal, J. R., and Janoff, A. (1982). Potential mechanism of emphysema: alpha 1-proteinase inhibitor recovered from lungs of cigarette smokers contains oxidized methionine and has decreased elastase inhibitory capacity. *Proc. Natl. Acad. Sci. USA*, *79*:2041-2045.
7. On oxidative inactivation of α1Pi in general, see: Abrams, W., Cohen, A. B., Damiano, V. (1981). A model of decreased functional alpha 1-proteinase inhibitor. Pulmonary pathology of dogs exposed to chloramine-T. *J. Clin. In-*

vest., *68*:1132-1139; Abrams, W. R., Weinbaum, G., Weissbach, L., Weissbach, H., Brot, N. (1981). Enzymatic reduction of oxidized α1-proteinase inhibitor restores biological activity. *Proc. Nat. Acad. Sci. (USA)*, *78*:7483-7486; Beatty, K., Robertie, P., Senior, R. M., Travis, J. (1982). Determination of oxidized alpha 1-proteinase inhibitor in serum. *J. Lab. Clin. Med.*, *100*:186-192; Cohen, A. B., James, H. L. (1982). Reduction of the elastase inhibitory capacity of alpha 1-antitrypsin by peroxides in cigarette smoke. An analysis of brands and filters. *Am. Rev. Respir. Dis.*, *126*:25-30; Dooley, M. M., Pryor, W. A. (1982). Free radical pathology: Inactivation of human α1-proteinase inhibitor by products from the reaction of nitrogen dioxide with hydrogen peroxide and the etiology of emphysema. *Biochem. Biophys. Res. Comm.*, *106*:981-987; Janoff, A., Dearing, R. (in press). Alpha 1-proteinase inhibitor is more sensitive to inactivation by cigarette smoke than leukocyte elastase. *Am. Rev. Respir. Dis.;* Ohlsson, K., Fryksmark, U., Tegner, H. (1980). The effect of cigarette smoke condensate on alpha 1-antitrypsin, antileukoprotease and granulocyte elastase. *Eur. J. Clin. Invest.*, *10*: 373-379; Stockley, R. A., Afford, S. C., Burnett, D. (1982). The electrophoretic mobility of α1-proteinase inhibitor: Effects of proteolysis and cigarette smoke. *Hoppe-Seyler's Z Physiol. Chem.*, *363*:387-393; Taylor, J. C., Oey, L. (1982). Ceruloplasmin: plasma inhibitor of the oxidative inactivation of alpha 1-proteinase inhibitor. *Am. Rev. Respir. Dis.*, *126*:476-482.

8. On cell-cell interactions increasing elastase "burden" of lung, see: Cohen, A. B., Chenoweth, D. E., Hugli, T. E. (1982). The release of elastase, myeloperoxidase, and lysozyme from human alveolar macrophages. *Am. Rev. Respir. Dis.*, *126*:241-247; Senior, R. M., Campbell, E. J., Landis, J. A., Cox, F. R., Kuhn, C., Koren, H. S. (1982). Elastase of U-937 monocyte-like cells. Comparisons with elastases derived from human monocytes and neutrophils and murine macrophagelike cells. *J. Clin. Invest.*, *69*:384-393.
9. On antiproteases of lower respiratory tract, see: Gadek, J. E., Fells, G. A., Zimmerman, R. L., Rennard, S. I., Crystal, R. G. (1981). Antielastases of the human alveolar structures. Implications for the protease-antiprotease theory of emphysema. *J. Clin. Invest.*, *68*:889-898.

8

Immunopharmacology of Lung Surfactant

BRADLEY J. BENSON, LELAND G. DOBBS,
and MICHAEL J. ANSFIELD

University of California
School of Medicine
San Francisco, California

I. Biochemistry and Physiological Functions of Lung Surfactant

Maintenance of normal alveolar function is generally considered to be modulated in part by a special mixture of compounds collectively termed pulmonary surfactant or surface active material (SAM). The ability of this surfactant lipoprotein complex to lower the surface tension at the alveolar air-liquid interface is its most commonly accepted role. This decrease in surface tension is thought to stabilize the alveoli by preventing their collapse at end expiration (Clements and Tierney, 1965; Clements, 1967; Scarpelli, 1968). While the physics and chemistry of the "detergent" properties of lung surfactant have been described most thoroughly, it is also important to consider factors that might control surfactant

Supported in part by grants from the National Institutes of Health (Program Project HL-24075 and AI-12296) and research funds from the Veterans Administration.

flux in the alveoli. There appears to be increasing interest by many investigators into the mechanisms by which SAM is synthesized, transported, packaged, secreted, and removed from the alveoli.

In addition, many new exciting avenues of research probing the immune mechanisms of lung are being explored. One of these—the role of SAM in lung lymphocyte regulation—will be discussed in this chapter. It is perhaps no longer appropriate to consider only the surface properties of surfactant in lung function but to consider how its presence is regulated and to discuss what regulatory capacities SAM itself fulfills in pulmonary biology.

A. Lipids of Lung Surfactant

Pulmonary SAM is generally isolated from endobronchial lavage fluid. In most cases the isolation involves differential or density gradient centrifugation in buffers containing sucrose (Frosolono, et al., 1970; Sawada and Kashiwamata, 1977) or salts (King and Clements, 1972a). The types of separations are designed to separate the soluble components of the lavage fluid, such as certain protein classes and carbohydrates, from the insoluble, cloudy surfactant fraction. Data from studies directed toward the investigation of some of the physicochemical properties of SAM indicate that the material has a density that would be attributed to a mixture containing a high proportion of lipid (King and Clements, 1972a). Investigators have studied the phospholipid components of this material most thoroughly, since these lipids seem to represent about 80-90% by weight of the SAM (King and Clements, 1972b).

The phospholipid compositions for SAM isolated from lungs of rats, dogs, and rabbits are shown in Table 1. The phospholipid compositions are very similar. This finding is perhaps not surprising if all mammalian lungs require a surfactant in order to function properly. Minor differences in composition probably reflect differences among laboratories in isolation, extraction, and analysis of surfactant as much as they reflect species variation. It is evident from many investigations that lung surfactant contains a large proportion of phosphatidylcholine, the predominant molecular species being dipalmitoylphosphatidylcholine (DPPC). The next most abundant phospholipid class is phosphatidylglycerol (PG) (Pfleger et al., 1972; Rooney et al. 1975). There are also small amounts of other acidic phospholipids including phosphatidylinositol, phosphatidylserine, and lysobisphosphatidic acid. This latter phospholipid is present in large quantities in alveolar macrophages (Mason et al., 1972). It has been shown to be specifically located in lysosomes (Brotherus and Renkonen, 1977) of cultured cells and can be synthesized from phosphatidylglycerol (Somerharju and Renkonen, 1980). There are also very small amounts of sphingomyelin and phosphatidylethanolamine. In addition to the phospholipids, the presence of cholesterol, glycerides, and fatty acids in SAM preparations has also been reported (King and Clements, 1972b). Certain glycolipids have also been isolated from the broncho-

Table 1 Phospholipid Composition of Lung Surfactant from Dog, Rat, and Rabbit

	% of Total Phosphorus		
	Dog[a]	Rat[b]	Rabbit[c]
Phosphatidylcholine	83.1	83.8	86.2
Phosphatidylglycerol	11.8	9.3	6.2
Phosphatidylethanolamine	1.9	1.9	3.0
Phosphatidylinositol	1.2	1.8	
Phosphatidylserine	0.3	0.2[d]	3.4[e]
Sphingomyelin	1.5	0.3	
Cardiolipin, lysobisphosphatidic acid	0.1	1.8	
Unknown	0.1	0.9	1.2

[a] B. J. Benson, unpublished observations.
[b] Compiled from Mason et al. (1977b).
[c] Adapted from Rooney et al. (1975).
[d] Phosphatidylserine and lysophosphatidylcholine were analyzed together.
[e] Phosphatidylinositol, phosphatidylserine, and sphingomyelin were combined.

alveolar lavage of patients with alveolar proteinosis (Sahu et al., 1976). Whether these minor lipids are integral components of SAM from normal lungs is unknown. Three other neutral glyceroglucolipids have been isolated from the lung lavage fluid of rabbits (Slomiany et al., 1979). Of the surfactant lipids, a physiologic role has been attributed to only one of them, DPPC. It is this molecular species of phosphatidylcholine that is almost universally accepted as being responsible for the maintenance of low surface tension in the alveoli (King, 1974) (see below).

The biologic function of the acidic phospholipids, particularly PG, in SAM has remained an intriguing mystery since their discovery. It has been suggested that these anionic lipids may have a significant effect on the structure and biologic activity of surfactant. Phosphatidylglycerol has been shown to activate specifically the enzyme CTP:phosphocholine cytidylyltransferase in rat lungs (Feldman et al., 1978). These investigators discussed the possibility that phosphatidylglycerol may have a regulatory function in the increase in phosphatidylcholine synthesis during development in fetal lungs. Godinez et al. (1975) suggested that PG might stabilize lung surfactant after secretion, or participate in some way in its storage. Using radioactive precursors, these investigators identified PG as an unusually metabolically active compound in that its specific activity was higher than any other phospholipid in isolated perfused rat lungs.

The absence of this phospholipid has also been implicated in respiratory distress syndrome (RDS) of the newborn human. Hallman et al. (1977) have shown that, in a number of babies with RDS, PG was always absent in the lung effluent. The acidic phospholipid present in material from these lungs was predominantly phosphatidylinositol. Physicochemical analyses in this study also reflected the hypothesis that PG was somehow important for lung stability. Surfactant without PG had surface-area relationships suggestive of lung instability compared with lung effluents rich in PG.

In the other systems, anionic phospholipids have been shown to facilitate important biochemical processes. These relate primarily to the ability of anionic phospholipids to bind to certain proteins and thereby modulate their biologic activity. For example, acidic phospholipids are required for normal hemostasis; all four vitamin K-dependent coagulation factors (II, VII, IX, X) bind avidly to aggregates of acidic phospholipids, presumably through calcium ion bridges (Benson and Hanahan, 1975; Stenflo et al., 1975). The phospholipid surface is thought to provide an appropriate interface for enzyme-zymogen interaction that serves to accelerate the coagulation reactions. Melitin, a small peptide extracted from bee venom, which has a direct lytic effect on living cells and on liposomes, binds to both neutral and acidic phospholipids. The binding is much greater when the liposomes carry a net negative charge resulting in enhanced lytic activity (Dufourcq and Faucon, 1977). In other invitro systems, anionic phospholipids apparently augment the rate of protein-mediated phosphatidylcholine exchange between intracellular membranes (Dicorleto et al., 1977). Certain membrane proteins have been shown to bind preferentially to anionic phospholipids. The nature of these interactions has been shown to be both hydrophobic and electrostatic. In the case of the N-2 protein in myelin (Boggs et al., 1977b), the binding is thought to be hydrophobic while for the basic protein in myelin the interactions with acidic lipids have been shown to be both electrostatic and hydrophobic (Boggs et al., 1977a). In this study, phosphatidylglycerol was bound most avidly compared with other acidic phospholipids. Striking changes in the thermodynamic properties of the phospholipids occur in the presence of these proteins and the changes are further enhanced by the presence of divalent cations (Papahadjopoulos et al., 1977). The addition of anionic phospholipids to amphipathic phospholipid liposomes results in marked changes in transition temperatures in the presence of calcium and magnesium ions (Papahadjopoulos et al., 1977). These changes in transition temperature are presumed to be a result of lateral phase separation of acid phospholipids. Similar phase separations may be largely responsible for membrane fusion between liposomes (Miller et al., 1976) and cell membranes (Poste and Papahadjopoulos, 1976). Whether PG and the other acidic phospholipids will be shown to serve similar roles in SAM structure and function remains to be investigated; however, the presence of PG in such unusually large amounts indirectly suggests a special function.

B. Proteins of Lung Surfactant

In well-characterized secretory systems in which the secretory product is lipid in nature, notably the liver and gut for serum lipoproteins, the lipids are associated with specific apoproteins. The role of these apoproteins ranges from that of a ligand for receptor-mediated uptake for the low-density lipoprotein (β-apoprotein) to that of cofactors for enzymes. Apoprotein C-II is a cofactor absolutely required for maximal activity of lipoprotein lipase; A-I is required for activity of the lecithin-cholesterol acyl transferase enzyme. (For review see Havel et al., 1980.)

Less is known about the protein components of the surfactant secretory system, although the isolation and study of these proteins is an area of active investigation. King et al. (1973) reported that two nonserum proteins were tightly associated with their isolated SAM. These had minimal molecular weights of 34,000 and 11,000 when analyzed by polyacrylamide gel electrophoresis under denaturing conditions. These proteins were hydrophobic, soluble only in detergent solutions, and the one with molecular weight 11,000, was shown to be soluble in organic solvents. Antibodies produced in rabbits against canine surfactant indicated that these two proteins shared partial antigenicity. These studies also indicated that the major antigen was the 34,000-molecular-weight protein. Other experiments with antibodies generated against these surfactant proteins indicated that they were present in the lung but in no other organ tested; Klass (1973) speculated that they might possibly be specific for SAM. Further studies with antisera raised against sheep SAM indicated that the larger protein was present in the tracheal fluid of fetal sheep (King et al., 1974; Gikas et al., 1977). The 34,000-molecular-weight species was present very early in gestation. The concentration of the protein increased concomitantly with the increase seen in phospholipids prior to birth. Further studies by King et al. (1977) and King and Martin (1980), using radiolabeled precursors in canine and murine lungs, gave evidence that the 34,000-molecular-weight protein was labeled and secreted with similar kinetics to that of the major surfactant phospholipid, DPPC. The labeling of the 11,000-dalton peptide occurred later in time, and its specific activity increased while the specific activity of the 34,000-molecular-weight protein was decreasing. These data led to the speculation that the 11,000-dalton peptide may be derived from the 34,000-dalton species. Proteins with similar molecular weights have also been demonstrated in cow lung surfactant (Sawada and Kashiwamata, 1977). Katyal and Singh (1979) also reported the presence of peptides of this molecular size in the surfactant obtained from rat lungs after removal of serum proteins by affinity chromatography.

Sueishi et al. (1977) and Williams and Benson (1981) used electron microscopic immunohistochemistry to define the cellular source of this protein. Both of these groups used horseradish peroxidase conjugates of Fab fragments of immunoglobulin molecules produced against isolated SAM to indicate that the alveolar type-II cell was the source of this protein. The only other cells containing reaction product indicating the presence of antigen were the alveolar macrophages and rarely type-I cells. The labeling pattern of these cell types was very different. The label was present in the lysosomal apparatus of the macrophages and type-I cells, indicative of uptake and possible degradation. The label was present in the endoplasmic reticulum and Golgi in type-II cells. These organelles are generally thought to be involved in the biosynthesis and packaging of secretory material.

A series of studies analyzing the proteins present in the lavage fluid of patients with alveolar proteinosis have indicated that three major proteins are present with molecular weights of 69,000, 62,000, and 36,000, respectively. These latter two proteins contained sugars and were insoluble. In addition they contain large percentages of the amino acids glycine and hydroxyproline (Passero et al., 1973; Bhattacharyya et al., 1976). Proteins with similar molecular weights were present in smaller quantities in lavage of certain animal species (Bhattacharyya et al., 1975, 1976) and in human amniotic fluid (Bhattacharyya and Lynn, 1978). Recently, Bhattacharyya and Lynn (1979) reported that the 62K and 36K peptides were derived from a soluble glycoprotein of molecular weight 80,000 found in substantial quantities in the lavage from patients with alveolar proteinosis. The relationship of these proteins to those characterized by King et al. (1973, 1977) is unknown. Since the methods of isolation of the starting material are very different, it is quite possible that these proteins are structurally and functionally different. Paciga et al. (1980) have reported that in addition to serum components, the SAM from rabbit lavage contains significant amounts of secretory IgA. Many hydrolases usually thought of as being derived from lysosomes were also reported to be present in the lavage fluid of rats (Hook, 1978). Hydrophobic proteins of relatively small molecular weights (11,500-16,500) were shown to be present in the lavage fluid of pig lungs (Phizackerley et al., 1979). Spitzer and Johnston (1978d), Johnston et al. (1978b) and Benson (1980) have shown that the enzyme phosphatidate phosphohydrolase was present in the surfactant isolated from porcine and canine lungs. The role of this enzyme in SAM awaits further investigation, but these authors have speculated that it may be involved in phsopholipid biosynthesis.

Indeed the cataloging and characterization of the proteins in lung washes has proved far less formidable than assigning a role to them. Of the proteins described so far, functional roles can be ascribed to none. There is speculation that some may be involved in modulation of the physicochemical properties of the surfactant phospholipids. This was based on adsorption experiments comparing isolated SAM to protein-poor phospholipids extracted from SAM. These data indicated that the phospholipids adsorbed faster in the presence of protein than without it (King and Clements, 1972b). More recently it has been demonstrated that the 34,000-dalton protein isolated from either dog (King and MacBeth, 1979) or cow (Sawada et al., 1977) SAM would bind to phospholipids in recombination experiments. King and McBeth (1979) showed that these recombinants would adsorb to an air-water interface more rapidly than the phospholipids alone. In contrast, Metcalfe et al. (1980) showed that the adsorption of phospholipids to an air-water interface occurred with the same rapidity in the presence or absence of any proteins. The basis for these discrepant results in unclear. The role of the glycoproteins found in small amounts in animal lungs and reasons for their accumulation in patients with alveolar proteinosis is also unknown. Likewise the function of the various enzymes and immunoglobins in lung wash remains unknown. Whether any or all of these proteins will ultimately be shown to have a role in normal or pathological lungs awaits further investigation. Since proteins in other biologic systems have been shown to be present for very specific reasons, it seems likely that continued interest in surfactant-associated proteins will provide further insights into their function in lung physiology and disease.

C. Physical Properties of Lung Surfactant

We have alluded to the surface chemistry of surfactant earlier in this discussion, since its most noted property is that of decreasing the surface tension at air-liquid interfaces. Indeed, the functional assay for lung washes and SAM studies is its ability to lower the surfact tension. The details of these types of measurements with respect to the lung have been extensively reviewed (Goerke, 1974) and are beyond the scope of this chapter. However, in order to discuss some of the more recent studies on the physical properties of lung surfactant, representative references from earlier work will be included. Pattle (1955) reported that bubbles made from surfactant extracts were very stable and hypothesized that a lining layer in the alveoli would generate surface tensions of near 0 mN/m. Using a surface balance, Clements (1957) reported low surface tensions (10 mN/m) on compression of surfactant-rich lung lavage fluid. He also described a marked hysteresis in the surface tension-surface area isotherms. Hysteresis and low surface tension have also been calculated from the pressure-volume characteristics of excised lungs (Bachofen et al., 1970). This was thought to result from decreasing surface tension with decreasing area during deflation. Steim et al. (1969) demonstrated that organic solvent extracts of lung washes would decrease surface tensions in a surface balance to very low levels. King and Clements (1972b) reported that isolated canine SAM had similar surface characteristics to those of a DPPC monolayer upon compression. Other investigators have disputed the hypothesis that surface tension in the alveoli is decreased to low levels. Reifenrath and Zimmerman (1973a,b) analyzed fluid withdrawn from the alveolar spaces by micropuncture. They demonstrated that the minimum surface tensions of these fluids were 18-20 nM/m. This data led investigators to speculate that not only were low alveolar surface tensions not required, but that surfactant could not stabilize the lung (Fung, 1975). A problem with all of these earlier studies was that they were indirect. Measurements were made on material removed from the lung. Schurch et al. (1976, 1978) recently considered the question of alveolar surface tension more directly. Their approach was to place by micropipette, droplets of various fluids of known surface tension into alveoli of cat and rat lungs. When observed through a dissecting microscope, these droplets assumed a characteristic shape depending on the surface tension of the monolayer on which they were resting. When the surface tension of the monolayer was equal to or less than the surface tension of the test liquid, the droplet spread to a lens, while the droplet remained hemispherical when the surface tension of the monolayer was greater than the droplet. Using various test fluids of varying surface tensions, they showed that at total lung capacity, the alveolar surface tension was 29.7 ± 1.4 mN/m. The surface tension decreased to below 9 mN/m at functional residual capacity. These studies also convincingly demonstrated that the surface tension in the alveoli at various points along the deflation limb of pressure-volume curves was very stable. Unfortunately, the test fluids used in these studies would not allow measurement of surface tensions below 9 mN/m. Extrapolation of these data do however indicate that the alveolar surface tension at functional residual capacity is well below 9 mN/m.

The realization that surface tensions in the alveoli are truly low and very stable has prompted further investigation of the properties of the monolayer in vitro. These studies have focused on the spreading, stability, removal, and the corresponding physical forms of SAM during the processes. There is universal agreement that the compressed monolayer film must be almost pure DPPC in order to generate low surface tension (Clements, 1973; Goerke, 1974; King, 1974). The observations that pure DPPC below its phase transition temperature does not adsorb or spread at an air-water interface within biologically relevant times (Villallonga, 1968; Gershfeld and Pagano, 1972; Pagano and Gershfeld, 1973) complicates our understanding. Clearly, other components are required for this adsorption, which has been suggested to be the rate-limiting step (Clements, 1973; King, 1974). Once films are formed, these extra components must in some way be removed. Hildebran et al. (1979) studying collapse rates of monolayer films have shown that only small amounts of other lipids could be present in a DPPC film in order for it to maintain stable, low surface tension. The segregation or phase separation and subsequent "squeeze-out" of certain components would be expected to occur during expiration in the alveoli or when monolayer films are compressed.

The structure of SAM during these events is also coming under scrutiny. It has been suggested that the intracellular precursors of SAM—lamellar bodies—

rearrange into a lattice called tubular myelin when they are secreted into the alveoli (Williams, 1977). This has been shown to occur in fetal rat lungs. These studies clearly showed secreted lamellar bodies undergoing transformation into tubular myelin. It might be argued that these studies were from fetal lungs which have fluid-filled alveoli and therefore no air-water interface. The phospholipid composition might be different from adult lungs as well. Goerke (1974) postulated that tubular meylin was the precursor to the active monolayer. Recently Paul et al. (1977a) have argued against the progression of secreted lamellar bodies to tubular myelin to surfactant monolayer. They suggested that part of the phospholipid in lamellar bodies formed tubular myelin while other portions formed the surface-active monolayer. Their hypothesis was based on the observations that preparations of purified tubular myelin were not surface active (Paul et al., 1977b). Thet et al. (1979) also invoked arguments against the hypothesis that tubular myelin was the precursor to the active monolayer, based on experiements with excised lungs. When excised lungs were ventilated at constant tidal volume, the lavage fluid contained more tubular myelin figures than those lungs that were ventilated at constant tidal volume followed by a large inflation. They observed that the increased amounts of tubular myelin were associated with an increase in atelectasis and with an increased alveolar surface tension and speculated that the monolayer might have collapsed. Therefore, according to their hypothesis the tubular myelin was inactivated surfactant. Another possible explanation might be that under ventilation at constant tidal volume the newly secreted tubular myelin formed from lamellar bodies cannot adsorb to the interface due to increased surface pressure. Following a large inflation with a concomitant decrease in surface pressure, the accumulated tubular myelin could then adsorb and spread thus alleviating the atelectasis. Other investigators have shown that increasing the surface area provides new interfacial areas for increased adsorption (Davies and Rideal, 1963). Directly related to these questions of the structure-function relationships of SAM, is that of the ionic requirements for adsorption and spreading. Gil and Reiss (1973) reported that they never observed tubular myelin in their surfactant preparations when the buffers contained a divalent cation chelator, EDTA. Sanders et al. (1980) also demonstrated that divalent cations were required for tubular myelin to form isolated lamellar bodies. They speculated that divalent cations serve not only to produce "surface activity" from lamellar bodies but cause rearrangements of the lipid and protein constituents of the lamellar bodies. How all of these observations pertain to the formation of the alveolar monolayer is open to conjecture.

The apparent dichotomy in requirements for adsorption and spreading versus low surface tension has compounded the difficulties in devising a "synthetic" SAM. Investigators in a number of laboratories are diligently trying to match some of the physical characteristics of natural lung surfactant with those of mixtures of purified phospholipids or lung extracts. This direction of SAM research is extremely important for considering future therapy of infants with RDS. Results from some of these studies are indeed hopeful. Fujiwara et al. (1980) instilled extracts of bovine lungs into the tracheas of infants with RDS. Clinically, the infants required less ventilatory assistance than those infants not receiving the treatment. A possible problem with extracts from animal lungs is the introduction of foreign proteins which might become antigens. Based on earlier experiments by Morley et al. (1978) suggesting that dry surfactant was required for optimal spreading, these investigators have devised a synthetic surfactant using DPPC and phosphatidylglycerol. This mixture was extensively dried and the resulting powder was instilled into infants suffering from RDS. These studies indicated that the infants receiving treatment had better clinical courses than did those infants not receiving the artificial surfactant (Morley et al., 1981). In another series of experiments using instillations of surfactant from adult rabbits, Enhorning and Robertson (1972), Enhorning et al. (1973), and Enhorning et al. (1978) were able to improve the pressure/volume characteristics in both fetal rabbit and primate lungs after treatment with the concentrated adult surfactant. It is to be hoped that further research on the physicochemical properties of SAM will invoke even more clinically useful material.

This discussion of the chemistry and physical properties of lung surfactant points out that while much has been learned, a great deal of information is still unavailable. The composition and role of the proteins in lung surfactant as well as the function of the more minor phospholipids are still an area of controversy. The function of the unique structures that SAM can assume with the participation of divalent cations eludes our understanding at present.

The next sections of this chapter also serve to illustrate the complexity of two other important and clinically relevant aspects of surfactant research: the regulation of its secretion and its possible role in immunologic modification.

II. Secretion of Lung Surfactant

While our understanding of the process of the secretion of surface-active material is greater than it was even 5 years ago, it is still far from complete. The difficulty in studying the secretion of SAM lies in the fact that SAM is not a defined chemical substance, but is composed of a variety of different substances, almost none of which are specific for SAM and very few of which are water-soluble. For these reasons, investigators have chosen to measure either the physical properties of SAM (such as inflation-deflation curves of isolated lungs or the surface tension of material obtained from lung lavage) or one of the various chemical constituents of SAM. From studies that depend on the measurement of physical properties of SAM, one cannot readily quantify the amount of secreted material. While components of SAM such as total phospholipid (PL), phosphatidylcholine, or disaturated phosphatidylcholine (DSPC) can be quantified, the lack of absolute specificity of these components makes interpretation of the data difficult.

The experimental models used have ranged from whole animal studies to studies with isolated alveolar type-II cells. Obviously, the model system chosen to study secretion of SAM affects the experimental results; each experimental system has advantages and disadvantages. Experiments with whole animals may more closely mimic the "natural" controls of secretion; the interrelationships of the more than 40 different types of lung cells are preserved, as is the influence of other organs (such as the adrenal glands, thyroid gland, or central nervous system). In the advantage of this approach lies the disadvantage, in that it is difficult to differentiate direct effects on alveolar type-II cells from effects that may be indirect. Studies on excised lungs share many of these problems as well; however, the effects of organ systems other than the lung are excluded, including neurally mediated effects secondary to disruption of the innervation of the lung. In addition, it is difficult to keep the isolated perfused lung functionally normal for a protracted period of time. The problem of deterioration of the model system with time is not solved by further subdivision of lung tissue, as there is a significant problem with necrosis in the lung explants or lung slices. Deterioration of the model system remains a problem in cell cultures. Both primary cultures of alveolar type-II cells and cloned "type-II cell lines" have been studied over the last 5 years. The advantage of such model systems is that one can study secretion directly, eliminating indirect effects. However, the primary cultures of type-II cells show signs of progressive dedifferentiation over the first 5 days in culture, and however good the characteristics of type-II cell "lines" appear when first isolated, several investigators (Schmidt-Sommerfeld and Borer, 1979; Mason and Williams, 1980) have reported such substantive morphologic and biochemical differences between these cell lines and primary cultures of type-II cells that the question must be raised whether these cell lines are similar enough to type-II cells to justify their use as type-II cell analogs.

The problem of the study of secretion of SAM in the fetus is even more complex, for in this model system there is a continuously changing cell constituency of the lung with the maturation of type-II cells. Although there is no evidence that secretion of SAM in the fetal state is controlled by different mechanisms than in the adult, this possibility certainly exists.

The following discussion will be centered around the various factors that have been shown to influence secretion and to describe the experimental model systems used.

A. General Factors

Although it has not been proven, it is generally assumed that most if not all components of surface-active material are, after synthesis, stored in the lamellar bodies. Secretion occurs by exocytosis, with fusion of the limiting membrane of the lamellar body with the cellular plasma membrane and extrusion of the contents of the lamellar body into the airspace. Secretion probably occurs continuously. There may well be different control pathways for basal secretion than for secretion stimulated above the basal rate. It is assumed that secretion in the alveolar type-II cell occurs by mechanisms that are similar to other exocytotic systems, with microtubules and calcium playing important roles. Colchicine and vinblastine, inhibitors of the microtubule system, have been shown to inhibit stimulated secretion in both lung slices (Delahunty and Johnson, 1976; Marino and Rooney, 1980), and isolated alveolar type-II cells (Dobbs and Mason, 1978).

B. Mechanical Factors

Many investigators have shown that ventilation affects surfactant. Wyszogrodski et al. (1975) provided convincing evidence that ventilation stimulates the secretion of SAM. They injected radiolabeled glycerol and palmitate into cats and allowed the labeled compounds to be incorporated for 17 hr following this, a 3-hr period of hyperventilation caused an increase in the specific activity of endobronchial lavage as compared with the specific activity of lung tissue. Other investigators have reported that air inflation causes an increase in the lecithin content of pulmonary lavage from excised lungs (Faridy, 1976) and from whole animals (Faridy, 1976; Oyarzún and Clements, 1978). The mechanisms by which increased ventilation cause secretion of surface-active material are not understood. The increase in phospholipid secretion caused by hyperventilation can be blocked by atropine (Oyarzún and Clements, 1977), β-adrenergic antagonists (Oyarzún and Clements, 1978), and inhibitors of prostaglandin synthetase (Oyarzún and Clements, 1978). Klass (1978) showed that hyperventilation caused an increase in lung tissue cGMP but not cAMP, raising the question whether hyperventilation may stimulate secretion by increasing the concentration of cGMP in some cells.

Of interest also is that the surfactant secreted in response to hyperventilation may be in an altered physical state. Faridy et al. (1966) and McClenahan and Urtnowski (1967) found that increased ventilation of isolated lungs decreased compliance. Wyszogrodski et al. (1975) showed that the addition of positive end-expiratory pressure to hyperventilation corrected the loss of compliance. Thet and coworkers (1979) showed that the surfactant in the pulmonary lavage from lungs ventilated at low constant tidal volume sedimented at a lower *g* force than the surfactant lavaged from freshly excised lungs. The lower-sedimenting material was predominantly tubular myelin. This study illustrates some of the complexities in the secretion of surface-active material: it was initially felt that, although hyperventilation stimulated the secretion of SAM, SAM was "inactivated" because the lungs had a lower compliance. Thet and coworkers' study supports the theoretical considerations of Clements and

Tierney (1965) and Williams et al. (1966) that at low lung volumes, the molecules are "squeezed out of the monolayer" and the low surface tension of the monolayer is lost. This finding raises the question once again of what is the nature and interrelationship of the various morphologic forms of surface-active material and also raises the question about the collection of surface-active material in secretion studies (a lower *g* force would tend to favor collection of tubular myelin and selective loss of other forms of surface-active materials). The whole area of possible feedback inhibition of secretion by specific forms (physical and chemical) of surface-active material and the influence of removal of such inhibition has not been studied.

C. Adrenergic Effects

β-Adrenergic Effects

It is now well established that β-adrenergic stimulation increases the secretion of SAM; this observation has been made in a variety of model systems. Olsen (1972), using morphometric techniques, reported that single injection of isoproterenol to a rat caused a decrease in the number of lamellar bodies per type-II cell and an increase in the amount of phosphorus (presumably phospholipid phosphorus) in lung lavage; this effect was blocked by propranolol. Kero et al. (1973) reported a very low incidence of respiratory distress syndrome in premature infants whose mothers had been treated with isoxuprine (a β-sympathomimetic agent) to prevent premature labor. These results were supported by a study (Wyszogrodski et al., 1974) of the effects of isoxsuprine in fetal rabbits. Oyarzún and Clements (1978) showed that one β-2 agonist, terbutaline, (but not isoproterenol) augmented the amount of phospholipid recovered from bronchoalveolar lavage; β-adrenergic antagonists inhibited the stimulation of secretion caused by hyperventilation (as did atropine and prostaglandin synthetase inhibitors, as mentioned earlier). Studies with isolated type-II cells in primary culture (Dobbs and Mason, 1979; Brown and Longmore, 1981) have demonstrated that β-adrenergic agonists stimulate the secretion of disaturated phosphatidylcholine; secretion is stimulated by analogs of cAMP and by inhibitors of the phosphodiesterase system as well. The kinetics of this stimulation are comparable with those of other β-adrenergic systems, as are the calculated binding constants for the cellular β-receptor. Intracellular concentrations of cAMP increase after treatment. The secretion is blocked by β-adrenergic antagonists but not by α-adrenergic or cholinergic antagonists. Therefore, it seems clear that β-adrenergic stimulation plays a direct role in stimulating the secretion of surface-active material. It should be noted that secretion is slow (occurring over hours) and the magnitude of the stimulation is relatively small (2.5-3.0 times baseline secretion).

α-Adrenergic Stimulation

Early experiments suggested that α-adrenergic effects may be important in the secretion of SAM because stimulation of the stellate ganglion in monkeys (Beckman and Mason, 1973) caused a decrease in lung compliance that could be blocked by α-adrenergic antagonists. Wyszogrodski and Taeusch (1975) were unable to reproduce these results. Studies in isolated cells (Dobbs and Mason, 1979; Brown and Longmore, 1981) showed that although α-adrenergic agonists caused a stimulation in the secretion of DSPC, this stimulation was observed at only very high concentrations of the agonists and could be inhibited by β-adrenergic antagonists but not by α-adrenergic antagonists. Therefore, the current evidence supports the view that α-adrenergic stimulation plays no direct role in the control of SAM secretion. It should be kept in mind, however, that overwhelming α-adrenergic stimulation could, by its crossover β-adrenergic stimulation be important (as for example, in cerebral trauma, as originally suggested by Beckman and Bean, 1970).

D. Cholinergic Effects

The precise influence of cholinergic stimulation on the secretion of SAM is not understood. Some of the earliest studies on secretion reported that cholinergic stimulation caused secretion. Goldenberg et al. (1969) reported that very large doses (150 mg/kg body weight) of pilocarpine, when injected into fasted rats, caused the alveolar type-II cells to secrete lamellar bodies. Oyarzún and Clements (1977) showed that both the infusion of acetylcholine into the pulmonary artery and efferent vagal stimulation caused an increase in alveolar phospholipid. Massaro (1975) found that a dose of 3 mg/kg body weight of pilocarpine given to rabbits stimulated the release of protein into the surface-active fraction of lung lavage and that this pilocarpine effect could be blocked by atropine. Pysher et al. (1977), working with hydrocortisone-pretreated explants from "late gestational" fetal rat lungs, also found that pilocarpine stimulated the release of phospholipid from explants. Klass (1978) showed rat dibutryl-cGMP (but not dibutyrl-cAMP) stimulates the release of PL from rat lungs. Problems occur when one tries to interpret the preceding data, since it has been known since 1912 that pilocarpine, in addition to its well-known stimulation of postsynaptic parasympathetic neurons, also stimulates the adrenal medulla to secrete catecholamines. Corbet et al. (1976, 1977) showed how important this dual stimulating effect of pilocarpine was by blocking the pilocarpine-induced stimulation of SAM not only with atropine but also with propranolol and phenoxybenzamine. (Corbet and coworkers did not try to block the effexts of isoxsuprine stimulation with atropine, but they did show that isoxsuprine stimulation was blocked with propranolol and not phenoxybenzamine.) These data were interpreted to mean that the pilocarpine effect was indirect rather than direct, acting via the sympathetic nervous system. Others (Dobbs and Mason, 1979) supported this concept with experiments utilizing alveolar type-II cells in primary culture, since the cells secreted disaturated phosphatidylcholine when treated with adrenergic agonists, but not when treated with pilocarpine or carbamylcholine. Brown and Longmore (1981) showed that isolated type-II cells were able to respond to exogenous cholinergic agonists in that the intracellular concentration of cGMP was increased, but once again there did not appear to be any stimulation of secretion of DSPC. Interestingly, the same authors showed that in the isolated perfused rat lung, pilocarpine and isoproterenol independently stimulated the recovery of DSPC from alveolar lavage and that the stimulation could be inhibited only by the appropriate antagonist (i.e., pilocarpine-induced stimulation could be inhibited by atropine and not by alprenolol).

We are left therefore with several observations whose interpretation is not understood. In isolated alveolar type-II cells, cholinergic agonists do not appreciably stimulate secretion, but in the isolated perfused lung or intact animal models, cholinergic agonists do stimulate secretion. In the isolated perfused rat lung model, the stimulation of secretion caused by pilocarpine is not blocked by β-adrenergic antagonists but in the fetal rabbit model, pilocarpine-induced stimulation is blocked by propranolol. It could well be that the process of isolating type-II cells in some ways alters the responsiveness of the cells to stimuli; on the other hand, it is possible that cholinergic effects are mediated via other organs, other lung cells, and/or other mediators and that the effect on type-II cells is therefore indirect.

E. Prostaglandins

The role of prostaglandins in the secretion of surface-active material has been the subject of only relatively recent study. Oyarzún and Clements (1978) showed that the release of phospholipid stimulated by hyperventilation could be blocked by indomethacin and sodium meclofenamate, inhibitors of prostaglandin synthetase. They failed to demonstrate any stimulation of secretion by intravenous injections of prostaglandins E_1, E_2, $F_{2\alpha}$ or arachidonic acid. In contrast, Marino and Rooney (1980), working with lung slices from newborn rabbits, demonstrated that secretion of phosphatidylcholine could be stimulated by prostaglandin E_2 (but not $PGF_{2\alpha}$) and that this stimulation could be inhibited by indomethacin and flufenamic acid. It is perhaps too early to evaluate these findings; there may be unique effects with both model systems, since the model system of Marino and Rooney did not secrete in response to treatment with β-adrenergic agonists and in the intact animal model there are a multitude of factors that could modulate an intravenous injection of prostaglandins.

F. Miscellaneous Effects

L-thyroxine

Redding et al. (1972) reported that L-thyroxine stimulates the secretion of surface-active material. Despite their convincing evidence of this effect, there has been little else published on the effect of L-thyroxine.

Calcium

It has been shown in primary cultures of type-II cells (Mason et al., 1977) and in lung slices (Marino and Rooney, 1980) that the calcium ionophore A23187 stimulates the secretion of phosphatidylcholine. Presumably this effect is mediated by calcium and the microtubular system.

TPA

The phorbol ester 12-*O*-tetradecanoyl-13-phorbol acetate (TPA) has been shown in primary cultures of type-II cells to be the most potent stimulant of secretion of disaturated phosphatidylcholine (Dobbs and Mason, 1978). The significance of this fact is unclear, since the mechanism of action of this compound (which has been shown to cause secretion in a number of other organ systems) is unknown.

G. Summary

Secretion of surface-active material occurs by exocytosis of lamellar bodies and is therefore presumably subject to regulation by the microtubular system and divalent cations. It has not been proven (although it is often assumed) that all components of surface active material are secreted in this manner. In vivo, ventilation appears to be a significant stimulus of secretion; the pathways by which this effect is achieved are unknown. There is now a substantial body of evidence from various model systems that β-adrenergic stimulation causes secretion of surface-active material; it is not known at this time exactly what role the cholinergic system has, that is, whether cholinergic stimulation causes secretion directly or only indirectly. Various other factors, such as prostaglandins and thyroxine, may be important in the regulation of secretion, but how all of these factors interact in vivo is a question that is very much still under investigation.

III. Immunosuppressive Effects of Lung Surfactant

The ability of surfactant to lower surface tension in the alveolus is a well-recognized physiologic function of this lung lipoprotein. Recently, however, it has been postulated that surfactant may have other functions in addition to main-

Table 2 Immunologic Responsiveness of Bronchoalveolar Lymphocytes (BAL)

Species	Stimulus[a]	BAL Response	Reference
Human	PHA, Con-A	Decreased	Daniele et al., 1975, 1977; Moore et al., 1980
Monkey	PHA, Con-A	Decreased	Kazmierowski et al. (1976)
Dog	PHA, Con-A, MLC	Markedly decreased	Kaltreider and Salmon (1973); Ansfield et al., 1979c, 1980
Guinea pig	PHA	Normal to decreased	Gorenberg and Daniele (1976); Hunninghake and Fauci (1976)
Mouse	PHA, Con-A,	Markedly	Caldwell and Kaltreider (1977)

[a] PHA, phytohemagglutinin; Con A, Concanavalin A; MLC, mixed lymphocyte culture.

taining alveolar stability. In particular, it appears that surfactant may influence the actions of the macrophages and lymphocytes that exist in the alveolar milieu. It has been shown, for example, that surfactant augments the bactericidal capacity of the alveolar macrophage in vitro, suggesting that it might contribute to the defense of the lung against pathogenic microorganisms (La Force et al., 1973; Juers et al., 1976). We have suggested recently that surfactant may play an important role in modulating the immunologic responsiveness of the bronchoalveolar lymphocyte. The basis for these considerations is discussed below.

A. Bronchoalveolar Lymphocyte Function

A number of investigators have studied the immunologic function of the bronchoalveolar lymphocytes resident in the distal airspaces of the lung. In general, lymphocytes have been harvested from the lung by lavage, washed, purified, and cultured in vitro with various T-lymphocyte-stimulating agents, such as mitogens or allogeneic cells. After appropriate periods of culture, the incorporation of tritiated thymidine into DNA is measured and used as an index of the lymphocyte proliferative response. The results of studies on the immunologic function of bronchoalveolar lymphocytes are outlined in Table 2. In most species, bronchoalveolar lymphocytes have been shown to be mildly to markedly hyporesponsive to T-lymphocyte stimulation when compared with lymphocytes harvested from blood or systemic lymphoid tissues. This hyporesponsiveness could not be attributed to a paucity of T lymphocytes since, in all species studied, T lymphocytes have been shown to be the predominant form of lymphocyte present in lavaged cell preparations. In detailed studies on canine bronchoalveolar lymphocytes, it has been shown that the hyporesponsiveness could not be attributed to decreased cell viability, to accessory cell dysfunction (Ansfield et al., 1980), to actions of suppressor macrophages or lymphocytes (Demenkoff et al., 1980), or to an abnormality in the number or affinity of lymphocyte mitogen receptors (Ansfield and Kaltreider, unpublished observations). In an attempt to elucidate the mechanism of the hyporesponsiveness of canine bronchoalveolar lymphocytes, the effects of surfactant on lymphocyte function were investigated. The impetus for these studies was the recent reports on the immunosuppressive effects of human serum lipoproteins (Curtiss and Edgington, 1976, 1977; Morse et al., 1977) (see below). Bronchoalveolar lymphocytes are unique in that they coexist in the alveolus with the lipoprotein mixture, surfactant. It was hypothesized that if surfactant could be shown to have immunosuppressive activity similar to that of other lipoproteins, it might help explain the diminished immune reactivity of bronchoalveolar lymphocytes.

B. Surfactant and Lymphocyte Function

The effects of surfactant on various aspects of lymphocyte function have been explored. In initial studies, canine surfactant was isolated from lavage fluid by differential and density gradient centrifugations and was added in graded concentrations to cultures of canine peripheral blood lymphocytes. The effect of added surfactant on the blood lymphocyte proliferative response to mitogens of allogeneic cells was assessed by measurements of tritiated thymidine incorporation or by cytologic determination of the number of mitotic cells. The results of a typical study are shown in Figure 1. Proliferative responses to two mitogens, concanavalin A (Con A) or pokeweed mitogen (PWM), and to allogeneic cells in mixed lymphocyte culture (MLC) were inhibited in a dose-related manner by canine surfactant (Ansfield et al., 1979a). The immunosuppressive effects of surfactant were similar whether proliferation was measured by thymidine incorporation or by mitotic index. This immunosuppressive activity was not due to a cytotoxic effect on lymphocytes or to inhibition of the initial binding of mitogen to its cell surface receptors (Ansfield and Benson, unpublished observations). Synthesis of protein and RNA were inhibited by surfactant, thus ruling out an isolated effect on DNA synthesis or cell division (Ansfield and Benson, 1980).

Surfactant exerted its maximum inhibitory effects when added to lymphocyte cultures either prior to or simultaneously with mitogen. If the addition of

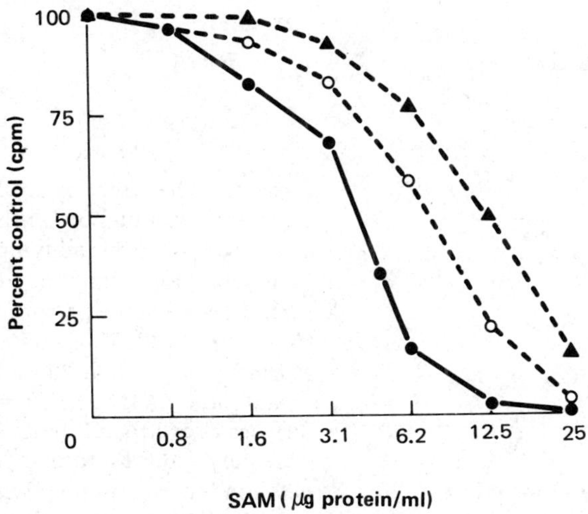

Figure 1 The effect of purified surfactant (SAM) on the proliferative response of blood lymphocytes. Peripheral blood lymphocytes were cultured in the presence of SAM in concentrations from 0.8 to 25 μg protein/ml. The net cpm incorporated by lymphocytes cultured with various concentrations of SAM and Con A (▲——▲), PWM (o —— o), or allogeneic cells (● —— ●) are expressed as a percent of the net cpm incorporated by similarly stimulated lymphocytes cultured in control media without added SAM. (From Ansfield et al., 1979a. © 1979 The Williams & Wilkins Co., Baltimore.)

surfactant was delayed for increasing periods of time after stimulation, it produced progressively less inhibition (Fig. 2). This suggests that surfactant may interfere with early events in the induction of an immune response. Surfactant does not however, have to be present at the time of stimulation to have immunosuppressive activity. Preincubation of lymphocytes with surfactant for 24 or 48 hr followed by washing to remove free surfactant before stimulation, resulted in suppression of the lymphocyte response to mitogenic or allogeneic stimulation. The degree of suppression of lymphocyte proliferation produced by preincubation was not as great as that produced by the continued presence of surfactant throughout the culture. Nevertheless, the persistently suppressed responses of preincubated lymphocytes indicate that this effect of surfactant is relatively irreversible (Ansfield et al., 1979b).

The immunosuppressive effects of surfactant are not species-specific (Ansfield et al., 1979a). Both dog and rat surfactant produced a dose-dependent suppression of lymphocyte proliferative responses to a variety of immunologic stimuli. The immunosuppressive activity of surfactant was similar regardless of

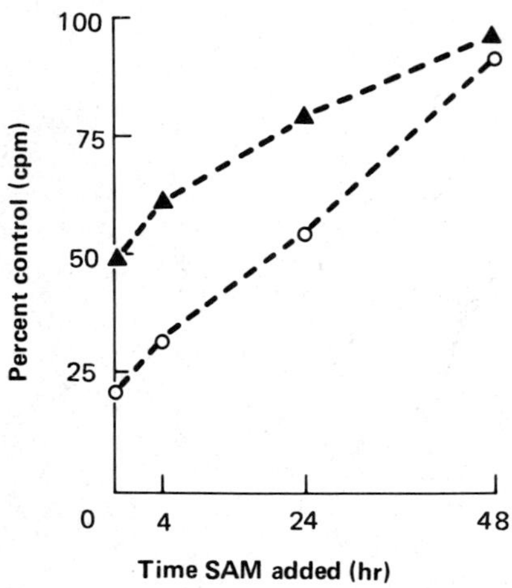

Figure 2 The effect of SAM at various times after stimulation on the proliferative response of blood lymphocytes. Peripheral blood lymphocytes were cultured in control media with Con A (▲——▲) or PWM (o——o) added at time zero. At 0, 4, 24 or 48 hr after stimulation, SAM (12.5 μg protein/ml) was added to cultures. All cells were cultured for a total of 72 hr. The net cpm incorporated by lymphocytes cultured with SAM added at various times after stimulation are expressed as a percent of the net cpm incorporated by lymphocytes in control media without added SAM. (From Ansfield et al., 1979a. © 1979 The Williams & Wilkins Co., Baltimore.)

the source of surfactant or the species from which the responding lymphocytes were obtained. Of the various immunologic stimuli studied, it appears that lymphocytes stimulated by allogeneic cells in mixed lymphocyte culture are more susceptible to suppression by surfactant than are lymphocytes stimulated by mitogen. Whether this reflects a differential sensitivity of various lymphocyte subpopulations to the suppressive effects of surfactant or is the result of the longer exposure of cells to surfactant in mixed lymphocyte cultures (7 days) than in mitogen-stimulated cultures (3 days) remains to be determined.

The T-lymphocyte response to mitogen, antigen, or allogeneic stimulation is accessory cell (macrophage)-dependent and is subject to suppression by a variety of regulatory cells. There is no evidence however, that surfactant exerts its immunosuppressive effects indirectly either by interfering with accessory cell function or by activating suppressor cells. In contrast, it appears most likely that surfactant acts directly to inhibit the responding lymphocyte itself (Ansfield et al., 1979a).

C. Immunosuppressive Components of Surfactant

Surfactant is a complex mixture of lipids and proteins (see above). In order to identify the components of surfactant that were responsible for its immunosuppressive effects, the suppressive activities of the isolated total protein or total

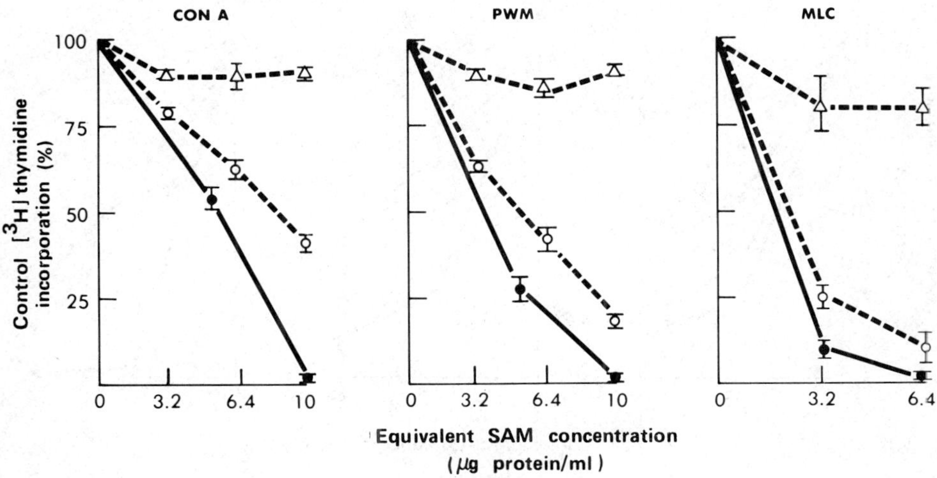

Figure 3 Immunosuppressive activities of the isolated protein and lipid fractions of SAM. Lymphocytes were cultured in medium alone (control) or in medium containing intact SAM (● —— ●), SAM-proteins (△ —— △), or total SAM-lipids (o —— o). Protein or lipid fractions of SAM were added to cultures in amounts equivalent to those present in the concentrations of intact SAM indicated on the *X* axis. The actual final concentrations of SAM-proteins were 3.2, 6.4, or 10 μg/ml and of total SAM-lipids were 37, 74, or 115 μg/ml. Each point represents the mean ± S.E.M. net cpm incorporated by triplicate cultures expressed as a per cent of control incorporation. (From Ansfield and Benson, 1980. © 1980 The Williams & Wilkins Co., Baltimore.)

lipid fractions of canine surfactant were compared with the suppressive activity of intact surfactant. The results of one such study is shown in Figure 3. The protein fraction of surfactant was shown to have a small degree of immunosuppressive activity. However, this effect was not dose-related and was not observed in all experiments. In contrast, the total lipid fraction of surfactant exhibited a dose-related immunosuppressive effect which accounted for most if not all of the suppressive activity of intact surfactant (Ansfield and Benson, 1980).

Several oxidized sterols have been shown to be potent immunosuppressive compounds (Humphries and McConnell, 1979). However, cholesterol or its oxidation products are not the active inhibitory lipids of surfactant, as no diminution in the immunosuppressive activity of surfactant was observed after removal of its sterol components.

Phospholipids comprise the majority of the lipids in surfactant. To determine whether one or more of the phospholipids accounted for the suppressive

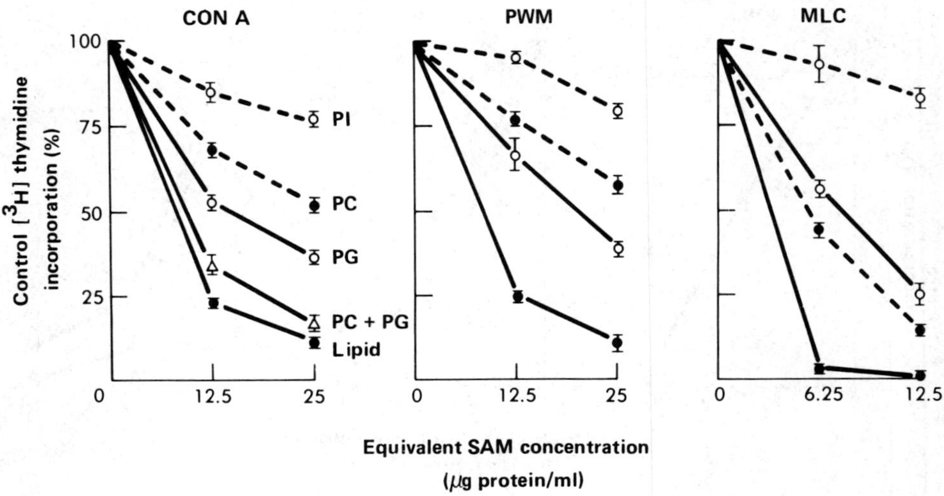

Figure 4 Immunosuppressive activities of the phospholipid components of SAM. Lymphocytes were cultured in medium alone (control) or in medium containing phosphatidylinositrol (PI), phosphatidylcholine (PC), phosphatidylglycerol (PG), PC + PG, or total SAM-lipids (lipid). Each SAM fraction was added to culture in an amount equivalent to that present in a concentration of 6.25, 12.5, or 25 μg protein/ml of intact SAM as indicated on the *X* axis. The actual final concentrations of each SAM fraction were: PI, 0.8, 1.6, and 3.2 μg/ml; PG, 7, 14, and 28 μg/ml; and lipid, 72, 144, and 288 μg/ml. Each point represents the mean ± S.E.M. net cpm incorporated by triplicate cultures expressed as a per cent of control incorporation. (From Ansfield and Benson, 1980. © 1980 The Williams & Wilkins Co., Baltimore.)

activity of srufactant, individual surfactant phospholipids were isolated in pure from and tested for immunosuppressive activity in mitogen (Con A, PWM)- or alloantigen (MLC)-stimulated lymphocyte cultures. Results of these studies are shown in Figure 4. Although all three phospholipids tested exhibited some suppressive activity, phosphatidylglycerol and phosphatidylcholine were the most suppressive and together accounted for most of the immunosuppressive activity of the surfactant lipid fraction. On a molar basis, phosphatidylglycerol was substantially more suppressive than phosphatidylcholine (Ansfield and Benson, 1980).

This suppressive activity is not unique to the phospholipids isolated from surfactant. A variety of phospholipids have been shown to have immunosuppressive activity in vitro. These include phosphatidylglycerol (Ansfield and Benson, 1980), phosphatidylserine (Ng et al., 1978; Kelly and Parker, 1979), phosphatidylethanolamine (Ng et al., 1978), phosphatidylinositol (Kelly and Parker, 1979), and several forms of phosphatidylcholine (lecithin) (Ng et al., 1978; Kelly and Parker, 1979; Ansfield and Benson, 1980; Ip et al., 1980). The suppressive effects of egg lecithin have been investigated in most detail; however, the mechanism of its immunosuppressive activity remains uncertain. Rivnay et al. (1978) attribute this effect of lecithin to its ability to alter lymphocyte membrane cholesterol/phospholipid ratios and therefore induce an alteration in membrane viscosity which inhibits the transmission of a mitogenic signal. In contrast, Chen and Keenan (1977) suggest that the efflux of membrane cholesterol induced by culture with lecithin lowers lymphocyte cholesterol to the extent that new membrane formation and blastogenesis are inhibited. Which, if either, of these mechanisms contributes to the immunosuppressive effects of the various surfactant phospholipids remains to be determined.

D. Immunosuppression by Serum Lipoproteins

All classes of human serum lipoproteins have been shown to have immunosuppressive activity in vitro (Morse et al., 1977). However, the most potent inhibitory lipoproteins are those with densities less than 1.063 g/ml. The suppressive actions of low-density lipoprotein (LDL) and a subfraction of LDL termed LDL-In have been studied in greatest detail. Like surfactant, LDL-In suppresses the lymphocyte response to mitogenic and allogeneic stiumlation (Curtiss and Edgington, 1976). This inhibitory activity, which is not due to cytotoxicity, is secondary to a direct effect of LDL-In on the resting, responding lymphocyte itself (Curtiss and Edgington, 1977). The specific lipids in LDL-In that are responsible for its immunosuppressive activity have not been identified. However, it does not appear as if cholesterol or an oxidation product of cholesterol is the primary inhibitory lipid in LDL-In (Curtiss and Edgington, 1980). The mechanism of this immunosuppressive action is unknown although the data suggest that LDL-In, like surfactant, interferes with processes involved in the prereplicative, triggering phase of the immune response.

Harmony and coworkers have studied the effects of LDL on the generation of the signals thought to mediate mitogen-induced lymphocyte activation. Results of their studies have shown that binding of LDL to the lymphocyte membrane inhibits the cellular accumulation of Ca^{2+} which normally occurs rapidly after interaction with mitogen (Hui et al., 1979). Subsequently, through its effects on Ca^{2+} transport, LDL inhibits the Ca^{2+}-dependent generation of cGMP, a putative second signal for the induction of lymphocyte proliferation (Hui and Harmony, 1980). These studies provide valuable insights on the effect of lipoproteins on lymphocyte function and should serve as a guide to further investigations on the mechanism of the immunosuppressive actions of surfactant.

The interaction between surfactant and lymphoid cells is an area which has only recently been subject to investigation. To date, our knowledge is limited to the studies described above. The results of these studies indicate that surfactant is a potent immunosuppressive factor in vitro, a brief exposure of lymphocytes to surfactant being sufficient to suppress their immunologic function relatively irreversibly. It is not yet clear, however, how this interaction between surfactant and lymphocytes influences immune responses in vivo. Additional information pertaining to both the mechanism of the immunosuppressive actions of surfactant and the immunologic function of pulmonary lymphocytes will be needed in order to assess the potential role of surfactant in modulating the expression of immune responses in the lung.

Acknowledgments

The authors are grateful to Drs. John A. Clements and Mary C. Williams for review of the manuscript. Special appreciation is extended to Ms. Barbara Ehrlich for her cooperation in preparation of the chapter.

References

Ansfield, M. J., and Benson, B. J. (1980). Identification of the immunosuppressive components of canine pulmonary surfact active material. *J. Immunol., 125*:1093-1098.

Ansfield, M. J., Benson, B. J., and Kaltreider, H. B. (1979a). Immunosuppression by surface-active material: Lack of species specificity. *Am. Rev. Respir. Dis., 120*:949-952.

Ansfield, M. J., Kaltreider, H. B., Benson, B. J., and Caldwell, J. L. (1979b). Immunosuppressive activity of canine pulmonary surface active material. *J. Immunol., 122*:1062-1066.

Ansfield, M. J., Kaltreider, H. B., Benson, B. J., and Shalaby, M. R. (1980). Canine surface active material and pulmonary lymphocyte function: studies with mixed-lymphocyte culture. *Exper. Lung Res., 1*:3-11.

Ansfield, M. J., Kaltreider, H. B., Caldwell, J. L., and Herskowitz, F. N. (1979c). Hyporesponsiveness of canine bronchoalveolar lymphocytes to mitogens: inhibition of lymphocyte proliferation by alveolar macrophages. *J. Immunol., 122*:542-548.

Bachofen, H., Hildebrandt, J., and Bachofen, M. (1970). Pressure-volume curves of air- and liquid-filled excised lungs—surface tension in situ. *J. Appl. Physiol., 29*:422-431.

Beckman, D. L., and Bean, J. W. (1970). Pulmonary pressure-volume changes attending head injury. *J. Appl. Physiol., 29*:631-636.

Beckman, D. L., and Mason, K. R. (1973). Sympathetic influence on the dynamic lung compliance. *Life Sci., 12*:43-48.

Benson, B. J. (1980). Properties of an acid phosphatase in pulmonary surfactant. *Proc. Natl. Acad. Sci. USA, 77*:808-811.

Benson, B. J., and Hanahan, D. J. (1975). Structural studies on bovine prothrombin. Isolation and partial characterization of the Ca^{2+}-binding and carbohydrate containing peptides of the N-terminus region. *Biochemistry, 14*:3265-3277.

Bhattacharyya, S. N., and Lynn, W. S. (1978). Isolation and characterization of a pulmonary glycoprotein from human amniotic fluid. *Biochim. Biophys. Acta 537*:329-335.

Bhattacharyya, S. N., and Lynn, W. S. (1979). Structural characterization of a glycoprotein isolated from alveoli of patients with alveolar proteinosis. *J. Biol. Chem., 254*:5191-5198.

Bhattacharyya, S. N., Sahu, S., and Lynn, W. S. (1976). Structural studies on a glycoprotein isolated from alveoli of patients with alveolar proteinosis. *Biochim. Biophys. Acta, 427*:91-106.

Bhattacharyya, S. N., Passero, M. A., DiAugustine, R. P., and Lynn, W. S. (1975). Isolation and characterization of two hydroxyproline-containing glycoproteins from normal animal lavage and lamellar bodies. *J. Clin. Invest., 55*:914-920.

Bhattacharyya, S. N., Rose, M. C., Lynn, M. C., MacLeod, C., Alberto, M., and Lynn, W. S. (1976). Isolation and characterization of a unique glycoprotein from lavage of chicken lungs and lamellar organelles. *Am. Rev. Respir. Dis., 114*:843-850.

Boggs, J. M., Moscarello, M. A., and Papahadjopoulos, D. (1977a). Phase separation of acidic and neutral phospholipids induced by human myelin basic protein. *Biochemistry, 16*:5420-5426.

Boggs, J. M., Wood, M. A., Moscarello, D. D., and Paphadjopoulos, D. (1977b). Lipid phase separation induced by a hydrophobic protein in phosphatidylserine-phosphatidylcholine vesicles. *Biochemistry, 16*:2325-2329.

Brotherus, J., and Renkonen, O. (1977). Subcellular distributions of lipids in cultured BHK cells: Evidence for the enrichment of lysobisphosphatidic acid and neutral lipids in lysosomes. *J. Lipid Res., 18*:191-202.

Brown, L. A. S., and Longmore, W. J. (1981). Adrenergic and cholinergic regulation of lung surfactant secretion in the isolated perfused rat lung and in the alveolar type II cell in culture. *J. Biol. Chem., 256*:66-72.

Caldwell, J. L., and Kaltreider, H. B. (1977). Response of murine pulmonary lymphocytes to mitogenic and allogeneic stimulation. *Am. Rev. Respir. Dis., 115*:49.

Chen, S. S., and Kennan, R. M. (1977). Effect of phosphatidylcholine liposomes on the mitogen-stimulated lymphocyte activation. *Biochem. Biophys. Res. Commun., 79*:852-858.

Clements, J. A. (1957). Surface tension of lung extracts. *Proc. Exp. Biol. Med., 95*:170-172.

Clements, J. A. (1967). The alveolar lining layer. In *Ciba Foundation Symposium, Development of the Lung.* Edited by A. V. S. de Reuck and R. Porter. London, Churchill, pp. 202-228.

Clements, J. A. (1973). Composition and properties of pulmonary surfactant. In *Respiratory Distress Syndrome.* Edited by C. A. Villee, D. B. Villee, and J. Zuckerman. New York, Academic Press, pp. 77-98.

Clements, J. A., and Tierney, D. F. (1965). Alveolar instability associated with altered surface tension. *Handbook Physiol., 3*:1565-1683.

Corbet, A. J. S., Flax, P., and Rudolph, A. J. (1976). Reduced surface tension in lungs of fetal rabbits injected with pilocarpine. *J. Appl. Physiol., 41*: 7-15.

Corbet, A. J. S., Flax, P., and Rudolph, A. J. (1977). Role of autonomic nervous system controlling surface tension in fetal rabbit lungs. *J. Appl. Physiol., 43*:1039-1045.

Curtiss, L. K., and Edgington, T. S. (1976). Regulatory serum lipoproteins: regulation of lymphocyte stimulation by a species of low density lipoprotein. *J. Immunol., 116*:1452-1458.

Curtiss, L. K., and Edgington, T. S. (1977). Effect of LDL-In, a normal immunoregulatory human serum low density lipoprotein, on the interaction of macrophages with lymphocytes proliferating in response to mitogen and allogeneic stimulation. *J. Immunol., 118*:1966-1970.

Curtiss, L. K., and Edgington, T. S. (1980). Differences in the characteristics of inhibition of lymphocyte stimulation by 25-hydroxycholesterol and by the immunoregulatory serum lipoprotein LDL-In. *J. Immunol., 125*:1470-1474.

Daniele, R. P., Altose, M. D., and Rowlands, D. T., Jr. (1975). Immunocompetent cells from the lower respiratory tract of normal human lungs. *J. Clin. Invest., 56*:986-995.

Daniele, R. P., Dauber, J. H., Altose, M. D., Rowlands, D. T., Jr., and Gorenberg, D. J. (1977). Lymphocyte studies in asymptomatic cigarette smokers: a comparison between lung and peripheral blood. *Am. Rev. Respir. Dis., 116*:997-1005.

Davies, J. T., and Rideal, E. K. (1963). *Interfacial Phenomena.* New York, Academic Press, pp. 154-216.

Demenkoff, J. H., Ansfield, M. J., Kaltreider, H. B., and Adam, E. (1980). Alveolar macrophage suppression of canine bronchoalveolar lymphocytes: The role of prostaglandin E_2 in the inhibition of mitogen-responses. *J. Immunol., 124*:1365-1370.

Dicorleto, P. E., Fakharzadeh, F. F., Searles, L. L., and Zilversmit, D. B. (1977). Stimulation by acidic phospholipid of protein-catalyzed phosphatidylcholine transfer. *Biochim. Biophys. Acta, 468*:296-304.

Dobbs, L. G., and Mason, R. J. (1978). Stimulation of secretion of disaturated phosphatidylcholine from isolated alveolar type II cells by 12-0-tetradecanoyl-13-phorbol acetate. *Am. Rev. Respir. Dis., 118*:705-713.

Dobbs, L. G., and Mason, R. J. (1979). Pulmonary alveolar type II cells isolated from rats: Release of phosphatidylcholine in response to β-adrenergic stimulation. *J. Clin. Invest., 63*:378-387.

Dufourcq, J., and Faucon, J.-F. (1977). Intrinsic fluorescence study of lipid-protein interactions in membrane models. Binding of mellitin, an amphipathic peptide, to phospholipid vescles. *Biochim. Biophys. Acta, 467*:1-11.

Enhorning, G., and Robertson, B. (1972). Lung expansion in the premature rabbit fetus after tracheal deposition of surfactant. *Pediatrics, 50*:58-66.

Enhorning, G., Grossman, G., and Robertson, B. (1973). Tracheal deposition of surfactant before the first breath. *Am. Rev. Respir. Dis., 107*:921-927.

Enhorning, G., Hill, D., Sherwood, G., Cutz, E., Robertson, B., and Bryan, C. (1978). Improved ventilation of prematurely delivered primates following tracheal deposition of surfactant. *Am. J. Obstet. Gynecol., 132*:529-536.

Faridy, E. E. (1976). Effect of distension on release of surfactant in excised dogs' lungs. *Resp. Physiol., 27*:99-114.

Faridy, E. E., Permutt, S., and Riley, R. L. (1966). Effect of ventilation on surface forces in excised dogs' lungs. *J. Appl. Physiol., 21*:1453-1462.

Feldman, D. A., Kovac, C. R., Dranginis, P. L., and Weinhold, P. A. (1978). The role of phosphatidylglycerol in the activation of CTP:phosphocholine cytidylyltransferase from rat lung. *J. Biol. Chem., 253*:4980-4986.

Fujiwara, T., Maeta, H., Chida, S., Morita, T., Watabe, Y., and Abe, T. G. (1980). Artificial surfactant therapy in hyaline membrane disease. *Lancet, I*:55-59.

Frosolono, M. F., Charmes, B. L., Pawlowski, R., and Slivka, S. (1970). Isolation, characterization and surface chemistry of a surface active fraction from dog lung. *J. Lipid Res., 11*:439-457.

Fung, Y. (1975). Does the surface tension make the lung inherently unstable? *Circulation Res., 37*:497-502.

Gershfeld, N. L., and Pagano, R. E. (1972). Physical chemistry of lipid films at the air-water interface. III. The condensing effect of cholesterol. A critical examination of mixed-film studies. *J. Phys. Chem., 76*:1244-1249.

Gikas, E. G., King, R. J., Mescher, E. J., Platzker, A. C. G., Kitterman, J. A., Ballard, P. L., Benson, B. J., Tooley, W. H., and Clements, J. A. (1977). Radioimmunoassay of pulmonary surface-active material in the tracheal fluid of the fetal lamb. *Am. Rev. Respir. Dis., 115*:587-593.

Gil, J., and Reiss, O. K. (1973). Isolation and characterization of lamellar bodies and tubular myelin from rat lung homogenates. *J. Cell Biol., 58*:152-171.

Godinez, R. I., Sanders, R. L., and Longmore, W. J. (1975). Phosphatidylglycerol in rat lung. I. Identification as a metabolically active phospholipid in isolated perfused rat lung. *Biochemistry, 14*:830-834.

Goerke, J. (1974). Lung surfactant. *Biochim. Biophys. Acta, 344*:241-261.

Goldenberg, V. E., Buckingham, S., and Sommers, S. C. (1969). Pilocarpine stimulation of granular pneumocyte secretion. *Lab. Invest., 20*:147-158.

Gorenberg, D. J., and Daniele, R. P. (1976). Characterization of immunocompetent cells recovered from the respiratory tract and tracheobronchial lymph node of normal guinea pigs. *Am. Rev. Respir. Dis., 114*:1099-1105.

Hallman, M., Feldman, B. H., Kirkpatrick, E., and Gluck, L. (1977). Absence of phosphatidylglycerol in respiratory distress syndrome in the newborn. *Pediat. Res., 11*:714-720.

Havel, R. J., Goldstein, J. L., and Brown, M. S. (1980). Lipoproteins and lipid transport. In *Metabolic Control and Disease, 8th Edition.* Edited by P. K. Bondy and L. E. Rosenberg. Philadelphia, W. B. Saunders, pp. 393-494.

Hildebran, J. N., Goerke, J., and Clements, J. A. (1979). Pulmonary film stability and composition. *J. Appl. Physiol., 47*:604-611.

Hook, G. E. R. (1978). Extracellular hydrolases of the lung. *Biochemistry, 17*: 520-528.

Hui, D. H., and Harmony, J. A. K. (1980). Inhibition by low density lipoproteins of mitogen-stimulated cyclic nucleotide production by lymphocytes. *J. Biol. Chem., 255*:1413-1419.

Hui, D. Y., Berebitsky, G. L., and Harmony, J. A. K. (1979). Mitogen-stimulated calcium ion accumulation by lymphocytes, influence of plasma lipoproteins. *J. Biol. Chem., 254*:4666-4673.

Humphries, G. M. K., and McConnell, H. M. (1979). Potent immunosuppression by oxidized cholesterol. *J. Immunol., 122*:121-126.

Hunninghake, G. W., and Fauci, A. S. (1976). Immunological reactivity of the lung. I. A guinea pig model for the study of pulmonary mononuclear cell subpopulations. *Cell. Immunol., 26*:89-97.

Ip, S. H. C., Abrahm, J., and Cooper, R. A. (1980). Enhancement of blastogenesis in cholesterol-enriched lymphocytes. *J. Immunol., 124*:87-92.

Johnston, J. M., Porter, J. C., and MacDonald, P. C. (1978). The biosynthesis and hormonal regulation of surfactant formation. *Adv. Exp. Med. Biol., 101*:327-329.

Juers, J. A., Rogers, R. M., McCurdy, J. B., and Cook, W. W. (1976). Enhancement of bactericidal capacity of alveolar macrophages by human alveolar lining material. *J. Clin. Invest., 58*:271-275.

Kaltreider, H. B., and Salmon, S. E. (1973). Immunology of the lower respiratory tract, functional properties of bronchoalveolar lymphocytes obtained from the normal canine lung. *J. Clin. Invest., 52*:2211-2217.

Katyal, S. L., and Singh, G. (1979). An immunologic study of the apoproteins of rat lung surfactant. *Lab. Invest., 40*:562-567.

Kazmierowski, J. A., Fauci, A. S., and Reynolds, H. Y. (1976). Characterization of lymphocytes in bronchial lavage fluid from monkeys. *J. Immunol., 116*: 615-618.

Kelly, J. P., and Parker, C. W. (1979). Effects of arachidonic acid and other unsaturated fatty acids on mitogenesis in human lymphocytes. *J. Immunol., 122*:1556-1562.

Kero, P., Hirvonen, T., and Valimaki, I. (1973). Prenatal and postnatal isoxsuprine and respiratory distress syndrome. *Lancet, II*:198.

King, R. J. (1974). The surfactant system of the lung. *Fed. Proc., 33*:2238-2247.

King, R. J., and Clements, J. A. (1972a). Surface active materials from dog lung. I. Method of isolation. *Am. J. Physiol., 223*:707-714.

King, R. J., and Clements, J. A. (1972b). Surface active materials from dog lung. II. Composition and physiological correlations. *Am. J. Physiol., 223*:715-726.

King, R. J., and MacBeth, M. C. (1979). Physicochemical properties of dipalmitoyl phosphatidylcholine after interaction with an apolipoprotein of pulmonary surfactant. *Biochim. Biophys. Acta, 557*:86-101.

King, R. J., and Martin, H. (1980). Intracellular metabolism of the apoproteins of pulmonary surfactant in rat lung. *J. Appl. Physiol., 48*:812-820.

King, R. J., Gikas, E. G., Ruch, J., and Clements, J. A. (1974). The radioimmunoassay of pulmonary surface active material in fetal sheep lung. *Am. Rev. Respir. Dis., 110*:273-281.

King, R. J., Klass, D. J., Gikas, E. G., and Clements, J. A. (1973). Isolation of apoproteins from canine surface active material. *Am. J. Physiol., 224*:788-795.

King, R. J., Martin, H., Mitts, D., and Holmstrom, F. M. (1977). Metabolism of the apoproteins in pulmonary surfactant. *J. Appl. Physiol., 42*:483-491.

Klass, D. J. (1973). Immunochemical studies of the protein fraction of pulmonary surface active material. *Am. Rev. Respir. Dis., 107*:784-789.

Klass, D. (1978). Lung tissue guanosine 3′, 5′-monophosphate: effects of ventilation and anesthesia. *J. Appl. Physiol., 45*:487-494.

LaForce, F. M., Kelly, W. J., and Huber, G. L. (1973). Inactivation of staphylococci by alveolar macrophages with preliminary observations on the importance of alveolar lining material. *Am. Rev. Respir. Dis., 108*:784-790.

Marino, P. A., and Rooney, S. A. (1980). Surfactant secretion in a newborn rabbit lung slice model. *Biochem. Biophys. Acta, 620*:509-519.

Mason, R. J., and Williams M. C. (1980). Phospholipid composition and ultrastructure of A549 cells and other cultured pulmonary epithelial cells of presumed type II cell origin. *Biochim. Biophys. Acta, 617*:36-50.

Mason, R. J., Stossel, T. P., and Vaughan, M. (1972). Lipids of alveolar macrophages, polymorphonuclear leukocytes, and their phagocytic vesicles. *J. Clin. Invest., 51*:2399-2407.

Mason, R. J., Williams, M. C., and Dobbs, L. G. (1977a). Secretion of disaturated phosphatidylcholine by primary cultures of type II alveolar cells. In *Pulmonary Macrophage and Epithelial Cells.* Edited by C. L. Sanders, R. P. Schneider, G. E. Dagle, and H. A. Ragan. Proc. of the 16th Annual Hanford Biology Symposium. Springfield, Virginia, Technical Information Center, Energy Research and Development Administration, pp. 280-297.

Mason, R. J., Dobbs, L. G., Greenleaf, R. D., and Williams, M. C. (1977b). Alveolar type II cells. *Fed. Proc., 36*:2697-2702.

Massaro, D. (1975). In vivo protein secretion by lung: evidence for active secretion and interspecies differences. *J. Clin. Invest., 56*:163-271.

McClenahan, J. B., and Urtnowski, S. (1967). Effect of ventilation on surfactant, and its turnover rate. *J. Appl. Physiol., 23*:215-220.

Metcalfe, I. L., Enhorning, G., and Possmayer, F. (1980). Pulmonary surfactant associated proteins: their role in the expression of surface activity. *J. Appl. Physiol., 49*:34-41.

Miller, C., Arvan, P., Telford, J. N., and Racker, E. (1976). Calcium-induced fusion of proteoliposomes: dependence of transmembrane osmotic gradient. *J. Membrane Biol., 30*:271-282.

Moore, V. L., Pedersen, G. M., Hauser, W. C., and Fink, J. N. (1980). A study of lung lavage materials in patients with hypersensitivity pneumonitis: in vitro response to mitogen and antigen in pigeon breeders' disease. *J. Allergy Clin. Immunol., 65*:365-370.

Morley, C. J., Miller, N., Bangham, A. D., and Davis, J. A. (1981). Dry artificial lung surfactant and its effect on very premature babies. *Lancet I*:64-68.

Morley, C. J., Bangham, A. D., Johnson, P., Thorburn, J. D., and Jenkin, G. (1978). Physical and physiological properties of dry lung surfactant. *Nature, 271*:162-163.

Morse, J. H., Witte, L. D., and Goodman, D. S. (1977). Inhibition of lymphocyte proliferation stimulated by lectins and allogeneic cells by normal plasma lipoproteins. *J. Exp. Med., 146*:1791-1799.

Ng, M. H., Ng, W. S., Ho, W. K. K., Fung, K. P., and Lamelin, J. P. (1978). Modulation of phytohemagglutinin-mediated lymphocyte stimulation by egg lecithin. *Exp. Cell Res., 116*:387-395.

Olsen, D. B. (1972). Neurohumoral-hormonal secretory stimulation of pulmonary surfactant in the rat. *Physiologist, 15*:230.

Oyarzún, M. J., and Clements, J. A. (1977). Ventilatory and cholinergic control of pulmonary surfactant in the rabbit. *J. Appl. Physiol., 43*:39-45.

Oyarzún, M. J., and Clements, J. A. (1978). Control of lung surfactant by ventilation, adrenergic mediators, and prostaglandins in the rabbit. *Am. Rev. Respir. Dis., 117*:879-891.

Paciga, J. E., Shelley, S. A., and Balis, J. U. (1980). Secretory IgA is a component of rabbit lung surfactant. *Biochim. Biophys. Acta, 631*:487-494.

Pagano, R. E., and Gershfeld, N. L. (1973). Phase separation in cholesteroldipalmitoyl lecithin mixed films and the condensing effect. *J. Colloid Interface Sci., 44*:382-383.

Papahadjopoulos, D., Poste, G., Schaeffer, B. E., and Vail, W. J. (1977). Membrane fusion and molecular segregation in phospholipid vesicles. *Biochim. Biophys. Acta, 352*:10-28.

Papahadjopoulos, D., Vail, W. J., Newton, E., Nir, S., Jacobson, K., Poste, G., and Lazo, R. (1977). Studies on membrane fusion. III. The role of calcium-induced phase changes. *Biochim. Biophys. Acta, 465*:579-598.

Passero, M. A., Tye, R. W., Kilburn, K. H., and Lynn, W. S. (1973). Isolation and characterization of two glycoproteins from patients with alveolar proteinosis. *Proc. Natl. Acad. Sci. USA, 70*:973-976.

Pattle, R. E. (1955). Properties, function and origin of the alveolar lining layer. *Nature, 175*:1125-1126.

Paul, G. W., Hassett, R. J., and Reiss, O. K. (1977a). Formation of lung surfactant films from intact lamellar bodies. *Proc. Natl. Acad. Sci. USA, 74*: 3617-3620.

Paul, G. W., Sanders, R. L., Hassett, R. J., and Reiss, O. K. (1977b). Kinetics of film formation and surface activity of lamellar bodies (LB), extracted lipids (ED), tubular myelin figures (TMF), and alveolar surfactant (AS) from rat lung. *Fed. Proc., 36*:615.

Pfleger, R. D., Henderson, R. F., and Waide, J. (1972). Phosphatidylglycerol—a major component of pulmonary surfactant. *Chem. Phys. Lipids, 9*:51-68.

Phizackerley, P. J. R., Town, M.-H., and Newman, G. E. (1979). Hydrophobic proteins of lamellated osmiophilic bodies isolated from pig lung. *Biochem. J., 183*:731-736.

Poste, G., and Papahadjopoulos, D. (1976). Lipid vesicles as carriers for introducing materials into cultured cells: influence of vesicle composition on mechanisms of vesicle incorporation into cells. *Proc. Natl. Acad. Sci. USA, 73*:1603-1607.

Pysher, T. J., Konrad, K. D., and Reed, G. B. (1977). Effects of hydrocortisone and pilocarpine on fetal rat lung explants. *Lab. Invest., 37*:588-593.

Redding, R. A., Douglas, W. H. J., and Stein, M. (1972). Thyroid hormone influence upon lung surfactant metabolism. *Science, 175*:994-996.

Reifenrath, R., and Zimmerman, I. (1973a). Blood plasma contamination of the lung alveolar surfactant obtained by various sampling techniques. *Resp. Physiol., 18*:238-248.

Reifenrath, R., and Zimmerman, I. (1973b). Surface tension properties of lung alveolar surfactant obtained by alveolar micropuncture. *Resp. Physiol., 19*:369-393.

Rivnay, E., Globerson, A., and Shinitzky, M. (1978). Perturbation of lymphocyte response to concanavalin A by exogenous cholesterol and lecithin. *Eur. J. Immunol., 8*:185-189.

Rooney, S. A., Page-Roberts, B. A., and Motoyama, E. K. (1975). Role of lamellar inclusions in surfactant production: studies on phospholipid composition and biosynthesis in rat and rabbit subcellular fractions. *J. Lipid Res., 16*:418-425.

Sahu, S., DiAugustine, R. P., and Lynn, W. S. (1976). Lipids found in pulmonary lavage of patients with alveolar proteinosis and in rabbit lung lamellar organelles. *Am. Rev. Respir. Dis., 114*:177-184.

Sanders, R. L., Hassett, R. J., and Vater, A. E. (1980). Isolation of lung lamellar bodies and their conversion to tubular myelin figures in vitro. *Anat. Rec., 198*:485-501.

Sawada, H., and Kashiwamata, S. (1977). Sodium dodecyl sulfate-disc gel electrophoresis patterns of bovine lung surfactant. *Biochim. Biophys. Acta, 490*:44-50.

Sawada, H., Okajima, Y., Hayashi, M., and Yamabayashi, H. (1977). Reassembly in vitro of lung surfactant apoprotein. *Biochem. Biophys. Res. Commun., 74*:1263-1267.

Scarpelli, S., Goerke, J., and Clements, J. A. (1976). Direct determination of surface tension in the lung. *Proc. Natl. Acad. Sci. USA, 73*:4698-4702.

Schurch, S., Goerke, J., and Clements, J. A. (1978). Direct determination of volume- and time-dependence of alveolar surface tension in excised lungs. *Proc. Natl. Acad. Sci. USA, 75*:3417-3421.

Slomiany, B. L., Smith, F. B., and Slomiany, A. (1979). The neutral glyceroglucolipids of alveolar lavage from rabbit. *Biochim. Biophys. Acta, 574*: 480-486.

Somerharju, P., and Renkonen, O. (1980). Conversion of phosphatidylglycerol lipids to bis(monoacylglycero)phosphate in vivo. *Biochim. Biophys. Acta, 618*:407-419.

Spitzer, H. L., and Johnston, J. M. (1978). Characterization of phosphatidate phosphohydrolase activity associated with isolated lamellar bodies. *Biochim. Biophys. Acta, 531*:275-285.

Steim, J. M., Redding, R. A., Hauck, C. T., and Steim, M. (1969). Isolation and characterization of lung surfactant. *Biochem. Biophys. Res. Commun., 34*: 434-440.

Stenflo, J., Fernlund, P., and Roepstorff, P. (1975). Structure of a vitamine K-dependent portion of prothrombin. In *Proteases and Biological Control.* Edited by E. Reich, D. B. Rifkin, and E. Shaw. Cold Spring Harbor, N.Y., Cold Spring Harbor Laboratory, vol. 2, pp. 111-122.

Sueishi, K., Tanaka, K., and Oda, T. (1977). Immunoultrastructural body of surfactant system. *Lab. Invest., 37*:136-142.

Thet, L. A., Clerch, L., Massaro, G. D., and Massaro, D. (1979). Changes in sedimentation of surfactant in ventilated excised rat lungs. *J. Clin. Invest., 64*:600-608.

Vilallonga, F. (1968). Surface chemistry of L-α-dipalmitoyl lecithin at the air-water interface. *Biochim. Biophys. Acta, 163*:290-300.

Williams, M. C. (1977). Conversion of lamellar body membranes into tubular myelin in alveoli of fetal rat lungs. *J. Cell. Biol., 72*:260-277.

Williams, M. C., and Benson, B. J. (1981). Immunocytochemical localization and identification of the major surfactant protein in adult rat lung. *J. Histochem. Cytochem., 29*:291-305.

Williams, J. V., Tierney, D. F., and Parker, H. R. (1966). Surface forces in the lung, atelectasis, and transpulmonary pressure. *J. Appl. Physiol., 21*: 819-829.

Wyszogrodski, I., and Taeusch, H. W., Jr. (1975). Prolonged sympathetic activation and pulmonary surfactant: absence of effect in anesthetized cats. *Am. Rev. Respir. Dis., 111*:619-622.

Wyszogrodski, I., Taeusch, H. W., Jr., and Avery, M. E. (1974). Isoxuprine-induced alterations of pulmonary pressure-volume relationship in premature rabbits. *Am. J. Obstet. Gynecol., 119*:1107-1111.

Wyszogrodski, I., Kyei-Aboagye, K., Taeusch, H. W., Jr., and Avery, M. E. (1975). Surfactant inactivation by hyperventilation: conservation by end-expiratory pressure. *J. Appl. Physiol., 38*:461-466.

9

Chemotactic Mechanisms in the Lung

JOSEPH C. FANTONE and PETER A. WARD

The University of Michigan Medical School
Ann Arbor, Michigan

I. Chemotactic Factors

A broad spectrum of pathologic changes can be observed in the lung after either an immunologic or nonimmunologic insult. These alterations are frequently the result of either the direct effects of a pathologic agent on resident lung cells or a consequence of an influx of inflammatory cells such as polymorphonuclear leukocytes, monocytes, eosinophils, or lymphocytes. Chemotaxis or cell-directed migration is the process in which a cell migrates in a chemical gradient towards an increasing concentration of the chemical stimulus. It is this process of cell movement that is generally accepted as the mechanism for the infiltration of tissues by inflammatory cells. The following discussion will examine what is currently understood about the mechanisms of inflammatory cell infiltration into the lung and the possible role of chemotactic factors in pulmonary diseases. Although there is an extensive literature covering the different sources of chemotactic factors and a wealth of information that describes the biochemical responses of individual cell types to various chemotactic agents (for review see, Ward, 1980), the relative importance of the different chemotactic factors in specific disease states is not yet clear.

Table 1 Physiological Properties of Human Complement Components

Protein	Serum concentration (approx.) (μg/ml)	Approximate molecular weight
Classical pathway		
C1q	190	400,000
Clr	—	167,000
Cls	100	108,000
C2	30	240,000
C4	400	117,000
C3	1200	185,000
C5	75	200,000
C6	60	125,000
C7	60	120,000
C8	80	150,000
C9	10	79,000
Alternate pathway		
Properidin (P)	25	190,000
Factor D (D)	1-5	25,000
Factor B (B)	200	100,000
Inhibitors		
C1-INH	180	90,000
C3-INA	25	100,000
B1H	133	100,000
SCPN	30-40	310,000
CFI-C5a	?	150,000

A. Complement-Derived Chemotactic Factors

The classical complement pathway is a series of 11 individual proteins that are present in human serum and can be grouped into three operational units (Table 1). Three distinct proteins (Clq, Clr, Cls) compose the trimolecular C1 complex of complement and serve as the recognition unit for the Fc component of certain classes of antibody (Andrews and Baillie, 1979; Hyslop et al., 1970; Muller-Eberhard, 1975; Sim et al., 1977). This is followed by sequential enzymatic activation of the complement components C4, C2, C3, and C5 with the generation of the products C3a (mw = 9000) and C5a (mw = 12,500) (Budzko and Muller-Eberhard, 1970; Dias Da Silva et al., 1967; Goldman et al., 1978; Hugli and Muller-Eberhard, 1978; Muller-Eberhard, 1978). After this activation unit is

COMPLEMENT DERIVED CHEMOTACTIC FACTORS

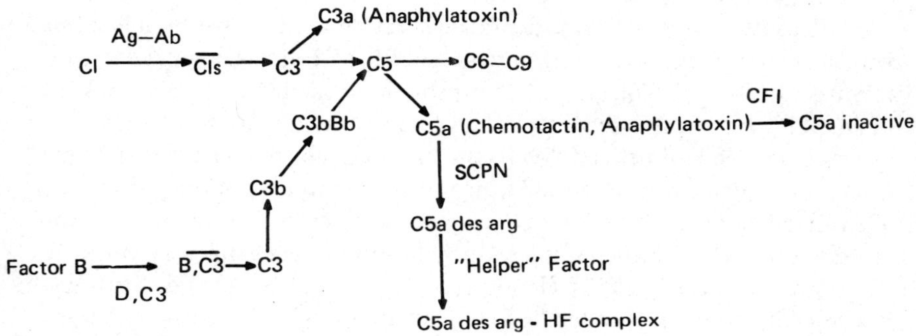

COMPLEMENT PRODUCTS

	Molecular Weight	Activity
C3a	9,000	Anaphylatoxin
C5a	12,500	Anaphylatoxin, Chemotactin Enzyme release, Aggregation
C5a des arg	12,300	Chemotaxis, ± "Helper" factor
"Helper" Factor	68,000	Binds to C5a des arg (Increases chemotactic activity)

Figure 1 Activation of complement pathways.

assembled on the cell membrane, a multimolecular membrane attack complex is assembled consisting of the additional binding of C6, C7, C8, and C9 to the membrane which results in cytolysis (Bhakdi et al., 1976; Podack and Muller-Eberhard, 1980). A second mechanism of activation of the complement system is the alternative (or properidin) pathway. This pathway consists of five unique proteins and six shared complement proteins that can be activated by a variety of immunologic and nonimmunologic factors, resulting in the generation of C3a and C5a (Fig. 1). These two biologically active products are known as the anaphylatoxins (Hugli and Muller-Eberhard, 1978). They are defined by their effects on the vasculature and their ability to cause release of vasoactive amines from mast cells and basophils (Vogt, 1974; Morrison et al., 1975; Siraganian and Hook, 1976). Of equal importance to its role as an anaphylatoxin, C5a has been shown to be the most potent serum-derived chemoattractant for neutrophils. In nanomolar concentrations, this peptide can cause unidirectional movement of neutrophils along a gradient (Ward and Newman, 1969; Damerau et al.,

1978; Fernandez et al., 1978). Other inflammatory cells, including peripheral monocytes (Ward, 1968a), eosinophils (Ward, 1968b, 1969), and basophils (Ward et al., 1975) have been shown to respond in a similar fashion to C5a.

Recently, a serum carboxypeptidase N (SCPN) activity has been identified with enzymatic activity resulting in removal of the C-terminal arginyl or lysyl residues from several biologically active peptides, including C3a, C5a, and bradykinin. SCPN is present in human plasma at a concentration of 30–40 μg/ml (Bokisch and Muller-Eberhard, 1970) and has been shown to cleave rapidly the C-terminal arginine from C5a producing C5a des arg which is much less active as an anaphylatoxin (Hugli, 1978; Chenoweth and Hugli, 1980) and, in the absence of other serum proteins, is less active (1/40) as a chemotactic agent (Chenoweth and Hugli, 1980). However, a small anionic polypeptide has been identified in serum that can bind C5a des arg, restoring its full chemotactic activity (Beebe et al., 1980; Perez et al., 1980). At this time, the precise biologic role of C5a des arg and its polypeptide "helper factor" is not known. However, the presence of large quantities of SCPN in serum suggests that the C5a des arg "helper" peptide complex may be responsible for the majority of the chemotactic activity generated by complement activation in vivo. Both the classical and alternative complement pathways and their biologically active produces are summarized in Figure 1.

Previous studies have suggested that C3a, like C5a, is chemotactically active for neutrophils (Ward et al., 1973; Damerau et al., 1978; and Ward and Becker, 1976). However, more recent studies with highly purified human C3a have failed to show any chemotactic activity at physiologically meaningful concentrations of C3a (Hugli, 1978). Therefore, if the complement cascade is activated within the lung parenchyma as a result of pulmonary injury, two complement-derived chemotactic activities can be generated, C5a and C5a des arg, which could cause tissue infiltration of peripheral leukocytes from the circulation.

B. Protease-Derived Chemotactic Factors

A second mechanism for generating chemotactic agents in the lung is the result of the action of leukocyte-derived products on both serum factors and structural components of the lung. Human neutrophils and alveolar macrophages are known to contain numerous proteinases, including elastase, cathepsins, collagenase, chymotrypsin, and plasminogen activator. Recent studies have shown that neutral proteases derived from leukocytes are capable of generating biologically active fragments from C3 and C5. In vitro incubation of C3 and C5 with elastase and cathepsin G, purified from human neutrophils, resulted in the generation of anaphylatoxin activity from C3 and chemotactic activity from C5 (Orr et al., 1979; Verge and Olsson, 1975). Additional evidence has demonstrated that in immune-complex-induced vasculitis in the dermis, greater than

90% of the C5-derived chemotactic activity is generated as a result of lysosomal enzyme cleavage of C5 and not from the local activation of the complement cascade (Ward and Hill, 1970).

Further evidence suggesting a significant role of leukocyte products in the generation of chemotactic factors is provided by several investigators. When rabbit serum is incubated in the presence of plasminogen and streptokinase (a plasmin-generating system) chemotactic activity for neutrophils is generated (Taylor and Ward, 1967; Ward, 1967). The data suggests that the chemotactic activity for neutrophils is derived from complement and offers another possible source for the generation of chemotactic factors in the lung. Not only will activation of the coagulation and fibrinolytic pathways result in plasmin generation, but neutrophils (Granelli-Piperno et al., 1977) and macrophages (Unkeless et al., 1974) have the ability to secrete plasminogen activator in response to a variety of stimuli.

Elastase and collagenase have the capacity to digest structural components of the lung; several recent reports suggest that, in the process, chemotactic factors are generated. Two studies have demonstrated chemotactic activity of collagen and collagen-derived peptides for monocytes and fibroblasts (Postlethwaite and Kang, 1976; Postlethwaite et al., 1978). In addition, human neutrophil elastase has been shown to generate biologically active fragments from human elastin that are chemotactic for monocytes, neutrophils, and alveolar macrophages (Senior et al., 1980). The molecular weight of the elastin-derived chemotactic activity is between 14,000 and 20,000 daltons and corresponds to elastin fragments with the highest density of desmosine cross-links. Alveolar macrophages from lungs of smokers as well as alveolar macrophages from non-smokers exposed to smoke in vitro are known to secrete increased quantities of elastase (Rodriguez et al., 1977). This suggests that the generation of chemotactic factors and the subsequent influx of inflammatory cells may in part be responsible for the structural changes in the lungs of smokers. In addition, activation of neutrophils, monocytes, and alveolar macrophages by various stimuli (including phagocytosis of inert particulate matter, bacteria, immune complexes, or stimulation with chemotactic factors) resulting in increased lysosomal enzyme release can cause additional generation of chemotactic factors by the action of the lysosomal proteases on tissue substrates. This could act either to initiate an inflammatory response or to amplify a preexisting inflammatory reaction.

C. Oxygen Metabolite-Derived Chemotactic Factors

During the last several years, a number of investigators have examined the possible role of oxygen metabolites and free radicals in initiating tissue injury. It is well established that both neutrophils and macrophages when stimulated with specific chemotactic agents or by phagocytic agents, secrete superoxide anion

(O_2^-) and hydorgen peroxide (H_2O_2) into the extracellular environment (Root et al., 1975; Becker et al., 1979; Curnutte and Babior, 1979). Additional free radicals may also be generated by the metal catalyzed nonenzymatic conversion of O_2^- (Haber-Weiss reaction)

$$M^{n+} + O_2^- = O_2 + M^{(n-1)+}$$

$$M^{(n-1)+} + H_2O_2 = OH^- + OH^{\cdot} + M^{n+}$$

$$\overline{O_2^- + H_2O_2 = O_2 + OH^- + OH}$$

and the myeloperoxidase-H_2O_2 oxidation of halide ions to hypohalite and the subsequent production of singlet oxygen ($O_2{}^1$) (Babior, 1978; Klebanoff, 1980). The generation of free radicals and their subsequent metabolites has also been implicated in tissue injury caused by exposure to toxic levels of oxygen (Saltzman and Fridovich, 1973; Rister and Baehner, 1976), antineoplastic drugs (Doroshow et al., 1980), herbicides and toxins including paraquat (Burls et al., 1980), as well as leukocyte-dependent tissue injury (Clark and Klebanoff, 1975; Kellogg and Fridovich, 1977; Nathan et al., 1979; Weiss et al., 1980; Johnson et al., 1981).

Recently, two investigators have reported the generation of chemotactic activity in plasma by superoxide-generating systems. When human plasma is incubated in vitro with the superoxide-generating system xanthine-xanthine oxidase, a chemotactic activity for neutrophils is generated (Petrone et al., 1980). This material is heat labile and appears to be a lipid bound to albumin. In separate experiments, Perez and Goldstein (1980) demonstrated the generation of a chemotactic lipid derived from the interaction of arachidonic acid and an O_2^--generating system. This product is chemotactically active at a concentration of 3.0 ng/ml and is chromatographically distinct from arachidonic acid. Thus, it appears that oxidants have the capability to generate chemotactic factors in plasma. These oxidants could possibly be derived from any of the sources noted above as well as noxious gases, including cigarette smoke, and serve to amplify the inflammatory response.

Additional studies have also suggested that oxidants may increase the local concentrations of chemotactically active materials by indirect means. Cigarette smoke, which has been shown to suppress serum elastase inhibitor (α_1-antiprotease) activity, could theoretically result in a local increase in chemotactic activity derived from interaction of leukocytic elastase in the lung (Senior et al., 1980). The inhibition of elastase inhibitor activity has been attributed to the presence of oxidants in smoke, since the phenolic antioxidants hydroquinone and thymol block the effects of the smoke-derived inactivator on α_1-antiprotease (Carp and Janoff, 1978). Also, purified α_1-protease inhibitor can be inactivated by oxygen-derived metabolites in vitro (Carp and Janoff, 1979). These data suggest that the local delivery or generation in lung of oxygen-derived metabolites may inactivate the serum-derived inhibitors of neutrophil- and monocyte-derived proteases, thereby the activity of the proteases. In addition to increasing their destructive effects on structural components of the lung, the production of chemotactic factors derived from these structural elements (e.g., elastin, collagen) would also be increased. Although the majority of recent evidence suggests that oxygen metabolites increase the local concentrations of chemotactic activity, a recent report suggests that the products of a myeloperoxidase halide system will inactivate chemotactic factors (Clark et al., 1980). In vitro studies have shown that when C5a and the synthetic chemotactic peptide (*N*-formyl-methionyl-leucyl-phenylalanine (f-Met-Leu-Phe) are exposed to a myeloperoxidase halide system, their chemotactic activities are abolished. The data suggest that the mechanism of inactivation involves the oxidation of methione residues in the chemotactic agents. Therefore, at this time it is difficult to define the precise role of oxygen-derived free radicals and metabolites in modulating inflammatory responses in the lung.

D. Cell-Derived Chemotactic Factors

Specific products of cell activation provide another possible source of chemotactic factors in the lung. One potential source of cell-derived chemotactic factor is the alveolar macrophage. Hemolytically active C5 has been identified in bronchial lavage fluids (Robertson et al., 1976; Henson et al., 1979) and, since mononuclear phagocytes have been shown to secrete several complement components, including C5 (Schrieber et al., 1973), it has been suggested that the alveolar macrophage may actively secrete C5 into the intraalveolar space. This would provide a source for the generation in the lung of C5-derived chemotactic peptides following alveolar insults from the environment. In this situation, prior vascular injury and exudation of plasma components would not be required for the generation of complement-derived chemotactic factors.

An additional mechanism by which neutrophils may be attracted to the lung is by the release of a chemotactic factor from alveolar macrophages. In vitro studies by several groups have demonstrated the secretion of a low molecular weight chemotactic factor from alveolar macrophages following stimulation by immune complexes, microorganisms, and noninfectious particulates (Kazmierowski et al., 1977; Roos et al., 1977; Hunninghake et al., 1978a; Merril et al., 1980). With human alveolar macrophages, the alveolar macrophage-derived chemotactic agent preferentially attracts neutrophils, has a molecular weight of between 400-600, and appears to be structurally related to a lipid component, that is distinctive from the hydroxy-derivatives of 5,8,10,14-eicosatetraenoic acid (Hunninghake et al., 1980b).

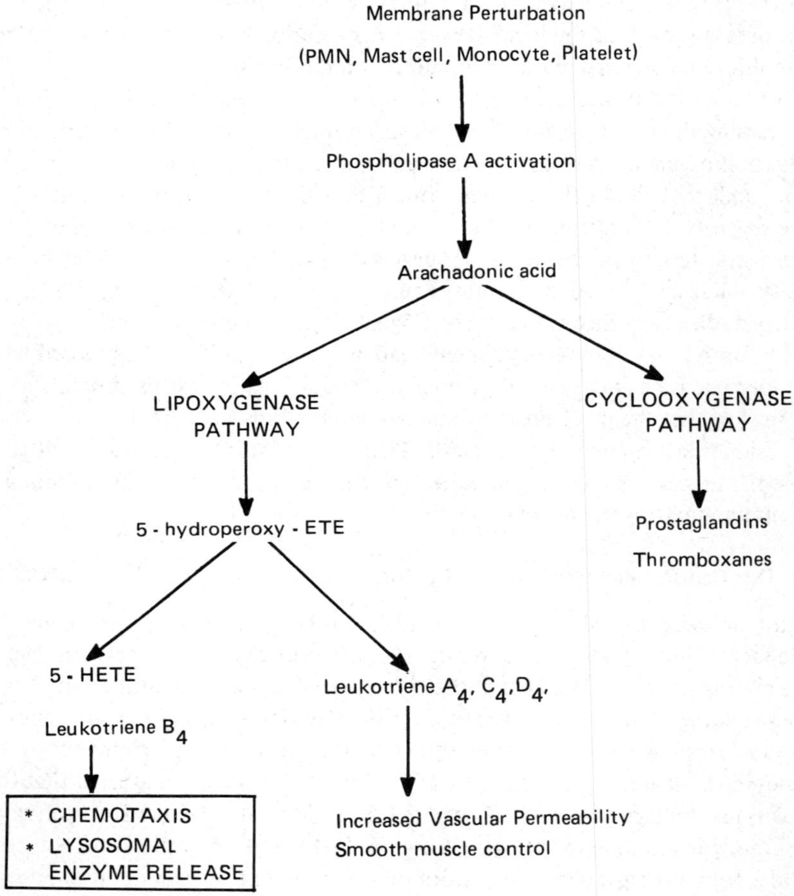

Figure 2 Metabolism of arachidonic acid.

Additional studies on stimulated alveolar macrophages have suggested that incubated macrophages release unsaturated fatty acids, primarily linoleic acid, which stimulate macrophage motility (Lynn and Mukherjee, 1979). In addition, phosphatidylglycerol, which is present in the mammalian airway, and linoleic acid, which is found in high concentration at certain inflammatory sites, have been shown to increase macrophage migration in Boyden chamber assays. Whether this represents a response of the macrophage to a specific stimulus is not clear, since macrophages show increased migrational activity in the presence of various proteins and peptides.

Another group of cell-derived chemotactic factors result from the lipoxygenation of arachidonic acid in a variety of inflammatory cells, including neutrophils (Goetzl and Sun, 1979), basophils (Goetzl, 1982), and mast cells (Roberts et al., 1979). Arachidonic acid released from the phospholipids of these activated cells is transformed by specific lipoxygenases into a series of biologically active hydroxy-eicosatetraenoic acids (HETES) and intermediate components (Fig. 2). The primary intermediate metabolite of arachidonic acid lipoxygenation that may participate in hypersensitivity responses is 5-hydroxy-eicosa-6,8, 11,14-tetraenoic acid (5-hydroperoxy-ETE) (Goetzl, 1980). The quantity and characteristics of subsequent products produced are distinct for different cell types and include a separate category of complex HETES, known as leukotrienes. Several of these arachidonic acid products have been demonstrated to have potent regulatory functions for neutrophils and eosinophils. The mono-HETES and complex HETES, including the leukotrienes, have been shown to be chemotactic for both neutrophils and eosinophils, the most potent of which are 5-HETE, 5,12-di-HETE, and leukotriene B_4 (Goetzl and Pickett, 1980). The latter two products possess chemotactic potency similar to that of C5a; however, they are much less potent than C5a in inducing lysosomal enzyme release. Therefore, the local activation of the lipoxygenase system in different cells can produce multiple products from arachidonic acid that have the ability to attract neutrophils and eosinophils to inflammatory sites. Under certain conditions, these lipid products may either be the principal mediators of the inflammatory response, or they may act to amplify an inflammatory response that is initiated by a chemotactic peptide such as C5a.

Certain classes of lymphocytes, when stimulated with either antigens or mitogens, respond by the secretion of nonantibody-soluble mediators collectively called "lymphokines." Although a large number of biologic activities of the lymphokines have been described in a number of species, the precise structure and biochemical behavior of the lymphokines have not been clearly defined. Of these various biologically active materials, several unique chemotactic activities have been described, including macrophage chemotactic factor (MCF), basophil chemotactic factor (BCF), eosinophil chemotactic factor (ECF), eosinophil stimulation promotor (ESP), lymphocyte (T cell) chemotactic factor (LCF), neutrophil chemotactic factor (NCF), and fibroblast chemotactic factor (FCF) (for review, see Altman, 1978). Although these activities have been defined in in vitro systems, it is believed that their production in vivo may be responsible for the mobilization of individual inflammatory cells leading to inflammation.

A distinct group of cell-derived chemotactic factors for eosinophils has also been defined. Neutrophils release small peptides that are chemotactic for eosinophils (Spillberg et al., 1977). These peptides are biochemically similar to the eosinophil chemotactic factor of anaphylaxis (ECF-A), which is released during IgE-mediated anaphylactic triggering of the mast cell. The ECF-A has been identified as a tetrapeptide with one of two chemical structures: Ala-Gly-Ser-Glu or Val-Gly-Ser-Glu (Kay and Austen, 1971; Goetzl and Austen, 1975). These peptides appear to react with a specific receptor on the cell membrane that triggers the locomotory response of the leukocyte. Initially thought to be specific for eosinophils, these peptides are also chemotactic for neutrophils. Although relatively high concentrations (circa 10^{-6} M) are required to induce a chemotactic response in vitro, current evidence suggests that ECF-A is responsible for the local infiltration of eosinophils associated with allergic reactions.

Histamine, another product released from mast cells during IgE-antigen activation, has also been shown to have limited chemotactic activity for eosinophils. However, the more important effect of histamine may be its ability to enhance the eosinophil responses to chemotactic factors by interaction with H_2 receptors (Clark et al., 1979).

E. Bacterial and Viral-Derived Chemotactic Factors

An additional source of chemotactic factor production in the lung includes infectious agents. Several strains of bacteria have been shown to elaborate small peptides (mol wt of approximately 1000) which are chemotactic for neutrophils (Ward et al., 1968; Schiffman et al., 1974). In addition, *Corynebacterium parvus*, which is capable of eliciting a granulomatous response in the lung, has been shown to secrete a chemotactic factor identified as a phospholipid (Russel et al., 1975). A second mechanism by which bacteria are capable of generating chemotactic agents is through the release of enzymes which are capable of cleaving C5 into active fragments (Ward et al., 1973). Similarly, viruses have been shown to induce the release of chemotactic factors which do not contain viral particles and are complement independent. Virus-infected cells also produce C5-cleaving enzymes which are most likely derived from host cell lysosomal granules (Brier et al., 1970; Ward et al., 1972). Therefore, there is substantial evidence that specific infectious agents are capable of directly and indirectly producing chemotactic activities in the lung and potentially initiate an inflammatory response.

II. Biological Effects of Chemotactic Factors on Lung

A. Effects of Intravascular Chemotactic Factors

The sequestration in lung vasculature of circulating neutrophils has been noted in extracorporal hemodialysis and is related to intravascular complement activation resulting in the generation of chemotactic factors (Craddock et al., 1977a,b). Also, circulating immune complexes, which have the ability to generate complement-derived chemotactic factors, have been associated with pulmonary injury. Neutrophils, when incubated in vitro in the presence of chemotactic factors, such as C5a or the synthetic chemotactic peptide *N*-formyl-methionyl-leucyl-phenylalanine (f-Met-Leu-Phe) respond with an increase in cell volume and the formation of multicellular aggregates (Jacob et al., 1980; for review see, O'Flaherty and Ward, 1978). Simultaneously, these leukocytes begin to produce active oxygen metabolites (Becker et al., 1979). In an in vitro system, oxygen-derived metabolites from complement-activated neutrophils have been shown to be cytotoxic for endothelial cells (Sacks et al., 1978; Weiss et al., 1981). It has been postulated that the sequestration of neutrophils in the lung results in endothelial cell injury caused by oxygen metabolites and is the mechanism of lung damage in patients with a variety of conditions associated with complement activation. Therefore, considerable effort has been devoted to examining the effects of lung complement activation products that have been preformed in vitro or formed in vivo. Several groups have shown that rabbits develop a marked, transient neutropenia with sequestration of neutrophils in the pulmonary vascular bed after infusion of the cobra venom factor (CVF), an activator of the alternative complement pathway (O'Flaherty et al., 1977, 1978). The evidence suggests that a low molecular weight complement-derived product may be responsible both for the resulting neutrophil aggregation and subsequent embolization in capillaries as well as an increased adherence of neutrophils to vessel endothelial cells (margination). In vivo, when a single intravenous infusions of f-Met-Leu-Phe, C5a, or complement-activated rabbit plasma is given, a rapid and marked neutropenia develops, reaching a nadir within 1 min with recovery of neutrophil counts to preinfusion levels within 30 min (O'Flaherty et al., 1977). This is frequently followed by an as yet unexplained neutrophilia (Gilbertson et al., 1980). However, in all cases, the neutropenia is transient and there is little evidence that the entrapment of neutrophils in the pulmonary capillary beds results in lung injury. In a recent report, zymosan-activated autologous serum reinfused into sheep produces marked pulmonary leukostasis and pulmonary edema (Craddock et al., 1977b). This represents one of the few reports in which infusion of activated complement components results in definitive lung injury. The discrepancy between the observations in sheep and rabbit experiments is puzzling. However, since the sheep neutrophils are not as well characterized as the rabbit, there may be species differences in their responses to chemotactic factors. The precise role that intravascular generation of chemotactic factors may play in initiating lung injury still remains to be clarified.

B. Effects of Intraalveolar Chemotactic Factors

Immune complexes (IC) have been implicated in a number of pulmonary diseases. In experimental models (see below), the phlogistic properties of IC have been attributed to their ability to activate complement and generate chemotactic peptides, resulting in neutrophil influx. In addition, the presence of complement

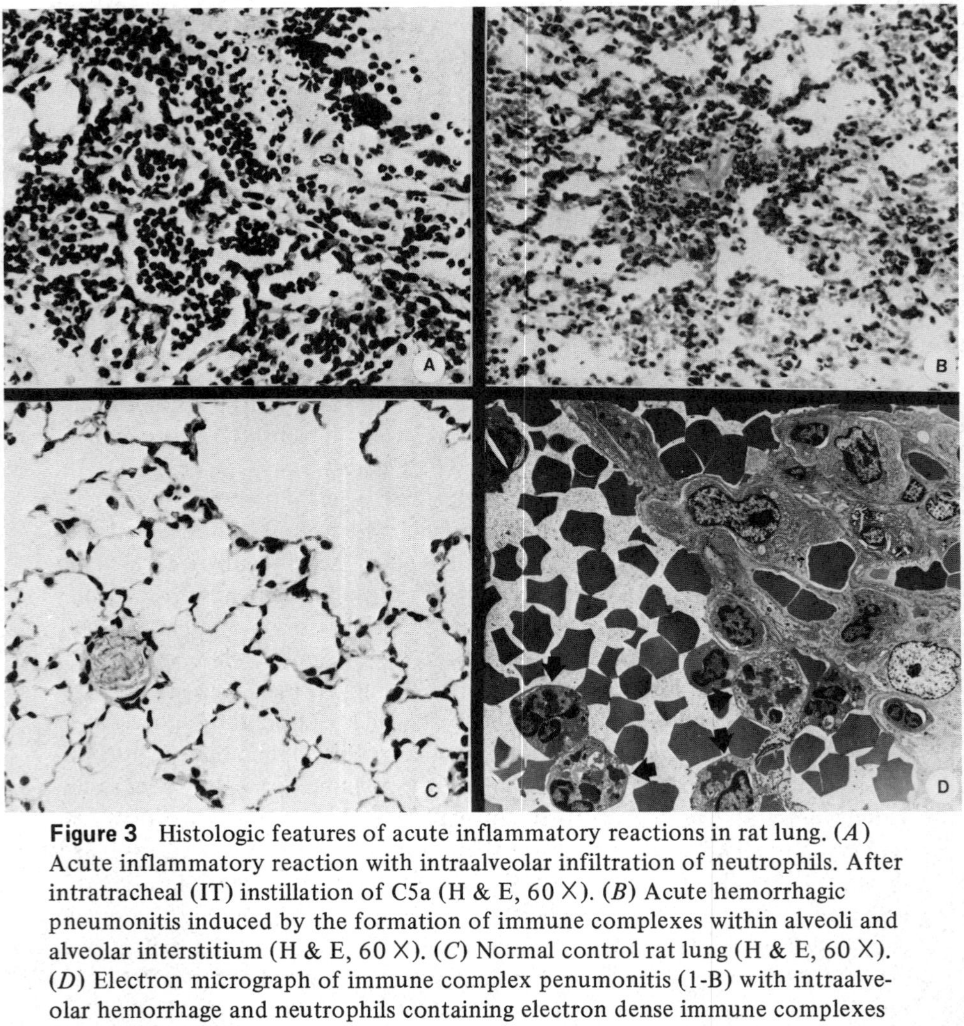

Figure 3 Histologic features of acute inflammatory reactions in rat lung. (*A*) Acute inflammatory reaction with intraalveolar infiltration of neutrophils. After intratracheal (IT) instillation of C5a (H & E, 60 X). (*B*) Acute hemorrhagic pneumonitis induced by the formation of immune complexes within alveoli and alveolar interstitium (H & E, 60 X). (*C*) Normal control rat lung (H & E, 60 X). (*D*) Electron micrograph of immune complex penumonitis (1-B) with intraalveolar hemorrhage and neutrophils containing electron dense immune complexes (arrows) (1250 X).

components, including C5, in bronchial lavage fluids has led to the investigation of the effects of intratracheal instillation of chemotactic factors into the lung.

Using highly purified preparations of C5, C5a, and C5a des arg, several groups have reported the production of acute lung injury after intratracheal instillation of the peptides. In hamsters, airway instillation of 200 mg of intact human C5 results in an intense, acute inflammatory reaction in the lung consisting of large numbers of neutrophils (Desai et al., 1979). This reaction appears to be the result of intrapulmonary cleavage of C5 into chemotactically active fragments by lung-derived proteases, possibly of alveolar macrophage origin. The intrapulmonary (airway) instillation into rabbits (Shaw et al., 1978) or hamsters (Kreutzer et al., 1979a) of small quantities (10-40 μg) of chemotactically active fragments derived from C5 produces a neutrophil-rich, diffuse inflammatory infiltrate which reaches a peak within 4 hr after instillation. This response is dose related and provides direct evidence for the phlogistic properties of C5a in the lung (Fig. 3).

Since C5a is rapidly converted to C5a des arg in vivo by SCPN, additional studies have been undertaken to investigate the inflammatory potential of C5a des arg in the lung (Stimler et al., 1980). After intratracheal instillation of C5a des arg (10-20 μg) into rabbit lungs, an intense acute inflammatory response develops, reaching a peak within 6 hr. In comparison with C5a, the rabbit lung was more susceptible to injury by C5a des arg, suggesting that in vivo C5a des arg may be the significant mediator of lung injury. Although C5a des arg is less active than C5a in in vitro systems, the possible formation of a C5a des arg-"helper" factor complex (discussed above) could explain the in vivo observations. These data demonstrate the strong phlogistic potential of C5-derived chemotactic peptides and support their potential role in inflammatory reactions in the lungs.

III. Experimental Studies Implicating a Role for Chemotactic Factors

A. Immune-Complex-Induced Alveolitis

There is abundant evidence in both in vivo and in vitro models suggesting that immune complexes have the ability to elicit an inflammatory response by the generation of chemotactic factors derived from complement activation. The first experimental studies that suggested a possible role of immune complexes in lung injury were described by Knicker and Cochrane (1965) in the model of acute ("one shot") serum sickness. They described reversible changes in medium-sized pulmonary arteries consisting of acute inflammatory reactions in the vessel wall with both medial and endothelial cell proliferation. Immunofluorescent studies of the vessel walls revealed the presence of both immunoglobulin (IgG), antigen, and complement components (C3). In a series of complement depletion experiments using CVF, the degree of vascular injury and neutrophil influx was markedly depressed despite the deposition of immune complexes. Although the intrapulmonary changes in these studies were limited to the vascular compartment, the data nevertheless implicate the role of complement in the initiation of neutrophil accumulation and tissue injury.

Currently, the only evidence that suggests that circulating immune complexes can directly cause irreversible lung injury is in the model of chronic serum sickness in rabbits. When antigen is injected daily over a period of weeks, an intense inflammatory response with irreversible changes of the alveolar interstitium and basement membrane develops (Brentjens et al., 1974). Electron microscopic and immunofluorescent studies reveal an inflammatory reaction with fibrin deposition, interstitial fibrosis, thickening of the capillary basement membrane, and deposits of immune complexes and complement in the vascular basement membrane. The most intense reaction is observed in those rabbits who have a marked and protracted antibody response and are maintained in a state of relative antigen-antibody equivalence. These conditions produce immune complexes whose size and complement-fixing activity are maximum. These studies suggest that circulating immune complexes can elicit inflammatory changes in the lung mediated by the local activation of complement and the generation of chemotactic factors. However, it is possible that other immune mechanisms are active in these models (e.g., cellular immune mechanisms) and may contribute to the inflammatory response and the development of interstitial fibrosis.

Immune complexes formed in the alveolar compartment are also capable of producing inflammatory reactions in the lung. In a model similar to the reversed passive Arthus reaction in the skin, an intense acute inflammatory reaction in rat lung is produced after the intratracheal administration of heterologous (rabbit IgG) antibody and the simultaneous intravascular injection of antigen (Johnson and Ward, 1974). This reaction produces a hemorrhagic, intra-alveolar, and interstitial reaction which is most intense 4-6 hr after antibody instillation (Fig. 3). The deposition of antibody, antigen, and complement components occurs in alveolar walls. The essential requirement for the participation of complement and neutrophils in the lung injury associated with these reactions has been demonstrated. The mechanism of neutrophil influx is thought to result from the diffusion of antibody and antigen from the alveoli and vascular compartments forming immune complexes within alveolar walls. Chemotactic peptides (e.g., C5a) are generated from the activation of the classical complement pathway, resulting in the chemotactic attraction of neutrophils from the circulation. The immune complexes are phagocytized by neutrophils, and they release proteolytic enzymes from lysosomal granules that are capable of both hydrolysis of the structural proteins (e.g., collagen and elastin) and generation of additional chemotactic factors from C5. In addition, oxygen-derived metabolites such as O_2^-, H_2O_2, $OH^\cdot$, and HOCl are also generated. These products have the capacity to augment the inflammatory response by generating chemotactic lipids (see above). In these inflammatory reactions, alveolar macrophages are theoretically capable of phagocytizing immune complexes and generating products similar to those described for the neutrophil (summarized, Fig. 4).

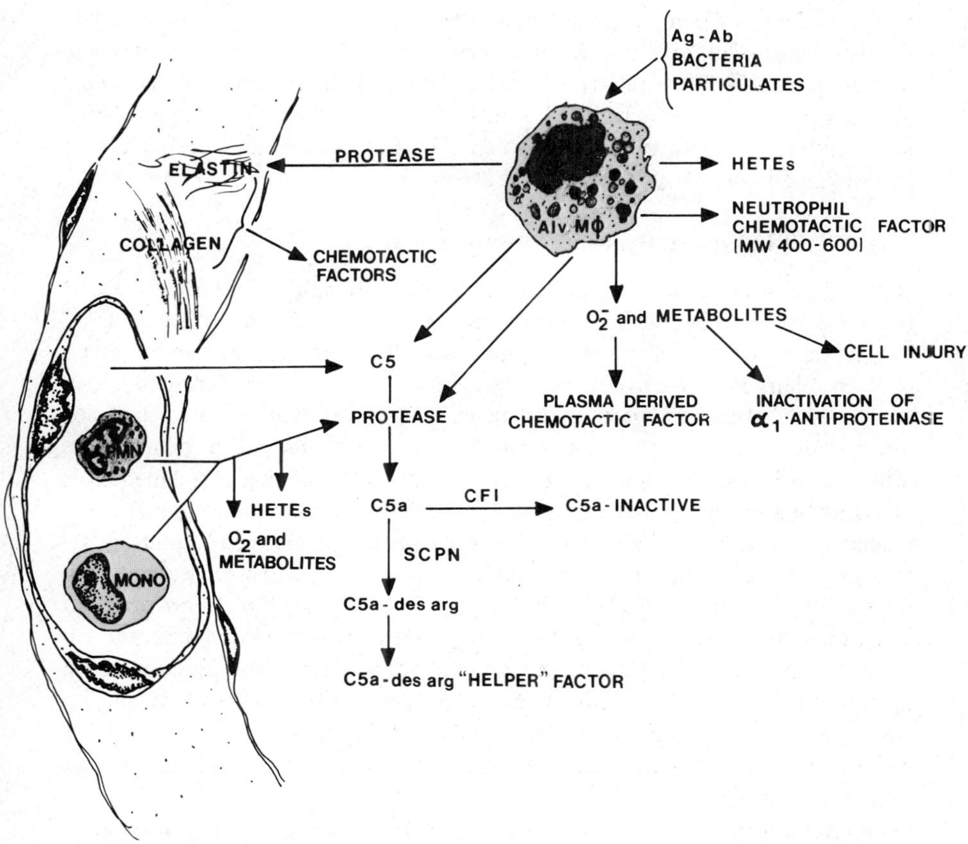

Figure 4 Local mechanisms of chemotactic factor generation in the lung.

A similar inflammatory response has been seen in the lung after the intratracheal administration of preformed immune complexes into rats (Scherzer and Ward, 1978a,b). An acute, hemorrhagic, inflammatory reaction with a pronounced neutrophil infiltrate is present in the lung after airway instillation of preformed immune complexes. The reaction resembles the reversed passive Arthus reaction in the lung (as described above) and is both neutrophil and complement dependent. The critical property in the initiation of the inflammatory reaction appears to be the ratio of antigen to antibody in the immune complexes. The most intense reaction occurs when the complexes are formed at equivalence, corresponding to complexes with the greatest complement-fixing activity. Complexes formed at six times antigen excess or greater are less phlogistic, smaller in size, and do not actively fix complement. This evidence supports the dependency of immune complex-induced lung injury on complement activation and neutrophil influx. Additional experimental models of immune-complex-mediated lung injury have demonstrated complement- and neutrophil-dependent mechanisms after aerosol challenge or intrapleural injection of antigen into actively immunized rabbits (Willoughby et al., 1979; Kaplan et al., 1980), and guinea pigs (Richerson, 1972; Roska et al., 1979).

B. Cell-Mediated Reactions—Lymphokines

It is well known that, in in vitro systems, sensitized lymphocytes have the ability to secrete lymphokines which appear to be the soluble mediators of delayed hypersensitivity (for review see, Rocklin et al., 1980). As described above, several distinct lymphocyte-derived chemotactic activities have been identified. However, in contrast to immune complex models of lung injury, there is a paucity of direct evidence that demonstrates a role for chemotactic factors in cell-mediated inflammatory reactions in the lung. Much of our understanding of the mediators of granulomatous lung disease must be inferred from in vitro data and cell-mediated reactions in other tissues. The mechanism of granuloma formation, at least in part, may involve the ingestion of insoluble antigen and subsequent slow release from macrophages of soluble antigen. The antigen is then "presented" to T lymphocytes resulting in "sensitization." After this initial period, effector T lymphocytes travel to the site of antigen, interacting with it, and produce a spectrum of lymphokines. Circulating monocytes, lymphocytes, neutrophils, and eosinophils are then recruited into the locale by the action of lymphokines with chemotactic activity. Quite clearly, the bulk of inflammatory cells in these reactions are antigen nonreactive.

Granulomas isolated from infected animals have been shown to secrete lymphokines in culture. Liver granulomas from mice with schistosomiasis have been shown to produce migration inhibitory factor (MIF) and an eosinophil chemotactic factor (ECF) (Boros et al., 1973; James and Colley, 1975). In mice infected with BCG organisms, MIF activity has been identified in the serum (Salvin et al., 1973), and a macrophage chemotactic factor (MCF) activity has been demonstrated in peritoneal exudates of sensitized guinea pigs challenged with antigen (Postlewaite and Snyderman, 1975). In vitro cultures of beryllium granulomas produce both MIF and lymphotoxin (Marx and Burrell, 1973) while lymphocytes isolated from sensitized guinea pigs produce MIF when incubated with *Micropolyspora faeni* antigen, the causative agent in farmer's lung disease (Marx et al., 1973). Recent studies have demonstrated the secretion of a chemotactic factor (mol wt approx. 11,000) for monocytes when T lymphocytes isolated from BCG granulomas in mice have been cultured in vitro (Schrier and Moore, personal communication). Finally, chemotactic lymphokines have been demonstrated in extracts of tissues of guinea pigs developing delayed hypersensitivity reactions in guinea pigs (Cohen et al., 1973). Thus, the evidence that chemotactic lymphokines play an essential role in lung inflammatory reactions is indirect. Much further study is required.

IV. Regulation of Chemotactic Factors of Lung

A. Inhibitors of Complement Activation

The regulation of chemotactic factor activity in the lung can occur by two different mechanisms. The first involves the inhibition of activation of the complement system. Spontaneous activation of the classical complement system is blocked by the presence of C1-esterase inhibitor (C1-INH) in serum. This α_2-globulin (mol wt approx. 100,000) forms an irreversible complex with activated C1 and inhibits the esterolytic sites of the C1 molecule (Pensky et al., 1961; Gigli et al., 1968). C1-INH has also been shown to block the proteolytic activity of kallikrein (McConnell, 1972), plasmin (Ratnoff et al., 1969; Schrieber et al., 1973), activated Hageman factor (factor XIIa), and factor XIa (Forbes et al., 1970). Thus, for successful activation of the classical complement pathway, the inhibitory activity of C1-INH must be overcome. This can occur if the activating stimulus is of sufficient intensity and adequate quantities of activated C1 are generated to react with C4 and C2. Also, C1-INH may be consumed by activation of the coagulation, fibrinolytic, or kinin-forming systems. A third mechanism involves a genetic deficiency of C1-INH that presents clinically as the syndrome of angioedema (Donaldson and Evans, 1963).

Spontaneous activation of the alternative complement pathway is inhibited by two serum proteins, B1H and C3b inactivator (C3b-INA). B1H blocks the formation of the C3 convertase (C3bBb) by competitively binding to C3b and blocking the binding to factor B (Pangburn and Muller-Eberhard, 1978; Kazatchkine et al., 1979). C3b-INA cleaves C3b into the inactive fragments C3c and C3d, which are from part of the complex that activates C5 (Ruddy and Austen, 1971; Gitlin et al., 1975). The presence of both these proteins is necessary to prevent spontaneous activation of the alternative pathway (Whaley and Ruddy, 1976a,b).

B. Inactivators of Chemotactic Factor

Two activities in serum have been identified with the ability to modulate the activity of chemotactic factors. The activities of the anaphylatoxin inactivator (serum carboxypeptidase N or SCPN) have been described above and appear to play an important role in modifying biologic responses to complement-derived chemotactic factors.

Another activity has been identified in serum defined as chemotactic factor inactivator activity (CFI). This represents a group of distinct activities present in serum that have the ability to irreversibly inactivate bacterial, lymphocyte, and complement-derived chemotactic factors (Berenberg and Ward, 1973; Till and Ward, 1975). The CFI, which inactivates the complement-derived chemotactic activities (i.e., C5a, C5a des arg), is distinct from SCPN and has a molecular weight of approximately 150,000 (Kreutzer et al., 1979a). At this time, its physical properties are not fully characterized, although it is believed to inactivate C5a by enzymatic cleavage. Studies of various disease states have shown the presence of altered levels of CFI activity in serum, suggesting that CFI may play an important role in modulating the inflammatory response. Elevated levels of serum CFI are found in patients with Hodgkin's disease (Ward and Berenberg, 1974), hepatic cirrhosis (Maderazo et al., 1975) sarcoidosis (Maderazo et al., 1976), and lepromatous leprosy (Ward et al., 1976). In general, the ability to mobilize acute inflammatory cells in these patients seems to be markedly impaired. Experimentally, the instillation of CFI purified from human serum into lungs of animals undergoing acute immune complex-induced injury markedly attenuates the intensity of the inflammatory reaction and resulting lung damage (Johnson et al., 1977), providing additional evidence that these reactions are mediated by C5 chemotactic factors.

V. Clinical Evidence for the Role of Chemotactic Factors in Lung Diseases

The experimental evidence presented above suggests that lung injury resulting from the accumulation of inflammatory cells, including neutrophils, eosinophils, lymphocytes, or macrophages, must in some way result from the local generation of chemotactic factors. However, there are only a few diseases in which chemotactic factors have been implicated in lung injury, and the evidence is usually of an indirect nature.

A role for chemotactic factors in lung injury is best supported in cases of idiopathic pulmonary fibrosis. In patients with active disease, immunofluorescent studies have revealed the presence of immunoglobulin and complement components in the lung interstitium (Dreisin et al., 1978). In addition, immune complexes capable of activating complement have been identified both in serum (Dreisin et al., 1978; Haslam et al., 1979) and in bronchial lavage fluids (Hunninghake et al., 1978b). The intensity of the inflammatory component in lung biopsy specimens has been shown to correlate with the presence of immune complexes in the lung and serum.

The inflammatory pneumonitis associated with systemic lupus erythematosis (SLE) is thought to be the result of immune complex deposition in the lung with activation of complement leading to an inflammatory infiltrate. Immunohistopathologic studies of lung tissue from patients with SLE pneumonitis have revealed deposits of IgG, C3, and antigen (DNA) in the alveolar and interstitial compartments (Brentjens et al., 1977; Pertschuck et al., 1977; Inoue et al., 1979). Analysis of pleural fluids from patients with SLE or rheumatoid arthritis (RA) have demonstrated the presence of immune complexes and decreased levels of complement activities (Hunder et al., 1972; Halla et al., 1980). In addition, the pleural fluid of one patient with RA has been shown to contain a substance capable of activating the classical complement pathway (Glovsky et al., 1976). Deposits of immune complexes with complement proteins has been reported in lung tissue of patients with eosinophilic granuloma of the lung (King et al., 1979). There are also selected reports of a decrease in serum complement levels after aerosol antigen challenge in asthmatic patients (Arroyave et al., 1982) and patients with farmer's lung (Edwards, 1976).

As emphasized above, there is a paucity of clinical evidence supporting the role of chemotactic factors in granulomatous lung inflammation. In vivo, T lymphocytes from patients with sarcoidosis (Hunninghake et al., 1979), farmer's lung disease (Caldwell et al., 1973), and pigeon breeder's disease (Hansen and Penny, 1974; Fink et al., 1975) show increased lymphokine production when stimulated with appropriate antigens. In one study, 60% of sarcoid patients showed circulating levels of MIF activity (Yoshida et al., 1979). Recent in vitro studies of T lymphocytes isolated from bronchoalveolar lavage fluids in patients with sarcoidosis have demonstrated that these cells secrete a factor chemotactic for monocytes (Hunninghake et al., 1980c). This factor also was secreted from peripheral blood lymphocytes in the same patients but in much smaller quantities. There are also rare reports of immunoglobulin and complement deposition in lung tissues of patients with hypersensitivity pneumonitis (Ghose et al., 1974b) and sarcoidosis (Ghose et al., 1974a). The precise significance of these findings as they relate to the clinical condition and treatment of the patients awaits further study.

References

Altman, L. C. (1978). Chemotactic lymphokines: A review. In *Leukocyte Chemotaxis, Methods, Physiology, and Clinical Implications.* Edited by J. I. Gallin and P. G. Quie, New York, Raven Press, pp. 267-289.

Andrews, J. M., and Baillie, R. D. (1979). The enzymatic nature of human C1r: A subcomponent of the first component of complement. *J. Immunol., 123*:1403.

Arroyave, C. M., Stevenson, D. D., Vaughan, J. H., and Tan, E. M. (1982). Plasma complement changes during provoked bronchospasm in asthmatic patients. *J. Clin. Allergy.* (In Press).

Babior, B. M. (1978). Oxygen-dependent microbial killing by phagocytes. Part I. *New Engl. J. Med., 298*:659-668.

Becker, E. L., Sigman, M., and Oliver, J. M. (1979). Superoxide production induced in rabbit polymorphonuclear leukocytes by synthetic chemotactic peptides and A23187. *Amer. J. Pathol., 95*:81-97.

Beebe, D. P., Ward, P. A., and Spitznagel, S. K. (1980). Isolation and characterization of an acidic chemotactic factor from complement activated human serum. *Clin. Immunol. Immunopathol., 15*:88-105.

Berenberg, J. L., and Ward, P. A. (1973). The chemotactic factor inactivator in normal human serum. *J. Clin. Invest., 52*:1200-1206.

Bhadki, S., Ey, P., and Bhakdi-Lehnen, B. (1976). Isolation of the terminal complement complex from target sheep erythrocyte membranes. *Biochim. Biophys. Acta, 419*:445.

Bokisch, V. A., and Muller-Eberhard, H. J. (1970). Anaphylatoxin inactivator of human plasma: Its isolation and characterization as a carboxypeptidase. *J. Clin. Invest., 49*:2427-2436.

Boros, D. L., Warren, K. S., and Pelley, R. P. (1973). The secretion of migration inhibitory factor by intact schistosome egg granulomas maintained in vitro. *Nature, 246*:224-231.

Brentjens, J. R., O'Connell, D. W., Pawlowski, I. B., Hsu, K. C., and Andres, G. A. (1974). Experimental immune complex disease of the lung. The pathogenesis of a laboratory model resembling certain human interstitial diseases. *J. Exp. Med., 140*:105-125.

Brentjens, J., Ossie, E., Albini, B., Sepulveda, M., Kano, K., Sheffer, J., Vasilion, P., Marine, E., Baliah, T., Jockin, H., and Andres, G. (1977). Disseminated immune deposits in lupus erythematosus. *Arthritis Rheum., 20*: 962-968.

Brentjens, J., Ossie, E., Albini, B. et al. (1977). Disseminated immune deposits in lupus erythematosus. *Arthritis Rheum., 20*:962-968.

Brier, A. M., Snyderman, R., Mergenhagen, J. E., and Notkins, A. L. (1970). Inflammation and herpes simplex virus: Release of a chemotaxis-generating factor from infected cells. *Science, 170*:1104-1106.

Budzko, D. B., and Muller-Eberhard, H. J. (1970). Cleavage of the fourth component of human complement (C4) by C1 esterases: Isolation and characterization of the low molecular weight product. *Immunochemistry, 7*: 227-234.

Burls, R. F., Lawrence, R. A., and Love, M. M. (1980). Liver necrosis and lipid peroxidation in the rat as a result of paraquot and diquot administration. Effect of selenium deficiency. *J. Clin. Invest., 65*:1024-1031.

Caldwell, J. R., Pearce, D. E., Spencer, C., Leder, R., and Waldman, R. H. (1973). Immunologic mechanisms in hypersensitivity pneumonitis: Evidence for cell-mediated immunity and complement fixation in pigeon breeder's disease. *J. Allergy Clin. Immunol., 52*:225-230.

Carp, H., and Janoff, A. (1978). Possible mechanisms of emphysema in smokers. In vitro suppression of serum elastase-inhibitory capacity by fresh cigarette smoke and its prevention by antioxidants. *Amer. Rev. Respir. Dis., 118*:617-621.

Carp, H., and Janoff, A. (1979). In vitro suppression of serum elastase inhitory capacity by reactive oxygen species generated by phagocytosing polymorphonuclear leukocytes. *J. Clin. Invest., 63*:793-797.

Chenoweth, D. E., and Hugli, T. F. (1980). Human C5a and C5a analogs as probes of the neutrophil C5a receptor. *Mol. Immunol., 17*:151-1588.

Clark, R. A., and Klebanoff, S. J. (1975). Neutrophil-mediated tumor cell toxicity: Role of the peroxidase system. *J. Exp. Med., 141*:1442-1447.

Clark, R. A., Sandler, J. A., Gallin, J. I., and Kaplan, A. P. (1979). Histamine modulation of eosinophil migration. *J. Immunol., 118*:137-146.

Clark, R. A., Szot, S., Venkatasubramanian, K., and Schiffman, E. (1980). Chemotactic factor inactivation by myeloperoxidase mediated oxidation of methionine. *J. Immunol., 124*:2020-2026.

Cohen, S., Ward, P. A., Yoshida, T., and Burek, C. L. (1973). Biologic activity of extracts of delayed hypersensitivity skin reaction sites. *Cell. Immunol., 9*:363-369.

Craddock, P. R., Fahr, J., Dalmasso, A. P., Brigham, K. L., and Jacob, H. S. (1977a). Pulmonary vascular leukostasis resulting from complement (C1) activation by dialyzer cellophane membranes. *J. Clin. Invest., 59*: 879-888.

Craddock, P. R., Fehr, J., Brigham, K. L., Kronenberg, R. S., and Jacob, H. S. (1977b). Complement and leukocyte-mediated pulmonary dysfunction in hemodialysis. *N. Engl. J. Med., 296*:769-774.

Curnette, J. T., and Babior, B. M. (1979). Biologic defense mechanisms. The effects of bacteria and serum on superoxide production of granulocytes. *J. Clin. Invest., 53*:1662-1674.

Damerau, B., Grunefeld, E., and Vogt, W. (1978). Chemotactic effects of the complement-derived peptides C3a, C3ai, and C5a (classical anaphylatoxin) on rabbit and guinea-pig polymorphonuclear leukocytes. *Naunyn-Schmiedeberg's Arch. Pharmacol., 305*:181-184.

Desai, U., Kreutzer, D. L., Showell, H. J., Arroyave, C. F., and Ward, P. A. (1979). Acute inflammatory pulmonary reactions induced by chemotactic factors. *Amer. J. Pathol., 96*:71-83.

Dias Da Silva, W., Eisele, J. W., and Lepow, I. H. (1967). Complement as a mediator of inflammation. III. Purification of the activity with anaphylatoxin properties generated by interaction of the first four components of complement and its identification as a cleavage produce of C3. *J. Exp. Med., 126*:1027-1048.

Donaldson, V. H., and Evans, R. R. (1963). A biochemical abnormality in hereditaroy angioneurotic edama. *Am. J. Med., 35*:37.

Doroshow, J. H., Locker, G. Y., and Myers, C. E. (1980). Enzymatic defenses of the mouse heart against reactive oxygen metabolites. Alterations produced by doxorubicin. *J. Clin. Invest., 65*:128-135.

Dreisen, R. B., Schwarz, M. I., Theofilopoulos, A. N., and Stanford, R. E. (1978). Circulating immune complexes in the idiopathic interstitial pneumonias. *New Engl. J. Med., 298*:353-357.

Edwards, J. H. (1976). A quantitative study in the activation of the alternative pathway of complement by mouldy hay dust and thermophilic actinomycetes. *Clin. Allergy, 6*:19-25.

Fernandez, H. N., Henson, P. M., Otani, A., and Hugli, T. E. (1978). Chemotactic response of human C3a and C5a anaplylatoxins. 1. Evaluation of C3a and C5a leukotaxis in vitro under simulated in vivo conditions. *J. Immunol., 120*:109-115.

Fink, J. N., Moore, V. L., and Barboriak, J. J. (1975). Cell-mediated hypersensitivity in pigeon breeders. *Int. Arch Allergy Appl. Immunol., 49*:831-836.

Forbes, C. D., Pensky, J., and Ratnoff, O. D. (1970). Inhibition of activated Hageman Factor and activated plasma thromboplastin antecedent by purified serum C1 inactivator. *J. Lab. Clin. Med., 76*:809-815.

Ghose, T., Landrigan, P., and Asif, A. (1974a). Localization of immunoglobulin and complement in pulmonary sarcoid granulomas. *Chest, 66*:264-268.

Ghose, T., Landrigan, P., Killeen, R., and Dill, J. (1974b). Immunopathological studies in patients with farmer's lung. *Clin. Allergy, 4*:119-126.

Gigli, I., Ruddy, S., and Austen, K. F. (1968). The stoichiometric measurement of the serum inhibitor of the first component of complement by the inhibition of immune hemolysis. *J. Immunol., 100*:1154-1164.

Gilbertsen, R. B., Carter, G. W., and Quinn, D. J. (1980). Effects of F-met-leu-phe and zymosan-activated serum on rat neutrophils in vivo. *J. Rect. Soc., 27*:485-494.

Gitlin, J. D., Rosen, F. S., and Lachman, P. J. (1975). The mechanism of action of the C3b inactivator (conglutinogen-activating factor) on its naturally occurring substrate, the major fragment of the third component of complement (C3b). *J. Exp. Med., 141*:1221-1229.

Glovsky, M. M., Louise, J. G., Pitts, W. H., and Alenty, A. (1976). Reduction of pleural fluid complement activity in patients with systemic lupus erythematosus and rheumetoid arthritis. *Clin. Immunol. Immunopathol., 6*: 31-41.

Goetzl, E. J. (1980). Mediators of immediate hypersensitivity derived from arachidonic acid. *N. Engl. J. Med., 303*:822-825.

Goetzl, E. J. (1982). The generation and secretion of hydroxyeicosatetranoic acids (HETES) by human basophils. In *Progress in Immunology IV.* (In Press).

Goetzl, E. J., and Austen, K. F. (1975). Purification and synthesis of eosinophilotactic tetrapeptides of human lung tissue: Identification as eosinophil chemotactic factor of anaphylaxis. *Proc. Natl. Acad. Sci. USA, 72*:4123-4127.

Goetzl, E. J., and Pickett, W. C. (1980). The human PMN leukocyte chemotactic activity of comples hydroxy-eicosatetranoic acids (HETES). *J. Immunol., 125*:1789-1791.

Goetzl, E. J., and Sun, F. F. (1979). Generation of unique mono-hydroxy-eicosatetranoic acids of arachidonic acid by human neutrophils. *J. Exp. Med., 150*:406-411.

Goldman, M. B., Bangalore, S., and Goldman, J. N. (1978). Functional and biochemical properties of the early classical complement system in mice. *J. Immunol., 120*:216-222.

Granelli-Piperno, A., Vassalli, J-D., and Reich, E. (1977). Secretion of plasminogen activator by human polymorphonuclear leukocytes modulation by glucocortivoids and other effectors. *J. Exp. Med., 146*:1693-1706.

Halla, J. T., Schrottenlotter, R. E., and Volankis, J. E. (1980). Immune complexes and other laboratory features of pleural effusions. A comparison of rheumatoid arthritis, systemic lupus erythematosus and other diseases. *Ann. Intern. Med., 92*:748-752.

Hansen, P. J., and Penny, R. (1974). Pigeon breeder's disease: Study of cell-mediated immune response to pigeon antigens by the lymphocyte culture technique. *Int. Arch. Allergy App. Immunol., 47*:498-507.

Haslam, D. L., Thompson, B., Mohammed, I., Townsend, P. J., Hodson, M. E., Holbrow, E. J., and Turner-Warwick, M. (1979). Circulating immune complexes in patients with cryptogenic fibrosing alveolitis. *Clin. Exp. Immunol., 37*:381-390.

Henson, P. M., McCarthy, K., Larsen, G. L., Webster, R. O., Gickas, P. C., Dreisin, R. B., King, T. E., and Shaw, J. O. (1979). Complement fragments, alveolar macrophages, and alveolitis. *Am. J. Pathol., 97*:93-110.

Hugli, T. E. (1978). Chemical aspects of the serum anaphylatoxins. *Contemp. Top. Mol. Immunol., 7*:181-214.

Hugli, T. E., and Muller-Eberhard. (1978). Anaphylatoxins: C3a and C5a. *Adv. Immunol., 26*:1

Hunder, G. G., McDuffie, F. C., and Hepper, N. G. G. (1972). Pleural fluid complement in systemic lupus erythematosis and rheumatoid arthritis. *Ann. Intern. Med., 76*:357-363.

Hunninghake, G., Gadek, J., and Crystal, R. (1980a). Mechanisms by which cigarette smoke attracts polymorphonuclear leukocytes to lung. *Chest, 77* (Suppl.):273.

Hunninghake, G. W., Gallin, J. I., and Fauci, A. S. (1978a). Immunologic reactivity of the lung: The in vivo and in vitro generation of a neutrophil chemotactic factor by alveolar macrophages. *Am. Rev. Respir. Dis., 117*: 15-23.

Hunninghake, G. W., Gadek, J. E., Fales, H. M., and Crystal, R. G. (1980b). Human alveolar macrophage-derived chemotactic factor for neutrophils. Stimuli and partial characterization. *J. Clin. Invest., 66*:473-483.

Hunninghake, G. W., Gadeh, J. E., Young, R. C., Kawanami, O., Ferran, N. J., and Crystal, R. (1980c). Maintenance of granuloma formation in pulmonary sarcoidosis by T-lymphocytes within the lung. *N. Engl. J. Med., 302*: 594-598.

Hunninghake, G. W., Fulmer, J. D., Young, R. C., Gadek, J. E., and Crystal, R. G. (1979). Localization of the immune response in sarcoidosis. *Am. Rev. Respir. Dis., 120*:49-57.

Hunninghake, G. W., Gadek, J. E., Lawly, T. J., Kelman, J., Fulmer, J. D., and Crystal, R. G. (1978b). Role of immune complexes in amplifying the alveolitis of idiopathic pulmonary fibrosis (IPF). *Clin. Res., 26*:446A (Abstract).

Hyslop, N. E., Dourmashkin, R. R., Green, N. M., and Porter, R. R. (1970). The fixation of complement and the activation first component of complement by complexes formed between antibody and divalent hapten. *J. Exp. Med., 131*:783-802.

Inoue, T., Kanayamu, Y., Ohe, Akiko, Kato, N., Horiguchi, T., Ishii, M., and Zshiota, K. (1979). Immunopathologic studies of pneumonitis in systemic lupus erythematosus. *Ann. Inter. Med., 91*:30-34.

Jacob, H. S., Craddock, P. R., Hammerschmidt, D. E., and Moldow, C. F. (1980). Complement-induced granulocyte aggregation. An unsuspected mechanism of disease. *N. Engl. J. Med., 302*:784-794.

James, S. C., and Colley, D. G. (1975). Eosinophils and immune mechanisms. Production of the Lymphokine eosinophil promotor (ESP) in vitro by isolated intact granulomus. *J. Reticuloendoth. Soc., 18*:283-293.

Johnson, K. J., and Ward, P. A. (1974). Acute immunologic pulmonary alveolitis. *J. Clin. Invest., 54*:349-357.

Johnson, K. J., Anderson, T. P., and Ward, P. A. (1977). Suppression of immune complex-induced inflammation by the chemotactic factor inactivator. *J. Clin. Invest., 59*:951-958.

Johnson, K. J., Fantone, J. C., Kaplan, J., and Ward, P. A. (1981). In vivo damage of rat lungs by oxygen metabolites. *J. Clin. Invest., 67*:983-992.

Kaplan, R. L., Schocket, A. L., King, T. E., Mawitz, R. M., Good, J. T., Stanford, R. E., and Sahn, S. A. (1980). A model of immune complex mediated pleuropulmonary injury. Evidence of deposition of circulating immune complexes in the lung. *Amer. J. Pathol., 100*:115-128.

Kay, A. B., and Austen, K. F. (1971). The IgE-mediated release of an eosinophil leukocyte chemotactic factor from human lung. *J. Immunol., 107*:899-902.

Kazlatchkine, M. D., Fearon, D. T., Silbert, J. E., and Austen, K. F. (1979). Surface-associated heparin inhibits zymosan-induced activation of the human alternative complement pathway by augmenting the regulating action of the control proteins on particle bound C3b. *J. Exp. Med., 150*: 1202-1215.

Kazmierowski, J. A., Gallin, J. I., and Reynolds, N. Y. (1977). Mechanism for the inflammatory response in primate lungs: Demonstration and partial characterization of an alveolar macrophage-derived chemotactic factor with preferential activity for polymorphonuclear leukocytes. *J. Clin. Invest., 59*:273-281.

Kellogg, E. W., and I. Fridovich. (1977). Liposome oxidation and erythrocyte lysis by enzymatically generated superoxide and hydrogen peroxide. *J. Biol. Chem., 252*:6721-6728.

King, T. E., Schwarz, M. I., Pratt, D. S., Dreisin, R. G., and Theofilopoulos, A. N. (1979). Circulating immune complexes with immunoglobulin and complement deposition in pulmonary tissue of patients with eosinophilic granuloma of the lung. *Ann. Intern. Med., 91*:397-399.

Klebanoff, J. J. (1980). Oxygen metabolism and the toxic properties of phagocytes. *Ann. Intern. Med., 93*:480-489.

Knicker, W. T., and Cochrane, G. G. (1965). Pathogenic factors in vascular lesions of experimental serum sickness. *J. Exp. Med., 122*:83-98.

Kolb, W. D., and Muller-Eberhard, H. J. (1975). The membrane attack mechanism of complement. Isolation and subunit composition of the C5d-9 complex. *J. Exp. Med., 141*:724-735.

Kreutzer, D. L., Claypool, W. D., Jones, M. L., and Ward, P. A. (1979a). Isolation by hydrophobic chromatography of the chemotactic factor inactivators from human serum. *Clin. Immunol. Immunopathol., 12*:162-176.

Kreutzer, D. L., Desai, U., Orr, W., Showell, H., and Ward, P. A. (1979b). Induction of acute inflammatory reactions in lung following intrapulmonary instillation of preformed chemotactic peptides and purified complement components. *Chest, 755*:2595-2625.

Levy, N. L., Snyderman, N., and Ladder, R. L. (1973). Cytogenetic engineering in vivo: Restoration of biologic complement activity to C5-deficient mice by intravenous innoculation of hybrid cells. *Proc. Natl. Acad. Sci. USA, 70*:3125-3129.

Lynn, W. S., and Mukherjee. (1979). Motility of rabbit alveolar cells. Role of unsaturated fatty acids. *Am. J. Pathol., 96*:663-672.

Maderazo, E. G., Ward, P. A., and Quintilliani, R. (1975). Defective regulation of chemotaxis in cirrhosis. *J. Lab. Clin. Med., 85*:621-624.

Maderazo, E. G., Ward, P. A., Woronick, C. L., Kubik, J., and DeGraff, A. C. (1976). Leukotactic dysfunction in sarcoidosis. *Ann Intern. Med., 84*:414-417.

Marx, J. J., Wenzel, F. J., Roberts, R. C., Fray, R. L., and Emanual, D. A.

(1973). Migration inhibition factor and farmer's lung antigens. *Clin. Res., 21*:852.

Marx, J. J., and Burrell, R. (1973). Delayed hypersensitivity to beryllium compounds. *J. Immunol., 111*:590-598.

McConnell, D. J. (1972). Inhibitors of kallikrein in plasma. *J. Clin. Invest., 51*: 1611.

Merrill, W. W., Naegel, G. P., Matthey, R. A., and Reynolds (1980). Alveolar macrophage-derived chemotactic factor. Kinetics of in vitro production and partial characterization. *J. Clin. Invest., 65*:268-276.

Morrison, D. C., Roser, J. R., Cochrane, C. G., and Henson, P. M. (1975). Two distinct mechanisms for the initiation of mast cell degranulation. *Int. Arch. Allergy, 49*:172-178.

Muller-Eberhard, N. J. (1975). Complement. *Ann. Rev. Biochem., 44*:697-724.

Muller-Eberhard, N. J. (1978). Complement: molecular mechanisms, regulation and biologic function. In *Molecular Basis of Biological Degradative Processes.* Edited by R. Berlin, H. Hermann, I. Lepow, and J. Tanzer. New York, Academic Press, p. 65.

Nathan, C. F., Brukner, L., Silverstein, S. C., and Cohn, Z. A. (1979). Extracellular cytolysis by activated macrophages and granulocytes. *J. Exp. Med., 149*:100-113.

O'Flaherty, J. T., Showell, H. J., and Ward, P. A. (1977). Neutropenia induced by systemic infusion of chemotactic factors. *J. Immunol., 118*: 1586-1589.

O'Flaherty, J. T., Craddock, P. R., and Jacob, H. S. (1978). Effect of intravascular complement activation on granulocyte adhesiveness and distribution. *Blood, 51*:731-739.

O'Flaherty, J. T., and Ward, P. A. (1978). Leukocyte aggregation induced by chemotactic factors. A Review *Inflammation, 3*:177-194.

Orr, F. W., Varani, J., Kreutzer, D. L., Senior, R. M., and Ward, P. A. (1979). Digestion of the fifth component of complement by leukocytic enzymes sequential generation of chemotactic activities for leukocytes and for tumor cells. *Am. J. Pathol., 94*:75-84.

Pangburn, M. K., and Muller-Eberhard, H. J. (1978). Complement C3 convertase: Cell surface restriction of B1H control and generation of restriction on neuraminidase-treated cells. *Proc. Natl. Acad. Sci. USA, 75*:2416-2420.

Pensky, J., Levy, L. R., and Lepow, I. H. (1961). Partial purification of a serum inhibitor of C'1-esterase. *J. Biol. Chem., 236*:1674.

Perez, H. D., and Goldstein, J. M. (1980). Generation of a chemotactic lipid from arachidonic acid by exposure to a superoxide generating system. *Fed. Proc., 39*:1170 (Abstract).

Perez, H. D., Goldstein, I. M., Chernoff, D., Webster, R. O., and Henson, P. M. (1980). Chemotactic Activity of C5a des arg: Evidence of a requirement for an Anionic peptide 'Helper factor' and inhibition by a cationic protein in serum from patients with systemic lupus erythematous. *Mol. Immunol.*, *17*:163-169.

Pertschuk, L. P., Morca, L. F., and Rosen, Y. (1977). Acute pulmonary complications in systemic lupus erythemetosis: immunofluorescence and light microscopic study. *Am. J. Clin. Pathol.*, *68*:553-557.

Petrone, W. F., English, D. K., Wong, K., and McCord, J. M. (1980). Free radicals and inflammation: The superoxide dependent activation of a neutrophil chemotactic factor in plasma. *Proc. Natl. Acad. Sci. USA*, *77*:1159-1163.

Podack, E. R., and Muller-Eberhard, N. J. (1980). SC5b-9 Complex of complement: Formation of the dimeric membrane attack complex by removal of 5-protein. *J. Immunol.*, *124*:1779-1783.

Postlethwaite, A. E., and Kang, A. H. (1976). Collagen and collagen peptide-induced chemotaxis of human blood monocytes. *J. Exp. Med.*, *143*:1299-1307.

Postlewaite, A. E., and Synderman, R. (1975). Characterization of chemotactic activity produced in vivo by a cell-mediated immune reaction in the guinea pig. *J. Immunol.*, *114*:274-278.

Postlewaite, A. E., Seyer, J. M., and Kang, A. H. (1978). Chemotactic attraction of human fibroblasts to type I, II and III collagens and collagen-derived peptides. *Proc. Natl. Acad. Sci. USA* *75*:871-875.

Ratnoff, O. D., Pensky, J., Ogston, D., and Naff, G. B. (1969). The inhibition of plasmin, plasma kallikrein, plasma permeability factor, and the C1r subcomponent of the first component of complement by serum C'1 esterase inhibitor. *J. Exp. Med.*, *129*:315-331.

Richerson, H. B. (1972). Acute experimental hypersensitivity pneumonitis in the guinea pig. *J. Lab. Clin. Med.*, *79*:745-757.

Rister, M., and Baehner, R. L. (1976). The alteration of superoxide dismutase, catalase, glutathione peroxidase, NAD(P)H, cytochrome C reductase in guinea pig polymorphonuclear leukocytes and alveolar macrophages during hyperoxia. *J. Clin. Invest.*, *58*:1174-1184.

Roberts, L. J. II, Lewis, R. A., Oates, J. A., and Austen, K. F. (1979). Prostaglandin, thromboxane, and 12-hydroxy-5,8,10,14-eicosatetraenoic acid production by ionophore-stimulated rat serosal mast cells. *Biochem. Biophys. Arch.*, *575*:185-192.

Robertson, J., Caldwell, J. R., Castle, J. R., and Waldman, R. I. I. (1976). Evidence for the presence of components of the alternative (properdin) pathway of complement activation in respiratory secretions. *J. Immunol.*, *117*:900-903.

Rocklin, R. E., Bendtzen, K., and Greinder, D. (1980). Mediators of immunity: Lymphokines and Monokines. *Adv. Immunol.*, *29*:55-136.

Rodriguez, R. J., White, R. R., Senior, R. M., and Levine, E. A. (1977). Elastase release from human alveolar macrophages: comparison between smokers and nonsmokers. *Science, 198*:313-314.

Root, R. K., Metcalf, J., Oshino, W., and Chence, B. (1975). H_2O_2 release from human granulocytes during phagocytosis. I. Documentation, quantitation and some regulating factors. *J. Clin. Invest., 55*:945-955.

Roska, A. K. B., Moore, V. L., and Abamoff, P. (1979). Immune complex disease in guinea pig lungs: Elicitation with pigeon serum. *Am. Rev. Respir. 120*:129-136.

Ruddy, S., and Austen, K. F. (1971). C3b inactivator of man. II. Fragments produced by C3b inactivator cleavage of cell-bound or fluid phase C3b. *J. Immunol., 107*:742-750.

Russel, R. J., McInroy, R. J., Wilkinson, P. C., and White, R. G. (1975). Identification of a lipid chemo-attractant (chemotactic) Factor for macrophages from anaerobic cornyeform bacteria. *Behring Inst. Mitt., 57*:103-109.

Sacks, T., Moldow, C. F., Craddock, P. R., Bowers, T. K., and Jacob, H. S. (1978). Oxygen radicals mediate endothelial cell damage by complement stimulated granulocytes. An in vitro model of immune vascular damage. *J. Clin. Invest., 61*:1161-1167.

Saltzman, H. A., and Fridovich, I. (1973). Oxygen toxicity. Introduction to a protective enzyme: Superoxide dismutase. *Circulation, 48*:921-923.

Salvin, S. B., Youngner, J. S., and Lederer, W. H. (1973). Migration inhibitory factor and interferon in the circulation of mice with delayed hypersensitivity. *Infect. Immunity, 7*:68-75.

Scherzer, H., and Ward, P. A. (1978a). Lung and dermal vascular injury produced by preformed immune complexes. *Amer. Rev. Respir. Dis., 117*: 551-557.

Scherzer, H., and Ward, P. A. (1978b). Lung injury produced by immune complexes of varying composition. *J. Immunol., 121*:947-952.

Schiffman, E., Showell, H., Corcoran, B., Smith, F., Ward, P. A., Tempel, T., and Becker, F. L. (1974). Isolation and characterization of the bacterial chemotactic factor. *Fed. Proc., 33*:631 (Abstract).

Schrieber, A. D., Kaplan, A. P., and Austen, K. F. (1973). Plasma inhibitors of the components of the fibrinolytic pathway in mon. *J. Clin. Invest., 52*: 1394-1401.

Senior, R. M., Griffin, G. L., and Mecham, R. P. (1980). Chemotactic activity of elastin-derived peptides. *J.Clin. Invest., 66*:859-862.

Shaw, J., Henson, J., Phillips, D., and Henson, P. M. (1978). Lung injury induced by intratracheal administration of a chemotactic fragment from the fifth component of complement. *Am. Rev. Respir. Dis., 117*:80

Sim, R. B., Porter, R. R., Reid, K. B., and Gigli, I. (1977). The Structure and

enzymatic activities of the C1r and C1s sub components of C1 the first component of human serum complement. *Biochem. J., 163*:219-227.
Siraganian, R. P., and Hook, W. A. (1976). Complement-induced histamine release from human basophils. II. Mechanism of the histamine release reaction. *J. Immunol., 116*:639-646.
Spillberg, I., Rosenberg, D., and Mandell, G. (1977). Induction of arthritis by purified cell-derived chemotactic factors. *J. Clin. Invest., 59*:582-585.
Stimler, N. P., Hugli, T. E., and Bloor, C. M. (1980). Pulmonary injury induced by C3a and C5a anaphylatoxins. *Am. J. Pathol., 100*:327-348.
Taylor, F. B., Jr., and Ward, P. A. (1967). Generation of chemotactic activity in rabbit serum by plasminogen streptokinase mixtures. *J. Exp. Med., 126*:149-160.
Till, G., and Ward, P. A. (1975). Two distinct chemotactic factor inactivators in human serum. *J. Immunol., 114*:843-847.
Unkeless, J., Gordon, S., and Reich, E. (1974). Secretion of plasminogen activator by stimulated macrophages. *J. Exp. Med., 139*:834-841.
Verge, P., and Olsson, I. (1975). Cationic proteins of human granuloyctes. VI. Effects on the complement system and mediation of chemotactic activity. *J. Immunol., 115*:1505-1508.
Vogt, W. (1974). Activation, activities, and pharmacologically active products of complement. *Pharmacol. Rev., 26*:125.
Ward, P. A. (1967). A plasmin split fragment of C'3 as a new chemotactic factor. *J. Exp. Med., 126*:189-206.
Ward, P. A. (1968a). Chemotaxis of mononuclear cells. *J. Exp. Med., 128*:1201-1220.
Ward, P. A. (1968b). Complement factors involved in chemotaxis of human eosinophils and a new chemotactic factor for neutrophils from C5. *J. Immunol., 101*:818-824.
Ward, P. A. (1969). Chemotaxis of human eosinophils. *Am. J. Pathol., 54*:121-128.
Ward, P. A. (1980). Chemotaxis. In *Textbook of Immunology*. Edited by C. W. Parker. Philadelphia, W. B. Saunders Co., vol. 1, pp. 272-297.
Ward, P. A., and Becker, E. L. (1976). Biology of Leukotaxis. *Rev. Physiol. Biochem. Pharmacol., 77*:125-148.
Ward, P. A., and Berenberg, J. L. (1974). Defective regulation of inflammatory mediators in Hodgkin's disease. Supernormal levels of chemotactic factor inactivator. *N. Engl. J. Med., 290*:76-78.
Ward, P. A., and Hill, J. H. (1970). C5 chemotactic fragments produced by an enzyme in lysosomal granules of neutrophils. *J. Immunol., 104*:535-543.
Ward, P. A., and Newman, L. J. (1969). A neutrophil chemotactic factor from human C5. *J. Immunol., 102*:93-99.

Ward, P. A., Cohen, S., and Fluragon, T. D. (1972). Leukotactic factors elaborated by virus infected tissues. *J. Exp. Med., 135*:1095-1103.

Ward, P. A., Goralnick, S., and Bullock, W. E. (1976). Defective leukotaxis in patients with lepromatous leprosy. *J. Lab. Clin. Med., 87*:1025-1029.

Ward, P. A., Lepow, I. H., and Newman, L. J. (1968). Bacterial factors chemotactic for polymorphonuclear leukocytes. *Am. J. Pathol., 52*:725-736.

Ward, P. A., Chapitis, J., Conroy, M. C., and Lepow, T. H. (1973). Generation by bacterial proteinases of leukotactic factors from human C3 and C5. *J. Immunol., 110*:1003-1009.

Ward, P. A., Dvorak, H. F., Cohen, S., Yoshida, T., Data, R., and Selvaggio, S. S. (1975). Chemotaxis of basophils by lymphocytes-dependent and lymphocyte-independent mechanisms. *J. Immunol., 114*:1423-1531.

Weiss, S. J., LoBuglio, A. F., and Kessler, H. B. (1980). Oxidative mechanisms of monocyte mediated cytotoxicity. *Proc. Natl. Acad. Sci. USA, 77*:584-587.

Weiss, S. J., Young, J., LoBuglio, A. F., Silvka, A., Wimek (1981). Role of hydrogen peroxide in neutrophil mediated destruction of cultured endothelial cells. *J. Clin. Invest., 68*:714-725.

Whaley, K., and Ruddy, S. (1976a). Modulation of C3b hemolytic activity by a plasma protein distinct form C3b inactivator. *Science, 193*:1011-1013.

Whaley, K., and Ruddy, S. (1976b). Modulation of the alternative complement pathway by B1H globulin. *J. Exp. Med., 144*:1147-1163.

Willoughby, W. F., Willoughby, J. B., Cantrell, B. B., and Wheelis, R. (1979). In vivo response to inhaled proteins. II. Induction of interstitial pneumonitis and enhancement of immune complex mediated alveolitis by inhaled concanavalin A. *Lab. Invest., 40*:399-414.

Yoshida, T., Siltzbach, L. E., Mashi, N., and Cohen, S. (1979). Serum-migration inhibitory activity in patients with sarcoidosis. *Clin. Immunol. Immunopathol., 13*:39-46.

10

In Vivo Immunopharmacology of the Lung

JAMES E. FISH and
HAROLD H. NEWBALL*

The Johns Hopkins University
School of Medicine
The Good Samaritan Hospital
Baltimore, Maryland

CLAUDE LENFANT

National Heart, Lung and Blood Institute
National Institutes of Health
Bethesda, Maryland

I. Introduction

Immunoglobulin (Ig) E-mediated hypersensitivity reactions are thought to play a significant role in the pathogenesis of certain respiratory disorders, most notably, bronchial asthma. The concept that immunologically activated mast cells secrete chemical mediators that are, either directly or indirectly, the agents responsible for the pathobiology of asthma, furnishes a working hypothesis for our efforts to explain the acute, subacute, and chronic abnormalities that are characteristic of this disorder. It seems very probable that some if not most cases of asthma are not triggered by IgE-dependent mechanisms. Nevertheless, there are compelling reasons for believing that mediators play a major role in nonallergic forms of asthma as well. Our understanding of the diversity of chemical mediators involved in immediate-hypersensitivity reactions as well as the mechanisms that control their generation and release has evolved largely from

---

Present Affiliation
*Institute of Chemical Defense, Edgewood, Maryland

Supported in part by NIH Grant No. HL24210, and Grant No. 1392 from The Council for Tobacco Research–U.S.A., Inc.

in vitro studies using isolated cell systems and lung tissue preparations. The knowledge derived from this work has facilitated the development of a meaningful approach for studying the immunopharmacology of the lung at the in vivo level, principally through immunologic and pharmacologic challenge studies in humans and animals. We seem, indeed, to be approaching a critical threshold wherein much of the enormous amount of basic science findings of the preceding decade will be tested and applied in vivo in experimental and clinical studies. In this chapter, we attempt to review both recent and historical advances related to the in vivo respiratory responses to immunologic and pharmacologic stimuli. Although the principal focus of this chapter is on work involving human subjects, animal studies are also considered, especially in relation to species variation and where information from human studies is either limited or unavailable.

II. Immediate-Type Immunologic Airway Reactions

Controlled studies of the effects of aerosolized or systemically administered antigens have not only contributed to our knowledge of the pathophysiology of IgE-mediated airway reactions, but also to a better understanding of the regulatory functions of pharmacologic and neurohumoral control mechanisms. Human studies, in particular, have afforded a unique capability, for they provide a species-relevant model of clinical allergic asthma. As with most experimental models, though, there are several features peculiar to the model itself that merit consideration. First, with respect to experimental airway reactions induced by ragweed pollen antigen, the dose of aqueous antigen required to evoke pulmonary function changes is several orders of magnitude greater than the amount of antigen an individual with autumnal asthma would be exposed to at any given time during the ragweed pollen season (Bruce et al., 1975). Second, immediate reactions of comparable magnitude can be induced by virtually equivalent doses of inhaled ragweed antigen in allergic asthmatic subjects and allergic nonasthmatic subjects with rhinitis (Fish et al., 1980). The ability to provoke such reactions in individuals who have never experienced a spontaneous attack of asthma with natural exposure is difficult to reconcile with the prevailing concept that asthmatic symptoms during the pollen season are related to the immediate effects of allergic reactions to pollen. Moreover, there are obvious differences in the general character of asthmatic reactions produced in the laboratory and those that occur spontaneously, for rarely is an episode that is so rapidly provoked or so easily reversed encountered under natural clinical conditions. Thus, there is the caveat that extrapolation from this experimental model to clinical reality is somewhat speculative on the basis of present information.

In this section, we will consider the pathophysiologic effects of inhaled antigen, the primary determinants of antigen-induced airway reactions, and the role of chemical mediators, and we will attempt to review recent information regarding neurohumoral and pharmacologic modulation of antigen responses in vivo.

A. Pathophysiology of Antigen-Induced Airway Reactions

The physiologic changes that occur in man after controlled antigen inhalation are virtually indistinguishable from the changes observed during spontaneous acute attacks of asthma. Characteristically, one observes a reduction in vital capacity, increases in residual volume and functional residual capacity, and abnormalities in virtually all pulmonary function measurements that reflect airflow limitation (Olive and Hyatt, 1972; Permutt, 1973a; Mansell et al., 1974; Fish et al., 1980; Ahmed et al., 1981). In an analysis of the effects of antigen broncho provocation on maximum expiratory flow-volume curves, Olive and Hyatt (1972) observed a reduction in expiratory flow at all volumes from total lung capacity to residual volume. The reduction in flow was noted to occur according to two distinct patterns. One pattern was characterized by increasing curvilinearity of the slope of the flow-volume curve, and the second was characterized by a parallel shift of the curve with an increase in residual volume. Mansell et al. (1974) reported similar observations and noted that an increase in curvilinearity of the slope was associated with a fall in elastic recoil pressure of the lung and a decrease in lung compliance. In contrast, changes in the lung pressure-volume relationship were not observed with a parallel shift. Because increasing curvilinearity implies inequality of time constants within the lung, Mansell suggested that an increase in the resistance of upstream airways was primarily responsible for flow limitation in this pattern. In a detailed study of the pressure-flow-volume relationship, Pride et al. (1967) postulated that a parallel shift in the curve was most likely the result of an increase in the critical closing pressure of the flow-limiting segment of airways owing to an increase in broncho motor tone, but with little change in the resistance between the alveoli and the site of flow limitation.

The fall in lung recoil pressure associated with a leftward shift of the pressure-volume curve noted by Mansell et al. (1974) occurs similarly in spontaneous attacks of asthma as well as in exercise-induced asthma (Gold et al., 1967; Woolcock and Read, 1968; Peress et al., 1976). Whether this phenomenon actually represents a change in the elastic properties of lung tissue or a change in the geometry of lung units, or whether it merely reflects complete closure of some units during expiration is uncertain. An increase in total lung capacity may also be observed in approximately 50% of subjects after antigen bronchoprovocation (Fish et al., 1980). Similar changes are found at about the same frequency in patients with spontaneous attacks of asthma (Woolcock and Read, 1966). Although the mechanism of this reversible increase in total lung capacity is poorly understood, an increase in the activity of inspriatory intercostal and accessory muscles of breathing may be responsible, in part, for the hyperinflation observed during acute airway obstruction (Martin et al., 1980b).

Other physiologic alterations reported after antigen challenge include hypoxemia secondary to intrapulmonary shunting and ventilation-perfusion inequalities; an increase in the physiologic dead space to tidal volume ratio; and an increase in pulmonary artery pressure relative to pleural pressure due to hyperinflation and the greater negativity of pleural pressure swings attendant with breathing at high volumes (Permutt, 1973a,b).

The airway obstruction induced by antigen is mediated in part by airway smooth muscle contraction as indicated by its rapid reversibility after the administration of an inhaled adrenergic bronchodilator (Fish et al., 1977). However, the cough and increased sputum production which persist for several days after an antigen-induced reaction and the direct observation of hyperemia and swelling of the airway mucosa after local instillation of antigen (Hutchcroft, 1977) suggest that mucous production and edema of the airway mucosa also contribute to the obstruction.

B. Determinants of Airway Reactions to Antigen

In many respects, airway reactions to inhaled antigen resemble other tests of allergic sensitivity. Reactions can be induced experimentally with the appropriate allergen in most individuals who possess antigen-specific IgE antibody. Lower respiratory tract symptoms with natural and environmental exposure are not a prerequisite, as allergic individuals who have never experienced atopic symptoms and those who experience symptoms of allergic rhinitis only are responsive also (Bruce et al., 1975; Bryant and Burns, 1976; Killian et al., 1976; Permutt et al., 1977; Fish et al., 1980). On this basis, it seems justified to view antigen-induced airway reactions as a form of localized anaphylaxis, much as we view skin tests as localized cutaneous anaphylaxis.

The dose of antigen required to provoke an airway response correlates with the degree of allergic sensitivity which is determined by circulating levels of specific IgE antibody, immediate skin reactivity, or in vitro leukocyte histamine release (Bruce et al., 1974; Bryant and Burns, 1976; Killian et al., 1976; Cockcroft et al., 1979). That this correlation is rather weak, however, suggests that other factors contribute. A number of investigators have shown that the response to inhaled antigen correlates also with the nonspecific (nonallergic) airway reactivity to chemical mediators, most notably histamine (Bryant and Burns, 1976; Killian et al., 1976; Cockcroft et al., 1979; Popa, 1980a). Thus, the pulmonary response to antigen is determined by the responsiveness of the target airway tissue to chemical mediators liberated during IgE-mediated reactions as well as allergic sensitivity (Fig. 1). An individual who is relatively unresponsive to inhaled histamine can sustain a significant airway reaction to antigen provided that the individual has sufficient allergic reactivity and that a sufficient dose of

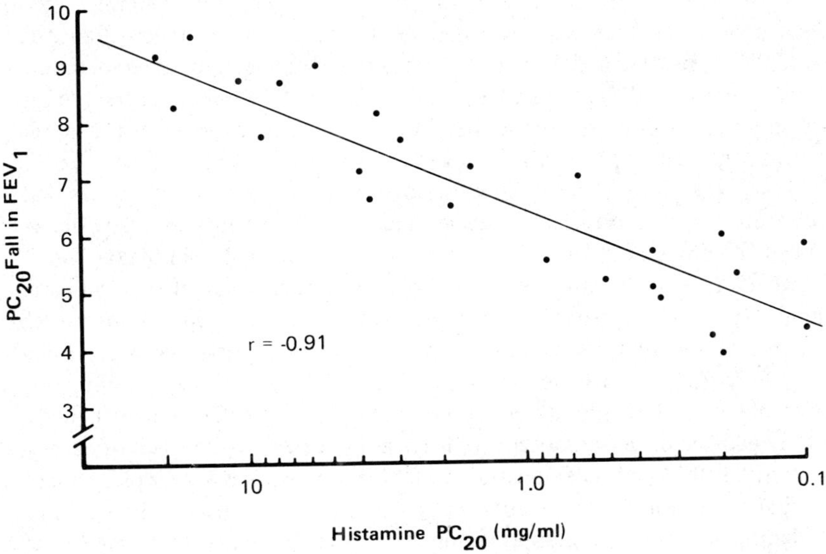

Figure 1 Relationship between nonspecific airway reactivity [determined by the histamine concentration causing 20% fall in forced expiratory volume in 1 sec (FEV_1) (PC_{20})] and allergic reactivity (determined by mean wheal diameter of the skin response to the antigen concentration which, when inhaled, caused a 20% fall in FEV_1). Relationship signifies that the airway response to antigen can be achieved in subjects with low nonspecific reactivity [higher histamine (PC_{20})] if skin reactivity is high. Conversely, the same can be achieved with low skin reactivity, if nonspecific airway reactivity is high. (From Cockcroft et al., 1979.)

antigen is administered. Conversely, individuals with exaggerated airway responses to histamine can demonstrate allergen-induced airway reactions in the presence of a modest degree of allergic reactivity. These same factors have been shown to determine airway responsiveness to antigen in various animal models of asthma, including dogs (Snapper et al., 1980b), monkeys (Patterson et al., 1976), and guinea pigs (Popa et al., 1976). However attractive it appears to view the airway response to antigen as a product of nonspecific airway reactivity and allergic reactivity as determined by skin tests or leukocyte histamine release, such a view is limited to the extent that it ignores organ-specific factors that may modulate the allergic response in lung but not in skin or circulating basophils.

C. Chemical Mediators

The evidence that chemical mediators derived from mast cells and perhaps other cell sources in the lung are principally responsible for the pathophysiologic changes in IgE-mediated airway reactions in man is largely circumstantial. Nevertheless, certain mediators such as histamine, slow-reacting substance of anaphylaxis (SRS-A), prostaglandins, and thromboxane are released or generated during allergic reactions and these substances are known to have direct contractile effects on bronchial smooth muscle. In addition, the acute hyperemia and swelling of the airway mucosa noted after antigen challenge in humans (Hutchcroft, 1977) suggest an important pathophysiologic role, not only for mediators that cause bronchospasm, but also for those capable of increasing vascular permeability and eliciting an inflammatory response by promoting chemotaxis.

In addition to the direct effects of chemical mediators, reflex vagal parasympathetic stimulation has also been implicated in the pathophysiology of airways obstruction induced by antigen. This is based on reports that parasympathetic blockade with atropine in humans (Yu et al., 1972) or vagal cooling in dogs (Gold et al., 1972) inhibited antigen responses. Indeed, chemical mediators are fully capable of initiating vagal reflexes as indicated by the work of Sampson and Vidruk (1979), who demonstrated that histamine stimulates rapidly adapting irritant receptors in canine airways by a direct H_1 receptor-mediated effect. The significance of these findings remains controversial, however, as others have shown little or no effect of parasympathetic blockade on the response to antigen in man (Itkin and Anand, 1970; Fish et al., 1977, 1980, 1981b; Rosenthal et al., 1977; Ruffin et al., 1978) or in other animal species (Krell et al., 1976; Patterson and Harris, 1976).

Histamine

As a first approach to understanding the role of chemical mediators, a number of investigators have attempted to relate in vivo mediator release to the physiologic abnormalities induced by inhaled antigen. Histamine has been the most extensively studied mast cell-derived mediator in man. While some laboratories have found increased plasma histamine levels after an antigen broncho provocation (Bhat et al., 1976; Martin et al., 1980a; Atkins et al., 1980), others have failed (Deal et al., 1980; Bleecker and Fish, unpublished observations 1981). Logically, we would expect histamine to be liberated from sensitized target cells in lung after antigen challenge. The failure to demonstrate increased levels in plasma in some studies, therefore, must be due to an insufficient quantity of histamine passing into the circulation from the tissue site of release. Alternatively, the metabolism of histamine may be too rapid to permit detection of appreciable quantities in the peripheral circulation at sites remote from the target organ. The disparity in results from different laboratories might also be explained by marked variability in the accuracy of plasma histamine measurements (Gleich and Hall, 1980). Because of this variability, much of the published information regarding histamine levels must be interpreted cautiously. Nevertheless, in other species antigen challenge has produced elevations in

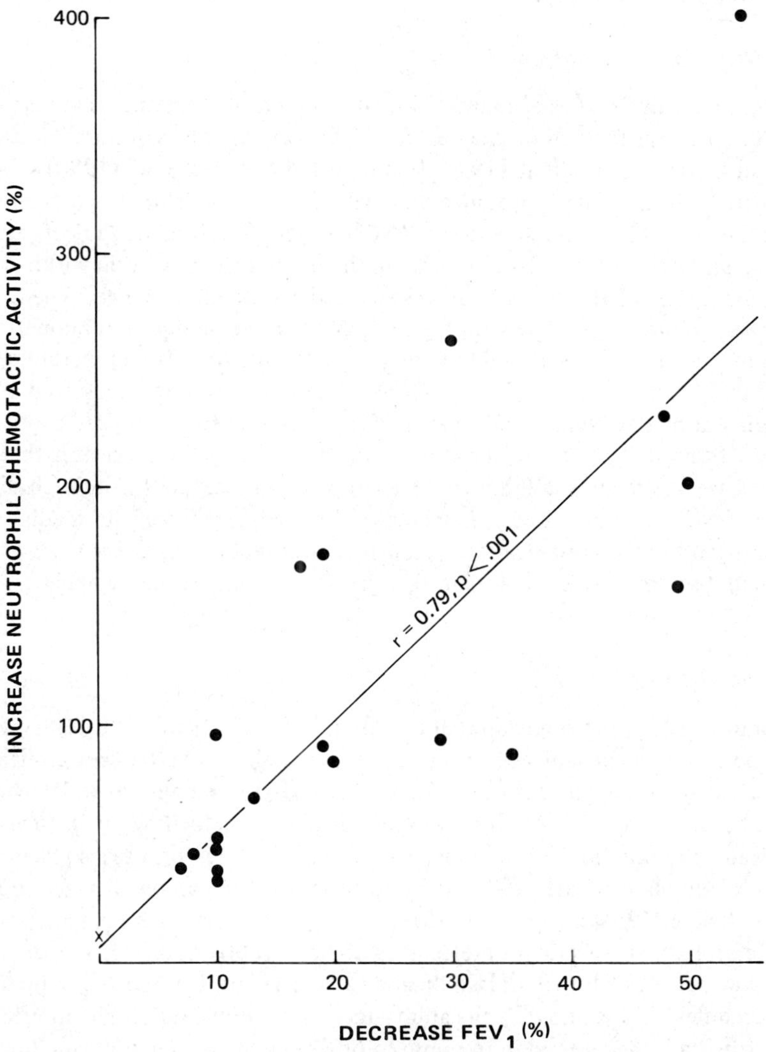

Figure 2 Correlation in 10 subjects of the mean percent increase in serum neutrophil chemotactic activity (*ordinate*) with mean percent decrease in forced expiratory volume in 1 sec (FEV_1) (*abscissa*) after antigen bronchoprovocation. (From Antigen-induced neutrophil chemotactic activity in man, P. C. Atkins, M. E. Norman, and B. Zweiman, *J. Allergy Clin. Immunol. 62*:149-155, 1978.)

circulating histamine levels for up to 10 min after challenge, and levels have corresponded to the severity of pulmonary function changes (Chiesa et al., 1975; Wanner et al., 1979).

Neutrophil Chemotactic Factor

Because of the difficulties encountered with histamine measurements in man, recent attention has focused on the detection of other mediators of immediate hypersensitivity. Atkins et al. (1977) first reported and Deal et al. (1980) subsequently confirmed the appearance of a high molecular weight, noncomplement derived, neutrophil chemotactic factor (NCF) in sera of asthmatic subjects after ragweed antigen challenge. NCF appears in the peripheral circulation within 1 min after antigen challenge and remains elevated for 30 min or longer. The increase was found to correlate with the severity of antigen-induced pulmonary function changes and it was inhibited by pretreatment with disodium cromoglycate (Fig. 2; Atkins et al., 1978). Similar elevations have not been observed after histamine or methacholine challenges or after cold- or exercise-induced bronchospasm (Atkins et al., 1978; Deal et al., 1980; Orr et al., 1980), suggesting that NCF release was related to IgE-mediated activation of mast cells. Although the source of NCF is unknown, the time course of the appearance of this mediator after antigen broncho provocation is similar to that reported in other mast cell-mediated disorders (Soter et al., 1980), suggesting the mast cell as a likely source.

Platelet Factor 4

McManus et al. (1979) demonstrated that plasma platelet factor 4 (PF4) levels could be used as a convenient marker of in vivo platelet-activating factor release from sensitized basophils during systemic anaphylaxis in rabbits. Acetylglyceryl ether phosphorylcholine (AGEPC), a synthetic platelet-activating factor identical chemically and functionally to rabbit platelet-activating factor, has also been shown to stimulate release of PF4 and serotonin from human platelets (Demopoulos et al., 1979; McManus et al., 1980, 1981). PF4 is an intrinsic, platelet-specific protein with a subunit molecular weight of 7800 daltons (Moore et al., 1975; Levine and Wohl, 1976; Handin and Cohen, 1976). It is located in platelet alpha granules. PF4 is noted for its ability to neutralize the anticoagulant effects of heparin, and it is released in response to other stimuli as well, inducing thrombin, collagen, and adenosine diphosphate (Youssef and Barkhan, 1968; O'Brien et al., 1970; Day et al., 1973; Rucinski et al., 1979). The relationship between IgE-mediated events in vivo and platelet-activating factor release in humans is largely unexplored, although platelet-activating factor has been isolated in vitro from a variety of human cell types, including basophils and human lung fragments (Benveniste, 1974; Lewis et al., 1975; Clark et al., 1980; Bogart and

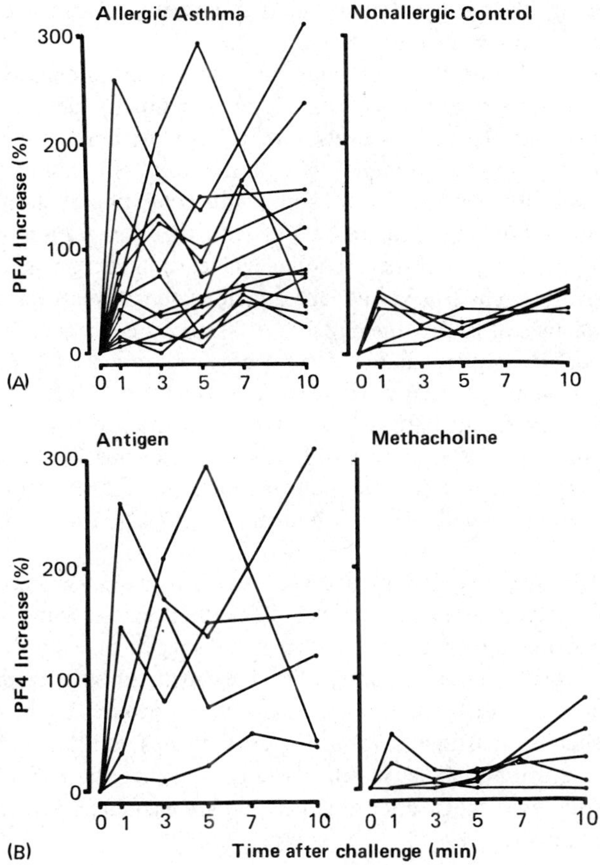

Figure 3 (*A*) Changes in plasma platelet factor 4 (PF4) levels after antigen challenge in allergic asthmatic and nonallergic control subjects. The percent increase in PF4 (*ordinate*) at each time point (*abscissa*) represents the mean of duplicate postchallenge samples and quadruplicate prechallenge samples. The maximum percent increase during the 10-min postchallenge period was significantly greater in the allergic asthmatic group ($p < 0.02$). (*B*) Changes in plasma PF4 levels during methacholine and antigen challenge in five allergic asthmatic subjects. Format is identical to *A*. PF4 levels were significantly higher after antigen ($p = 0.031$, by paired analysis). PF4 levels after methacholine were no higher than levels observed in non-allergic control subjects (see *A*). (Adapted from Knauer et al., 1981, by permission of *The New England Journal of Medicine 304*:1405, 1406).

Stechschulte, 1974). Moreover, AGEPC was recently recovered from human lung mast cells of 98% purity after stimulation with anti-IgE antibody (Pinckard and Newball, unpublished data).

We recently demonstrated elevated PF4 levels in the circulation of allergic asthmatic subjects after antigen broncho-provocation (Knauer et al., 1981). Elevations in venous plasma PF4 levels were observed within 1 min after antigen challenge, corresponding temporally with the onset of pulmonary function changes as well as with subjective complaints consisting of chest tightness and a sensation of "itching in the throat." The further observation that PF4 elevations did not occur after methacholine challenge in allergic asthmatic subjects or after antigen challenge in nonallergic, nonasthmatic subjects indicated that the appearance of PF4 in the circulation was not a consequence of bronchospasm per se or a non-IgE-mediated effect of the antigen material (Fig. 3). While it is tempting to speculate that the PF4 increase is related to release of a basophil/mast cell chemical mediator which activates platelets, other factors, such as thromboxane A_2, prostaglandins, or lung-derived coagulation factors which have been shown to be released from lung parenchymal cells in vitro, may also be involved (Adkinson et al., 1980; Schulman et al., 1981, 1982; Newball et al., 1981a,b,c).

Although further studies are necessary to clarify the mechanisms of PF4 release in these experiments, the results indicate that platelet activation occurs during IgE-mediated airway reactions in man and suggest that the measurement of PF4 levels provides a useful marker of such events. Although there is no current evidence that PF4, itself, is a mediator or contributes to the pathophysiologic changes in asthma, a recent report indicates that human PF4 enhances the effects of human leukocyte elastase on hamster lung elastin, causing morphologic and physiologic abnormalities that are characteristic of emphysema (Lonky and Wohl, 1981).

D. Pharmacologic Modulation of Antigen Reactions

Histamine Antagonists

A further approach to the study of mediators at the in vivo level involves studies of the effects of various pharmacologic agents on the immediate hypersensitivity response. Studies of the role of histamine, in particular, have been examined by testing the effects of specific histamine type 1 (H_1) and histamine type 2 (H_2) receptor antagonists on antigen-induced airway reactions. In a guinea pig model, the H_2-blocking agents, metiamide and burimamide, potentiated the respiratory response to intravenous antigen (Drazen et al., 1978). While cimetidine had no effect in the studies of Drazen et al. (1978), others have reported potentiation of antigen reactions with high concentrations of cimetidine using the same model (Dulabh and Vickers, 1978). In dogs, however, metiamide had no effect on antigen-induced bronchospasm (Krell and Chakrin, 1977). Because H_2-blocking agents failed to cause significant enhancement of the pulmonary response to exogenous histamine in guinea pigs (Drazen et al., 1978), the most likely explanation for the enhanced response to antigen is that it occurs through the prevention of H_2 receptor-mediated feedback inhibition of anaphylactic mediator release. The concept of an autoregulatory role for histamine via H_2-receptor-mediated feedback inhibition of further mediator release has been demonstrated under certain experimental conditions in cells and tissues from several species, and this is presumably the result of increased intracellular levels of cAMP (Lichtenstein and Gillespie, 1973, 1975; Chakrin et al., 1974; Holroyde and Eyre, 1978).

Published information regarding the effects of H_2 receptor antagonists on antigen-induced airway reactions in man is scant. Eiser et al. (1979) reported slight but significant inhibition with a 200-mg dose of cimetidine given intravenously. These findings clearly conflict with the effects of other H_2-blocking agents in guinea pigs (Drazen et al., 1978) and in sensitized human bronchus in vitro (Dunlop and Smith, 1977). The fact that Eiser et al. (1979) failed to observe inhibition with a higher dose of cimetidine (400 mg), however, suggests that the unexpected finding of inhibition with lower doses should be interpreted cautiously. Although H_2-receptor-mediated feedback inhibition of histamine release has been demonstrated in passively sensitized monkey lung fragments challenged with antigen (Chakrin et al., 1974), a similar phenomenon could not be demonstrated in sensitized human lung fragments (Kaliner, 1978) or in dispersed, purified human lung mast cells (Newball, unpublished observations). Therefore, the finding of enhanced contractile responses in antigen-challenged human bronchi treated with H_2 receptor antagonists in vitro (Dunlop and Smith, 1977) is most likely due to inhibition of receptors mediating smooth muscle relaxation, or perhaps inhibition of anti-inflammatory H_2 receptors on cell types other than the mast cell. Further studies are needed to clarify the role of H_2 receptors at the in vivo level.

The effects of H_1 antihistamines on antigen-induced bronchoconstriction in man has also been examined and, in general, the results are consistent with in vitro studies. Popa (1980b) reported that an intravenous dose of chlorpheniramine (15 mg) sufficient to produce a four-fold decrease in sensitivity to inhaled histamine also produced a two-fold decrease in sensitivity to inhaled antigen in allergic asthmatic subjects. Varying degrees of protection against antigen-induced bronchoconstriction have also been reported with H_1 antihistamines by other investigators (Herxheimer, 1949; Nakazawa et al., 1976; Eiser et al., 1979), although Schiller and Lowell (1947) failed to demonstrate inhibition with low doses of intravenous tripelennamine. H_1 antihistamines have well-known anticholinergic effects (Pandit et al., 1973) and are thus capable of inhibiting the airway response to inhaled cholinergic agonists (Woenne et al., 1978; Popa, 1980b).

Nevertheless, because protection against the effects of antigen could be obtained with chlorpheniramine and not atropine (Popa, 1980b), the inhibitory effects of H_1 antihistamines are best explained on the basis of specific blocking activity at the H_1 receptor. The relatively small degree of protection afforded by these agents is consistent with previous in vitro findings (Schild et al., 1951; Adams and Lichtenstein, 1979) and evinces the importance of chemical mediators other than histamine.

β-Adrenergic Drugs

It is well documented that β-adrenergic agonists inhibit IgE-mediated mediator release from sensitized basophils and mast cells (Lichtenstein and Margolis, 1968; Ishizaka et al., 1971; Orange et al., 1971; Bourne et al., 1972). The fact that the kinetics and dose-response relationships of drug-induced inhibition of mediator release correspond to drug-induced changes in cAMP levels provides suggestive evidence that the cAMP system is responsible for negatively modulating histamine release from mast cells and basophils. Evidence that similar pharmacologic control mechanisms operate in vivo is provided by recent work wherein oral and inhaled β-adrenergic agents were shown to inhibit antigen-induced airway reactions in asthmatic subjects (Rosenthal, 1978; Ruffin et al., 1978; Martin et al., 1980a). The suggestion that β-adrenergic agents inhibit antigen-induced airway reactions at the in vivo level by preventing mediator release is conjectural, however, since these drugs can exert similar effects by inhibiting airway smooth muscle contraction. Although it is clearly difficult to separate the effects of adrenergic agents on the secretory process and airway smooth muscle, several lines of evidence suggest that inhibition of mediator release may be at least partially responsible for the in vivo effects of β-adrenergic agents. Rosenthal (1978) demonstrated significant inhibition of antigen-induced airway constriction when isoproterenol was given at least 30 min prior to antigen aerosol. These findings paralleled the short-term protective effects of isoproterenol in inhibiting IgE-mediated histamine release from basophils taken from the same group of subjects. When basophils were incubated with isoproterenol in vitro, there was a rapid increase in cAMP, which returned to control levels within 20 min; the inhibition of IgE-mediated histamine release paralleled this increase in cAMP levels. Moreover, Martin et al. (1980a) recently reported that both theophylline and terbutaline decrease airway responsiveness to antigen in asthmatic subjects with a corresponding fall in postchallenge neutrophil chemotactic factor and histamine levels in plasma. Although these studies suggest that inhibition of antigen responsiveness was associated with prevention of mediator release, the possibility that these drugs prevent the reaction by inhibiting smooth muscle contraction cannot be excluded. These investigators also found that significant changes in pulmonary function could be produced by extremely high doses of antigen after terbutaline pretreatment, even when histamine and NCF levels in plasma were still suppressed. This interesting observation remains unexplained at present, although it suggests that other mediators from either primary or secondary target cells may not be affected by drugs which increase cAMP levels (Martin et al., 1980a).

IgE-mediated activation of primary target cells in the lung can itself alter cyclic nucleotide levels at the in vivo level. Lazarus et al. (1977) demonstrated increased lung tissue concentrations of cAMP and cGMP in dogs challenged with *Ascaris* antigen. These findings are consistent with in vitro studies of antigen-challenged sensitized guinea pig lung (Mathé et al., 1974) and human lung (Platshon and Kaliner, 1978). The cell source of the elevated cyclic nucleotides, the significance of these elevations with respect to modulation of further IgE-mediated release, and the effects of cyclic nucleotides on secondary mediators, target cells, or effector tissue remain outstanding questions.

Ouellette and Reed (1967) found a significant increase in the airway responsiveness of hay fever subjects to ragweed aerosol after pretreatment with propranolol (5 mg, iv). Here, too, the data are difficult to interpret. Gold (1977) found that propranolol decreased tissue cAMP levels in vivo in dogs and suggested that basal cAMP concentrations in lung tissue were under the control of circulating catecholamines acting on the β-receptor. Although it is tempting to speculate that Ouellette and Reed (1967) demonstrated enhanced antigen responsiveness in their subjects by virtue of decreased tissue cAMP levels, the evidence for this is circumstantial. Furthermore, if altered cyclic nucleotide metabolism were in fact responsible for the change in antigen responsiveness, it is not clear whether the effect was a consequence of inhibition of mediator release or protection of airway smooth muscle from the contractile effects of chemical mediators.

Arachidonic Acid Metabolism

The role of arachidonic acid metabolism in the modulation of immediate-type immunologic airway responses is a matter of increasing interest and complexity. In vitro studies have shown that cyclooxygenase products of arachidonic acid are generated from human lung fragments after antigen stimulation (Piper and Walker, 1973; Adkinson et al., 1980; Schulman et al., 1980,1981,1982), and that these products can exert direct effects on airway smooth muscle (Sweatman and Collier, 1968; Hyman et al., 1978; Hedqvist et al., 1978), as well as modulate the release or activity of other chemical mediators of immediate hypersensitivity (Lichtenstein and Henney, 1972; Engineer et al., 1978a; Lewis et al., 1981). Moreover, recent work indicates that lipoxygenase products of arachidonic acid are perhaps even more potent and fundamentally important mediators of hypersensitivity reactions. In particular, leukotrienes are potent bronchoconstrictor agents and may contribute to changes in vascular permeability (Drazen et al., 1980). Other lipoxygenase products can augment preformed mediator release

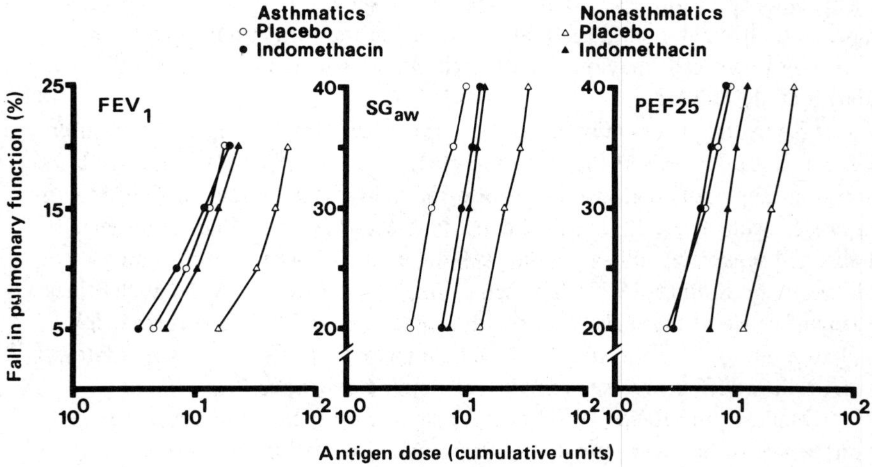

Figure 4 Antigen dose-response curves after placebo and indomethacin in allergic asthmatic and allergic nonasthmatic subjects. Each point represents the mean dose of antigen required to produce a specified fall in pulmonary function for each group [e.g., the mean dose of antigen required to produce a 5, 10, 15, or 20% fall in forced expiratory volume in 1 sec (FEV_1). After placebo asthmatics had approximately a 3.5-fold greater sensitivity to antigen than nonasthmatic subjects. After indomethacin, non-asthmatic subjects demonstrated a significant increase in sensitivity by all measurements. Asthmatic subjects had no change in sensitivity by FEV_1 or by peak expiratory flow at 25% of the vital capacity (PEF25) measurements, and had a slight but significant decrease in sensitivity with specific airway conductance (SGaw) measurements.

from human basophils and guinea pig lung (Adcock et al., 1978; Marone et al., 1979, 1980), and several mono- and dihydroxy-eicosatetraenoic acid derivatives of the lipoxygenase pathway possess chemotactic properties for human polymorphonuclear leukocytes and eosinophils (Goetzel et al., 1977; Goetzel and Pickett, in press).

In vitro studies have shown that cyclooxygenase inhibitors enhance mediator release from sensitized leukocytes and lung tissue and augment antigen-induced contraction of isolated guinea pig smooth muscle (Walker, 1973; Engineer et al., 1978c; Schulman et al., 1980; Marone et al., 1980). These findings prompted us to examine the effects of indomethacin on antigen-induced airway reactions in vivo in allergic subjects. Although a previous report by Smith and Dunlop (1975) indicated that indomethacin had no effect on antigen challenge in allergic asthmatic subjects, Patterson et al. (1978) had shown that indomethacin increased the airway response of rhesus monkeys to

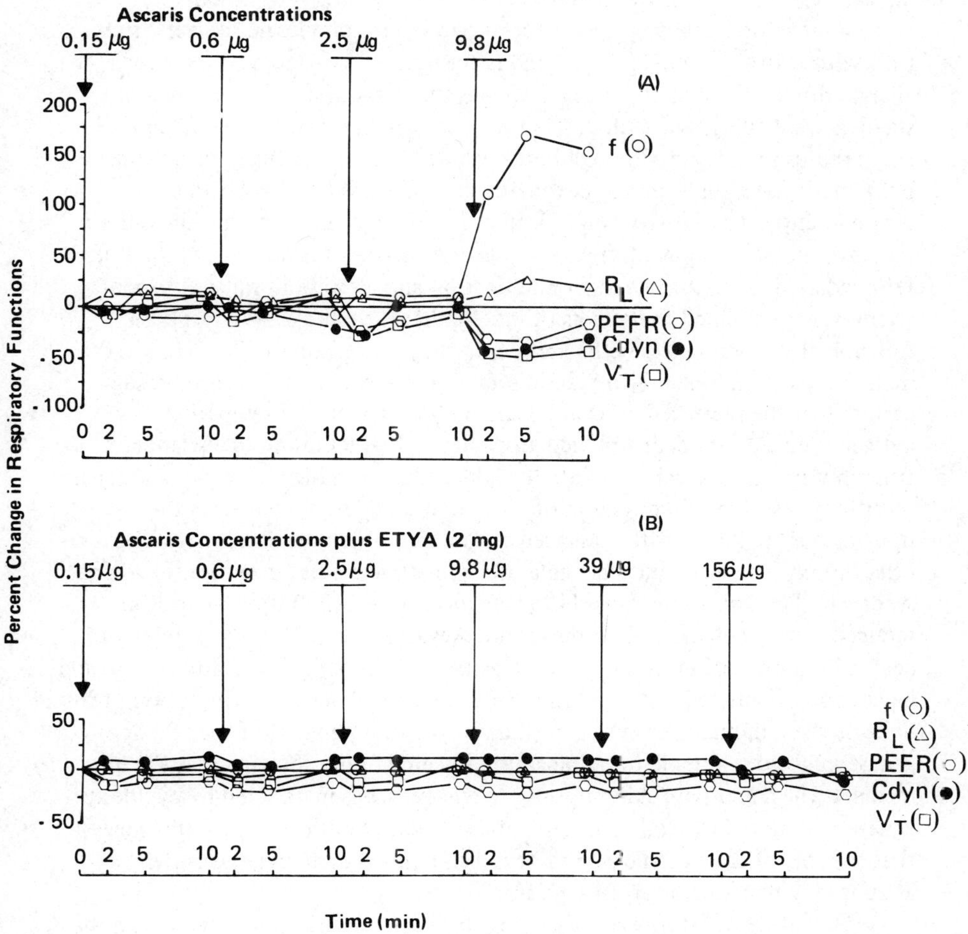

Figure 5 (*A*) Airway response of a rhesus monkey to increasing concentrations of *Ascaris* antigen alone. (*B*) Response of the same monkey after receiving increasing concentrations of *Ascaris* antigen mixed with 5, 8, 11, 14-eicosatetraenoic acid (ETYA) in 40% ethanol. ETYA prevented the response to a 16-fold higher antigen concentration. f, Respiratory frequency; R_L, pulmonary resistance; PEFR, peak expiratory flow rate; V_T, tidal volume; Cdyn, dynamic compliance. (From Inhigition of immunoglobin E-mediated, antigen-induced monkey asthma and skin reactions by 5, 8, 11, 14-eicosatetraenoic acid, R. Patterson and K. E. Harris, *J. Allergy Clin. Immunol.* 67:146-152, 1981.)

inhaled *Ascaris* antigen. We therefore compared the effects of indomethacin on antigen inhalation challenge responses in two groups of allergic subjects: subjects with ragweed allergic asthma and nonasthmatic subjects with ragweed allergic rhinitis (Fish et al., 1981a). The results in the allergic nonasthmatic subjects were consistent with previous in vitro findings and the results in allergic rhesus monkeys: Although indomethacin failed to change prechallenge pulmonary function in the nonasthmatic group, it produced a 2.5-fold increase in antigen sensitivity (Fig. 4). In order to determine whether the indomethacin-induced augmentation of antigen sensitivity was due to an effect on IgE-mediated mediator release or an effect on airway smooth muscle responsiveness, we examined the effects of indomethacin on the airway response to a nonallergic stimulus, methacholine. In the same group of allergic nonasthmatic subjects, indomethacin had no effect on methacholine sensitivity, suggesting that the increased antigen sensitivity was related to modulation of antigen-induced IgE-mediated mediator release. It is tempting to extrapolate from in vitro studies and speculate that the mechanism of the increased antigen sensitivity was due to redirection of arachidonic acid metabolism via the lipoxygenase pathway with enhanced production of leukotrienes as well as other lipoxygenase products capable of augmenting mediator release. Further studies by Patterson and Harris (1981) demonstrating inhibition of antigen-induced airway constriction in rhesus monkeys by 5, 8, 11, 14-eicosatetraenoic acid, an inhibitor of both the cyclooxygenase and lipoxygenase pathways, would be consistent with this interpretation (Fig. 5). Experimental confirmation of this hypothesis in humans, however, must await the development of specific lipoxygenase inhibitors suitable for clinical use. Recent studies showing that the immediate wheal and flare skin response to allergens was unaffected by cyclooxygenase inhibitors in allergic nonasthmatic subjects (Smith et al., 1980b) suggest that the role of arachidonic acid metabolism in immediate hypersensitivity reactions may be tissue or organ specific.

One of the most intriguing findings in this study was the difference in the effects of indomethacin on antigen response in asthmatic and nonasthmatic subjects. In contrast to the result in nonasthmatics, indomethacin had no effect on antigen sensitivity in the asthmatic group (Fig. 4). One possible explanation for these group differences takes into consideration the possibility of differences in the relative metabolism of arachidonate by the lipoxygenase and cyclooxygenase pathways. We demonstrated that antigen responses of nonasthmatic subjects were increased after indomethacin and suggested that this could be due to an increase in lipoxygenase metabolism. In this context it could also be postulated that asthmatics have a preexisting alteration in arachidonic acid metabolism giving rise to a greater ratio of lipoxygenase to cyclooxygenase metabolism compared with nonasthmatics. Although there is no direct evidence for excessive synthesis of lipoxygenase products in asthmatic subjects, such an alteration could account for the lack of further enhancement.

Miscellaneous Pharmacologic Agents

Other pharmacologic agents that have been evaluated to determine their effect on antigen-induced airway reactions include corticosteroids and agents whose putative mechanism of action is to inhibit mediator release from mast cells. There have been surprisingly few well-controlled studies of the effects of corticosteroids. Martin et al. (1980a) demonstrated partial inhibition of the immediate airway response to pollen antigens with oral prednisone, but others have failed to demonstrate similar inhibition of the immediate response to antigens from flour and house dust (Booij-Noord et al., 1972; Nakazawa et al., 1976). Although steroids failed to provide protection against the immediate bronchoconstrictor effects of antigen in the latter studies, they furnished uniform protection against the late airway response that occurred 6–8 hr after antigen challenge. Although the mechanism of action of corticosteroids in immediate hypersensitivity reactions remains unknown, the protective effect of steroids on the late airway response suggests a possible mode of action for the beneficial effects of steroids clinically. Cockcroft et al. (1977b) demonstrated that late airway responses to antigen were associated with an increase in nonallergic bronchial reactivity to agents such as histamine and methacholine. Subjects who were placed on topical inhaled corticosteroids prior to challenge failed to develop an increase in nonallergic airway reactivity after antigen exposure. Thus, it is conceivable that by inhibiting the delayed or prolonged inflammatory effects of antigen, corticosteroids may prevent or partially inhibit the development of increased bronchial sensitivity to nonallergic stimuli.

While disodium cromoglycate (DSCG), a putative inhibitor of mediator release, has been studied extensively at the in vivo level, these studies have shed little light on pathophysiologic mechanisms of immediate hypersensitivity reactions or on the mode of action of the drug itself. There is strong evidence that DSCG inhibits the immediate airway response to inhaled antigen (Altounyan, 1979). Although the mechanism responsible for protection is classically thought to be related to inhibition of mast cell mediator release, the evidence for this in man is largely circumstantial. Inconsistent with this notion is the fact that DSCG is remarkably effective in inhibiting exercise-induced asthma (Eggleston et al., 1972), a condition wherein a role for mediators has not been established (Deal et al., 1980). Recent evidence suggests that DSCG may inhibit airway reactions by a direct effect on either bronchial irritant receptors or on airway smooth muscle (Dixon et al., 1980; Harries et al., 1981). Other studies by Bryant (1977) have indicated that the effectiveness of DSCG in preventing antigen-induced bronchospasm in man may depend in part on antigen-specific IgE levels and that DSCG may be ineffective in reactions mediated by other homocytotropic antibodies such as short-term sensitizing antibody (IgG4). Considering the remarkable protection that DSCG and other similar agents such as lodoxamide provide (Katcher and Reed, 1980), it seems clear that a better understanding of the mode of action of these agents will furnish vital information concerning pathophysiologic mechanisms of allergic reactions in the lung. Whereas the lung mast cell may not be the sole source of mediators responsible for the pathobiology of acute allergic reactions, it is conceivable that these putative inhibitors of mediator release exert protective effects by acting on other cell types within the lung.

E. Late Asthmatic Responses to Antigen

In addition to the immediate airway reaction, some subjects demonstrate a biphasic response to antigen, that is, an immediate fall in pulmonary function within the first 30 min followed by a return to baseline, and then a subsequent fall in lung function between 4 and 12 hr after the initial antigen challenge. The late response is characterized by physiologic evidence of airway obstruction, clinical evidence of wheezing, and subjective symptoms of chest tightness and occasionally dyspnea. In contrast to the delayed physiologic changes produced by the inhalation of organic antigens associated with hypersensitivity pneumonitis, such as pigeon breeder's lung, late responses due to inhaled allergens are not associated with pyrexia, leukocytosis, hypoxemia, or abnormal radiologic findings (Booij-Noord et al., 1972; Robertson et al., 1974).

Late-phase reactions may also be observed in skin sites after the intradermal injection of allergen in sensitized individuals. Because of similarities between late-phase skin and airway reactions, it has been suggested that they have a common underlying mechanism. For example, both late-phase skin and airway reactions can be induced with greater frequency using increasing concentrations of antigen, and both types of late reactions can be inhibited by prednisone (Robertson et al., 1974; Poothullil et al., 1976). Evidence that the late-phase skin reaction is mediated by IgE-dependent mechanisms is derived from studies showing that the reaction can be induced by intradermal injection of monospecific antiserum to IgE (Dolovich et al., 1973) and that the response can be abolished in passive transfer tests by heating atopic serum at 56°C or by removal of IgE from atopic serum by solid-phase anti-IgE immunoabsorbent (Solley et al., 1976). Histologic studies of late-phase skin lesions have demonstrated edema and mixed cellular infiltrates consisting of lymphocytes, eosinophils, neutrophils, and basophils (Dolovich et al., 1973; Solley et al., 1976; de Shazo et al., 1979), but as Richerson et al. (1979) and deShazo et al. (1979) have pointed out, these histologic features are qualitatively similar to those seen 6 or 24 hr after an immediate wheal and flare reaction in volunteers who fail to demonstrate a late-phase reaction. Studies by deShazo et al. (1979), however, demonstrated fibrin deposition in the absence of immunoglobulin or complement by fluorescent microscopy in the late-phase reactions only. Thus, activation of the intrinsic coagulation system may in some way be involved (see Sec. VII).

III. Histamine

Histamine (β-imidazolylethylamine) is formed by the enzymatic decarboxylation of L-histidine. In most speices, it is stored as a heparin complex in secretory granules of tissue mast cells and blood basophils. It is reported that histamine is also found as a nonstored mediator in epidermal tissue, the gastro-intestingal mucosa, and the central nervous system (Douglas, 1980). Since Dale and Laidlaw (1910, 1911) first described the physiologic effects of histamine as characteristic of those observed in anaphylaxis, numerous other biologic functions have been ascribed to this mediator; these include regulation of gastric secretory function, control of the microcirculation (Shayer, 1963), as well as a role in tissue growth and repair (Kahlson and Rosengren, 1968). That the physiologic effects of histamine are mediated by two distinct receptor subtypes was first suggested by Ash and Schild (1966) who demonstrated that mepyramine, an H_1 antagonist, selectively inhibited the contractile effects of histamine on guinea pig ileum and guinea pig or human airway smooth muscle, but failed to block stimulation of gastric acid secretion and tachycardia or histamine-induced relaxation of rat uterus. Black et al. (1972) subsequently established the existence of H_2 receptors by demonstrating selective antagonism of histamine effects on guinea pig heart rate and gastric acid secretion with the synthetic compound, burimamide.

A. In Vitro Effects of Histamine

In spite of extensive research with this mediator, the pathophysiologic role of histamine in immediate-type hypersensitivity reactions in the lung remains poorly defined. Our understanding of this role has been confounded in part by marked variability in the reported physiologic effects of this mediator. This variability is manifest in species differences, in dissimilarities between in vitro and in vivo studies within the same species, and in discrepancies in the reported in vivo effects of histamine in human studies. Species differences are clearly illustrated by the results of in vitro studies of the effects of histamine on lung tissue. Whereas histamine via H_1 receptor stimulation produces contraction of guinea pig, sheep, dog, and human tracheal and bronchial tissue (Persson and Ekman, 1976; Dunlop and Smith, 1977; Eyre, 1977; Drazen and Schneider, 1978; Chand et al., 1979), it produces relaxation of monkey, rabbit, and cat tracheal smooth muscle preparations that have been previously contracted by cholineric stimulation (Fleisch and Calkins, 1976; Eyre, 1977; Chand et al., 1980). The latter relaxant effects on tracheal smooth muscle are thought to be due to a predominant H_2 receptor effect in monkeys (Chand et al., 1980) and by a combined effect of H_1, H_2 and β-adrenergic receptor stimulation in cats (Maengwyn-Davies, 1968; Eyre, 1973). Similar species variation is observed in the effects of histamine on peripheral airway or parenchymal tissue. For example, histamine contracts guinea pig parenchymal tissue by an H_1 effect (Drazen and Schneider, 1978) but relaxes ovine peripheral airway tissue by an H_2 receptor mechanism (Eyre, 1977). Pharmacologic nonuniformity is further illustrated by the contrasting effects of histamine on tissues from different sites of the lung from the same species. For example, in sheep histamine causes contraction of the bronchi and trachea and relaxation of bronchioles (Eyre, 1969); in rabbits it causes relaxation of trachea and contraction of bronchi (Somlyo and Somlyo, 1970). The potency of H_1-mediated activity also varies with different tissues; thus, histamine is a more potent agonist in parenchyma as compared with trachea in guinea pigs and monkeys (Drazen and Schneider, 1978; Chand et al., 1980).

B. In Vivo Effects of Histamine on Airway Physiology

At the in vivo level histamine acts as a bronchoconstrictor in most species. This has been demonstrated with aerosolized or intravenous histamine in guinea pigs (Douglas et al., 1973; Drazen and Austen, 1975), dogs (DeKock et al., 1966; Krell et al., 1976; Dixon et al., 1979b), and humans (Newball and Keiser, 1973; Laitinen et al., 1976; Habib et al., 1979). In species where both contraction and relaxation were observed in isolated in vitro preparations of different airway generations, the net response to histamine in vivo is constriction of the airways. In sheep, for example, histamine contracts strips of trachea, major bronchi, and lung parenchyma and relaxes strips of smaller bronchi and bronchioles, but in the intact animal the net effect of intravenous or aerosolized histamine is an increase in airway resistance (Alexander et al., 1967; Ahmed et al., 1980). Similar increases in airway resistance have been observed in monkeys, cats, and rabbits (Colebatch, et al., 1966; Mills et al., 1969; Michoud et al., 1978), even though histamine caused relaxation of tracheal smooth muscle in vitro in these species.

In addition to changes in airway resistance, histamine induces profound changes in other mechanical properties of the lung that reflect alterations in the function of peripheral lung tissue. For example, Colebatch (1970) observed a marked increase in the static elastic recoil pressures of the lung corresponding to bronchiolar and alveolar duct constriction in cats after histamine infusion. These alterations were potentiated by adrenalectomy and unchanged by vagotomy. Evidence for peripheral airway effects in vivo may be found in other species also, including guinea pigs (Drazen and Austen, 1975), dogs (DeKock et al., 1966; Krell, Chakrin and Wardell, 1976), and humans (Newball and Keiser, 1973; Brown et al., 1977; Ploy-Song-Sang et al., 1978). In the animal studies cited, this evidence was based primarily on the demonstration of greater changes in dynamic compliance (as reflecting small airways) relative to changes in pulmonary resistance (as reflecting large airways), whereas in human studies this evidence is based on changes in closing volume (Newball and Keiser, 1973), density dependence of maximum expiratory flow (Ploy-Song-Sang et al., 1978), or selective changes in dynamic compliance and frequency dependence of compliance (Brown et al., 1977). In human studies, the peripheral effects of intravenous histamine appear to involve smooth muscle of alveolar ducts and bronchioles as suggested by a reduction in static lung compliance (Laitinen et al., 1976; Ploy-Song-Sang et al., 1978). It should be noted, however, that histamine does not preferentially affect peripheral airways in man if it is administered by aerosol (Brown et al., 1977; Habib et al., 1979). Thus, the observed physiologic effects depend largely on the route of administration.

Although these studies describe the net physiologic response to histamine in vivo, they do not, in most instances, discriminate between the direct and indirect effects of this agonist. It is clear that histamine-induced alterations in lung mechanics are subject to modulation by a variety of humoral and neural factors and by the interaction of H_1 and H_2 receptor activities as well. For example, histamine may induce prostaglandin generation in lung tissue (Steel et al., 1979); it may stimulate catecholamine release from adrenal and nonadrenal sources (Trendelenburg, 1954; Piper et al., 1967); and it may induce changes in lung mechanics indirectly by stimulating vago-vagal reflexes (Widdicombe, 1963).

C. Reflex Effects of Histamine

Animal Studies

A number of investigators have reported that the bronchoconstrictor effects of histamine in vivo can be abolished or decreased by atropine (Herxheimer, 1956; DeKock et al., 1966; Douglas et al., 1973; Drazen and Austen, 1975; Nadel, 1980) or by cervical vagotomy (DeKock et al., 1966; Mills et al., 1969; Mills and Widdicombe, 1970). There is substantial evidence that the reflex effects of histamine are due to stimulation of rapidly adapting irritant receptors located in the airway epithelium which then triggers reflex efferent parasympathetic stimulation via afferent and efferent fibers of the vagus nerve (DeKock et al., 1966; Mills and Widdicombe, 1970; Sellick and Widdicombe, 1971; Vidruk et al., 1977). Originally, it was proposed that histamine stimulated irritant receptors by virtue of local deformation of tissue surrounding receptors as a result of airway smooth muscle contraction (Sellick and

Widdicombe, 1971). Later studies, however, revealed that the histamine-induced increase in ventilation in dogs was independent of changes in bronchomotor tone and it was therefore suggested that histamine had a direct effect on irritant receptors (Bleecker et al., 1976). Recent studies by Vidruk et al. (1977) confirmed this hypothesis by demonstrating that histamine applied locally in the vicinity of the receptor increased the rate of receptor discharge in the absence of changes of bronchomotor tone and that a similar increase in receptor discharge did not obtain after local application of acetylcholine. Further studies by Sampson and Vidruk (1979) established that irritant receptor stimulation by histamine was in fact mediated specifically by H_1 receptors.

Although histamine appears to have both direct, H_1-receptor-mediated histaminergic and indirect, reflex-mediated cholinergic effects on bronchomotor tone, the relative contribution of the cholinergic component seems to vary, however, depending on species and experimental conditions, such as type of anesthesia used, route of histamine administration, and which physiologic measurements are employed to evaluate the response. For example, Dennis and Douglas (1970) found that urethane anesthesia decreased histamine sensitivity in guinea pigs and demonstrated that this effect was due to anesthesia-related inhibition of reflex-mediated cholinergic stimulation. Subsequent experiments by Jackson and Richards (1977) revealed that pentobarbitone also inhibited the vagal component of histamine-induced bronchoconstriction in dogs either by blocking transmission through postganglionic parasympathetic fibers or by preventing the release of acetylcholine from postganglionic nerve endings. The route of histamine administration was shown to be an important determinant of the relative contribution of reflex effects by DeKock et al. (1966), who demonstrated greater reflex effects on bronchomotor tone in dogs with bronchial artery injections than with pulmonary artery injections. These findings were consistent with the predominant localization of irritant receptors in larger bronchi in dogs (Mortola et al., 1975). That the relative contribution of vagal reflexes is also dependent on the type of physiologic measurements used to evaluate histamine responses is indicated by the fact that vagal blockade or atropine has a greater inhibitory effect on histamine-induced pulmonary resistance changes than on dynamic compliance changes in dogs and guinea pigs (Drazen and Austen, 1975; Krell et al., 1976; Jackson and Richards, 1977). Recent work has shown that for similar changes in pulmonary conductance induced by either electrical stimulation of the vagi or histamine aerosols, dead space volume is reduced with the former but not with histamine (Drazen et al., 1979b). This suggests that the effects of vagal stimulation as compared with histamine are more prominent in large airways. The reflex effects of histamine on mechanical function are therefore more likely to be demonstrated by pulmonary function tests that reflect resistance changes in large airways as opposed to tests of small airway dysfunction, or changes in the elastic properties of the lungs. This interpretation is supported by the fact that there are few parasympathetic ganglia in small airways (Larsell, 1922) and that vagal stimulation constricts large- and intermediate-sized airways, having little effect on airways less than 0.8 mm in diameter (Woolcock et al., 1969; Nadel et al., 1971).

Loring et al. (1978) recently offered an alternative explanation for the partial inhibition of histamine responses observed after vagal interruption or anti-cholinergic drug administration. On the basis of dog studies in which they observed supra-additive effects of histamine and vagal stimulation on airway resistance changes, they postulated that the interaction between these stimuli was due to synergism between the effects of histamine and postganglionic efferent vagal activity, rather than a simple reflex increase of vagal impulse traffic. Whether this hypothetical interaction involves histamine potentiation of muscarinic activity or vice-versa is unknown.

Human Studies

Simonsson et al. (1967) demonstrated inhibition of the response to histamine aerosols in asthmatic subjects with atropine sulfate. Similarly, Holtzman et al. (1980) reported decreased histamine responsiveness in atopic, nonasthmatic subjects after administration of a ganglionic blocker (hexamethonium). In both of these studies the effects of cholinergic blockade were evaluated by plethysmographic measurements of airway resistance. In contrast, several other investigators have failed to demonstrate inhibition of the histamine-induced fall in FEV_1 in allergic asthmatic subjects with atropine (Itkin and Anand, 1970; Casterline et al., 1976; Woenne et al., 1978). Although differences in the types of patients used in these studies may in part explain this discrepancy, it is also conceivable that these discordant results reflect differences in the specificity of different tests for measuring changes in large versus small airway function. Thus, if the previous interpretation is correct and the reflex effects of histamine are more readily manifest by changes of central airway tone, atropine modification of histamine responses may be best demonstrated by changes in airway resistance as compared with measurements of forced expiration. On the other hand, the demonstration of greater inhibition of histamine-induced changes with measurements of airway resistance may be a consequence of the pattern of aerosol deposition; inhaled atropine may be preferentially deposited in large central airways.

D. Modulation of Histamine-Induced Bronchoconstriction

Catecholamines

Adrenergic modulation of histamine-induced bronchoconstriction has been described in several species including man. McCulloch et al. (1967) and Douglas et al. (1973) have demonstrated potentiation of the airway response to histamine in guinea pigs with propranolol, indicating that the bronchomotor effects of this agonist are partially inhibited by the in vivo release of catecholamines from adrenal or nonadrenal sources. Drazen (1978) extended these observations in guinea pigs by demonstrating that adrenalectomy prolonged the recovery time of histamine-induced bronchoconstriction, but that propranolol and not adrenalectomy potentiated the airway response during the course of histamine infusion. He further demonstrated that α-adrenergic blockade with phentolamine inhibited the airway response during histamine infusion, and that in the presence of both α- and β-adrenergic blockade the airway response to histamine was equivalent to the response observed without adrenergic blockade. Adrenergic regulation of histamine effects on lung mechanics has also been demonstrated in cats by Colebatch (1970) who reported potentiation of the histamine-induced fall in dynamic compliance after adrenalectomy. He also observed a histamine-induced fall in airway resistance in cats whose airways were previously constricted with neostigmine. In the presence of propranolol or after bilateral adrenalectomy, however, histamine caused a rapid and sustained increase in airway resistance. These findings were consistent with the in vitro observation of histamine-induced relaxations of contracted cat trachealis muscle, which was partially inhibited by β-adrenergic blockade (Eyre, 1973).

Evidence for adrenergic modulation of histamine effects in man is not strong, but in its favor are the findings of Ploy-Song-Sang et al. (1978) who demonstrated a reduction in maximum expiratory flow rates in normal subjects during histamine infusion after intravenous propranolol pretreatment but not with histamine alone. Other investigators, however, have failed to demonstrate a similar effect of oral propranolol on mechanical alterations induced by an intravenous bolus injection of histamine (Laitinen et al., 1976). Whereas histamine itself stimulates adrenal catecholamine release (Staszewska-Barczak and Vane, 1965), differences in plasma histamine concentrations recirculated to the adrenal glands may have accounted for differences in the effects of propranolol in these experiments. Thus, because of its rapid metabolism in the circulation, effectively greater plasma histamine concentrations may have been achieved by continuous infusion than by bolus injection. Studies of the effects of inhaled histamine in normal subjects have also failed to reveal a significant effect of propranolol (Habib et al., 1979), although this, too, may be due to insufficient quantities of histamine reaching the circulation from the airways.

H_2 Receptor Modulation

The functional role of H_2 receptors in airway smooth muscle has also been examined in vivo and the results of these studies are in general agreement with in vitro observations. Studies showing that 4-methylhistamine, a specific H_2 agonist, had no effect on pulmonary mechanics in the guinea pig and that specific H_2 antagonists, burimamide and metiamide, failed to alter histamine-induced alterations in lung mechanics suggest that there are no functional H_2 receptors on airway smooth muscle in this species (Drazen et al., 1978). Similarly, in dogs, specific H_2 antagonists, metiamide and cimetidine, had no effect or produced only slight enhancement of histamine-induced changes in lung mechanics (Krell and Chakrin, 1977; Dixon et al., 1979a; Snapper et al., 1980a). By contrast, metiamide potentiated histamine-induced increases in airway resistance in sheep and monkeys (Ahmed et al., 1980; Greenberger et al., 1979).

The results of studies examining the role of H_2 receptor modulation of histamine responses in man are inconclusive. Nathan et al. (1979) reported slight potentiation of the airway response to histamine in asthmatic subjects with cimetidine (300 mg orally). Eiser et al. (1979), in contrast, found a slight decrease in histamine sensitivity in a similar group of subjects with cimetidine (400 mg iv), while Maconochie et al. (1979) found no alteration of the histamine response in healthy, nonasthmatic subjects with cimetidine (400 mg orally and 200 mg iv). The decrease in histamine sensitivity reported by Eiser et al. (1979) is difficult to interpret in light of our understanding of the role of H_2 receptors as mediators of relaxation in some species. However, it is conceivable that in high concentrations cimetidine may possess H_1-blocking activity. The smaller dose of cimetidine used by Nathan et al. (1979) resulted in slight potentiation of the bronchoconstrictor effects of histamine and these findings are consistent with in vitro observations in human bronchi of 2-3 mm diameter (Dunlop and Smith, 1977).

E. Airway Reactivity to Histamine

Clinical studies have uniformly revealed a characteristic increase in the airway responsiveness to inhaled and parenteral histamine in asthmatic subjects as compared with nonasthmatic individuals (Curry, 1946; Herxheimer, 1951; Tiffeneau, 1958; Townley et al., 1965; Makino, 1966; Cockcroft et al., 1977a). This exaggerated airway responsiveness in asthmatics also occurs with other agonists, including methacholine and $PGF_{2\alpha}$. The mechanisms responsible for this phenomenon are unknown and constitute one of the most important outstanding questions in our understanding of the pathogenesis of asthma. Although potential mechanisms are discussed briefly, a detailed review of airway hyperreactivity is beyond the scope of this chapter. For further discussion, the reader is referred to a recent, extensive review by Boushey et al. (1980).

It should be noted that an increase in airway reactivity to histamine has been noted in conditions other than asthma. For example, nonasthmatic individuals who are atopic, as demonstrated by skin sensitivity to common allergens and elevated serum IgE levels, demonstrate a slight increase in histamine responsiveness compared with nonatopic normals. This increase is less than that observed in asthmatic subjects (Bryant and Burns, 1976; Cockcroft et al.,

1977, 1977a; Townely et al., 1965), but the finding nevertheless, suggests that the allergic diathesis may be a factor in the pathogenesis of hyperreactivity. Viral respiratory infections and exposure to toxic substances such as ozone have also been shown to produce a transient increase in histamine responsiveness in normal subjects (Empey et al., 1976; Golden et al., 1978; Holtzman et al., 1979). The increase in reactivity observed under these conditions is also somewhat less than that found in most asthmatic subjects. Moreover, some investigators have shown that the increased responsiveness attending viral infections or ozone exposure can be inhibited with atropine sulfate (Empey et al., 1976; Holtzman et al., 1979), whereas others have failed to obtain similar inhibition of histamine reactivity in asthmatic subjects (Itkin and Anand, 1970; Casterline et al., 1976; Woenne et al. , 1978). Thus, there is reason to belive that different mechanisms may be responsible for increased histamine reactivity seen in asthma and after infections or toxic exposure. Several mechanisms have been postulated for the increase in reactivity observed with the latter, including increased permeability of the respiratory mucosa due to damage of the airway epithelium (Pare, 1980) and lowering of the stimulation threshold of irritant receptors secondary to epithelial damage (Empey et al., 1976). This topic is considered further in Section VI of this chapter.

IV. Prostaglandins, Endoperoxides, and Thromboxane

The major cyclooxygenase products of arachidonic acid–prostaglandins (PGs), PG endoperoxides, prostacyclin (PGI_2), and thromboxane (Tx)–are generated by the lung at the time of a physiologic stimulus and are inactivated or converted to other active metabolites by various enzymatic mechanisms. Although there is compelling evidence that cyclooxygenase products play a significant role in immediate hypersensitivity reactions and are thus involved in the pathophysiology of allergic asthma, the significance of this role has not been established at the in vivo level in clinical or experimental studies in humans. Attempts to define the importance of cyclooxygenase products at the in vivo level have involved several experimental approaches: (1) studies of the effects of exogenous prostaglandins on airway function; (2) studies of prostaglandin levels in the circulation of patients under natural clinical conditions or after experimentally induced asthma attacks; and (3) studies of the effects of cyclooxygenase inhibitors on the physiologic response to various bronchoconstrictor stimuli. With respect to the first of these approaches, the effects of exogenous $PGF_{2\alpha}$, PGE, and PGI_2 have been examined in man, while the effects of PGD_2, endoperoxide analogs, and TxB_2 (the stable metabolite of TxA_2) have been evaluated in other animal species.

Table 1 Effects of Anticholinergic Agents on $PGF_{2\alpha}$ Airway Responses

Reference	Subjects studied	Anticholinergic pretreatment	$PGF_{2\alpha}$ dose inhaled[a]	Pulmonary function tests	Results
Smith et al. (1975)	Normals	Atropine (1.0 mg inhaled)	48-96 μ g	Airway conductance	No significant inhibition
Newball and Lenfant (1977)	Normals and asthmatics	Atropine (2.5 mg iv)	150-300 μg	Airway conductance Spirometry Closing volume	No significant inhibition
Mathé and Hedqvist (1975)	Normals and asthmatics	Atropine (0.5 mg iv; 0.5 mg subcutaneous)	0.008-500 μg	Airway conductance	Bronchodilation after atropine but no change in threshold dose or absolute fall in conductance after $PGF_{2\alpha}$
Alanko and Poppius (1973)	Asthmatics	Ipratropium bromide (80 μg aerosol)	<400 μg	Peak flow rate	Partial inhibition
Patel (1975)	Asthmatics	Atropine (1.2 mg aerosol)	25 μg	Airway conductance Spirometry	Significant inhibition
Orehek et al. (1977)	Asthmatics	Ipratropium bromide (1000 μg aerosol)	1-30 μg	Airway resistance	Significant inhibition

[a]Estimated from published description of inhalation challenge methods.

A. Effects of Cyclooxygenase Products on Airway Function

Prostaglandin $F_{2\alpha}$

In man, inhaled $PGF_{2\alpha}$ evokes a dose-dependent increase in airway resistance and fall in vital capacity which is not inhibited by DSCG, cyclooxygenase inhibitors, or α-adrenergic blocking agents (Smith et al., 1975; Patel, 1975; Newball and Lenfant, 1977). Most studies indicate that inhaled $PGF_{2\alpha}$ acts as a local respiratory tract irritant, producing cough. Accordingly, it has been suggested that the bronchoconstrictor effects of inhaled $PGF_{2\alpha}$ are in part mediated by irritant-induced reflex vagal parasympathetic stimulation, although there is some disagreement concerning the relative magnitude of reflex versus direct effects. Some investigators have reported moderate to marked inhibition of the airway response to $PGF_{2\alpha}$ with cholinergic blocking agents, while others have noted little or no inhibition. A summary of the effects of anticholinergic agents on $PGF_{2\alpha}$ responses from different laboratories is provided in Table 1. The reasons for the disparity in these results are unclear, but variation in the concentration of $PGF_{2\alpha}$ used as well as the dose and route of administration of anticholinergic agents may be responsible. Despite a potential to induce reflex bronchoconstriction under certain experimental conditions, it seems clear that $PGF_{2\alpha}$ has direct contractile effects on airway smooth muscle at the in vivo level. This interpretation is consistent with the failure to demonstrate a corelation between $PGF_{2\alpha}$ and carbachol sensitivity in asthmatics (Orehek et al., 1977), for one might expect to find such a correlation if the principal mechanism of $PGF_{2\alpha}$-induced bronchoconstriction was related to reflex cholinergic stimulation.

Compared with normal subjects, asthmatic individuals are more responsive to the bronchoconstrictor effects of inhaled $PGF_{2\alpha}$ (Fig. 6) (Mathé and Hedqvist, 1975; Newball and Lenfant, 1977; Newball et al., 1980a). Although the mechanism of this hyperreactivity is unknown, as it is for histamine and methacholine, the persistence of increased $PGF_{2\alpha}$ sensitivity in the presence of atropine sulfate suggests that cholinergic mechanisms are not responsible (Mathé and Hedqvist, 1975; Newball and Lenfant, 1977). Several investigators have examined $PGF_{2\alpha}$ hyperreactivity in relation to various types of bronchial asthma. For example, Szczeklik et al. (1977) found that atopic asthmatics were more sensitive to $PGF_{2\alpha}$ than patients with asthma provoked by nonsteroidal, anti-inflammatory agents or viral respiratory infections. Orehek et al. (1977), on the other hand, failed to find differences in the sensitivity of aspirin-sensitive asthmatics and those with so-called "common asthma," but the causes and clinical features of disease in the latter group were not characterized.

Although there is a consensus that asthmatic subjects demonstrate enhanced responsiveness to inhaled $PGF_{2\alpha}$, there are conflicting reports concerning

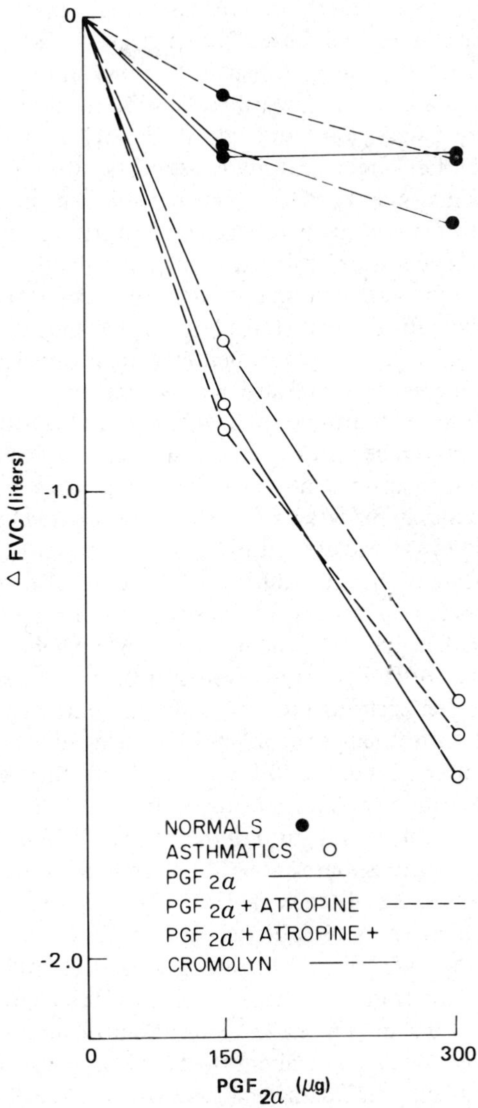

Figure 6 Influence of atropine and atropine plus cromolyn on aerosolized $PGF_{2\alpha}$-induced FVC changes in asthmatics (dose-response relationships of aerosolized $PGF_{2\alpha}$ on the FVC of 6 normals and 7 asthmatics). The dose-response curves were not plotted beyond the 300-μg dose because some asthmatics were unable to reach higher doses. Asthmatic subjects demonstrate significantly greater sensitivity which persists after atropine pretreatment. (From Newball and Lenfant, 1977.)

the relative sensitivity of asthmatic and nonasthmatic subjects to $PGF_{2\alpha}$ administered by the intravenous route. Brown et al. (1978) demonstrated comparable changes in vital capacity, maximum flow, and increases in residual volume in asthmatic and nonasthmatic subjects after the intravenous infusion of $PGF_{2\alpha}$ (1.5 μg/kg·min). In contrast, Newball et al. (1980a) observed a significantly greater fall in vital capacity in asthmatics than in nonasthmatics after a bolus injection of 4 μg/kg $PGF_{2\alpha}$. One possible explanation for this discrepancy is the differences in prechallenge pulmonary function status of the populations studied. Whereas prechallenge pulmonary function values were relatively normal in both the asthmatic and nonasthmatic groups studied by Brown et al. (1978), the asthmatic subjects studied by Newball et al. (1980a) demonstrated marked prechallenge airway obstruction as compared with the normals. Under conditions of laminar flow through airways, resistance to airflow is inversely proportional to the fourth power of the radius. Therefore, for a given change in radius, there will be a greater change in resistance in airways that are already narrowed than in airways of normal dimension. Thus, the greater response of the asthmatics in the latter study may have resulted in part from geometric considerations (Mead et al., 1967).

A striking feature of the asthmatic sensitivity to inhaled $PGF_{2\alpha}$ is a wide intersubject variation in responsiveness to this agonist compared with histamine or methacholine (Mathé et al., 1973; Smith et al., 1975; Orehek et al., 1977). Similarly, a wide range of $PGF_{2\alpha}$ responsiveness was observed in dogs by Snapper et al. (1979). By demonstrating that the range of sensitivity was not decreased by vagal blockade, Snapper et al. (1979) concluded that the variation was not related to differences in the contribution of efferent vagal interaction. Other factors, however, such as individual differences in the time course of the response and differences in the role of tachyphylaxis to $PGF_{2\alpha}$ could contribute to the wide distribution of responsiveness. Variation in the time course of the response has been reported by Orehek et al. (1977), who described two patterns, the first characterized by peak bronchoconstrictor effects within the first minute after inhalation of $PGF_{2\alpha}$ with a return to baseline levels within 10-15 min and the second characterized by a slower onset of bronchoconstriction, peak effects between 10 and 20 min and a return to basal levels within 35 min. Tachyphylaxis to the bronchoconstrictor effects of $PGF_{2\alpha}$ has also been demonstrated in asthmatic subjects (Mathé and Hedqvist, 1975) and in isolated human bronchial smooth muscle as well (Sweatman and Collier, 1968). The demonstration of progressively diminished responses with repeated $PGF_{2\alpha}$ administration was observed in only some of the asthmatic subjects, though, and none of the normal subjects. Although peculiarities in the pattern of response have been reported as incidental findings, these factors would seem to merit further consideration as they may have a significant bearing on the degree of sensitivity as well as the relative importance of $PGF_{2\alpha}$ at the clinical level.

Prostaglandin E

Early studies indicated that prostaglandins of the E series relaxed airway smooth muscle, suggesting a potential therapeutic role for these substances. PGE_1, a monoenoic PG, as well as a number of synthetic PGE analogs relax tracheal or bronchial smooth muscle of serveral species including man in vitro (Main, 1964; Sweatman and Collier, 1968; Gardiner and Collier, 1980). PGE_2 also relaxes airway smooth muscle in vitro, but contractile activity has been observed in some experiments in guinea pig and human airway tissue (Mathé et al., 1971; Gardiner and Collier, 1980). At the in vivo level, PGE_1 and PGE_2 have both been shown to antagonize nonspecifically the bronchoconstrictor effects of cholinergic agonists, histamine, $PGF_{2\alpha}$, serotonin, and bradykinin in a variety of animal species (Rosenthale et al., 1970, 1971; Patterson and Harris, 1977). Early studies in man established that inhaled PGE_1 and PGE_2 produced bronchodilation in both normals and asthmatics and that the bronchoconstrictor effects of $PGF_{2\alpha}$ could be reversed by the subsequent inhalation of either PGE_1 or PGE_2 (Cuthbert, 1971; Smith and Cuthbert, 1972). Although the bronchodilator effects of PGE in man have been confirmed by others (Kawakami et al., 1973), Mathé and Hedqvist (1975) observed bronchoconstriction after PGE_2 inhalation in some asthmatic patients. Moreover, when administered intravenously for termination of pregnancy, large doses of PGE_2 increased lung resistance in healthy women (Smith, 1973). Bronchoconstriction has been observed in other species in vivo as well (James, 1969; Piper and Vane, 1969).

There are several possible explanations for the variable effects of PGE_2, although there is little supporting evidence. At low doses, inhaled PGE_2 could elicit reflex vagally mediated bronchoconstriction, especially in asthmatic subjects who have hyperreactive airways. Such a mechanism, however, would not explain contractile responses observed at low concentrations of PGE_2 in isolated guinea pig or human airway smooth muscle (Gardiner and Collier, 1980). Lambley and Smith (1975) suggested that the response to PGE_2 was dependent on the initial state of bronchomotor tone, although a recent study of the effects of PGs under varying states of airway tone by Gardiner and Collier (1980) failed to support this contention. Other possibilities include the release of other bronchoactive mediators or the existence of different receptor subtypes that determine the effects of PGE_2. Indeed, there is evidence that PGE_2 can stimulate both $PGF_{2\alpha}$ and PGE_1 receptors of isolated human bronchial smooth muscle in vitro (Gardiner, 1975).

Prostacyclin

Prostacyclin (PGI_2) acts as a local and circulating hormone, as it is generated in vivo by lung tissue and released into the arterial circulation (Gryglewski et al., 1978; Moncada et al., 1978). Although it has potent antiaggregatory effects on platelets and potent vasodepressor activity in man (Szczeklik et al., 1978a), on the basis of current studies, PGI_2 appears to have limited activity in the control of bronchomotor tone. Intravenous and aerosolized PGI_2 had no effect on resting pulmonary function in healthy volunteers or in patients with bronchial asthma at doses that caused significant inhibition of adenosine diphosphate-induced platelet aggregation (Szczeklik et al., 1978b; Bianco et al., 1978). Despite the lack of effect on resting bronchomotor tone, Bianco et al. (1978) reported that PGI_2 afforded slight but significant protection against the bronchoconstrictor effects of an inhaled irritant (ultransonic mist) and exercise in asthmatic patients. The mechanism responsible for this protection is unknown. That PGI_2 and its metabolite (6-keto-PGE_1) can function as a bronchodilator under certain experimental conditions, however, is suggested by animal studies in which these substances reversed serotonin-induced bronchoconstriction (Spannhake et al., 1980, 1981). Other investigators have shown, however, that the bronchoconstrictor activity of PGD_2 in rhesus monkeys was enhanced by aerosolized PGI_2 (Patterson et al., 1980), suggesting that the activity of PGI_2 and/or its metabolites are species-specific or perhaps dependent on an interaction with other mediators.

Prostaglandin D_2, Endoperoxides, and Thromboxane

PGD_2 was recently reported to be the major cyclooxygenase product generated by immunologically activated human lung mast cells (Lewis et al., 1980b; Schulman et al., 1981). Although the in vivo effects of PGD_2 on human lung function are unknown, PGD_2 causes an increase in airway resistance and fall in dynamic compliance in rhesus monkeys and in dogs (Wasserman et al., 1977; Spannhake et al., 1978a; Patterson et al., 1980). In the dog, PGD_2-induced bronchoconstriction was attenuated by vagotomy, indicating that functional alterations were partially mediated by cholinergic stimulation (Spannhake et al., 1978a). With respect to potency, PGD_2 is considerably more potent than $PGF_{2\alpha}$ in contracting guinea pig trachea (Hamberg et al., 1975). Moreover, the contractile effects of PGD_2 were shown to be greater in guinea pig lung parenchyma than trachea (Schneider and Drazen, 1980).

Limited animal studies have been carried out to examine the in vivo effects of the endoperoxides (PGG_2, PGH_2) and a stable endoperoxide analog (15S-hydroxy-9α, 11α-(epoxymethano) prosta-5z, 13e-dienoic acid). These indicate that endoperoxides cause an increase in airway resistance and a fall in dynamic compliance that is not inhibited by vagotomy in dogs (Spannhake et al., 1978b). Moreover, the endoperoxides are more potent than $PGF_{2\alpha}$ in producing bronchoconstriction in guinea pigs and cats (Hedqvist et al., 1978). In vitro studies of human bronchus have shown that PGG_2 and PGH_2 to be of equivalent potency to $PGF_{2\alpha}$ (Hedqvist et al., 1978).

Thromboxane B_2 (TxB_2), the stable metabolite of TxA_2, is released following antigen challenge of sensitized guinea pig and human lung (Dawson et al., 1976; Schulman et al., 1982). In addition, TxA_2 activity is increased in arterial blood after histamine and bradykinin challenge in guinea pigs (Rossoni et al., 1980). Whether thromboxanes contribute to functional alterations induced by challenge with antigen or other autocoid agents, however, is unknown. Relevant in vivo studies do indicate that TxA_2 is more potent than $PGF_{2\alpha}$ in producing bronchoconstriction in guinea pigs (Svensson et al., 1977), and others have shown that TxB_2 is slightly less potent than $PGF_{2\alpha}$ in causing airway constriction in anesthetized dogs (Wasserman and Griffin, 1976).

B. Circulating Levels of Cyclooxygenase Products

Investigations of PG levels in the circulation of man under natural or experimental conditions have yielded provocative but inconclusive observations. Nemoto et al. (1976) reported elevated PGE_1 and $PGF_{2\alpha}$ levels in the sera of asthmatic patients as compared with nonasthmatic normal subjects. In a similar study using plasma, Okazaki et al. (1978) confirmed the finding of elevated PGE levels, but failed to demonstrate higher plasma $PGF_{2\alpha}$ levels, suggesting that PGF elevations found by Nemoto et al. (1976) were a result of increased release from blood cells rather than lung tissue. Green et al. (1974) reported up to an eight-fold increase in plasma levels of the $PGF_{2\alpha}$ metabolite (15-keto-13, 14-dihydro-$PGF_{2\alpha}$) within 30 min after antigen-induced airway reactions in five allergic asthmatic subjects. Because the increase in $PGF_{2\alpha}$ metabolite levels corresponded to the severity of the airway reaction, it was suggested that $PGF_{2\alpha}$ played a significant role in the pathogenesis of the response. However, control studies were not carried out to determine whether similar increases would occur in the absence of an airway response in challenged nonallergic subjects or after similar physiologic reactions were produced by nonallergenic substances such as histamine or methacholine. Recent advances in the development of specific assays for the various prostaglandins and TxB_2 should permit a more detailed analysis of the relationship between induced or spontaneously occurring ashtmatic attacks and circulating levels of cyclooxygenase products.

C. Effects of Cyclooxygenase Inhibitors

Although the major cyclooxygenase products of arachidonate have appreciable effects on airway function, the results of in vivo studies using cyclooxygenase inhibitors have failed to clarify the importance of these mediators in naturally occurring or experimentally induced asthma. With the exception of a select population of patients wherein asthma is provoked by aspirin or similar analgesic drugs, nonsteroidal anti-inflammatory agents have no demonstrable clinical effects in most cases of asthma (Pearson, 1963). Moreover, in asthmatic subjects, cyclooxygenase inhibitors fail to alter the airway response to a number of provocative stimuli including exercise and inhaled allergens (Rudolf et al., 1975; Schachter et al., 1978; Smith and Dunlop, 1975; Fish et al., 1981a).

Cyclooxygenase inhibitors have been employed to investigate the importance of prostaglandins in the regulation of normal resting airway smooth muscle tone. In guinea pigs, for example, indomethacin caused a fall in basal pulmonary resistance (Michoud et al., 1976). This effect on airway resistance was consistent with the fall in resting tension observed in guinea pig tracheal smooth muscle in vitro (Orehek et al., 1975), and illustrates the role of prostaglandins as a determinant of resting airway caliber in this particular species. A fall in resting tension has also been reported in indomethacin-treated isolated human airway preparations (Dunlop and Smith, 1975). However, several investigators have failed to demonstrate an indomethacin effect on resting pulmonary function at the in vivo level in asthmatic and nonasthmatic subjects (Fish et al., 1981a; Ogilvy et al., 1981). The discrepancy between the in vivo effects of indomethacin on resting airway function in guinea pigs and humans could be explained by species-related differences in the relative contribution of cholinergic factors as a determinant of resting airway tone. Whereas parasympathetic activity is a major determinant of resting airway tone in humans (Nadel, 1973), it appears to contribute little to resting tone in guinea pigs (Michoud et al., 1976). Thus, the failure of indomethacin to alter resting airway function in humans could be explained by the fact that, relative to parasympathetic factors, prostaglandins have little, if any, influence on resting bronchomotor tone. The fall in resting tension in indomethacin-treated isolated human airway preparations is consistent with this explanation since these preparations lacked parasympathetic innervation.

The augmentation of antigen-induced airway reactions with indomethacin in nonasthmatic allergic humans and rhesus monkeys (Fish et al., 1981a; Patterson et al., 1978), furnishes evidence that products of arachidonic acid metabolism participate in the modulation of in vivo respiratory responses to immediate-type immunologic stimuli in humans. Moreover, the lack of indomethacin-related enhancement in allergic asthmatic subjects suggests that the role of arachidonic acid metabolism in the modulation of allergic responses in the lung differs in asthmatic and nonasthmatic individuals. Whether these differences relate to a disparity in the relative metabolism of arachidonate by the lipoxygenase and cyclooxygenase pathways in these groups, or whether there are qualitative and quantitative differences in the effects of the various cyclooxygenase products must yet be established.

V. Slow-Reacting Substance of Anaphylaxis

Among the biologically active materials released during immediate-type hypersensitivity reactions, slow-reacting substance of anaphylaxis (SRS-A) has received perhaps the most attention in recent years. SRS-A was first described by Kellaway and Trethewie (1940) as a smooth muscle-contracting activity released during the perfusion of sensitized guinea pig lungs with antigen. Brocklehurst (1960) demonstrated that this activity could be distinguished from the effects of histamine by the inability of antihistamines to inhibit the contractile response of guinea pig ileum. Subsequent studies have shown SRS-A to have a unique profile of activity that distinguishes it from other mediators including bradykinin, prostaglandins, and serotonin (Orange and Austen, 1969). In contrast to histamine and other preformed, stored mediators of anaphylaxis, SRS-A appears to be generated from precursors derived from the cell membrane after cell activation. SRS-A activity has been derived from a variety of human sources including lung fragments and cell suspensions (Orange et al., 1971; Lewis et al., 1974; Paterson et al., 1976), nasal polyp fragments (Kaliner et al., 1973), and mixed peripheral leukocytes (Grant and Lichtenstein, 1974), as well as from cells and tissues from a number of other species. Although SRS-A can be generated during IgE-mediated activation of cells, the full spectrum of stimuli capable of initiating release in vivo are unknown, nor is the major cell source for lung SRS-A known. SRS-A release has been demonstrated in the rat peritoneal cavity by IgGa-neutrophil complement-dependent mechanisms (Morse et al., 1968); in guinea pig lung fragments by activation with anti-IgG_1 antibodies (Watanabe and Koda, 1979); in human leukocytes and rat basophilic leukemia cells by the divalent calcium ionophore A23187 (Conroy et al., 1976; Jakschick et al., 1977); and in the perfused cat paw by the histamine-releasing agent compound 48/80 (Strandberg and Uvnas, 1971). Moreover, recent work showing that contraction of isolated guinea pig trachea induced by the split product of the fifth component of the complement system (C5A peptide) was inhibited by the SRS-A antagonist, FPL-55712, suggest that anaphylatoxins are also capable of initiating SRS-A release (Regal and Pickering, 1981).

Only recently has SRS-A been characterized structurally. It has been established that several leukotrienes—these are complex hydroxy-eicosatetraenoic acid (HETEs) derivatives of the lipoxygenase pathway of arachidonic acid metabolism—constitute the major functional components of SRS-A (Hammarstrom et al., 1979; Murphy et al., 1979; Lewis et al., 1980a; Orning et al., 1980). Although the development of synthetic leukotrienes has facilitated an analysis of the specific functional activities of SRS-A, at this writing only limited information is available (further details are discussed elsewhere in this text). In preliminary studies leukotriene (LT) C4 and D4, respectively, were found to be 200-fold and 20,000-fold more potent than histamine in contracting guinea pig tracheal spirals (Drazen et al., 1980). In addition, LTC4 and LTD4 selectively caused greater contraction of guinea pig peripheral airway tissue than guinea pig tracheal spirals, confirming the results of previous studies using partially purified native SRS-A preparations (Drazen et al., 1979a). A discussion of previous in vivo studies of crude and partially purified SRS-A preparations merits some consideration, although it should be clear that these results are subject to reinterpretation as new evidence is brought to bear on the subject.

A. Animal Studies

Because of limited availability of native material, our knowledge of the in vivo effects of SRS-A is scant and most of this is derived from studies in guinea pigs using relatively impure preparations. Both crude and partially purified, native SRS-A preparations have been shown to alter pulmonary mechanics when injected intravenously in guinea pigs (Berry et al., 1963; Berry and Collier, 1964; Collier and James, 1967; Drazen and Austen, 1974; Mathé et al., 1977). Some of these studies are complicated, however, by the fact that the pulmonary response to intravenously administered SRS-A was inhibited by aspirin and other nonsteroidal anti-inflammatory agents (Berry and Collier, 1964; Mathé et al., 1977). This suggested that at least some of the effects of SRS-A were indirectly mediated by cyclooxygenase products of arachidonic acid metabolism. Subsequent studies confirmed that crude SRS-A induced release of TxA2 and prostaglandins from guinea pig and human lung tissue and that the release of these substances was inhibited by nonsteroidal anti-inflammatory agents (Mathé et al., 1977; Engineer et al., 1978b).

Several investigators failed to demonstrate changes in pulmonary mechanics in guinea pigs when crude SRS-A was given by aerosol (Herxheimer and Stressman, 1963; Collier and James, 1967). On the other hand, Sheard et al., (1977) furnished evidence for a significant direct effect of SRS-A on guinea pig airways by demonstrating that the specific SRS-A antagonist, FPL-55712, partially inhibited pulmonary mechanical alterations induced by intravenous and inhaled antigen in sensitized guinea pigs.

Discrepancies in the pulmonary effects of crude SRS-A in guinea pig studies are most likely a reflection of differences in the biologic activity or purity of the preparations used. Nevertheless, differences in the route of administration and differences in the measurements used to assess the physiologic response may account for some of the discordancy as well. For example, using partially purified rat SRS-A as well as synthetic and highly purified native rat and human

LTC4 and LTD4, Drazen observed remarkable selectivity of SRS-A in producing contraction of peripheral guinea pig lung tissue as compared with tracheal spirals (Drazen and Austen, 1974; Drazen et al., 1979a, 1980). Thus, an accurate assessment of the direct effects of SRS-A on guinea pig lungs may require the use of physiologic tests designed to examine peripheral airway effects as opposed to measurements of the total pulmonary response that were used in many previous studies.

In contrast to the results obtained with guinea pigs, partially purified rat SRS-A administered directly into the airways produced pulmonary mechanical changes in vivo in *Ascaris*-sensitive monkeys (Patterson et al., 1978; Michoud et al., 1979). Michoud and co-workers demonstrated a preferential effect on peripheral airways by directly instilling SRS-A into the trachea. In contrast, when SRS-A was administered by aerosol, Patterson demonstrated a predominant central effect in some monkeys, suggesting that the observed physiologic effects depend to some extent on the route of administration. In both studies, SRS-A produced mechanical alterations of slower onset and longer duration than either histamine or *Ascaris* antigen alone. In addition, for comparable changes in pulmonary resistance, Patterson found minimal SRS-A-induced changes in respiratory frequency as compared with antigen, histamine, or $PGF_{2\alpha}$. These findings suggested that aerosolized SRS-A, unlike histamine, $PGF_{2\alpha}$ or antigen, did not evoke reflex tachypnea mediated by vagal afferent pathways in monkeys (Patterson et al., 1978b; Patterson and Harris, 1978). On the other hand, that crude SRS-A is capable of producing reflex-mediated changes in bronchomotor tone in guinea pigs is indicated by the fact that atropine partially inhibits SRS-A-induced bronchoconstriction (Drazen and Austen, 1975).

B. Human Studies

The in vivo effects of partially purified guinea pig SRS-A in man were evaluated by Herxheimer and Stressman (1963), who demonstrated a fall in vital capacity in asthmatic patients but not in normal controls. Because these studies failed to discriminate between the direct effects of SRS-A and the potential irritant-induced reflex effects of the preparation used, the results cannot be given a meaningful interpretation. On the basis of preliminary studies using highly purified or synthetic leukotrienes, however, SRS-A appears to have potent contractile activity in isolated human airway tissue (Dahlen et al., 1980). The significance of the role played by this mediator in IgE-mediated as well as other nonallergic forms of airways dysfunction must await the development of specific SRS-A antagonist as well as specific inhibitors of the lipoxygenase pathway that are suitable for in vivo human experimentation.

VI. Cholinergic Agonists

Although acetylcholine is not properly considered a primary chemical mediator of anaphylaxis, there is evidence implicating the parasympathetic system in the response to antigens and chemical mediators. This evidence, in addition to the consistent finding of cholinergic hyperreactivity in asthma, suggests that cholinergic factors are potentially important as an effector system in allergic reactions of the lung. Various aspects of cholinergic pharmacology and the role of the parasympathetic system in the response of the lung to various stimuli have recently been reviewed in detail (Nadel, 1980) and are briefly discussed elsewhere in this chapter.

A. Effects of Cholinergic Agonists on Airways

Cholinergic agonists contract parenchymal strips as well as tracheobronchial smooth muscle in a variety of species (Drazen and Schneider, 1978; Chand et al., 1979; Chand et al., 1980). The sensitivity of these tissues differs, however, as carbachol is more potent in contracting tracheobronchial smooth muscle than parenchymal tissue in monkeys and guinea pigs (Drazen and Schneider, 1978; Chand et al., 1980). The relative potency of cholinergic agonsists as compared with other bronchoconstrictor stimuli varies, not only with the type of tissue studied, but also with species. For example, cholinergic agonists are less potent than histamine in causing contraction of guinea pig parenchymal strips but more potent than histamine in causing contraction of parenchyma from monkeys (Drazen and Schneider, 1978; Chand et al., 1980).

Exogenous cholinergic agonists and vagal stimulation cause central and peripheral airways obstruction in vivo, and are thought to produce alveolar duct constriction, as suggested by an increase in the elastic recoil pressure of the lung (Colebatch et al., 1966; Woolcock et al., 1969). Emmanuel et al. (1968) studied the effects of intravenous acetylcholine in humans and reported that arterial oxygen tension fell before airway resistance changes occurred; instead, the fall in oxygen tension corresponded temporally to a fall in lung compliance. Because the hypoxemia was not corrected by breathing 100% oxygen, it was concluded that acetylcholine produced closure of small peripheral lung units, presumably at the level of alveolar ducts, causing shunting of pulmonary capillary blood through airless areas of the lung. Woolcock et al. (1969), on the other hand, failed to demonstrate gas trapping in dogs with peripheral airways obstruction induced by vagal stimulation. Although they interpreted these findings as indicating that cholinergic stimulation did not produce airway closure, Murtagh et al. (1971) have provided direct morphologic evidence of closure of lobar bronchi with methacholine in excised canine lungs.

B. Cholinergic Hyperreactivity

Since Starr first reported that small doses of methacholine could provoke bronchospasm in an asthmatic patient (Starr et al., 1933), it has been firmly established that asthma is associated with an exaggerated responsiveness of the airways to cholineric stimuli. On the basis of early studies showing that extrapulmonary reactions to methacholine, such as flushing, sweating, salivation, and tachycardia, were of no greater magnitude in asthmatic subjects than nonasthmatic subjects (Moll, 1940; Curry, 1947), it was suggested that cholinergic hyperreactivity of the airways in asthma was due to a local tropism confined to the lung, in contrast to a systemic hypersensitivity. This interpretation was supported by recent studies showing that pupillary sphincter muscle and eccrine sweat responses to cholinergic stimuli in asthmatic and nonasthmatic subjects with skin sensitivity to common aeroallergens were comparable in magnitude (Kaliner, 1976; Smith et al., 1980a) in spite of well-established group differences in cholinergic airway reactivity (Curry, 1947; Townley et al., 1965; Parker et al., 1965; Fish et al., 1976). Allergic nonasthmatic subjects, however, were noted to have greater systemic cholinergic reactivity than nonallergic individuals. This finding was compatible with previous observations of slight but significantly greater airway responses to methacholine in allergic rhinitis subjects as compared to nonallergic normal subjects (Townley et al., 1965; Fish et al., 1976), although the significance of this phenomenon is unclear.

In spite of recent advances in our understanding of airway physiology and pharmacology, we remain largely ignorant of the cause or causes of cholinergic airway hyperreactivity in asthma. A number of mechanisms have been proposed to account for this phenomenon. These include decreased airway caliber, an imbalance in the autonomic regulation of bronchomotor tone, alterations in the intrinsic properties of airway smooth muscle, and abnormalities in the nonadrenergic inhibitory nervous system (Boushey et al., 1980). Although there is compelling evidence to support each of these theories, because of contradictory data or a lack of sufficient information, none, by itself, has gained general acceptance as a satisfactory explanation. It seems unlikely that decreased baseline airway caliber is exclusively responsible, since hyperreactivity can be demonstrated in asthmatics with normal as well as abnormal pulmonary function (Fish et al., 1976; Permutt et al., 1977). Conversely, normal responses to methacholine may be observed in some patients with chronic irreversible airway obstruction (Parker et al., 1965). Pharmacologic β-adrenergic blockade with propranolol was shown to increase methacholine responsiveness in nonasthmatic subjects in one study (Townley et al., 1976), but the resultant degree of reactivity was modest in comparison with the reactivity observed in asthmatic subjects without propranolol treatment. This and other evidence of virtually no effect of β-adrenergic blockade on methacholine or histamine sensitivity in normal subjects (Ouellette and Reed, 1967; Zaid and Beall, 1966; Ryo and Townley, 1976) mitigate the case for natural β-adrenergic receptor dysfunction as the principal cause.

One approach to the investigation of airway hyperreactivity has involved studies of conditions in which an increase in reactivity is acquired in association with damage to the airway epithelium. Viral respiratory infections and exposure to agents such as ozone, sulfur dioxide, and nitrogen dioxide have been shown to induce a transient and sometimes striking increase in airway responsiveness to methacholine or histamine (Islam et al., 1972; Empey et al., 1976; Orehek et al., 1976; Golden et al., 1978; Little et al., 1978). Empey et al. (1976) demonstrated that increased histamine responsiveness after viral infections could be abolished by atropine and speculated that the increase was due to epithelial irritant receptor sensitization and potentiation of the reflex-mediated parasympathetic component of the response. It seems unlikely that methacholine hyperreactivity attending viral infections is also the product of exaggerated reflex activity, however, since cholinergic agents, unlike histamine, do not stimulate afferent epithelial irritant receptors (Vidruk et al., 1977). Indeed, the fact that cholinergic hyperreactivity can be demonstrated with parenteral methacholine (Curry, 1947) and with cholinesterase inhibitors as well (Miller et al., 1977) suggests that abnormal responsiveness is the result of a postjunctional abnormality of smooth muscle. Thus, the greater response to both agonists could be explained by an increase in responsiveness of target airway smooth muscle to both the direct cholinergic effects of methacholine and the indirect cholinergic effects of histamine. The reason for the increase is unclear, although several possibilities merit consideration.

Damage to the epithelial lining could alter permeability of the respiratory mucosa and, thereby, facilitate penetration of greater amounts of agonist to the level of smooth muscle. The principal basis for this hypothesis is the observation that damage to the airway mucosa facilitates transport of proteins, ions, and small hydrophilic solutes across the epithelial barrier (Boucher et al., 1980; Hogg and Hulbert, 1980; Pare, 1980). Although this hypothesis offers an attractive explanation for the increase in methacholine reactivity, it cannot be fully reconciled with the results of experiments using histamine. Because mucosal permeability to histamine would also be expected to increase, there should be a predictable increase in the bronchomotor response to the direct effects of histamine. The data of Empey et al. (1976) suggest that this is not the case, however, since in their experiments atropine completely abolished the increased histamine response.

A further explanation considers the possibility that either the binding affinity or the number of cholinergic receptors on smooth muscle is increased after a viral respiratory infection. Although there is no direct evidence to support this, such a hypothesis is consistent with the enhanced direct effects of

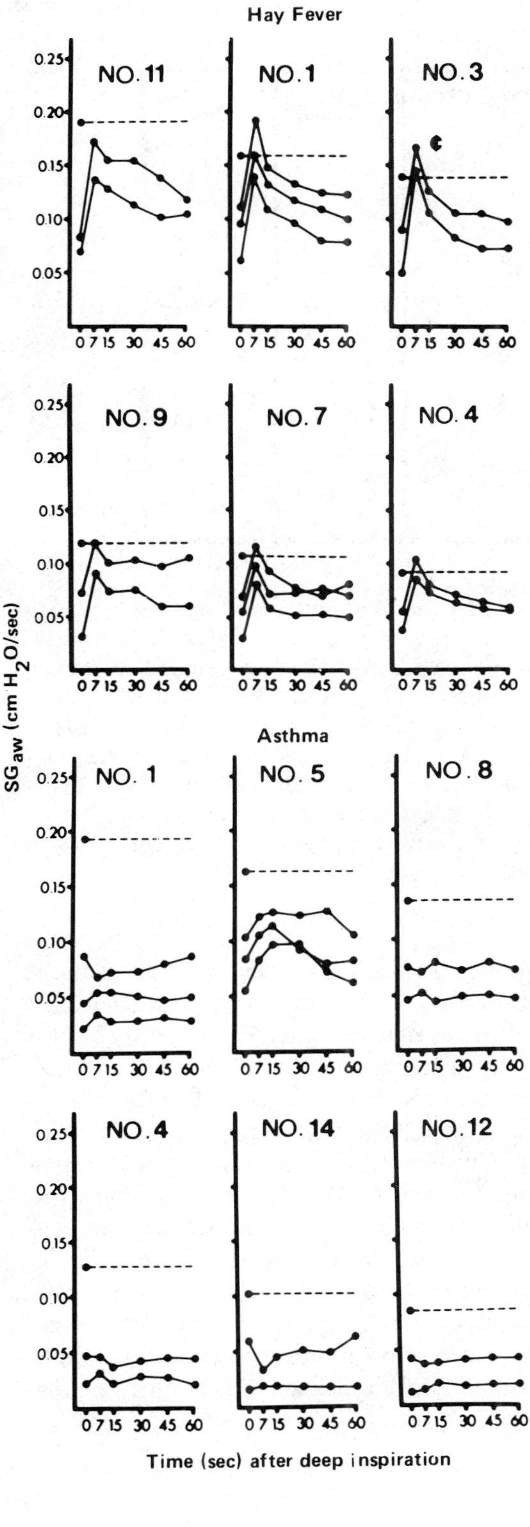

Figure 7 Effect of deep inspiration on specific airway conductance (SGaw) at varying levels of methacholine induced obstruction in six asthmatic subjects and six nonasthmatic subjects with hay fever. Horizontal dashed lines (- - - - - -) represent prechallenge baseline SGaw values. Points connected by solid lines were obtained after methacholine, before deep inspiration (zero sec) and at varying times after inspiration. Each solid line represents a different methacholine dose. SGaw increased after inspiration in all hay fever subjects with maximum improvement at 7 sec and a gradual return toward preinspiration levels during the 60-sec observation period. No appreciable changes in SGaw were observed in asthmatic subjects after inspiration. Subjects were matched vertically according to prechallenge SGaw levels and the degree of obstruction produced with methacholine. (From Fish et al., 1981b.)

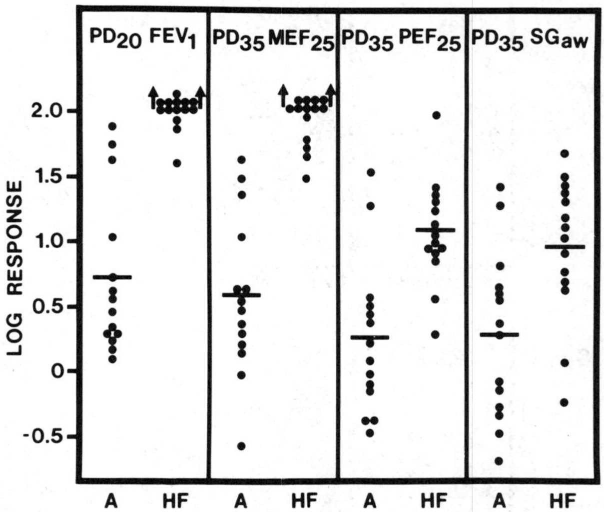

Figure 8 Comparison of methacholine sensitivity in nonasthmatic subjects with hay fever (HF) and asthmatic subjects (A) using different tests of lung function. Sensitivity is defined as the common logarithm of the dose required to produce a 20% forced expiratory volume in 1 sec (FEV_1), and a 35% fall in MEF25, PEF25, and specific airway conductance (SGaw). MEF25 and PEF25 signify flow at 25% of the vital capacity (above residual volume) from maximum and partial expiratory flow-volume curves, respectively. Whereas groups were markedly different with tests requiring a preceding deep inspiration (FEV_1 or MEF25), group differences were reduced when using tests with no preceding inspiration (SGaw or PEF25). (From Fish et al., 1981b.)

methacholine as well as the increase in the vagal component of the histamine response. Holtzman et al. (1980) have shown that parasympathetic ganglionic blockade with hexamethonium abolishes enhanced histamine reactivity but has no effect on methacholine reactivity in atopic nonasthmatic subjects. As these results indicate that increased histamine reactivity was due to enhanced cholinergic responsiveness at some level distal to the parasympathetic ganglion, they tend to support the possibility that hyperreactivity is the result of an increased sensitivity of cholinergic receptors. The problem with this interpretation is that there remains a persistent increase in histamine reactivity in asthmatic subjects even after the administration of atropine (Casterline et al., 1976; Woenne et al., 1978). It should be noted that the increase in reactivity acquired as a result of infections or toxic exposures is usually of smaller magnitude than the increase observed in patients with asthma. Clearly, more information is needed to determine whether the mechanisms responsible for acquired hyperreactivity are the same as for endogenous reactivity. It is curious that interruption of reflex pathways abolishes histamine hyperreactivity in atopic subjects without asthma but fails to block hyperreactivity in atopic asthmatic subjects. Since both groups of subjects are presumed to have endogenous hyperreactivity, the possibility that different mechanisms are involved should be considered.

With respect to differences in cholinergic reactivity between asthmatic and nonasthmatic subjects, we recently demonstrated that the normal capacity to reverse the bronchoconstrictor effects of methacholine by an active change in lung volume (i.e., a deep breath) was diminished or absent in asthmatic subjects (Fig. 7; Fish et al., 1977; Fish and Kelly, 1979; Fish et al., 1980, 1981b). Because commonly reported differences in bronchial sensitivity to methacholine are based primarily on measurements that require an antecedent maximum inspiration to total lung capacity, we suggested that airway hyperreactivity was perhaps not so much a reflection of increased end-organ responsiveness to a stimulus as a reflection of an impaired ability to modify changes in bronchomotor tone by lung inflation. In our studies, we found that marked differences in methacholine sensitivity between asthmatic and nonasthmatic individuals were more readily demonstrated with tests requiring a maximum inflation to total lung capacity (Fig. 8). Intrigued by the possibility that the ability to abolish or diminish increases in airway tone by inflation was a normal means of regulating airway caliber and thus represented a protective mechanism against the bronchoactive effects of endogenous and environmental stimuli, we have postulated that a loss of this regulatory capacity could potentially result in unopposed bronchoconstriction and thus could be a potential cause of abnormal airway reactivity. Further studies are needed to establish this as a possible mechanism and to determine the underlying causes that may impair volume regulation of bronchomotor tone.

In recent years, a number of animal models have been developed for the study of allergic asthma. While some investigators have reported increased cholinergic airway reactivity in monkeys with skin and respiratory sensitivity to *Ascaris suum* (Patterson et al., 1976), others have failed to confirm these findings in the monkey model (Michoud et al., 1978) or in a similar canine model (Krell and Chakrin, 1976). These models may indeed provide a potential opportunity for studying airway reactivity, but attempts to extrapolate from these models to human asthma should be regarded with caution. Although sensitized monkeys and dogs can develop acute airway obstruction after exposure to antigen in the laboratory, these animals usually do not develop spontaneous attacks of asthma. Similarly, nonasthmatic humans with skin sensitivity and symptoms of allergic rhinitis only also develop airway reactions after laboratory exposure, but they, too, do not develop spontaneous attacks of asthma with natural environmental exposure (Fish et al., 1980). Thus, the human counterpart to these animal models may very well be the nonasthmatic individual with positive skin tests, rather than the individual with asthma.

VII. The Kallikrein-Kinin System and the Lung

Among the biologically active agents that are putative mediators of acute, subacute, and chronic allergic and/or inflammatory disorders of the lung, bradykinin has also been implicated as a mediator in bronchial asthma (Aas, 1972). This hypothesis was strengthened by the observations of Abe et al. (1967) who observed a tenfold elevation from normal of blood kinin levels in severe asthmatic patients. Although these studies suggest a relationship between the severity of symptoms and kinin levels in plasma, a cause and effect relationship between kinins and asthma remains circumstantial.

There is, however, other evidence to support the participation of kinins and the kallikrein-kinin system in disorders of the cardiopulmonary systems. In a study of human anaphylaxis (induced by the sting of a yellow jacket), patients were noted to experience breathlessness with wheezing, in addition to systemic hypotension. These studies showed that there was depletion of plasma kininogen during the acute anaphylactic event, suggesting the participation of the kallikrein-kinin system in the anaphylactic reaction in man (Smith et al., 1980c). Other studies in a rabbit model of anaphylaxis showed depletion of coagulation factors XII, XI, and IX during the acute reaction. These studies suggest that during IgE-mediated anaphylaxis there is, by virtue of the activation of Hageman factor (factor XII), the potential for the activation of the kallikrein-kinin system and the generation of bradykinin (Pinckard et al., 1975).

There are also in vitro data to support the activation of the Hageman factor-dependent pathways (and thus the generation of bradykinin) during IgE-mediated reactions of human lungs. We have demonstrated that three distinct proteases in supernatants from passively sensitized, antigen challenged human lungs directly cleave three proteins of the human Hageman factor (HF)-dependent systems (HF, prekallikrein, kininogen). The first protease, like plasma kallikrein, is a lung Hageman factor activator (LHFA). It not only cleaves but also activates human plasma Hageman factor (Newball et al., 1981a). The second protease is a lung prekallikrein activator (LPKA) and it is also released by lung fragments as a functionally active molecule and converts prekallikrein to its active form, kallikrein, which, in turn, generates bradykinin from human plasma kininogen (Newball et al., 1981b). The third protease observed in lung supernatants is a kininogenase and it directly cleaves human plasma kininogen to generate a kinin (Newball et al., 1981c). Further studies utilizing the in vitro basophil model also demonstrate the IgE-mediated release of a kininogenase and an activator of human Hageman factor (Newball et al., 1975; Newball et al., 1979a,b,c; Newball et al., 1979b; Newball et al., 1980b).

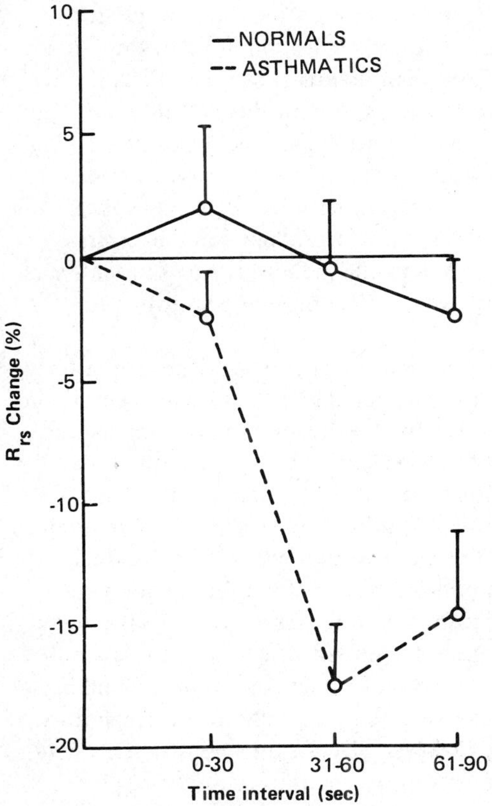

Figure 9 Effects of intravenous bradykinin on the respiratory resistance (Rrs) of normals and asthmatics. Normal subjects show how a small but progressive decrease of the Rrs, which did not reach levels of significance. Asthmatics showed a significant decrease of the Rrs, indicating that bronchdilation had occurred. (From Newball et al., 1975.)

A. In Vivo Effects of Bradykinin

Intravenous Bradykinin

Since bradykinin had been implicated as a mediator of the acute asthmatic event (Aas, 1972), studies were designed to determine the effects of intravenous bradykinin on human airways. Single bolus injections of bradykinin (1 μg/kg body weight) were given intravenously to both normal and asthmatic subjects, and we determined their effects on the respiratory system (Newball and Keiser, 1973; Newball, 1974; Newball et al., 1975). In all subjects, intravenous bradykinin produced systemic reactions while placebo (normal saline) had no effects. None of the normal subjects experienced wheezing at any time while some asthmatics developed transient wheezing. Some asthmatics also developed breathlessness and symptoms of tightness in the chest. The symptoms of respiratory distress were transient, persisting for about a minute only. Several asthmatics stated that, after the initial transient but often severe respiratory distress, they could breath easier than before the injection of bradykinin. Bradykinin is known to release adrenalin from the cat adrenal medulla (Feldburg and Lewis, 1964) and also to release prostaglandins from the lung (Moncada et al., 1972). Our data is compatible with the hypothesis that bradykinin does induce contraction of respiratory smooth muscle (probably predominantly alveolar duct constriction) with decreases of the vital capacity (Newball and Keiser, 1973). However, the direct contractile effects of bradykinin on the respiratory system were transient, perhaps due to bradykinin-induced release of agents such as adrenalin, which lead to secondary bronchodilation (Fig. 9; Newball et al., 1975).

Our data supported the claim of most asthmatics who found that, after the transient initial respiratory distress, they could breath easier than before the bradykinin injection. The greater sensitivity of asthmatics to bronchodilators is probably a result of an initial higher intrinsic bronchial tone, and this may explain the secondary bronchodilation observed in asthmatics, but not in normals. Intravenous bradykinin in vivo (1 μg/kg body weight) failed to produce constriction of normal human airways (Newball and Keiser, 1973; Newball, 1974). There did not appear to be a principal constrictor effect of bradykinin on the large airways of asthmatics (vide infra). When given intravenously to human subjects, bradykinin probably exerts its primary effects at the level of alveolar ducts. It is unlikely, however, that alveolar duct constriction would increase the work of breathing sufficiently to account totally for the respiratory distress described by the asthmatics. However, alveolar duct constriction could lead to stimulation of intrapulmonary receptors and thus cause the respiratory distress described.

In a guinea pig preparation, James (1969) found that intravenous bradykinin had a dual effect on the airways, dilating the trachea indirectly through an adrenergic mechanism (abolished by propranolol), and constricting intrathoracic airways perfused by pulmonary arteries. On the basis of these observations, we suggest that intravenous bradykinin has a similar dual effect on the airways of man, dilating the conducting airways (airways proximal to the respiratory bronchiole), while predominantly constricting peripheral airways served by the pulmonary artery (respiratory bronchioles and the alveolar ducts).

Aerosolized Bradykinin

The importance of bradykinin as an agonist of human airways has been extensively disputed, primarily because of the contradictory data that have been reported. Peak expiratory flow was measured in normal and asthmatic children before and after the administration of aerosolized bradykinin. There were no effects on the normals, but the asthmatic children demonstrated a significant

Table 2 Bradykinin Relaxes or Contracts Isolated Human Bronchial Muscle

Patient diagnosis	Age	Sex	Effective dose of bradykinin: Contraction μg/ml	Relaxation μg/ml
Lung cancer	58	M	5	
Lung cancer, emphysema	67	M	10	
Lung cancer, emphysema	52	F		3
Lung cancer		M		10
Lung cancer	54	F	10	
Lung cancer	78	F		10
Lung cancer	66	M	10	3
Lung cancer		F		10

Isolated human bronchi varying in diameter from 3-7 mm were cut spirally and suspended in a tissue bath containing Krebs-Henseleit solution at 36°C aerated with 95% oxygen and 5% carbon dioxide. Tension (1.3-1.6 *g*) was applied; and, after an equilibrium period of about 1 hr, BK was added to the bath for 10 min. *Source*: Newball et al. (1977).

decrease of peak expiratory flow rates (Varonier and Panzani, 1968). However, Simonsson et al. (1973) suggested that aerosolized bradykinin-induced bronchoconstriction merely reflects a nonspecific vagus-dependent irritant effect. Further studies are clearly required to clarify the mechanism of bradykinin-induced human airway constriction.

B. In Vitro Effects of Bradykinin

Pieces of human bronchi recovered from lungs excised for carcinoma were exposed to bradykinin in vitro in a tissue bath. Bradykinin in concentrations up to 667 μg/ml did not contract isolated human bronchi, while histamine in concentrations of 0.067 to 0.67 μg/ml did (Bhoola et al., 1962). Other studies on human bronchi have shown that bradykinin occasionally induces a weak contraction (Simonsson et al., 1973). In our studies, however, bradykinin, in the dose range of 3-10 μg/ml, induced both contraction and relaxation of human bronchi (Table 2). In most tissues, the initial response, whether contraction or relaxation, could be repeated for a period of 3-6 hr, but attempts to quantitate the contractile response were unsuccessful. In one tissue specimen, an initial high contractile response was followed by a prolonged period where only relaxation could be elicited (Newball et al., 1977). This data is similar to that described by Iorio and Constantine (1969) for the effects of bradykinin on guinea pig trachea. The responses of the human bronchus to bradykinin are most likely due to the release of secondary substances which, in turn, induce either relaxation or contraction. Prostaglandins are potential secondary mediators, since bradykinin is known to induce their synthesis (Moncada et al., 1972). What determines whether a constricting or a relaxing prostaglandin is synthesized, however, is unknown.

VIII. Serotonin

Although the pharmacologic actions of serotonin (5-hydroxytryptamin, 5-HT) have been extensively characterized since its discovery in the late 1940s, the importance of this substance as a mediator of bronchial asthma remains unknown. 5-HT causes bronchoconstriction in a number of species. In cats, guinea pigs, rabbits, and rats this activity is mediated in part by direct stimulation of the airways and in part by enhanced cholinergic stimulation (Comroe et al., 1953; Herxheimer, 1955; Konzett, 1956; Jankala and Virtama, 1961; Colebatch et al., 1966). Several investigators reported that in dogs 5-HT-induced bronchoconstriction was almost completely abolished with atropine or by interruption of the vagi and concluded that the constrictor effects of this mediater were predominantly reflex mediated (Islam et al., 1974; Krell et al., 1976). Recent studies by Hahn et al. (1978), however, suggest that a more complex interaction exists between 5-HT and efferent vagal impulses. They found that doses of 5-HT that were too low to have a direct effect on bronchomotor tone greatly increased the bronchoconstriction induced by electrical stimulation of the vagus, and that local application of 5-HT to one lung caused unilateral bronchoconstriction. Because bilateral bronchoconstriction would be the predicted response if a classic parasympathetic reflex were involved, they postulated that there was a direct, nonreflex interaction between 5-HT and efferent vagal activity whereby 5-HT potentiated the effects of the latter. The site and mechanims of this interaction are unknown.

Brocklehurst (1958) reported that 5-HT relaxed human airway tissue in vitro. At the in vivo level, however, aerosolized 5-HT caused bronchoconstriction in patients with bronchial asthma, although similar responses were not observed in nonasthmatic individuals (Herxheimer, 1953; Panzani, 1962; Girard and Moret, 1963; Marcelle et al., 1968; Booij-Noord et al., 1969). A number of observations suggest that the bronchoconstrictor activity of 5-HT in man may be due to reflex parasympathetic stimulation rather than a consequence of the direct effects of 5-HT on airways. Herxheimer (1966) reported that 5-HT-induced bronchoconstriction in asthmatic patients was related to the acidity or irritant properties of the aerosol solution, and others found that the bronchoconstrictor effects were correlated with nonspecific airway reactivity as determined by the response to inhaled histamine (Booij-Noord et al., 1969). In addition, when 5-HT was administered intravenously, it failed to produce bronchoconstriction in asthmatic as well as nonasthmatic subjects (Michelson et al., 1958). Although most evidence indicates that 5-HT has minor, if any, direct effects on airway smooth muscle function in man, other actions of this agonist may prove relevant. For example, in some species 5-HT produces pre- and postcapillary pulmonary vasoconstriction (Comroe et al., 1953), and in man intravenous 5-HT can stimulate hyperpnea and tachypnea (Michelson et al., 1958).

The basis for suggesting that 5-HT has a relevant function in asthma is not strong,but in its favor is the emerging role of platelets in immediate hypersensitivity reactions. The bulk of 5-HT in many species, including man, originates in the enterochromaffin cells of the gastrointestinal tract. After release into the circulation, it is taken up by platelets through an active transport mechanism and stored in the dense granules (Drummond, 1976). During IgE-mediated anaphylaxis in rabbits, platelets become activated, sequester in the lung, and release their granular constituents (Pinckard et al., 1977; McManus et al., 1979). This reaction is caused by a basophil/mast cell-derived platelet-activating factor recently characterized as the lipid mediator, acetylglyceryl ether phosphorycholine (AGEPC) (Demopoulus et al., 1979; McManus et al., 1979; Pinckard et al., 1979). Recent studies showing that AGEPC infusion causes bronchoconstriction in rabbits and guinea pigs and that these effects can be abolished by prior immune platelet depletion suggest that 5-HT and/or other platelet mediators play a role in the pathophysiology of IgE-mediated airway reactions (Pinckard et al., 1977; Vargaftig et al., 1980). Although the significance of AGEPC, platelets, and platelet-derived mediators during IgE-mediated events in man is unknown, our recent work demonstrating platelet activation during allergen-induced airway reactions in ragweed allergic asthmatic subjects indicates the need for further investigation of this subject (Knauer et al., 1981).

Acknowledgment

The authors acknowledge with gratitude the invaluable contribution of Ms. Judy M. Mason who assisted in the preparation of this chapter.

References

Aas, B. (1972). *The Biochemical and Immunological Basis of Bronchial Asthma.* Springfield, Charles C. Thomas, pp. 115-130.

Abe, K., Watanabe, N., Kumagai, Mouri T., Seki, T., and Yosinga, K. (1967). Circulating plasma kinin in patients with bronchial asthma. *Experimentia, 22*:626-627.

Adams, G. K., and Lichtenstein, L. (1979). In vitro studies of antigen-induced bronchospasm: Effect of antihistamine and SRS-A antagonist on response to sensitized guinea pig and human airways to antigen. *J. Immunol., 122*: 555-562.

Adcock, J. J., Garland, L. G., Moncada, S., and Salmon, J. A. (1978). The mechanism of enhancement by fatty acid hydroperoxides of anaphylactic mediator release. *Prostaglandins, 16*:179-187.

Adkinson, N. F., Newball, H. H., Findlay, S., Adams, K., and Lichtenstein, L. M. (1980). Anaphylactic release of prostaglandins from human lung *in vitro. Am. Rev. Respir. Dis. 121*:911-920.

Ahmed, T., Fernandez, R. J., and Wanner, A. (1981). Airway responses to antigen challenge in allergic rhinitis and allergic asthma. *J. Allergy Clin. Immunol., 67*:135-145.

Ahmed, T., Eyre, P., Januszkiewicz, A. J., and Wanner, A. (1980). Role of H_1 and H_2-receptors in airway reactions to histamine in conscious sheep. *J. Appl. Physiol., 49*:826-833.

Alanko, K., and Poppius, H. (1973). Anticholinergic blocking of prostaglandin-induced bronchoconstriction. *Br. Med. J., 1*:294.

Alexander, F., Eyre, P., Head, K. W., and Sanford, J. (1967). Effect of histamine and 5-hydroxytryptamine on sheep. *J. Comp. Pathol., 77*:1-14.

Altounyan, R. E. C. (1979). Review of the clinical activity and modes of action of sodium cromoglycate. In *The Mast Cell.* Edited by J. Pepys and A. M. Edwards. Kent, England, Pitman Medical Publishing Co., Ltd., pp. 199-216.

Ash, A. S. F., and Schild, H. O. (1966). Receptors mediating some actions of histamine. *Br. J. Pharmacol., 27*:427-439.

Atkins, P. C., Norman, M. E., and Zweiman, B. (1978). Antigen-induced neutrophil chemotactic activity in man. *J. Allergy Clin. Immunol., 62*:149-155.

Atkins, P. C., Norman, M., Weiner, H., and Zweiman, B. (1977). Release of neutrophil chemotactic activity during immediate hypersensitivity reactions in humans. *Ann. Int. Med., 86*:415-418.

Atkins, P. C., Rosenblum, F., Dunsky, E. H., Coffey, R., and Zweiman, B. (1980). Comparison of plasma histamine and cyclic nucleotides after antigen and methacholine inhalation in man. *J. Allergy Clin. Immunol., 66*: 478-485.

Benveniste, J. (1974). Platelet activating factor, a new mediator of anaphylaxis and immune complex deposition from rabbit and human basophils. *Nature, 249*:581-582.

Berry, P. A., and Collier, H. O. J. (1964). Bronchoconstrictor action and antagonism of a slow-reacting substance from anaphylaxis of guinea pig isolated lung. *Br. J. Pharmacol., 23*:201-216.

Berry, P. A., Collier, H. O. J., and Holgate, J. A. (1963). Bronchoconstrictor action in vivo of slow reacting substance in anaphylaxis (SRS-A) and its antagonism. *J. Physiol. 165*:41-42P.

Bhat, K. N., Arroyave, C. M., Marney, S. R., Jr., Stevenson, D. D., and Tan, E. M. (1976). Plasma histamine changes during provoked bronchospasm in asthmatic patients. *J. Allergy Clin. Immunol., 58*:647-656.

Bhoola, K. D., Collier, H. O. J., Schachter, M., and Shorley, P. G. (1962). Actions of some peptides on bronchial muscle. *Br. J. Pharmacol., 19*:190-197.

Bianco, S., Robuschi, M., Ceserani, R., Gandolfi, C., and Kamburoff, P. L. (1978). Prevention of aspecifically induced bronchoconstriction by PGI_2 and 20-methyl-PGI_2 in asthmatic patients. *Pharmacol. Res. Commun., 10*: 657-674.

Black, J. W., Duncan, W. A. M., Durant, C. J., Ganellin, C. R., and Parsons, E. M. (197). Definition and antagonism of histamine H_2 receptors. *Nature, 236*:385-390.

Bleecker, E. R., Cotton, D. J., Fischer, S. P., Graf, P. D., Gold, W. M., and Nadel, J. A. (1976). The mechanism of rapid, shallow breathing after inhaling histamine aerosol in exercising dogs. *Am. Rev. Resp. Dis., 114*: 909-916.

Bogart, D. B., and Stechschulte, D. J. (1974). Release of platelet activating factor from human lung. *Clin. Res. 22*:652.

Booij-Noord, H., Orie, N. G. M., and deVries, K. (1969). Serotonin (5-hydroxytryptamine) inhalation in patients with chronic non-specific lung disease. *Scand. J. Respir. Dis., 50*:301-308.

Booij-Noord, H., deVries, K., Sluiter, H. J., and Orie, N. G. M. (1972). Late bronchial obstructive reaction to experimental inhalation of house dust extract. *Clin. Allergy 2*:43-61.

Boucher, R. C., Bromberg, P. A., and Gatzy, J. T. (1980). Airway mucosal permeability. In *Airway Reactivity, Mechanisms and Clinical Relevance.* Edited by F. E. Hargreave. Canada, Astra Pharmaceuticals Canada Ltd., pp. 40-48.

Bourne, H. R., Lichtenstein, L. M., and Melmon, K. L. (1972). Pharmacologic control of allergic histamine release *in vitro*: Evidence for an inhibitory role of 3′,5′-adenosine monophosphate in human leukocytes. *J. Immunol., 108*:695-705.

Boushey, H. A., Holtzman, M. J., Shellar, J. R., and Nadel, J. A. (1980). Bronchial hyper-reactivity. *Am. Rev. Respir. Dis. 121*:389-413.

Brocklehurst, W. E. (1958). Histamine and other mediators in hypersensitivity reactions. Paris, *Proc. III Intern. Congr. Allergol.*, pp. 361-371.

Brocklehurst, W. E. (1960). The release of histamine and formation of a slow reacting substance (SRS-A) during anaphylactic shock. *J. Physiol., 151*:416.

Brown, N. E., McFadden, E. R., Jr., and Ingram, R. H., Jr. (1977). Airway responses to inhaled histamine in asymptomatic smokers and nonsmokers. *J. Appl. Physiol., 42*:508-513.

Brown, R., Ingram, R. H., Jr., and McFadden, E. R., Jr. (1978). Effects of prostaglandin $F_{2\alpha}$ on lung mechanics in non-asthmatic and asthmatic subjects. *J. Appl. Physiol., 44*:150-155.

Bruce, C. A., Rosenthal, R. R., Lichtenstein, L. M., and Norman, P. S. (1974). Diagnostic tests in ragweed-allergic asthma. *J. Allergy Clin. Immunol., 53*: 230-239.

Bruce, C. A., Rosenthal, R. R., Lichtenstein, L. M., and Norman, P. S. (1975). Quantitative inhalation bronchial challenge in ragweed hay fever patients: A comparison with ragweed allergic asthmatics. *J. Allergy Clin. Immunol., 56*:331-337.

Bryant, D. H. (1977). Role of IgE in human asthma. In *Asthma: Physiology, Immunopharmacology, and Treatment.* Second International Symposium. Edited by L. M. Lichtenstein and K. F. Austen. New York, New York, Academic Press, Inc., pp. 315-325.

Bryant, D. H., and Burns, M. W. (1976). Bronchial histamine reactivity: Its relationship to the reactivity of the bronchi to allergens. *Clin. Allergy, 6*: 523-532.

Casterline, C. L., Evans, R., and Ward, G. W., Jr. (1976). The effect of atropine and albuterol aerosols on the human bronchial response to histamine. *J. Allergy Clin. Immunol., 58*:607-613.

Chakrin, L. W., Krell, R. D., Mengel, J., Young, D., Zaker, C., and Wardell, J. R., Jr. (1974). Effect of histamine H_2 receptor antagonist on immunologically induced mediator release *in vitro. Agents Actions, 4*:297-303.

Chand, N., Deroth, L., and Eyre, P. (1979). Pharmacology of Schultz-Dale reaction in canine lung strip *in vitro*: Possible model for allergic asthma. *Br. J. Pharmacol., 66*:511-516.

Chand, N., Dhawaan, B. N., Srimal, R. C., Rahmani, N. H., Shukla, R. K., and Altura, B. M. (1980). Reactivity of trachea, bronchi, and lung strips to histamine and carbachol in rhesus monkeys. *J. Appl. Physiol., 49*:729-734.

Chiesa, A., Dain, D., Meyers, G. L., Kessler, G. F., and Gold, W. M. (1975). Histamine release during antigen inhalation in experimental asthma in dogs. *Am. Rev. Respir. Dis., 111*:148-156.

Clark, P. O., Hanahan, D. J., and Pinckard, R. N. (1980). Physical and chemical properties of platelet activating factor obtained from human neutrophils and monocytes and rabbit neutrophils and basophils. *Biochem. Biophys. Acta., 628*:69-75.

Cockcroft, D. W., Killian, D. N., Mellon, J. J. A., and Hargreave, F. E. (1977a). Bronchial reactivity to inhaled histamine: A method and clinical survey. *Clin. Allergy, 7*:235-243.

Cockcroft, D. W., Ruffin, R. E., Dolovich, J., and Hargreave, F. E. (1977b). Allergen-induced increase in non-allergic bronchial reactivity. *Clin. Allergy, 7*:503-513.

Cockcroft, D. W., Ruffin, R. E., Frith, P. A., Cartier, A., Juniper, E. F., Dolovich, J., and Hargreave, F. E. (1979). Determinants of allergen-induced asthma: Dose of allergen, circulating IgE antibody concentration, and bronchial responsiveness to inhaled histamine. *Am. Rev. Respir. Dis., 120*:1053-1058.

Colebatch, H. J. H. (1970). The humoral regulation of alveolar ducts. In *Airway Dynamics: Physiology and Pharmacology.* Edited by A. Bouhuys. Springfield, Illinois, Thomas, pp. 169-189.

Colebatch, H. J. H., Olsen, C. R., and Nadel, J. A. (1966). Effects of histamine, serotonin, and acetylcholine on the peripheral airways. *J. Appl. Physiol., 21*:217-226.

Collier, H. O. J., and James, G. W. L. (1967). Humoral factors affecting pulmonary inflation during acute anaphylaxis in the guinea pig *in vivo. Br. J. Pharmacol., 30*:283-301.

Comroe, J. H., Jr., VanLingen, B., Stroud, R. C., and Roncoroni, A. (1953). Reflex and direct cardiopulmonary effects of 5-OH-Tryptamine (serotonin). *Am. J. Physiol., 173*:379-386.

Conroy, M. C., Orange, R. P., and Lichtenstein, L. M. (1976). Release of slow reacting substance of anaphylaxis (SRS-A) from human leukocytes by the calcium ionophore A23187. *J. Immunol., 116*:1677-1681.

Curry, J. J. (1946). The action of histamine on the respiratory tract in normal and asthmatic subjects. *J. Clin. Invest., 25*:785-791.

Curry, J. J. (1947). Comparative action of acetyl-beta-methyl choline and histamine on the respiratory tract in normals, patients with hay fever and subjects with bronchial asthma. *J. Clin. Invest., 26*:430-438.

Cuthbert, M. F. (1971). Bronchodilatory activity of aerosols of prostaglandins E_1 and E_2 in asthmatic subjects. *Proc. R. Soc. Med., 64*:15-16.

Dahlen, S. E., Hedqvist, P., Hammarstrom, S., and Samuelsson, B. (1980). Leukotrienes are potent constrictors of human bronchi. *Nature, 288*:484-486.

Dale, H. H., and Laidlaw, P. P. (1910). The physiological action of β-imidazolylethylamine. *J. Physiol., 41*:318-344.

Dale, H. H., and Laidlaw, P. P. (1911). Further observations on the action of β-imidazolylethylamine. *J. Physiol., 43*:182-195.

Dawson, W., Boot, J. R., Cockerill, A. F., Mallen, D. N. B., and Osborne, D. J. (1976). Release of novel prostaglandins and thromboxanes after immunological challenge of guinea pig lung. *Nature, 262*:699-702.

Day, H. J., Stormorken, H., and Holmsen, H. (1973). Subcellular localization of platelet factor 3 and platelet factor 4. *Scand. J. Haematol., 10*:254-260.

Deal, E. C., Jr., Wasserman, S. I., Soter, N. A., Ingram, R. H., Jr., and McFadden, E. R. Jr. (1980). Evaluation of the role played by mediators of immediate hypersensitivity in exercise-induced asthma. *J. Clin. Invest., 65*:659-665.

DeKock, M. A., Nadel, J. A., Zwi, S., Colebatch, H. J. H., and Olsen, C. R. (1966). New method for perfusing bronchial arteries: Histamine bronchoconstriction and apnea. *J. Appl. Physiol., 21*:185-194.

Demopoulos, C. A., Pinckard, R. N., and Hanahan, D. J. (1979). Platelet activating factor: Evidence for 1-0-alkyl-2-acetyl-sn-glyceryl-3-phosphorylcholine as the active component (a new class of lipid chemical mediators). *J. Biol. Chem., 254*:9355-9358.

Dennis, M. W., and Douglas, J. S. (1970). Control of bronchomotor tone in spontaneously breathing, unanesthetized guinea pigs. In *Airway Dynamics: Physiology and Pharmacology*. Edited by A. Bouhuys. Springfield, Illinois, Charles C. Thomas, pp. 253-262.

deShazo, R. D., Levinson, A. I., Dvorak, H. F., and Davis, R. W. (1979). The late phase skin reaction: Evidence for activation of the coagulation system in an IgE-dependent reaction in man. *J. Immunol., 122*:692-698.

Dixon, M., Jackson, D. M., and Richards, I. M. (1979a). The effects of H_1 and H_2 receptor antagonists and antagonists on total lung resistance, dynamic lung compliance and instant receptor discharge in the anesthetized dog. *Br. J. Pharmacol., 66*:203-209.

Dixon, M., Jackson, D. M., and Richards, I. M. (1979b). The effect of a respiratory tract infection on histamine-induced changes in lung mechanics and irritant receptor discharge in dogs. *Am. Rev. Respir. Dis., 120*:843-848.

Dixon, M., Jackson, D. M., and Richards, I. M. (1980). The action of sodium cromoglycate on "C" fiber endings in the dog lung. *Br. J. Pharmacol., 70*:11-13.

Dolovich, J., Hargreave, F. E., Chalmers, R., Shier, K. J., Gauldie, J., and Bienenstock, J. (1973). Late cutaneous allergic responses in isolated IgE-dependent reactions. *J. Allergy Clin. Immunol., 52*:38-46.

Douglas, J. S., Dennis, M. W., Ridgway, P., and Bouhuys, A. (1973). Airway constriction in guinea pigs: Interaction of histamine and autonomic drugs. *J. Pharmacol. Exp. Ther., 184*:169-179.

Douglas, W. W. (1980). Histamine and 5-hydroxytryptamine (serotonin) and their antagonists. In *The Pharmacologic Basis of Therapeutics.* Edited by A. G. Gilman, L. S. Goodman and A. Gilman. New York, MacMillan Publishing Co., pp. 609-696.

Drazen, J. M. (1978). Adrenergic influences on histamine-mediated bronchoconstriction in the guine pig. *J. Appl. Physiol., 44*:340-345.

Drazen, J. M., and Austen, K. F. (1974). Effects of intravenous administration of slow-reacting substance of anaphylaxis, histamine, bradykinin, and prostaglandin $F_{2\alpha}$ on pulmonary mechanics in the guinea pig. *J. Clin. Invest., 53*:1679-1685.

Drazen, J. M., and Austen, K. F. (1975). Atropine modification of the pulmonary effects of chemical mediators in the guinea pig. *J. Appl. Physiol., 38*: 834-838.

Drazen, J. M., and Schneider, M. W. (1978). Comparative responses of tracheal spirals and parenchymal strips to histamine and carbachol *in vitro. J. Clin. Invest., 61*:1441-1447.

Drazen, J. M., Venugopalan, C. S., and Soter, N. A. (1978). H_2 receptor mediated inhibition of immediate type hypersensitivity reactions *in vivo. Am. Rev. Respir. Dis., 117*:479-484.

Drazen, J. M., Loring, S. H., Jackson, A. C., Snapper, J. R., and Ingram, R. H., Jr. (1979b). Effects of volume history on airway changes induced by histamine or vagal stimulation. *J. Appl. Physiol., 47*:657-665.

Drazen, J. M., Lewis, R. A., Wasserman, S. I., Orange, R. P., and Austen, K. F. (1979a). Differential effects of a partially purified preparation of slow-reacting substance of anaphylaxis on guinea pig tracheal spirals and parenchymal strips. *J. Clin. Invest., 63*:1-5.

Drazen, J. M., Austen, K. F., Lewis, R. A., Clark, D. A., Goto, G., Marfat, A., and Corey, E. J. (1980). Comparative airway and vascular activities of leukotrienes C-1 and D *in vivo* and *in vitro. Proc. Natl. Acad. Sci., 77*:4354-4358.

Drummond, A. H. (1976). Interactions of blood platelets with biogenic amines: Uptake, stimulation and receptor binding. In *Platelets in Biology and Pathology.* Edited by J. L. Gordon. New York, North-Holland Publishing Co., pp. 203-239.

Dulabh, R., and Vickers, M. R. (1978). The effects of H_2 receptor antagonists on anaphylaxis in the guinea pig. *Agents Actions, 8*:559-565.

Dunlop, L. S., and Smith, A. P. (1975). Reduction of antigen-induced contraction of sensitized human bronchus *in vitro* by indomethacin. *Br. J. Pharmacol., 54*:495-497.

Dunlop, L. S., and Smith, A. P. (1977). The effect of histamine antagonists on antigen-induced contractions of sensitized human bronchus *in vitro. Br. J. Pharmacol., 59*:475P (Abstract).

Eggleston, P. A., Bierman, W., and Pierson, W. (1972). A double-blind trial of the effect of cromolyn sodium on exercise-induced bronchospasm. *J. Allergy Clin. Immunol., 50*:57-62.

Eiser, N. M., McRae, K. D., Snashall, P. D., and Guz, A. (1979). Histamine receptors in normal and allergic studies. In *The Mast Cell.* Edited by J. Pepys and A. M. Edwards. Kent, England, Pitman Medical Publishing Co., Ltd., pp. 262-264.

Emmanuel, G. E., Rosenbluth, A., Ansari, I., Villano, R., and Carducci, R. (1968). Evidence of active alveolar closure in the human lung. In *Current Research in Chronic Respiratory Disease. Proceedings of the Eleventh Aspen Emphysema Conference.* Edited by R. S. Mitchell. Arlington, Virginia, pp. 287-296.

Empey, D. W., Laitinen, L. A., Gold, W. M., and Nadel, J. A. (1976). Mechanisms of bronchial hyper-reactivity in normal subjects after upper respiratory tract infection. *Am. Rev. Respir. Dis., 113*:131-139.

Engineer, D. M., Jose, P. J., Piper, P. J., and Tippins, J. R. (1978a). Modulation of slow-reacting substance of anaphylaxis and histamine release by prostacyclin and thromboxanes. *J. Physiol., 281*:42P.

Engineer, D. M., Morris, H. R., Piper, P. J., and Sirois, P. (1978b). The release of prostaglandins and thromboxanes from guinea pig lung by slow-reacting substance of anaphylaxis, and its inhibition. *Br. J. Pharmacol., 64*:211-218.

Engineer, D. M., Niederhauser, U., Piper, P. J., and Sirois, P. (1978c). Release of mediators of anaphylaxis: Inhibition of prostaglandin synthesis and the modification of release of slow-reacting substance of anaphylaxis and histamine. *Br. J. Pharmacol., 62*:61-66.

Eyre, P. (1969). The pharmacology of sheep tracheobronchial muscle: A relaxant effect of histamine on the isolated bronchi. *Br. J. Pharmacol., 36*: 409-417.

Eyre, P. (1973). Histamine H_2 receptors in the sheep bronchus and cat trachea: The action of burimamide. *Br. J. Pharmacol., 48*:321-323.

Eyre, P. (1977). Pulmonary histamine H_1 and H_2 receptor studies. In *Asthma II: Physiology, Immunopharmacology, and Treatment.* Edited by K. F. Austen and L. Lichtenstein. New York, Academic Press, Inc., pp. 169-177.

Feldberg, W., and Lewis, G. P. (1964). Release of adrenalin by bradykinin and angiotensin. *J. Physiol., 171*:98-108.

Fish, J. E., and Kelly, J. F. (1979). Measurements of responsiveness in bronchoprovocation testing. *J. Allergy Clin. Immunol., 64*:592-596.

Fish, J. E., Peterman, V. I., and Cugell, D. W. (1977). Effect of deep inspiration on airway conductance in subjects with allergic rhinitis and allergic asthma. *J. Allergy Clin. Immunol., 60*:41-46.

Fish, J. E., Ankin, M. G., Adkinson, N. F., Jr., and Peterman, V. I. (1981a). Indomethacin modification of immediate-type immunologic airway responses in allergic asthmatic and non-asthmatic subjects. *Am. Rev. Respir. Dis., 123*:609-614.

Fish, J. E., Ankin, M. G., Kelly, J. F., and Peterman, V. I. (1980). Comparison of responses to pollen extract in subjects with allergic asthma and non-asthmatic subjects with allergic rhinitis. *J. Allergy Clin. Immunol., 65*:154-161.

Fish, J. E., Ankin, M. G., Kelly, J. F., and Peterman, V. I. (1981b). Regulation of bronchomotor tone by lung inflation in asthmatic and non-asthmatic subjects. *J. Appl. Physiol., 50*:1079-1086.

Fish, J. E., Rosenthal, R. R., Summer, W. R., Menkes, H., Norman, P. S., and Permutt, S. (1977). The effect of atropine on acute antigen-mediated airway constriction in subjects with allergic asthma. *Am. Rev. Respir. Dis., 115*:371-379.

Fish, J. E., Rosenthal, R., Menkes, H., Summer, W., Batra, G., Permutt, S., and Norman, P. (1976). Airway responses to methacholine in allergic and nonallergic subjects. *Am. Rev. Respir. Dis., 113*:579-586.

Fleisch, J. H., and Calkins, P. J. (1976). Comparison of drug-induced responses of rabbit trachea and bronchus. *J. Appl. Physiol., 41*:62-66.

Gardiner, P. J. (1975). The effects of some natural prostaglandins on isolated human circular bronchial muscle. *Prostaglandins, 10*:607-616.

Gardiner, P. J., and Collier, H. O. J. (1980). Specific receptors for prostaglandins in airway. *Prostaglandins, 19*:819-841.

Girard, J. P., and Moret, P. (1963). Action de la serotonine et de la bradykinine en aerosols chez les asthmatiques. *Helv. Med. Acta., 30*:520-526.

Gleich, G. J., and Hall, M. (1980). Measurement of histamine: A quality control study. *J. Allergy Clin. Immunol., 66*:295-298.

Goetzl, E. J., and Pickett, W. C. (1982). The human PMN leukocyte chemotactic activity of complex hydroxy-eicosatetraenoic acids (HETEs). *J. Immunol.*, (In Press).

Goetzl., E. J., Woods, J. M., and Gorman, R. R. (1977). Stimulation of human eosinophil and neutrophil polymorphonuclear leukocyte chemotaxis and random migration of 12-L-hydroxy-5, 8, 10, 14-eicosatetraenoic acid (HETE). *J. Clin. Invest., 59*:179-183.

Gold, W. M. (1977). Neurohumoral interactions in airways. *Am. Rev. Respir. Dis., 115*:127-137.

Gold, W. M., Kaufman, H. S., and Nadel, J. A. (1967). Elastic recoil of the lungs in chronic asthmatic patients before and after therapy. *J. Appl. Physiol., 23*:433-438.

Gold, W. M., Kessler, G. F., and Yu, D. Y. C. (1972). Role of vagus nerves in experimental asthma in allergic dogs. *J. Appl. Physiol., 33*:719-725.

Golden, J. A., Nadel, J. A., and Boushey, H. A. (1978). Bronchial hyperirritability in healthy subjects after exposure to ozone. *Am. Rev. Respir. Dis., 118*:287-294.

Grant, J. A., and Lichtenstein, L. M. (1974). Release of slow-reacting substance of anaphylaxis from human leukocytes. *J. Immunol., 112*:897-904.

Green, K., Hedqvist, P., and Svanborg, N. (1974). Increased plasma levels of 15-keto-13, 14-dihydro-prostaglandin $F_{2\alpha}$ after allergen-provoked asthma in man. *Lancet, ii*:1419-1421.

Greenberger, P., Harris, K., and Patterson, R. (1979). The effect of histamine-1 and histamine-2 antagonists on airway responses to histamine in the rhesus monkey. *J. Allergy Clin. Immunol., 64*:189-196.

Gryglewski, R. J., Korbut, R., and Ocetkiewicz, A. (1978). Generation of prostacyclin by lungs *in vivo* and its release into the arterial circulation. *Nature, 273*:765-767.

Habib, M. P., Paré, P. D., and Engel, L. A. (1979). Variability of airway responses to inhaled histamine in normal subjects. *J. Appl. Physiol., 47*: 51-58.

Hahn, H. L., Wilson, A. G., Graf, P. D., Fischer, S. P., and Nadel, J. A. (1978). Interaction between serotonin and efferent vagus nerves in dog lungs. *J. Appl. Physiol., 44*:144-149.

Hamberg, M., Hedqvist, P., Strandberg, K., Svensson, J., and Samuelsson, B. (1975). Prostaglandin endoperoxides. IV. Effects on smooth muscle. *Life Sciences, 16*:451-462.

Hammarstrom, S., Murphy, R. C., Samuelsson, B., Clark, D. A., Mioskowski, C., and Corey, E. J. (1979). Structure of leukotriene C: Identification of the amino acid part. *Biochem. Biophys. Res. Commun., 91*:1266-1272.

Handin, R. I., and Cohen, H. J. (1976). Purification and binding properties of human platelet factor 4. *J. Biol. Chem., 251*:4273-4279.

Harries, M. G., Parkes, P. E. G., Lessof, M. H., and Orr, T. S. C. (1981). Role of bronchial irritant receptors in asthma. *Lancet, i*:5-7.

Hedqvist, P., Strandberg, K., and Hamberg, M. (1978). Bronchial and cardiovascular actions of prostaglandin endoperoxides and an endoperoxide analogue. *Acta. Physiol. Scand., 103*:299-307.

Herxheimer, H. (1949). Antihistamines in bronchial asthma. *Br. Med. J., 4*: 901-905.

Herxheimer, H. (1951). Bronchial obstruction induced by allergens, histamine and acetyl-β-methylcholine chloride. *Int. Arch. Allergy, 2*:27-39.

Herxheimer, H. (1953). Further observations on the influence of 5-hydroxytryptamine on bronchial functions. *J. Physiol., 122*:49-53.

Herxheimer, H. (1955). The 5-hydroxytryptamine shock in the guinea pig. *J. Physiol., 128*:435-445.

Herxheimer, H. (1956). Bronchoconstrictor agents and their antagonists in the intact guinea pig. *Arch. Int. Pharmacodyn. Ther., 106*:371-380.

Herxheimer, H. (1966). Antihistamines–Serotonin. *Ann. Allergy, 24*:382-384.

Herxheimer, H., and Stresemann, E. (1963). The effect of slow-reacting substance (SRS-A) in guinea pigs and in asthmatic patients. *J. Physiol., 165*: 78-79P.

Hogg, J. C., and Hulbert, W. (1980). Anatomic aspects of bronchial mucosal permeability. In *Airway Reactivity, Mechanisms and Clinical Relevance.* Edited by F. E. Hargrave. Canada, Astra Pharmaceuticals Canada Ltd., pp. 35-39.

Holroyde, M. C., and Eyre, P. (1978). Histamine enhances anaphylactic histamine release from bovine lung and leukocytes via histamine H_2 receptor. *J. Pharmacol. Exp. Ther., 204*:183-186.

Holtzman, M. J., Cunningham, J. H., Sheller, J. R., Irsigler, G. B., Nadel, J. A., and Boushey, H. A. (1979). Effect of ozone on bronchial reactivity in atopic and nonatopic subjects. *Am. Rev. Respir. Dis., 120*:1059-1067.

Holtzman, M. J., Sheller, J. R., Dimeo, M., Nadel, J. A., and Boushey, H. A. (1980). Effect of ganglionic blockade on bronchial reactivity in atopic subjects. *Am. Rev. Respir. Dis., 122*:17-25.

Hutchcroft, B. J. (1977). In *Asthma: Physiology, Immunopharmacology, and Treatment.* Edited by L. M. Lichtenstein and K. F. Austen. New York, Academic Press, pp. 14-15.

Hyman, A. L., Spannhake, E. W., and Kadowitz, P. J. (1978). Prostaglandins and the lung. *Am. Rev. Respir. Dis., 117*:111-136.

Iorio, L. C., and Constantine, J. W. (1969). Bradykinin on isolated guinea pig tracheal muscle. *J. Pharmacol. Exp. Ther., 160*:264-270.

Ishizaka, T., Ishizaka, K., Orange, R. P., and Austen, K. F. (1971). Pharmacologic inhibition of the antigen-induced release of histamine and slow-reacting substance of anaphylaxis (SRS-A) from monkey lung tissues mediated by human IgE. *J. Immunol., 106*:1267-1273.

Islam, M. S., Melville, G. N., and Ulmer, W. T. (1974). Role of atropine in antagonizing the effect of 5-hydroxytryptamine (5-HT) on bronchial and pulmonary vascular systems. *Respiration, 31*:47-59.

Islam, M. S., Vastag, E., and Ulmer, W. T. (1972). Sulphur dioxide induced bronchial hyper-reactivity against acetylcholine. *Int. Arch. Arbeitsmed., 29*:221-232.

Itkin, I. H., and Anand, S. C. (1970). The role of atropine as a mediator blocker of induced bronchial obstruction. *J. Allergy, 45*:178-186.

Jackson, D. M., and Richards, I. M. (1977). The effects of pentobarbitone and chloralose anesthesia on the vagal component of bronchoconstriction produced by histamine aerosol in the anesthetized dog. *Br. J. Pharmacol., 61*:251-256.

Jakschik, B. A., Kulczycki, A., Jr., MacDonald, H. H., and Parker, C. W. (1977). Release of slow-reacting substance (SRS) from rat basophilic leukemia (RBL-1) cells. *J. Immunol., 119*:618-622.

James, C. W. L. (1969). The use of the *in vivo* trachea preparation of the guinea pig to assess drug action on lung. *J. Pharm. Pharmacol., 21*:379-386.

Jankala, E. O., and Virtama, P. (1961). On the bronchoconstrictor effect of serotonin. Bronchographic studies on rabbits and guinea pigs. *J. Physiol., 159*:381-383.

Kahlson, G., and Rosengren, E. (1968). New approaches to the physiology of histamine. *Physiol. Rev., 48*:155-196.

Kaliner, M. (1976). The cholinergic nervous system and immediate hypersensitivity. I. Eccrine sweat responses in allergic patients. *J. Allergy Clin. Immunol., 58*:308-311.

Kaliner, M. (1978). Human lung tissue and anaphylaxis: The effects of histamine on the immunologic release of mediators. *Am. Rev. Respir. Dis., 118*: 1015-1022.

Kaliner, M., Wasserman, S. I., and Austen, K. F. (1973). Immunologic release of chemical mediators from human nasal polyps. *N. Engl. J. Med., 289*:277-281.

Katcher, M. L., and Reed, C. E. (1980). Prevention of antigen-induced bronchoconstriction by lodoxamide ethyl, a new orally active antiallergic drug. *J. Allergy Clin. Immunol., 66*:223-226.

Kawakami, Y., Uchiyama, K., Irie, T., and Murao, M. (1973). Evaluation of aerosols of prostaglandins E_1 and E_2 as bronchodilators. *Eur. J. Clin. Pharmacol., 6*:127-131.

Kellaway, C. H., and Trethewie, E. R. (1940). The liberation of a slow-reacting smooth muscle stimulating substance in anaphylaxis. *Q. J. Exp. Physiol., 30*:121-127.

Killian, D., Cockcroft, D. W., Hargreave, F. E., and Dolovich, J. (1976). Factors in allergen-induced asthma: Relevance of the intensity of the airways allergic reaction and non-specific bronchial reactivity. *Clin. Allergy, 6*:219-225.

Knauer, K. A., Lichtenstein, L. M., Adkinson, N. F., Jr., and Fish, J. E. (1981). Platelet activation during antigen-induced airway reactions in asthmatic subjects. *N. Engl. J. Med., 304*:1404-1407.

Konzett, H. (1956). The effects of 5-hydroxytryptamine and its antagonists on tidal air. *Br. J. Pharmacol., 11*:289-291.

Krell, R. D., and Chakrin, D. W. (1976). Canine airway responses to acetylcholine, prostaglandin $F_{2\alpha}$, histamine, and serotonin after chronic antigen exposure. *J. Allergy Clin. Immunol., 58*:664-675.

Krell, R. D., and Chakrin, L. W. (1976). Canine airway responses to acetylcho- and *in vivo* canine models of Type I hypersensitivity reactions. *Eur. J. Pharmacol., 44*:35-44.

Krell, R. D., Chakrin, L. W., and Wardell, J. R., Jr. (1976). The effect of cholinergic agents on a canine model of allergic asthma. *J. Allergy Clin. Immunol., 58*:19-30.

Laitinen, L. A., Empey, D. W., Poppius, H., Lemen, R. J., Gold, W. M., and Nadel, J. A. (1976). Effects of intravenous histamine on static lung compliance and airway resistance in normal man. *Am. Rev. Respir. Dis., 114*: 291-295.

Lambley, J. E., and Smith, A. P. (1975). The effects of arachidonic acid, indomethacin and SCI9220 on guinea pig tracheal muscle tone. *Eur. J. Pharmacol., 30*:148-153.

Larsell, O. (1922). The ganglia, plexuses and nerve-terminations of the mammalian lung and pleura pulmonalis. *J. Comp. Neurol., 35*:97-101.

Lazarus, S. C., Chesrown, S. E., Reed, B. R., Frey, M. J., and Gold, W. M. (1977). Experimental canine anaphylaxis: Effects of cyclic AMP (cAMP), cyclic GMP (cGMP), histamine, and function in the periphery of the lung. *Am. Rev. Respir. Dis., 115*:62 (Abstract).

Levine, S. P., and Wolh, H. (1976). Human platelet factor 4: Purification and characterization by affinity chromatography. *J. Biol. Chem., 251*:324-329.

Lewis, R. A., Soter, N. A., Corey, E. J., and Austen, K. F. (1981). Local effects of synthetic leukotrienes (LTs) on monkey (M) and human (H) skin. *Clin. Res., 29*:492A (Abstract).

Lewis, R. A., Wasserman, S. I., Goetzl, E. J., and Austen, K. F. (1974). Formation of slow reacting substance of anaphylaxis in human lung tissue and cells before release. *J. Exp. Med., 140*:1133-1146.

Lewis, R. A., Goetzl, E. J., Wasserman, S., Valone, F. H., Rubin, R. H., and Austen, K. F. (1975). The release of four mediators of immediate hypersensitivity from human leukemia basophils. *J. Immunol., 114*:87-95.

Lewis, R. A., Roberts, L. J., Holgate, S. T., Oates, J. A., and Austen, K. F. (1980b). Prostaglandin D_2 production by rat and human mast cells activated by reversed anaphylaxis. *Fed. Proc., 39*:305 (Abstract).

Lewis, R. A., Austen, K. F., Drazen, J. M., Clark, D. A., Marfat, A., and Corey, E. J. (1980a). Slow reacting substances of anaphylaxis: Identification of leukotrienes C-1 and D from human and rat sources. *Proc. Natl. Acad. Sci. USA 77*:3710-3714.

Lichtenstein, L. M., and Gillespie, E. (1973). Inhibition of histamine release by histamine is controlled by an H_2 receptor. *Nature 244*:287-288.

Lichtenstein, L. M., and Gillespie, E. (1975). The effects of the H_1 and H_2 antihistamines on "allergic" histamine release and its inhibition by histamine. *J. Pharmacol. Exp. Ther., 192*:441-450.

Lichtenstein, L. M., and Henney, C. S. (1972). Prostaglandin inhibition of immediate and delayed hypersensitivity in vitro. In *Prostaglandins in Cellular Biology.* Edited by P. W. Ramwell and B. B. Phariss. New York, Plenum Publishing Corp. pp. 293-308.

Lichtenstein, L. M., and Margolis, S. (1968). Histamine release *in vitro*: Inhibition by catecholamines and methylxanthines. *Science, 161*:902-903.

Little, J. W., Hall, W. J., Douglas, R. G., Jr., Mudholkar, G. S., Speers, D. M., and Patel, K. (1978). Airway hyperreactivity and peripheral airway dysfunction in influenza A injection. *Am. Rev. Respir. Dis., 118*:295-303.

Lonky, S. A., and Wohl, H. (1981). Stimulation of human leukocyte elastase by platelet factor 4. *J. Clin. Invest., 67*:817-826.

Loring, S. H., Drazen, J. M., Snapper, J. R., and Ingram, R. H., Jr. (1978). Vagal and aerosol histamine interactions on airway responses in dogs. *J. Appl. Physiol., 45*:40-44.

McCulloch, M. W., Proctor, C., and Rand, M. J. (1967). Evidence for an adrenergic homeostatic bronchidilator reflex mechanism. *Eur. J. Pharmacol., 2*: 214-223.

McManus, L. M., Hanahan, D. J., and Pinckard, R. N. (1981). Human platelet stimulation by acetyl glyceryl ether phosphorylcholine. *J. Clin. Invest., 67*:903-909.

McManus, L., Hanahan, D. J., Demopoulos, C., and Pinckard, R. N. (1980). Pathobiology of the intravenous infusion of acetyl glyceryl ether phosphorylcholine (AGEPC), a synthetic platelet-activating factor (PAF), in the rabbit. *J. Immunol., 124*:2919-2926.

McManus, L. M., Morley, C. A., Levine, S. P., and Pinckard, R. N. (1979). Platelet activating factor (PAF) induced release of platelet factor 4 (PF4) *in vitro* and during IgE anaphylaxis in the rabbit. *J. Immunol., 123*:2835-2841.

Maconochie, J. G., Woodings, E. P., and Richards, D. A. (1979). Effects of H_1 and H_2-receptor blocking agents on histamine-induced bronchoconstriction in nonasthmatic subjects. *Br. J. Clin. Pharmacol., 7*:231-236.

Maengwyn-Davies, G. D. (1968). The dual mode of action of histamine in the cat isolated tracheal chain. *J. Pharm. Pharmacol., 20*:572-573.

Main, I. H. M. (1964). The inhibitory actions of prostaglandins on respiratory smooth muscle. *Br. J. Pharmacol., 22*:511-519.

Makino, S. (1966). Clinical significance of bronchial sensitivity to acetylcholine and histamine in bronchial asthma. *J. Allergy, 38*:127-142.

Mansell, A., Dubrawsky, D., Levison, H., Bryan, A. C., Langer, H., Collins-Williams, C., and Orange, R. P. (1974). Lung mechanics in antigen-induced asthma. *J. Appl. Physiol., 37*:297-301.

Marcelle, R., Bottin, R., Juchmes, J., and Petit, J. M. (1968). Evaluation de l' activite bronchomotrice de la 5-hydroxytryptamine (5-HT) chez les sujets normaux et asthmatiques. *Acta. Allerg.* (Kobenhavn), *23*:1-12.

Marone, G., Hammarstrom, S., and Lichtenstein, L. M. (1980). An inhibitor of lipoxygenase inhibits histamine release from human basophils. *Clin. Immunol. and Immunopathol., 17*:117-122.

Marone, G., Kagey-Sobotka, A., and Lichtenstein, L. M. (1979). Effects of arachidonic acid and its metabolites on antigen-induced histamine release from human basophils *in vitro*. *J. Immunol.*, *123*:1669-1677.

Martin, G. L., Atkins, P. C., Dunsky, E. H., and Zweiman, B. (1980a). Effects of theophylline, terbutaline, and prednisone on antigen-induced bronchospasm and mediator release. *J. Allergy Clin. Immunol.*, *66*:204-212.

Martin, J., Powell, E., Shore, S., Emrich, J., and Engel, L. A. (1980b). The role of respiratory muscles in the hyperinflation of bronchial asthma. *Am. Rev. Respir. Dis.*, *121*:441-445.

Mathé, A. A., and Hedqvist, P. (1975). Effect of prostaglandins $F_{2\alpha}$ and E_2 on airway conductance in healthy subjects and asthmatic patients. *Am. Rev. Respir. Dis.*, *111*:313-320.

Mathé, A. A., Strandberg, K., and Astrom, A. (1971). Blockade by polypholoretin phosphate of the prostaglandin $F_{2\alpha}$ action on isolated human bronchi. *Nat. New Biol.*, *230*:215-216.

Mathé, A. A., Strandberg, K., and Yen, S-S. (1977). Prostaglandin release by slow reacting substance from guinea pig and human lung tissue. *Prostaglandins 14*:1105-1115.

Mathé, A. A., Volicer, L., and Puri, S. K. (1974). Effect of anaphylaxis and histamine, pyrilamine and burimamide on levels of cyclic AMP and cyclic GMP in guinea pig lung. *Res. Commun. Chem. Pathol. and Pharmacol.*, *8*: 635-651.

Mathé, A. A., Hedqvist, P., Holmgren, A., and Svanborg, N. (1973). Bronchial hyper-reactivity to prostaglandin $F_{2\alpha}$ and histamine in patients with asthma. *Br. Med. J.*, *1*:193-196.

Mead, J., Turner, J. M., Macklem, P. T., and Little, J. B. (1967). Significance of the relationship between lung recoil and maximum expiratory flow. *J. Appl. Physiol.*, *22*:95-108.

Michelson, A. L., Hollander, W., and Lowell, F. C. (1958). The effect of 5-hydroxytryptamine (serotonin) on the respiration of non-asthmatic and asthmatic subjects. *J. Lab. Clin. Med.*, *51*:57-62.

Michoud, M. C., Fraser, R. S., Paré, P. D., and Hogg, J. C. (1976). Effect of indomethacin and atropine in experimental asthma in conscious guinea pigs. *J. Appl. Physiol.*, *40*:889-894.

Michoud, M. C., Paré, P. D., Boucher, R., and Hogg, J. C. (1978). Airwar responses to histamine and methacholine in *Ascaris suum*-allergic rhesus monkeys. *J. Appl. Physiol.*, *45*:846-851.

Michoud, M. C., Paré, P. D., Orange, R. P., and Hogg, J. C. (1979). Airway sensitivity to slow-reacting substance of anaphylaxis, histamine, and antigen in *Ascaris* sensitive monkeys. *Am. Rev. Respir. Dis.*, *119*:419-424.

Miller, M. M., Fish, J. E., and Patterson, R. (1977). Methacholine and physostigmine airway reactivity in asthmatic and non-asthmatic subjects. *J. Allergy Clin. Immunol., 60*:116-120.

Mills, J. E., and Widdicombe, J. G. (1970). Role of the vagus nerves in anaphylaxis and histamine-induced bronchoconstrictions in guinea pigs. *Br. J. Pharmacol., 39*:724-731.

Mills, J. E., Sellick, H., and Widdicombe, J. G. (1969). Activity of lung irritant receptors in pulmonary microembolism, anaphylaxis and drug-induced bronchoconstrictions. *J. Physiol. 203*:337-357.

Moll, H. H. (1940). The action of parasympathetic-mimetic drugs in asthma. *Q. J. Med., 35*:229-240.

Moncada, S., Ferreira, S. H., and Vane, J. R. (1972). *Report of the Fifth International Congress on Pharmacology.* New York, Albert J. Phiebig, Inc., pp. 160.

Moncada, S., Korbut, R. Bunting, S., and Vane, J. R. (1978). Prostacyclin is a circulating hormone. *Nature, 273*:767-768.

Moore, S., Pepper, D. S., and Cash, J. D. (1975). Platelet antiheparin activity. The isolation and characterization of platelet factor 4 released from thrombin-aggregated washed human platelets and its dissociation into subunits and the isolation of membrane-bound antiheparin activity. *Biochem. Biophys. 379:*370-380.

Morse, H. C., Block, K. J., and Austen, K. F. (1968). Biologic properties of rat antibodies. *J. Immunol., 101*:658-663.

Mortola, J., Sant'Ambrogio, G., and Clement, M. G. (1975). Localization of irritant receptors in the airways of the dog. *Respir. Physiol., 24*:107-114.

Murphy, R. C., Hammarstrom, S., and Samuelsson, B. (1979). Leukotriene C: A slow reacting substance from murine mastocytoma cells. *Proc. Natl. Acad. Sci. USA, 76*:4275-4279.

Murtagh, P. S., Proctor, D. F., Permutt, S., Kelly, B., and Evering, S. (1971). Bronchial closure with mecholyl in excised dog lobes. *J. Appl. Physiol., 31*:409-415.

Nadel, J. A. (1973). Neurophysiologic aspects of asthma. In *Asthma: Physiology, Immunopharmacology, and Treatment.* Edited by L. M. Lichtenstein and K. F. Austen. New York, Academic Press, pp. 29-37.

Nadel, J. A. (1980). Autonomic regulation of airway smooth muscle. In *Physiology and Pharmacology of the Airways.* Edited by J. A. Nadel. New York, Marcel Dekker, Inc., pp. 217-257.

Nadel, J. A., Cabezas, G. A., and Austin, J. H. M. (1971). *In vivo* roentgenographic examination of parasympathetic innervation of small airways: Use of powdered tantalum and a fine focal spot x-ray tube. *Invest. Radiol., 6*:9-17.

Nakazawa, T., Toyoda, T., Furukawa, M., Taya, T., and Kobayashi, S. (1976). Inhibitory effects of various drugs on dual asthmatic responses in wheat flour-sensitive subjects. *J. Allergy Clin. Immunol., 58*:1-9.

Nathan, R. A., Segall, N., Glover, G. C., and Schocket, A. L. (1979). The effects of H_1 and H_2 antihistamines on histamine inhalation challenges in asthmatic patients. *Am. Rev. Respir. Dis., 120*:1251-1258.

Nemoto, T., Aoki, H., Ike, A., Yamada, K., Kondo, T., Kobayashi, S., and Inagawa, T. (1976). Serum prostaglandin levels in asthmatic patients. *J. Allergy Clin. Immunol., 57*:89-94.

Newball, H. H. (1974). Response of asthmatic airways to intravenous bradykinin and histamine. *Med. Annals of the District of Columbia, 43*:111-114.

Newball, H. H., and Keiser, H. R. (1973). Relative effects of bradykinin and histamine on the respiratory system of man. *J. Appl. Physiol., 35*:552-556.

Newball, H. H., and Lenfant, C. (1977). The influence of atropine and cromolyn on human bronchial hyper-reactivity to aerosolized prostaglandin $F_{2\alpha}$. *Resp. Physiol., 30*:125-136.

Newball, H. H., Keiser, H. R., and Lenfant, C. (1980a). Prostaglandin $F_{2\alpha}$ functions as a local hormone on human airways. *Respir. Physiol., 41*:183-197.

Newball, H. H., Keiser, H. R., and Pisano, J. J. (1975). Bradykinin and human airways. *Respir. Physiol., 24*:139-146.

Newball, H. H., Meier, H. L., and Lichtenstein, L. M. (1980b). Basophil mediators and their release, with emphasis on BK-A. *J. Invest. Derm., 74*:344-348.

Newball, H. H., Talamo, R. C., and Lichtenstein, L. M. (1975). Release of a leukocyte kallikrein mediated by IgE. *Nature, 254*:635-636.

Newball, H. H., Talamo, R. C., and Lichtenstein, L. M. (1979b). Anaphylactic release of a basophil kallikrein-like activity. II. A mediator of immediate hypersensitivity reactions. *J. Clin. Invest., 64*:466-475.

Newball, H. H., Berninger, R. W., Talamo, R. C., and Lichtenstein, L. M. (1979a). Anaphylactic release of a basophil kallikrein-like activity. I. Purification and characterization. *J. Clin. Invest., 64*:457-465.

Newball, H., Berninger, R., Talamo, R., and Lichtenstein, L. (1979d). Basophil kallikrein of anaphylaxis (BK-A). In *Kinins II, Part B.* New York, Plenum Press Publishing Co., pp. 233-247.

Newball, H. H., Keiser, H. R., Webster, M. E., and Pisano, J. J. (1977). The effects of bradykinin on human airways. In *Chemistry and Biology of the Kallikrein-Kinin System in Health and Disease.* Edited by J. Pisano and K. F. Austen. USDHEW, PHS, NIH, pp. 505-511.

Newball, H. H., Revak, S. D., Cochrane, C. G., Griffin, J. H., and Lichtenstein, L. M. (1979c). Activation of human Hageman factor by a leukocytic protease. In *Kinins II, Part B.* New York, Plenum Press Publishing Co., pp. 139-151.

Newball, H. H., Meier, H. L., Kaplan, A. P., Revak, S. D., Cochrane, C. G., and Lichtenstein, L. M. (1981a). Activation of Hageman factor by proteases released during antigen challenge of human lung. In *Transactions of the Association of American Physicians, 94*:126-133.

Newball, H. H., Meier, H. L., Kaplan, A. P., Revak, S. D., Cochrane, C. G., and Lichtenstein, L. M. (1981b). Activation of the Hageman factor-dependent systems during IgE-mediated reactions of the human lung. *Int. Arch. Allergy Appl. Immunol., 66*:165-167.

Newball, H. H., Meier, H. L., Kaplan, A. P., Revak, S. C., Cochrane, C. G., and Lichtenstein, L. M. (1981c). Activation of Hageman factor by a protease released during antigen challenge of human lung. *Clin. Res., 29*:516 (Abstract).

O'Brien, J. R., Finch, W., and Clark, E. (1970). Platelet-bound and soluble platelet factor 4: Effects of aggregating agents, of aggregation and of aspirin. *Proc. Soc. Exp. Biol. Med., 134*:1128-1131.

Ogilvy, C. S., DuBois, A. B., and Douglas, J. S. (1981). Effects of ascorbic acid and indomethacin on the airways of healthy male subjects with and without induced bronchoconstriction. *J. Allergy Clin. Immunol., 67*:363-369.

Okazaki, T., Johnson, T. F., Reisman, R. E., Arbesman, C. E., and Middleton, E., Jr. (1978). Plasma prostaglandin concentrations in allergic bronchial asthma. *Int. Archs. Allergy Appl. Immunol., 57*:279-281.

Olive, J. T., Jr., and Hyatt, R. E. (1972). Maximal expiratory flow and total respiratory resistance during induced bronchoconstriction in asthmatic subjects. *Am. Rev. Respir. Dis., 106*:366-376.

Orange, R. P., and Austen, K. F. (1969). Slow reacting substance of anaphylaxis. In *Advances in Immunology.* Edited by F. J. Dixon and H. G. Kunkel. New York, Academic Press, p. 106.

Orange, R. P., Austen, W. G., and Austen, K. F. (1971). Immunologic release of histamine and slow-reacting substance of anaphylaxis from human lung. I. Modulation by agents influencing cellular levels of cyclic 3′, 5′-adenosine monophosphate. *J. Exp. Med., 134*:136S-148S.

Orehek, J., Douglas, J., and Bouhuys, A. (1975). Contractile responses of the guinea pig trachea *in vitro*: Modification by prostaglandin synthesis-inhibiting drugs. *J. Pharmacol. Exp. Ther., 194*:554-564.

Orehek, J., Gayrard, P., Grimaud, C., and Charpin, J. (1977). Bronchial response to inhaled prostaglandin $F_{2\alpha}$ in patients with common or aspirin-sensitive asthma. *J. Allergy Clin. Immunol., 59*:414-419.

Orehek, J., Massari, J. P., Gayrard, P., Grimaud, C., and Charpin, J. (1976). Effect of short-term, low level nitrogen dioxide exposure on bronchial sensitivity of asthmatic patients. *J. Clin. Invest., 57*:301-307.

Orning, L., Hammarstrom, S., and Samuelsson, B. (1980). Leukotriene D: A slow reacting substance from rat basophilic leukemia cells. *Proc. Natl. Acad. Sci. USA, 77*:2014-2017.

Orr, T. S. C., Elliott, E. V., Altounyan, R. E. C., and Stern, M. A. (1980). Modulation of release of neutrophil chemotactic factor (NCF). *Clin. Allergy 10*: 491-496.

Ouellette, J. J., and Reed, C. E. (1967). The effect of partial beta adrenergic blockade on the bronchial response of hay fever subjects to ragweed aerosol. *J. Allergy 39*:160-166.

Pandit, P. R., Kulkarni, S. D., and Jogleker, A. Y. (1973). Study on the relationship between antihistamine, anticholinergic and central depressant properties of various antihistamines. *Indian J. Med. Sci., 27*:920-929.

Panzani, R. (1962). 5-Hydroxytryptamine (serotonin) in human bronchial asthma. *Ann. Allergy 20*:721-732.

Paré, P. (1980). Bronchial reactivity in animals and its relationship to bronchial permeability. In *Airway Reactivity, Mechanisms and Clinical Relevance.* Edited by F. E. Hargreave. Canada, Astra Pharmaceuticals Canada Ltd., pp. 49-53.

Parker, C. D., Bilbo, R. E., and Reed, C. E. (1965). Methacholine aerosol as test for bronchial asthma. *Arch. Intern. Med., 115*:452-458.

Patel, K. R. (1975). Atropine, sodium cromoglycate, and thymoxamine in $PGF_{2\alpha}$–induced bronchoconstriction in extrinsic asthma. *Br. Med. J., 2*:360-362.

Paterson, N. A. M., Wasserman, S. I., Said, J. W., and Austen, K. F. (1976). Release of chemical mediators from partially purified human lung mast cells. *J. Immunol., 117*:1356-1361.

Patterson, R., and Harris, K. E. (1976). The effect of cholinergic and anticholinergic agents on the primate model of allergic asthma. *J. Lab. Clin. Med., 87*:65-72.

Patterson, R., and Harris, K. E. (1977). Effect of PGE_1 on immediate-type immunologic and pharmacologic respiratory responses of the rhesus monkey. *J. Lab. Clin. Med., 90*:18-24.

Patterson, R., and Harris, K. E. (1978). The qualitative evaluation of airway responses to immunologic and pharmacologic stimuli in rhesus monkeys. *J. Allergy Clin. Immunol., 61*:261-267.

Patterson, R., and Harris, K. E. (1981). Inhibition of immunoglobulin E-mediated, antigen-induced monkey asthma and skin reactions by 5,8,11, 14-eicosatetraenoic acid. *J. Allergy Clin. Immunol., 67*:146-152.

Patterson, R., Harris, K. E., and Greenberger, P. A. (1978a). The effect of arachidonic acid on airway responses of rhesus monkeys. *Life Sci., 22*:389-400.

Patterson, R., Harris, K. E., and Greenberger, P. A. (1980). Effect of prostaglandin D_2 and I_2 on the airways of rhesus monkeys. *J. Allergy Clin. Immunol., 65*:269-273.

Patterson, R., Orange, R., and Harris, K. E. (1978b). A study of the effect of slow-reacting substances of anaphylaxis on the rhesus monkey airway. *J. Allergy Clin. Immunol., 62*:371-377.

Patterson, R., Harris, K. E., Suszko, I. M., and Roberts, M. (1976). Reagin-mediated asthma in rhesus monkeys and relation to bronchial cell histamine release and airway reactivity to carbacholine. *J. Clin. Invest., 57*: 586-593.

Pearson, R. S. B. (1963). Hypersensitivity to aspirin. In *Salicylates: An International Symposium.* Edited by A. S. Dixon, B. K. Martin, M. J. H. Smith, and P. H. N. Wood. Boston, Little, Brown and Company, pp. 170-173.

Peress, L., Sybrecht, G., and Macklem, P. T. (1976). The mechanism of increase in total lung capacity during acute asthma. *Am. J. Med., 61*:165-169.

Permutt, S. (1973a). Physiologic changes in the acute asthmatic attack. In *Asthma: Physiology, Immunopharmacology, and Treatment.* Edited by F. Austen and L. M. Lichtenstein. New York, Academic Press, Inc., pp. 15-27.

Permutt, S. (1973b). Relation between pulmonary arterial pressure and pleural pressure during the acute asthmatic attack. *Chest, 63*:255-285.

Permutt, S., Rosenthal, R. R., Norman, P. S., and Menkes, H. A. (1977). Bronchial challenge in ragweed-sensitive patients. In *Asthma: Physiology, Immunopharmacology, and Treatment.* Edited by L. M. Lichtenstein and K. F. Austen. New York, Academic Press, pp. 265-281.

Persson, C. G. A., and Eckman, M. (1976). Contractile effects of histamine in large and small respiratory airways. *Agents Actions 6*:389-393.

Pinckard, R. N., Farr, R. S., and Hanahan, J. (1979). Physicochemical and functional identity of rabbit platelet-activating factor (PAF) released *in vivo* during IgE anaphylaxis with PAF released *in vitro* from IgE sensitized basophils. *J. Immunol., 123*:1847-1857.

Pinckard, R. N., Tanigawa, C., and Halonen, M. (1975). IgE-induced blood coagulation alterations in the rabbit: Consumption of coagulation factors XII, XI, and IX *in vivo. J. Immunol., 115*:525-532.

Pinckard, R. N., Halonen, M., Palmer, J. D., Butler, C., Shaw, J. O., and Henson, P. M. (1977). Intravascular aggregation and pulmonary sequestration of platelets during IgE-induced systemic anaphylaxis in the rabbit: Abrogation of lethal anaphylactic shock by platelet depletion. *J. Immunol., 119*: 2185-2193.

Piper, P. J., and Vane, J. R. (1969). Release of additional factors in anaphylaxis and its antagonism by anti-inflammatory drugs. *Nature, 233*:29-36.

Piper, P. J., and Walker, J. L. (1973). The release of spasmogenic substances from chopped human lung tissue and its inhibition. *Br. J. Pharmacol., 47*: 291-304.

Piper, P. J., Collier, H. O. J., and Vane, J. R. (1967). Release of catecholamines in the guinea pig by substance involved in anaphylaxis. *Nature, 213*:838-840.

Platshon, L. F., and Kaliner, M. (1978). The effects of the immunologic release of histamine upon human lung cyclic nucleotide levels and prostaglandin generation. *J. Clin. Invest., 62*:1113-1121.

Ploy-Song-Sang, Y., Corbin, R. P., and Engel, L. A. (1978). Effects of intravenous histamine lung mechanics in man after beta-blockade. *J. Appl. Physiol., 44*:690-695.

Poothullil, J., Umenoto, L., Dolovich, J., Hargreave, F. E., and Day, R. P. (1976). Inhibition by prednisone of late cutaneous allergic responses induced by antiserum to human IgE. *J. Allergy Clin. Immunol., 57*:164-167.

Popa, V. T. (1980a). Respiratory allergy to ragweed: Correlation of bronchial responses to allergen with bronchial responses to histamine and circulating immunoglobulin E. *J. Allergy Clin. Immunol., 65*:389-397.

Popa, V. T. (1980b). Effect of an H_1 blocker, chlorpheniramine, on inhalation tests with histamine and allergen in allergic asthma. *Chest, 78*:442-451.

Popa, V., Douglas, J. S., and Bouhuys, A. (1976). Airway responses to histamine, acetylcholine and antigen in sensitized guinea pigs. *J. Lab. Clin. Med., 4*:225-231.

Pride, N. B., Permutt, S., Riley, R. L., and Bromberger-Barnea, B. (1967). Determinants of maximal expiratory flow from the lungs. *J. Appl. Physiol., 23*: 646-662.

Regal, J. F., and Pickering, R. J. (1981). C5a-induced tracheal contraction: Effect of an SRS-A antagonist and inhibitors of arachidonate metabolism. *J. Immunol., 126*:313-316.

Richerson, H. B., Rajtora, D. W., Penick, G. D., Dick, F. R., Yoo, T. J., Kammermeyer, J. K., and Anuras, J. S. (1979). Cutaneous and nasal allergic responses in ragweed hay fever: Lack of clinical and histopathologic correlations with late phase reactions. *J. Allergy Clin. Immunol., 64*:67-77.

Robertson, D. G., Kerigan, A. T., Hargreave, F. E., Chalmers, R., and Dolovich, J. (1974). Late asthmatic responses induced by ragweed pollen allergen. *J. Allergy Clin. Immunol., 54*:244-250.

Rosenthal, R. R. (1978). Effect of beta adrenergic agents on *in vitro* histamine release and bronchial challenge responses. *Chest, 73*:977-979.

Rosenthal, R. R., Norman, P. S., Summer, W. R., and Permutt, S. (1977). Role of parasympathetic system in antigen-induced bronchospasm. *J. Appl. Physiol., 42*:600-606.

Rosenthale, M. E., Dervinis, A., and Kassarich, J. (1971). Bronchodilator activity of the prostaglandins E_1 and E_2. *J. Pharmacol. Exp. Ther., 178*:541-548.

Rosenthale, M. E., Dervinis, A., Begany, A. J., Lapidus, M., and Glickman, M. S. (1970). Bronchodilator activity of PGE_2 when administered by aerosol to three species. *Experimentia, 26*:1119-1127.

Rossoni, G., Omini, C., Vigano, T., Mandelli, V., Folco, G. C., and Berti, F. (1980). Bronchoconstriction by histamine and bradykinin in guinea pigs:

Relationship to thromboxane A_2 generation and the effect of aspirin. *Prostaglandins, 20*:547-557.

Rucinski, B., Niewiarowski, S., James, P., Walz, D. A., and Budzynski, A. Z. (1979). Anti-heparin proteins secreted by human platelets. Purification, characterization, and radioimmunoassay. *Blood, 53*:47-53.

Rudolf, M., Grant, B., Saunders, K. B., Brostoff, J., Salt, P. J., and Walker, D. S. (1975). Aspirin in exercise-induced asthma. *Lancet, i*:450-460.

Ruffin, R. E., Cockcroft, D. W., and Hargreave, F. E. (1978). A comparison of the protective effect of fenoterol and Sch1000 on allergen-induced asthma. *J. Allergy Clin. Immunol., 61*:42-47.

Ryo, U. Y., and Townley, R. G. (1976). Comparison of respiratory and cardiovascular effects of isoproterenol, propranolol, and practolol in asthmatic and normal subjects. *J. Allergy Clin. Immunol., 57*:12-24.

Sampson, S. R., and Vidruk, E. H. (1979). The nature of the receptor mediating stimulant effects of histamine on rapidly adapting vagal afferents in the lungs. *J. Physiol., 287*:509-518.

Schachter, E. N., Kreisnian, H., and Bouhuys, A. (1978). Prostaglandin synthesis inhibition and exercise bronchospasm. *Ann. Int. Med., 89*:287-288.

Schayer, R. W. (1963). Induced synthesis of histamine, microcirculatory regulation and the mechanism of action of the glucocorticoid hormones. *Prog. Allergy* 7:187-212.

Schild, H. O., Hawkins, D. F., Mongar, J. L., and Herxheimer, H. (1951). Reactions of isolated human asthmatic lung and bronchial tissue to a specific antigen. Histamine release and muscular contraction. *Lancet ii*:376-382.

Schiller, I. W., and Lowell, F. C. (1947). The effects of drugs in modifying the response of asthmatic subjects to inhalation of pollen extracts determined by vital capacity measurements. *Ann. Allergy, 5*:564-569.

Schneider, M. W., and Drazen, J. M. (1980). Comparative *in vitro* effects of arachidonic acid metabolites on tracheal spiral and parenchymal strips. *Am. Rev. Respir. Dis., 121*:835-842.

Schulman, E. S., Adams, G. K., III, and Lichtenstein, L. M. (1980). Inhibition of antigen-induced bronchospasm *in vitro* by 5,8,11,14-eicosatetraenoic acid. *Am. Rev. Respir. Dis. 121*:92 (Abstract).

Schulman, E. S., Newball, H. H., Demers, L. M., Fitzpatrick, F. A., and Adkinson. N. F., Jr. (1981). Anaphylactic release of thromboxane A_2, prostaglandin D_2, and prostacyclin from human lung parenchyma. *Am. Rev. Respir. Dis., 124*:402-406.

Schulman, E. S., Adkinson, N. F., Jr., Newball, H. H. (1982). Cyclooxygenase metabolites in human lung anaphylaxis: Airway vs. parenchyma. *J. Appl. Physiol., 53*:589-595.

Sellick, H., and Widdicombe, J. G. (1971). Stimulation of lung irritant receptors by cigarette smoke, carbon dust, and histamine aerosol. *J. Appl. Physiol., 31*:15-19.

Sheard, P., Lee, T. B., and Tattersall, M. L. (1977). Further studies on the SRS-A antagonist FPL 55712. *Monogr. Allergy, 12*:245-249.

Simonsson, B. G., Jacobs, F. M., and Nadel, J. A. (1967). Role of autonomic nervous system and the cough reflex in the increased responsiveness of airways in patients with obstructive airway disease. *J. Clin. Invest., 48*: 1812-1818.

Simonsson, B. G., Skoogh, B. E., Beigh, N. P., Anderson, R., and Svedmyr, N. (1973). *In vivo* and *in vitro* effect of bradykinin on bronchial motor tone in normal subjects and patients with airways obstruction. *Respiration, 30*: 378-388.

Smith, A. P. (1973). The effects of intravenous infusion of graded doses of prostaglandins $F_{2\alpha}$ and E_2 on lung resistance in patients undergoing termination of pregnancy. *Clin. Sci., 44*:17-19.

Smith, A. P., and Cuthbert, M. F. (1972). Antagonistic action of aerosols of prostaglandins $F_{2\alpha}$ and E_2 on bronchial muscle tone in man. *Br. Med. J., 3*:212-213.

Smith, A. P., and Cuthbert, M. F. (1973). Anticholinergic blocking of prostaglandin-induced bronchoconstriction. *Br. Med. J., 1*:294-296.

Smith, A. P., and Dunlop, L. (1975). Prostaglandins and asthma. *Lancet i*:39-44.

Smith, A. P., Cuthbert, M. F., and Dunlop, L. S. (1975). Effects of inhaled prostaglandins E_1, E_2, and $F_{2\alpha}$ on the airway resistance of healthy and asthmatic man. *Clin. Sci. Mole. Med., 48*:421-430.

Smith, L. J., Shelhamer, J. H., and Kaliner, M. (1980a). Cholinergic nervous system and immediate hypersensitivity. *J. Allergy Clin. Immunol., 66*:374-378.

Smith, J. A., Mansfield, L. E., deShazo, R. D., and Nelson, H. S. (1980b). An evaluation of the pharmacologic inhibition of the immediate and late cutaneous reaction to allergen. *J. Allergy Clin. Immunol., 65*:118-121.

Smith, P. L., Kagey-Sobotka, A., Bleecker, E. R., Traystman, R., Kaplan, A. P., Gralnick, H., Valentine, M. D., Permutt, S., and Lichtenstein, L. M. (1980c). Physiologic manifestations of human anaphylaxis. *J. Clin. Invest., 66*:1072-1080.

Snapper, J. R., Braasch, P. S., Ingram, R. H., Jr., Loring, S. H., and Drazen, J. M. (1980a). *In vivo* effect of cimetidine on canine pulmonary responsiveness to aerosol histamine. *J. Allergy Clin. Immunol., 66*:70-74.

Snapper, J. R., Braasch, P. S., Loring, S. H., Ingram, R. H., Jr., and Drazen, J. M. (1980b). Comparison of the responsiveness to histamine and to *Ascaris suum* challenge in dogs. *Am. Rev. Respir. Dis., 122*:775-780.

Snapper, J. R., Drazen, J. M., Loring, S. H., Braasch, P. S., and Ingram, R. H., Jr. (1979). Vagal effects on histamine, carbachol, and prostaglandin $F_{2\alpha}$ responsiveness in the dog. *J. Appl. Physiol., 47*:13-16.

Solley, G. O., Gleich, G. J., Jordon, R. E., and Schroeter, A. L. (1976). The late phase of the immediate wheal and flare skin reaction. Its dependence upon IgE antibodies. *J. Clin. Invest., 58*:408-420.

Somlyo, A. P., and Somlyo, A. V. (1970). Biophysics of smooth muscle excitation and contraction. In *Airway Dynamics: Physiology and Pharmacology.* Edited by A. Bouhuys. Springfield, Illinois, Charles C. Thomas, pp. 209-227.

Soter, N. A., Wasserman, S. I., Austen, K. F., and McFadden, E. R., Jr. (1980). Release of mast cell mediators and alterations in lung function in patients with cholinergic urticaria. *N. Engl. J. Med., 302*:604-608.

Spannhake, E. W., Levin, J. L., Hyman, A. L., and Kadowitz, P. J. (1981). 6-keto-PGE_1 exhibits more potent bronchodilatory activity in the cat than its precursor, PGI_2. *Prostaglandins, 21*:267-275.

Spannhake, E. W., Lemen, R. J., Wegmann, M. J., Hyman, A. L., and Kadowitz, P. J. (1978a). Effects of arachidonic acid and prostaglandins on lung function in the intact dog. *J. Appl. Physiol., 44*:397-405.

Spannhake, E. W., Lemen, R. J., Wegemann, M. J., Hyman, A. L., and Kadowitz, P. J. (1978b). Analysis of airway effects of a PGH_2 analog in the anesthetized dog. *J. Appl. Physiol., 44*:406-415.

Spannhake, E. W., Levin, J. L., Million, B. T., Gruetter, C. A., Hyman, A. L., and Kadowitz, P. J. (1980). Reversal of 5HT-induced bronchoconstriction by PGI_2: Distribution of central and peripheral actions. *J. Appl. Physiol., 49*:521-527.

Starr, S., Jr., Elsom, K. A., and Reisinger, J. A. (1933). Acetyl-β-methylcholine. I. The action on normal persons. *Am. J. Med. Sci., 186*:313-322.

Staszewska-Barczak, J., and Vane, J. R. (1965). The release of catecholamines from the adrenal medulla by histamine. *Br. J. Pharmacol., 25*:728-742.

Steel, L., Platshon, L., and Kaliner, M. (1979). Prostaglandin generation by human and guinea pig lung tissue: Comparison of parenchymal and airway responses. *J. Allergy Clin. Immunol., 64*:287-293.

Strandberg, K., and Uvnas, B. (1971). Purification and properties of the slow reacting substance formed in the cat paw perfused with compound 48/80. *Acta Physiol. Scand., 82*:358-374.

Svensson, J., Strandberg, K., Tuvemo, T., and Hamberg, M. (1977). Thromboxane A_2: Effects on airway and vascular smooth muscle. *Prostaglandins, 14*:425-436.

Sweatman, W. J. F., and Collier, H. O. J. (1968). Effects of prostaglandins on human bronchial muscle. *Nature, 217*:69-76.

Szczeklik, A., Nizankowska, E., and Nizankowski, R. (1977). Bronchial reactivity to prostaglandins $F_{2\alpha}$, E_2, and histamine in different types of asthma. *Respiration, 34*:323-331.

Szczeklik, A., Gryglewski, R. J., Nizankowski, R., Musial, J., Pieton, R., and Mruk, J. (1978a). Circulatory and anti-platelet effects of intravenous prostacyclin in healthy man. *Pharmacol. Res. Commun., 10*:545-556.

Szczeklik, A., Gryglewski, R. J., Nizankowska, E., Nizankowski, R., and Musial, J. (1978b). Pulmonary and anti-platelet effects of intravenous and inhaled prostacyclin in man. *Prostaglandins, 16*:651-660.

Tiffeneau, R. (1958). Cholinergic and histamine hypersensitivity of lung of the asthmatic. *Acta Allergy (Kobenhavn)* Suppl. *5*:187-221.

Townley, R. G., Dennis, M., and Itkin, S. H. (1965). Comparative action of acetyl-beta-methylcholine, histamine, and pollen antigens in subjects with hayfever and patients with bronchial asthma. *J. Allergy, 36*:121-126.

Townley, R. G., McGeady, S., and Bewtra, A. (1976). The effectof beta adrenergic blockade on bronchial sensitivity to acetyl-beta-methacholine in normal and allergic rhinitis subjects. *J. Allergy Clin. Immunol., 57*:358-366.

Trendelenburg, U. (1954). The action of histamine and pilocarpine on the superior cervical ganglion and the adrenal glands of the cat. *Br. J. Pharmacol., 9*:481-487.

Vargaftig, B. B., Lefort, J., Chignard, M., and Benveniste, J. (1980). Platelet-activating factor induces a platelet-dependent bronchoconstriction unrelated to the formation of prostaglandin derivatives. *Eur. J. Pharmacol., 65*:185-192.

Varonier, H. S., and Panzani, R. (1968). The effect of inhalations of bradykinin on healthy and atopic (asthmatic) children. *Intern. Arch. Allergy, 34*:293-296.

Vidruk, E. H., Hahn, H. L., Nadel, J. A., and Sampson, S. R. (1977). Mechanisms by which histamine stimulates rapidly adapting receptors in dog lungs. *J. Appl. Physiol., 43*:397-402.

Walker, J. L. (1973). The regulatory function of prostaglandins in the release of histamine and SRS-A from passively sensitized human lung tissue. In *Advances in the Biosciences* (*Vol. 9*), *International Conferences on Prostaglandins.* Edited by S. Bergstiom and S. Bernhard. Vieiveg, Braunschweig, Pergamon Press, pp. 235-240.

Wanner, A., Mezey, R. J., Reinhart, M. E., and Eyre, P. (1979). Antigen-induced bronchospasm in conscious sheep. *J. Appl. Physiol., 47*:917-922.

Wasserman, M. A., DuCharme, D. W., Griffin, R. L., DeGraaf, G. L., and Robinson, F. G. (1977). Bronchopulmonary and cardiovascular effects of prostaglandin D_2 in the dog. *Prostaglandins, 13*:255-269.

Wasserman, M. A., and Griffin, R. L. (1976). In vivo and in vitro bronchoconstriction responses to prostaglandin $F_{2\alpha}$, cyclic endoperoxide analogs, and thromboxane B_2. In *Lung Cells in Disease.* Edited by A. Bouhuys. Amsterdam, North-Holland Publishing Co., pp. 309-312.

Watanabe, S., and Koda, A. (1979). Purification and some physiochemical properties of slow reacting substance of anaphylaxis (SRS-A) from sensitized guinea pig lung. *Microbiol. Immunol., 23*:1009-1012.

Widdicombe, J. G. (1963). Regulation of tracheobronchial smooth muscle. *Physiol. Rev., 43*:1-37.

Woenne, R., Kattan, M., Orange, R. P., and Levison, H. (1978). Bronchial hyperreactivity to histamine and methacholine in asthmatic children after inhalation of SCH 1000 and chlorpheniramine maleate. *J. Allergy Clin. Immunol., 62*:119-124.

Woolcock, A. J., and Read, J. (1966). Lung volumes in exacerbations of asthma. *Am. J. Med., 41*:259-273.

Woolcock, A. J., and Read, J. (1968). The static elastic properties of the lungs in asthma. *Am. Rev. Respir. Dis., 98*:788-794.

Woolcock, A. J., Macklem, P. T., Hogg, J. C., Wilson, N. J., Nadel, J. A., Frank, N. R., and Brain, J. (1969). Effect of vagal stimulation on central and peripheral airways in dogs. *J. Appl. Physiol., 26*:806-813.

Youssef, A., and Barkhan, P. (1968). Release of platelet factor 4 by adenosine diphosphate and other platelet aggregating agents. *Br. Med. J., 1*:746-752.

Yu, D. Y. C., Galant, S. P., and Gold, W. M. (1972). Inhibition of antigen-induced bronchoconstriction by atropine in asthmatic patients. *J. Appl. Physiol., 32*:823-828.

Zaid, G., and Beall, G. N. (1966). Bronchial response to beta-adrenergic blockade. *N. Engl. J. Med., 275*:580-584.

11

In Vitro Immunopharmacology of Airway Contractile Tissues

Histamine and Slow-Reacting Substance of Anaphylaxis (Leukotrienes)

JEFFREY M. DRAZEN

Harvard School of Public Health
Brigham and Women's Hospital
Harvard Medical School
Boston, Massachusetts

ROBERT A. LEWIS

Harvard Medical School
Boston, Massachusetts

K. FRANK AUSTEN

Harvard Medical School
Brigham and Women's Hospital
Boston, Massachusetts

I. Introduction

The in vitro immunopharmacology of the contractile tissues of the lung involves two separate and distinct considerations. First the mediators that become available during immunologic activation of target tissues must be identified chemically and the mechanisms that control their synthesis, release, and metabolism understood. Second, the contractile activity and mechanisms of action of the various mediators on airway tissues at different loci within the lung must be appreciated. Since the first of these considerations forms the basis for a number of the preceding chapters in this text, we will limit our analysis to selected aspects of the second, i.e., specifically examination of the effects of histamine and the leukotriene constituents of slow-reacting substance of anaphylaxis (SRS-A) on airway tissues. We will examine the contractile activity of these

---

Supported in part by National Institutes of Health Grants HL0059 and HL17382.

two substances both when applied directly on appropriate tissue assays and when synthesized or released in direct contact with the contractile tissue in an in vitro anaphylactic response.

II. Contractile Tissue Assays

A. General Considerations

The contractile activity of immunopharmacological mediators has been studied on a wide variety of tissue preparations. The major differences among these preparations include variation in the anatomic location from which the contractile tissues are taken within the lung, the method of tissue preparation, and the physical mode of contraction (isometric versus isotonic). It is now well appreciated that the most important factor in determining the variability of contractile response appears to be the anatomic location in the lung from which the contractile tissues were taken. For example, Golla and Symes (1913) demonstrated a differential response of tracheal and bronchiolar smooth muscle from cats to adrenaline, nicotine, and tyramine. They concluded that muscle from each location may subserve different physiological functions. Although the physiological function of smooth muscle from various anatomic locations within the lung has not been determined, many workers have repeatedly confirmed the observation that contractile elements from various anatomic lung regions have different contractile profiles (Somylo and Somylo, 1970; Persson and Eckman, 1976; Fleisch and Calkins, 1976; Lullich et al., 1976; Drazen and Schneider, 1978). Thus, the response of a given airway contractile tissue preparation cannot be considered representative of contractile tissues throughout the tracheobronchial tree. Further the contractile activity of a given airway preparation in vitro reflects the relative activity attributed to a given airway level in vivo (Drazen and Schneider, 1978).

We will first consider preparative and technical differences in two classes of airway contractile tissue assays; tracheal, bronchial and bronchiolar assays, and lung strip assays. Subsequently, we will consider the different pharmacological responses of each of these tissue preparations to immunopharmacologic mediators.

B. Tracheal, Bronchial, and Bronchiolar Assays

Tracheal Preparations

There are two general categories of commonly used tracheal preparations: (1) tracheal chains or spirals and (2) isolated tracheal smooth muscle. The former preparation was originally described by Castillo and DeBeer (1947) and consists of a number of tracheal rings that are cut from the trachea and sewn together to form a chain such that when the chain is stretched the membranous portions of the tracheal rings are parallel to the long axis of the chain. The entire chain is placed in an organ bath and attached to a force transducer in an apparatus where its resting length can be varied (isometric case) or attached to a fixed weight and motion transducer such that variations in its total length can be detected (isotonic case). When passively stretched, the smooth muscle in the membranous portion of the trachea, which connects the ends of tracheal cartilage, is placed under tension such that an increase in active tension resulting from smooth muscle constriction is reflected as an increase in total tension of the chain. Akcasu (1952) introduced a modification of this preparation in which the cartilagenous portion of each ring is cut. This results in a more substantial fractional increment in total tension for a given pharmacologic stimulus than does the simple chain preparation. However, as these chains are somewhat time consuming to prepare, a modification was originally introduced by Patterson (1958) and later more fully described by Constantine (1965) in which the trachea is cut spirally from the larynx to the carina. When the spirally cut trachea is passively stretched, the long axis of the tracheal smooth muscle becomes oriented toward the direction of passive stretch such that an increase in active tension of the smooth muscle is reflected as an increase in the total tension of the spiral.

The nature of these preparations restricts their use to tracheae from small animals. Further they are not suited for the study of smooth muscle physiology because the contribution of the tracheal cartilage to the tension developed with passive stretch cannot be separated from stretching elastic elements within the muscle itself. The utility of these preparations rests in their ease of preparation, and reproducibility of results from many different laboratories. For example, if the active contractile response to 100 μM histamine is assigned an arbitrary value of 100, then many different workers have shown that a response of one-half this magnitude can be achieved with histamine solutions of 3-6 μM concentration (Ushinski et al., 1971; Douglas et al., 1977; Hanna and Roth, 1978; Drazen and Schneider, 1978). As the concentration-effect relationships obtained with these preparations are reproducible from laboratory to laboratory, they are useful for comparative pharmacological testing (i.e., testing one contractile agonist, against the response of a standard agonist such as histamine).

In contrast to these preparations, which contain both muscle and cartilage, the tracheal smooth muscle from larger species, such as dog, is easily prepared free of its surrounding cartilage and epithelial surfaces (Stephens et al., 1969; Russell, 1978). Using such preparations extensive information concerning the biochemistry and physiology of canine tracheal smooth muscle has been gathered and recently reviewed (Stephens and Kroeger, 1980). The major advantage of these preparations over the tracheal chain and spiral preparations from smaller animals, for use in pharmacological studies, is that their optimal length for mechanical response to a given stimulus can be determined with relative ease. Thus, the muscle can be "tuned" to maximize contractile action for a given stimulus. In addition, descriptions of the mechanical behavior of the muscle other than tension gathered after exposure to a given agent can be obtained (Stephens et al., 1969). The disadvantage of these preparations is that their physical size may limit the diffusion of contractile agonists into the tissues and thus diminish the response to a given stimulus (Dale and Gaddum, 1930).

Bronchial Preparations

The contractile response of bronchi and bronchioles has been studied in a variety of species using a preparative technique similar to the tracheal spiral (Golla and Symes, 1913; Persson and Eckman, 1976; Russell, 1978). An airway of a given size is located in the lung by placing a stylus of rod through it and dissecting away the surrounding pulmonary parenchyma. The tissue is then cut spirally including both contractile and noncontractile elements and mounted for tension recording in a manner similar to that employed for guinea pig tracheal preparations. This technique has been employed to study contractile activity of airways as small as canine bronchioles of approximately 1-mm diameter (Krell, 1978; Russell, 1978). Recently Evans (1979) has developed a preparation for the study of even smaller airways. This technique involves the isolation of circular segments of airways initially 300-500 μm in diameter. Airway sections are then placed in an apparatus which allows them to be passively stretched while the resulting tension is measured with specially constructed microtransducers. When appropriate, the active tension resulting from addition of pharmacologic agents can be determined. Although this apparatus does not differ conceptually from that used by others to study larger muscle strips (Stephens and Kroeger, 1980), it is technically complex and its use has not been widely disseminated.

C. Lung Strip Preparations

Strips of pulmonary parenchyma have also been used to examine the contractile activity of elements in the lung periphery. Although the existence of smooth muscle in the lung periphery has been appreciated since the early observations reported by Miller (1921), investigators did not take advantage of this observation until the pioneering work of Kapanci and colleagues (1974), who proposed that there were contractile cells in the lung interstitium that could be responsible for contractile activity of isolated lung parenchyma.

Although Kapanci and coworkers (1974) demonstrated that lung strips could constrict, Lulich et al. (1976) were the first to use the lung strip as a pharmacologic tool. These investigators demonstrated that a subpleural strip of feline parenchyma could constrict in response to a number of pharmacologic agonists including histamine, carbachol, and serotonin. Further, the contractile responses obtained differed from those of tracheal smooth muscle preparations from the same animals. Although the lung strips used by these investigators contained both bronchi and muscular blood vessels, the authors provided evidence that these structures were not the ones primarily responsible for the active tension developed in response to pharmacologic agonists. These authors demonstrated that lung strips of equivalent overall size cut from near the hilum, where there is an abundance of large airways and conducting vessels, and those from just under the pleura, containing fewer of such structures, had similar contractile profiles. Drazen and Schneider (1978) also demonstrated that strips of pulmonary parenchyma could be made to contract in response to pharmacologic stimulation and they also provided two additional insights into the nature of the contractile responses of these strips. First they demonstrated that strips without histologically identifiable conducting airways or blood vessels had similar profiles of activity as strips containing substantial numbers of such structures. This observation is consistent with the idea that the component of the strip most likely responsible for the contractile activity observed is in the parenchyma and most probably represents alveolar duct smooth muscle (Miller, 1921) or interstitial contractile cells (Kapanci, 1974). Second, (although they could not conclusively identify the exact tissue responsible for the contractile responses of the strip) they demonstrated that the comparative response of the tracheal spirals and parenchymal strips was similar to that attributed to central and peripheral airways in vivo (Colebatch et al., 1966). Thus, the comparative response of the two tissues in vitro could be used to predict the relative contractile potential of agonists in vivo.

Evans and coworkers (1978) have suggested that the contractile activity of rabbit lung strips is not due to alveolar duct smooth muscle but due to contractile interstitial cells. The basis of their arguments is that if alveolar duct smooth muscle and 300 μm diameter airways have similar profiles of pharmacologic activity, then lung strips and 300-μm diameter airways should exhibit similar profiles of pharmacologic activity. The demonstration that these two tissues do not have similar profiles of activity suggested that rabbit lung strips contain nonairway contractile tissues. Alternatively, the data could be interpreted to mean that small and very peripheral contractile elements have different pharmacologic profiles of activity. It is clearly important to establish the precise nature of the contractile tissues in lung strips and it seems unlikely that pharmacological methods will allow a conclusive identification.

D. Relationship of In Vivo and In Vitro Contractile Activity

Although a number of smooth muscle assays have been in use to assess by in vitro techniques the contractile potential of various agonists, a fundamental question not only remains unanswered but also remains relatively unexplored. Specifically, what fraction of maximum in vitro contractile potential is realized in vivo and how is this reflected in the severity of the in vivo reaction? For example, it is easy to reach a maximal contractile response to histamine in vitro, but in vivo death occurs before the maximal response is reached. When death occurs what fraction of the potential contractile response had been achieved? For example, if 20% of a maximal in vitro response leads to death then attention should be focused on low drug concentrations in the concentration-effect relationship; however if death coincided with a near maximal in vitro response then attention would have to be paid to the entire concentration-effect relationship. Full appreciation of the in vivo consequences of the in vitro assays will require an understanding of this as yet unresolved problem.

III. Specific Mediators

A. Introduction

Each of these smooth muscle assays has been used to examine the effects of various contractile agonists alone and on the contractile response of appropriately sensitized tissue to the addition of specific antigen—the so-called Schultz-Dale response (Schultz, 1910; Dale, 1913). In this response, the tissues are thought to contract in response to mediators released and synthesized as a result of events initiated by the addition of antigen. Although, as detailed elsewhere in this volume (Chap. 1-4, 6), many mediators participate in this contractile response, histamine and slow-reacting substance of anaphylaxis (SRS-A) have received the most attention in the literature. In the remainder of this chapter, we will consider the comparative in vitro pharmacology of these two moieties and the contractile response to addition of specific antigen.

B. Histamine

Histamine (β-imidazolylethylamine) was synthesized by Windus and Vost (1907) and originally noted by Dale and Laidlaw (1910) to be a potent agonist mediating smooth muscle constriction as well as a number of other effects. Classic antihistamines [latter shown to be H_1-receptor antagonists (Arunklashana and Schild, 1959; Ash and Schild, 1966)] were originally shown to inhibit the contractile effects of histamine on guinea pig bronchial preparations, demonstrating that histamine mediated its effects on this preparation through stimulation of H_1-subclass receptors. With the recent availability of H_2-receptor antagonists (Arunklashana and Schild, 1959; Black et al., 1972; Durant et al., 1975; Ganellin et al., 1976), it has been demonstrated that the airways of some species contain H_2-subclass receptors which when stimulated mediate airway relaxation (Eyre, 1977; Drazen et al., 1979). The availability and activity of H_1- and H_2-subclass receptors varies both among species and also within a given species with the location of the airway within the lung.

Tracheal and Bronchial Histamine Receptors

Guinea Pigs

In the original descriptions of the guinea pig tracheal chain (Castillo and DeBeer, 1947; Akcasu, 1952) and spiral (Patterson, 1958; Constantine, 1965), histamine was shown to be a contractile agonist. Arunkshlana and Schild (1959) demonstrated that this was due to histamine's action at H_1-subclass receptors in the guinea-pig trachea. Since these original descriptions, many workers have demonstrated that the guinea pig trachea constricts in response to histamine exposure (Ushinski et al., 1971; Douglas et al., 1977; Drazen et al., 1979; Hanna and Roth, 1978; Okpako et al., 1978; Mitchell and Denoborough, 1979; Souhrada and Loader, 1979). In the majority of these studies, a maximal contractile response is reached at a bath concentration of histamine between 30 and 100 μM and a half maximal response is achieved at bath concentrations of 3-6 μM.

In addition to H_1-subclass receptors that mediate airway constriction, guinea pig airways have been shown to contain H_2-subclass receptors that mediate airway relaxation. Okpako et al. (1978) demonstrated that metiamide (a selective H_2-receptor antagonist) enhanced the response of tracheal spirals to histamine and that 4-methyl histamine (a selective H_2-receptor agonist) relaxed previously constricted tracheal spirals. Drazen and coworkers (1978) confirmed these findings in vitro and extended them by demonstrating the presence of an H_2 inhibitory mechanism in vivo in guinea pig airways. Thus, guinea pig airways possess both contractile H_1-subclass receptors and inhibitory H_2-subclass receptors. Since the effects of histamine administered without receptor antagonists are clearly contractile in the guinea pig, H_1 receptor stimulation is of greater consequence than the effects of H_2 receptor stimulation.

Hanna and Roth (1978) demonstrated that guinea pig bronchial spirals had slightly greater responses to histamine than tracheal spirals, both in terms of the maximal tension developed and the concentration required to achieve a one-half maximal response. In addition to contractile H_1 receptors, Okpako et al. (1978) demonstrated that H_2-receptor antagonism by metiamide enhanced the histamine response and that stimulation with an H_2 agonist resulted in relaxation of previously constricted bronchial strips. Thus, both lobar and segmental bronchi (Kliment, 1973) of guinea-pigs, in addition to the trachea, contain H_2-subclass inhibitory receptors, but as in the trachea H_1-subclass receptors dominate.

Cat

Histamine does not constrict the cat trachea, rather it induces relaxation of previously constricted feline tracheal chains (Maengwyn-Davies, 1978). This may be in part due to release of catecholamines from intratracheal stores, since the relaxation is in part inhibited by prior treatment with reserpine. However, it has recently been demonstrated that both H_1- and H_2-receptor antagonists prevent this inhibitory action of histamine (Eyre, 1973). The observations are consistent with the hypothesis that the airway relaxation is mediated by stimulation of both H_1- and H_2-subclass receptors and that cat trachea does not contain H_1-subclass contractile receptors.

Dog

Histamine constricts isolated canine trachealis muscle by interaction at H_1-subclass receptors (Yamatake et al., 1978; Stephens and Kroeger, 1980; Antonissen et al., 1980). In contrast to guinea pig tracheal smooth muscle where histamine and acetylcholine are almost equipotent contractile agonists on a molar concentration basis (Drazen and Schneider, 1978), the maximal tension achieved with histamine on canine trachealis muscle is less than one-half that achieved with acetylcholine (Yamatake et al., 1978). Further, the effective histamine bath concentration for a one-half maximal contraction is 10 times that required to achieve a similar relative response of the guinea pig trachea (Yamatake et al., 1978; Drazen and Schneider, 1978; Antonissen et al., 1980). H_2-subclass receptor antagonists do not enhance the contractile effects of histamine on canine trachea, thus the relative insensitivity of this tissue to histamine cannot be attributed to stimulation of H_2-subclass inhibitory receptors (Antonissen et al., 1980). Compared with canine trachea, canine bronchi (Yamatake et al., 1978) and bronchioles (Krell, 1978; Yamatake et al., 1978) show a greater contractile response to histamine compared with acetylcholine in terms of the maximal tension achieved and the concentration of histamine required to achieve this tension.

Other Nonhuman Species

Somylo and Somylo (1970) and Fleisch and Calkins (1976) demonstrated that histamine constricted both tracheal and bronchiolar smooth muscle from rabbits by interaction at H_1-subclass receptors. However, the tracheal contractile response to histamine was only a small fraction of the maximally achievable response, while the bronchial response was a substantial fraction of its possible maximal response. It is not known if rabbit trachea or bronchi contain H_2-subclass receptors.

Sheep bronchi do not possess H_1 contractile or inhibitory receptors, however H_2-receptor antagonists prevent histamine-induced relaxation of the previously constricted sheep bronchus (Eyre, 1975). This observation suggests that sheep bronchi possess only H_2-subclass inhibitory receptors.

Bovine trachea and bronchi constrict in response to histamine (Burka and Eyre, 1977), although the exact receptor population mediating this constriction has not been clearly defined. Swine trachea and bronchus (Chand and Deroth, 1978) constrict in response to histamine by action at H_1-subclass receptors. Swine airways (both trachea and bronchus) also contain H_2 inhibitory receptors that mediate airway relaxation when H_1 receptors are inhibited. Horse trachea and bronchus are somewhat similar to swine airways (Chand and Eyre, 1975, 1978) in that they contain both H_1 contractile and H_2 inhibitory receptors. It is of interest that the relaxation mediated by histamine in horse airways cannot be completely antagonized by combined H_1 and H_2 receptor antagonism.

In the rhesus monkey, histamine does not constrict tracheal smooth muscle and is only a weak agonist for bronchial smooth msucle by its action at H_1-subclass receptors (Chand et al., 1980). Both trachea and bronchi, if constricted with carbachol, will relax upon addition of histamine and this relaxation can be antagonized by H_2 receptor antagonists. Thus, the bronchi of the rhesus monkey resemble those of the guinea pig, swine, and horse in that they contain both H_1 contractile and H_2 inhibitory receptors.

Human Airways

There is only limited data on the responses of isolated human airways. Bronchi (lobar or segmental) from human subjects obtained at surgery or at autopsy constrict in response to addition of histamine through action at H_1-subclass receptors (Adams and Lichtenstein, 1979; Thulesius et al., 1978; Dunlop and Smith, 1977). In the presence of H_1 receptor antagonists, histamine mediates airway relaxation, consistent with the hypothesis that human airways contain H_2-subclass inhibitory receptors (Dunlop and Smith, 1977).

Lung Strips

Lung strips from guinea pigs (Drazen and Schneider, 1978; Mitchell and Denoborough, 1979; Chand, 1979), cat (Lulich et al., 1976), dog (Chand et al., 1979), cow (Mirbahar and Eyre, 1980), rabbit (Chand and Deroth, 1979), and monkey (Chand et al., 1980) constrict in response to histamine by action at H_1-subclass receptors. If H_1-subclass receptors are antagonized, histamine will weakly relax the previously constricted guinea pig lung strip (Drazen et al., 1979), but not the dog, monkey, or rabbit lung strip.

Summary

Although there are species variations, these findings establish the presence of both H_1 contractile and H_2 inhibitory receptors in the lung. In the trachea, both H_1-subclass receptors and H_2 inhibitory receptors may be found, and either may dominate. The dominance in humans is not known. Bronchi of most species contain both H_1 and H_2 receptors, although the H_1 contractile receptors dominate. This is true in human airways. Parenchymal strips in contrast contain predominantly H_1 contractile receptors, with only the guinea pig having demonstrable H_2 receptors.

C. Slow-Reacting Substance of Anaphylaxis

SRS-A – Identification of Chemical Structure

Although this subject has been recently reviewed both elsewhere (Lewis and Austen, 1981) and in this text (Chap. 3), a brief synopsis is included. Kelleway and Trethewie (1940) identified a material of unknown chemical structure in anaphylactic perfusates from sensitized, antigen-challenged guinea pig lungs which resulted in a slow-onset prolonged constriction of the guinea pig ileum; they called this material slow-reacting substance or SRS. Brocklehurst (1953, 1960) demonstrated that the contractile activity of SRS was distinct from that of histamine by showing that contractions of the guinea pig ileum induced by SRS were resistant to the effects of (H_1) antihistamines and designated the material formed during anaphylaxis—slow-reacting substance of anaphylaxis, or SRS-A. SRS-A was shown to possess a unique profile of contractile activity with its most substantial activity being on the guinea pig ileum, rabbit stomach and human bronchus (Chakravarty, 1959; Brocklehurst, 1960, 1962). Although the accepted standard in vitro assay for SRS-A, the slow, sustained constriction of the guinea pig ileum in the presence of mepyramine (an H_1 receptor antagonist) and atropine eliminated from consideration histamine or cholinergic agonists, many mediators such as prostaglandins or bradykinin could induce slow ileal constriction under these conditions. Thus, the definition of SRS-A was more sharply focused by Orange and Austen (1969) to exclude other mediators whose structures were known. An initial purification procedure for SRS-A based on a partial physicochemical characterization (Orange et al., 1973) and the isolation of a semispecific SRS-A antagonist, FPL-55712 (Augstein et al., 1973), made identification of SRS-A activity in diffusates more conclusive. The analysis of the chemical structure of SRS-A was further aided by the observation that it contained a sulfur moiety (Orange et al., 1974) and that radiolabeled arachidonic acid could be incorporated into a slow-reacting substance produced by ionophore stimulation of rat mastocytoma cells (Bach et al., 1977; Jakschik et al., 1977). As the ionophore-induced SRS had the isolation and physiochemical characteristcs of SRS-A (Orange et al., 1973, 1974; Morris et al., 1978) this SRS was used for chemical definition as 5(*S*)-hydroxy-6(R)-*S*-glutathionyl-7,9,-*trans*, 11,13-*cis* eicosatetraenoic acid, designated leukotriene C or LTC_4 (Murphy et al., 1979; Corey et al., 1980). With the aid of material prepared by total synthesis the major chemical components of SRS-A have been identified to be LTC_4, and its 6-sulfido-cysteinylglycine and 6-sulfido-cysteinyl analogs designated LTD_4 and LTE_4, respectively (Lewis et al., 1980a,b; Orning et al., 1980).

Since the identification of the chemical structure of these components of SRS-A has occurred within the past 2 years, only limited information has become available concerning their in vitro airway pharmacology. Therefore, in addition to reviewing the in vitro airway pharmacology of leukotrienes C_4, D_4, and E_4, we will also include selected studies on the in vitro pharmacology of biologically produced and purified SRS-A.

In Vitro Airway Pharmacology of SRS-A

Brocklehurst (1960, 1962) was the first to point out that 1 unit/ml of guinea pig SRS-A was a potent constrictor of human bronchial tissues; 1 unit/ml of SRS-A eliciting a contraction equal in magnitude to that resulting from 10 μg/ml of histamine. Berry and Collier (1964) demonstrated that SRS-A constricted the guinea pig trachea with a force equal in magnitude to the contraction resulting from 50 μg/ml acetylcholine. Strandberg and Uvnas (1971) and Mathe and Strandberg (1971) demonstrated that a partially purified preparation of cat paw SRS was also a potent constrictor of human bronchi in vitro. Drazen et al. (1979) working with rat SRS-A, purified by high-performance liquid chromatography, and also using silicic acid-purified SRS-A, demonstrated that these SRS-A preparations were more potent contractile agonists for parenchymal strips than tracheal spirals when compared to histamine. Mitchell and Denborough (1979) also confirmed these findings. In these experiments, the contractile effects of SRS-A on guinea pig lung strips were shown to be inhibited by FPL-55712. Coleman and co-workers (1980) used partially purified SRS-A to constrict guinea pig lung strips and computed a pA_2 for FPL-55712 of 7.04. Burka and Eyre (1977) provided additional data for the selective peripheral airway action of SRS-A by demonstrating that bovine bronchial strips were more sensitive to the contractile effects of SRS-A than isolated bovine trachealis muscle. These in vitro findings were consistent with the hypothesis that SRS-A is a relatively selective peripheral airway constrictor; a hypothesis which had been proposed based upon in vivo findings in guinea pigs (Drazen and Austen, 1974) and confirmed in rhesus monkeys (Michoud et al., 1979).

Synthetic LTC_4 constricts both guinea pig tracheal spirals and parenchymal strips, but compared with histamine is 200 times more active on the parenchymal strip and only 10 times more active in tracheal spirals (Drazen et al., 1980; Lewis et al., 1980a). On the pulmonary parenchymal strip, 1 unit of SRS-A (defined conventionally as the amount yielding a contraction equivalent to that produced by 5.0 ng/ml histamine on the guinea pig ileum has the same contractile activity as 0.43 pmol of LTC_4. Thus, LTC_4 is an extremely potent, relatively selective constrictor of peripheral airways in vitro. LTD_4 is 10 to 20 times more potent (on a molar basis) than LTC_4 in effecting contractions of the guinea pig pulmonary parenchymal strip (Drazen et al., 1980) but equiactive with LTC_4 on the tracheal spirals—making it an even more selective peripheral airway contractile agonist in vitro, than LTC_4. Contractions of the guinea pig parenchymal strip initiated by LTC_4 are not antagonized in a concentration-related manner by FPL-55712, however, the responses of this tissue

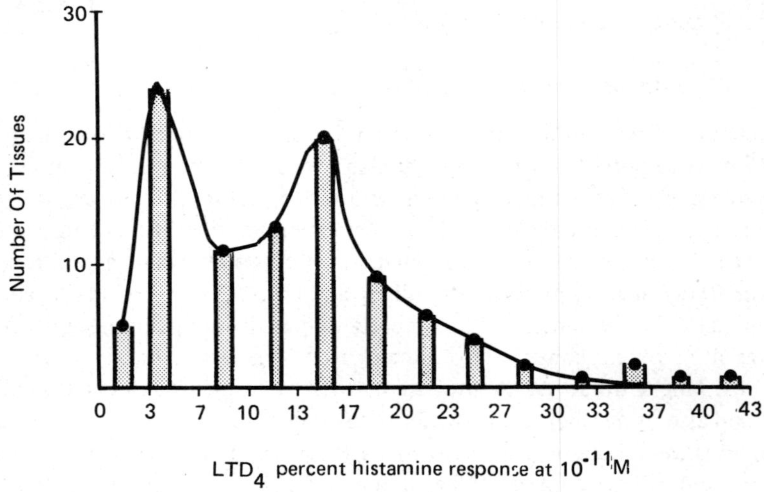

Figure 1 Histogram showing the contractile response of guinea pig pulmonary parenchymal strips to 10 picomolar concentrations of leukotriene D_4. The response is bimodal with peaks at 5% and 16% of the maximal histamine contractile response.

to LTD_4 at low response levels are effectively antagonized by FPL-55712 with a pA_2 of 7.0 (Drazen et al., 1980). This value compares favorably with the pA_2 for FPL-55712 versus SRS-A on pulmonary parenchymal strips of 7.04 calculated by Coleman and workers (1980). At higher response levels, FPL-55712 did not antagonize LTD_4 constrictions (Drazen et al., 1980). This may reflect the fact that with the availability of synthetic material, larger constrictions are being realized than were possible with biologically derived material. A possible interpretation is that there are two leukotriene receptors in guinea pig pulmonary parenchymal strips, a low-activity, high-affinity receptor antagonized by FPL-55712 and activated specifically by LTD_4 and a low-affinity, high-activity receptor activated by all leukotrienes but not antagonized by FPL-55712. In a series of 99 guinea pig pulmonary parenchymal strips, the distribtution of responses to a 10 picomolar solution of LTD was bimodal with peaks at 5% and 16% of maximal histamine activity (Fig. 1), suggesting that activity of the high affinity receptor can be appreciated only in tissue removed from selected animals. Evidence that animal-to-animal variability accounted for the distribution shown in Figure 1 was obtained in an experiment with synthetic LTD_4, in which a pulmonary parenchymal strip from one animal demonstrated

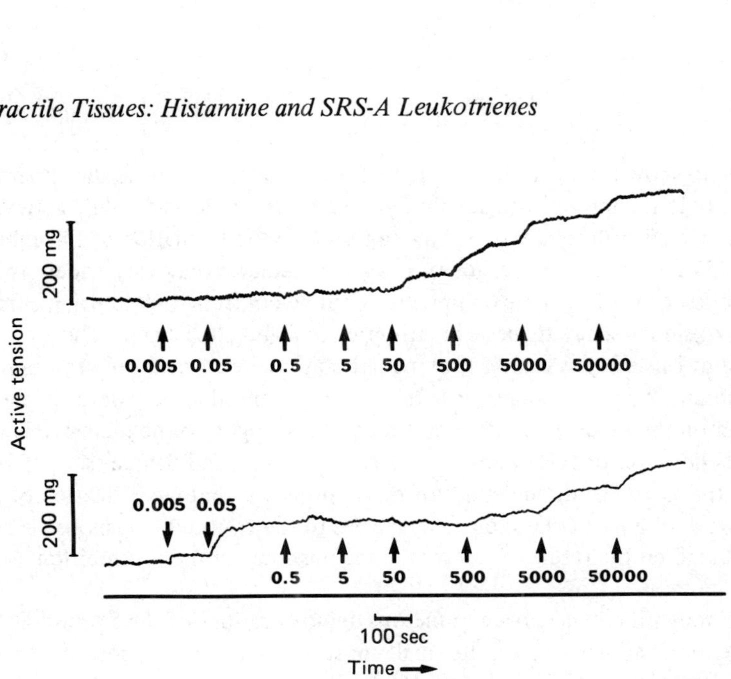

Figure 2 Tracing of an experimental record showing in vitro constriction of guinea pig pulmonary parenchymal strips from two animals with leukotriene D4. The bath concentration of leukotriene D4 (pg/ml) is shown at the arrows. Note that the upper tracing fails to show low-dose contractile effect while the lower tracing demonstrates the presence of a low-dose effect.

the low-concentration activity while a simultaneously run strip from a second animal did not show evidence for this activity (Fig. 2). The factors controlling the expression of this receptor and its relevance to the in vivo response to the various leukotrienes are not known. LTE4, the most recently identified leukotriene component of SRS-A, is also a selective peripheral airway agonist and is of similar potency on a molar basis as LTC4 (Lewis et al., 1980b).

D. Schultz-Dale Response—In Vitro Airway and Airspace Anaphylaxis

It has been appreciated since the early 1900s that addition of specific antigen to sensitized contractile tissues results in a contractile response (Schultz, 1910; Dale, 1913). Thus, in vitro the tissue under examination both produces or releases various mediators and serves as the assay tissue for these mediators. The response is far more complex than that resulting from addition of an identified mediator on a specific contractile tissue for three reasons: (1) The number and availability of sensitized target cells may vary from tissue to tissue. (2) The enzymatic apparatus needed for synthesis and degradation of secondary mediators may vary from tissue to tissue. For example, Gryglewski and co-workers

(1976) have shown that the guinea pig trachea contains the metabolic apparatus to form predominantly prostaglandin E_2 from arachidonic acid, while activation of the guinea pig pulmonary parenchyma results in the formation of thromboxane A_2. (3) The contractile response to a given mediator may vary widely from tissue to tissue. Most of these complexities can be controlled by limiting comparisons to similar assay tissues similarly prepared and challenged. The great potential of this assay system is that mediators that are formed only transiently or are present in small amounts near their receptor and that may have substantial effect on the tissue response even though they might not be identifiable in anaphylactic diffusates (Dawson et al., 1976; Hamburg and Samuelsson, 1976) can be expressed. The disadvantage of this approach is that identification of the contribution of a particular molecular species to the contractile response is necessarily based on the result of receptor antagonism or synthesis inhibition studies.

Although there have been numerous demonstrations of the Schultz-Dale phenomenon in airway tissues, the single most important early contribution was made by Brocklehurst (1953, 1960). He demonstrated that antigen-induced contractions of guinea-pig airways were substantially resistant to the effects of the H_1-subclass receptor antagonist, mepyramine, and suggested (on the basis of this observation) that SRS-A plays a substantial role in anaphylactic airway constriction. His observations have been repeated on numerous occasions as outlined in the recent extensive review by Chand and Eyre (1978).

H_2 Receptors and In Vitro Anaphylaxis

Chand (1979) demonstrated that the guinea pig lung strip contained H_2-subclass receptors which when antagonized by metiamide (10^{-5} M and 5×10^{-5} M) resulted in an enhanced response to antigen. However he was unable to determine if this enhancement resulted from lack of H_2 receptor-mediated lung strip relaxation or from lack of H_2 receptor-mediated inhibition of mediator release (Lichtenstein and Gillespie, 1975; Drazen et al., 1978). Similar findings were reported by Dunlop and Smith (1977) in sensitized human bronchial strips. H_2 receptor-mediated inhibition of the Schultz-Dale phenomenon appears to be quite species specific, since neither canine lung strips nor canine trachealis muscle exhibits an enhanced response after treatment with H_2 receptor antagonists (Antonissen et al., 1980).

Role of Lipoxygenase Products in the Schultz-Dale Response

Brocklehurst (1960) first suggested that SRS-A was important in antigen-induced airway constriction in vitro. Adams and Lichtenstein (1978) demonstrated that the prolonged constriction of sensitized guinea pig tracheal spirals or human bronchial strips induced by antigen (which was not inhibited by H_1-subclass receptor antagonism) could be partially blocked by the SRS-A antagonist FPL-55712. Mitchell and Denoborgh (1979) extended their findings to include the Schultz-Dale response of guinea pig lung strips. Recently Burka and Paterson (1980a,b,c) demonstrated that indomethacin and sodium meclofenamate [inhibitors of the cyclooxygenase pathway of arachidonic acid (AA) metabolism] enhanced antigen-induced constriction of guinea pig tracheal spirals, while addition of the combined cyclooxygenase and lipoxygenase inhibitors eicosatetrayinoic acid (ETYA) or phenidone prevented this enhancement. They interpreted these observations to mean that during anaphylactic smooth muscle constriction available AA was metabolized to both dilator (cyclooxygenase) and constrictor (lipoxygenase) products respectively and that addition of a cyclooxygenase inhibitor prevented the synthesis of inhibitory compounds and enhanced the synthesis of contractile compounds. In contrast, addition of a combined cyclooxygenase and lipoxygenase inhibitor prevented formation of AA metabolic products from both either pathways and thus prevented further enhancement due to the SRS-A leukotrienes generated by the lipoxygenase pathway.

Understanding of the in vitro immunopharmacology of the airways is still very limited. However, with the identification and characterization of the interactive effects of the secondary mediators generated by the oxidative metabolism of arachidonate by smooth muscle, our understanding is greatly enhanced.

References

Adams, G. K., III, and Lichtenstein, L. (1978). *In vitro* studies of antigen-induced bronchosapsm: Effect of antihistamine and SRS-A antagonist on response of sensitized guinea pig and human airways to antigen. *J. Immunol., 122*:555-562.

Akcasu, A. (1952). The actions of drugs on the isolated trachea. *J. Pharm. Pharmacol., 4*:671.

Antonissen, L. A., Mitchell, R. W., Kroeger, E. A., Kepron, W., Stephens, N. L., and Bergen, J. (1980). Histamine pharmacology in airway smooth muscle from a canine model of asthma. *J. Pharmacol. Exper. Therap., 213*:150-155.

Arunlakshana, O., and Schild, H. O. (1959). Some quantitative uses of drug antagonists. *Br. J. Pharmacol., 14*:45-58.

Ash, A. S., and Schild, H. O. (1966). Receptors mediating some actions of histamine. *Br. J. Pharmac. Chemother., 27*:427-439.

Augstein, J., Farmer, J. B., Lee, T. B., Sheard, P., and Tattersall, M. L. (1973). Selective inhibitor of slow-reacting substance of anaphylaxis. *Nat. New Biology, 245*:215-217.

Bach, M. K., Brashler, J. R., and Gorman, R. G. (1977). On the structure of slow-reacting substance of anaphylaxis: evidence of biosynthesis from arachidonic acid. *Prostaglandins, 14*:21-38.

Berry, P. A., and Collier, H. O. J. (1964). Bronchoconstrictor action of a slow-reacting substance from anaphylaxis of guinea-pig isolated lung. *Br. J. Pharmacol., 23*:201-216.

Black, J. W., Duncan, W. A. M., Durant, C. J., Ganellin, C. R., and Parsons, E. J. (1972). Definition and antagonism of histamine H_2-receptors. *Nature, 236*:385-390.

Brocklehurst, W. E. (1953). Occurrence of an unidentified substance during anaphylactic shock in cavy lung. *J. Physiol., 120*:16P-17P.

Brocklehurst, W. E. (1960). The release of histamine and formation of a slow reacting substance (SRS-A) during anaphylactic shock. *J. Physiol., 151*: 416-435.

Brocklehurst, W. E. (1962). Slow-reacting substance and related compounds. *Progr. Allergy, 6*:339-558.

Burka, J. F., and Eyre, P. (1977). Effects of bovine SRS-A (SRS-A bov) on bovine respiratory tract and lung vasculature *in vitro. Eur. J. Pharmacol., 44*:169-177.

Burka, J. F., and Paterson, N. A. M. (1980a). Inhibition of antigen-induced release of prostaglandin-like material from guinea-pig trachea by antihistamine, FPL55712 and atropine. *J. Pharm. Pharmacol., 32*:869-870.

Burka, J. F., and Paterson, N. A. M. (1980b). Evidence for lipoxygenase pathway involvement in allergic tracheal contraction. *Prostaglandins, 19*:499-515.

Burka, J. F., and Paterson, N. A. M. (1980c). Enhancement of antigen-induced tracheal contraction by cyclooxygenase inhibition, In *Advances in Prostaglandin Thromboxane Research,* vol. 8. Edited by B. Samuelsson, P. W. Ramwell, and R. Paoletti. New York, Raven Press, pp. 1755-1758.

Castillo, J. C., and De Beer, E. J. (1947). The tracheal chain, a preparation for the study of antispasmodics with particular reference to bronchodilator drugs. *J. Pharmacol. Exp. Therap., 90*:104-109.

Chakravarty, N. (1959). A method for the assay of "slow reacting substances." *Acta Physiologica Acand., 46*:298-313.

Chand, N. (1979). *In vitro* anaphylaxis histamine H_2-receptors. *Eur. J. Pharmacol., 55*:337-339.

Chand, N., and DeRoth, L. (1978). Actions of histamine and other substances on the airway smooth muscle of swine (*in vitro*). *Veterminary Sci. Comm., 2*:151-155.

Chand, N., and DeRoth, L. (1979). Pharmacological characterization of the rabbit lung strip, *Research Comm. Chem. Pathol. Pharmacol., 23*:223-232.

Chand, N., DeRoth, L., and Eyre, P. (1979). Pharmacology of Schultz-Dale reaction in canine lung strip *in vitro*: possible model for allergic asthma. *Br. J. Pharmacol., 66*:511-516.

Chand, D., and Eyre, P. (1975). Classification and biological distribution of histamine receptor sub-types. *Agents Actions, 5*:277-295.

Chand, N., and Eyre, P. (1978). The Schultz-Dale Reaction: A Review. *Agents Actions, 8*:171-184.

Chand, N., and Eyre, P. (1978). Spasmolytic action of histamine in airway smooth muscle of horse. *Agents Actions, 8*:191-198.

Chand, N., Dhawan, B. H., Srimal, R. C., Rahmani, N. H., Schukla, R. K., and Altura, B. M. (1980). Reactivity of trachea, bronchi, and lung strips to histamine and carbachol in rhesus monkeys. *J. Appl. Physiol., 49*:729-734.

Colebatch, H. J. H, Olsen, C. R., and Nadel, J. A. (1966). Effect of histamine, serotonin and acetylcholine on the peripheral airways. *J. Appl. Physiol., 21*:217-226.

Coleman, R. A., Kennedy, I., and Whelan, C. J. (1980). The contractile action of slow-reacting substance of anaphylaxis (SRS-A) on guinea-pig isolated lung strip. *Br. J. Pharmacol., 68*:83-P.

Constantine, J. W. (1965). The spirally cut tracheal strip preparation, *J. Pharm. Pharmacol., 17*:834-838.

Corey, E. J., Clark, D. A., Goto, G., Marfat, A., Mioskowski, C., Samuelsson, B., and Hammerstron, S. (1980). Stereospecific total synthesis of a "slow-reacting substance of anaphylaxis" (SRS), leukotrene C-1. *J. Am. Chem. Soc., 102*:1436-1439.

Dale, H. H. (1913). The anaphylactic reaction of plain muscle in the guinea pig, *J. Pharmacol. Exp. Therap., 4*:167-223.

Dale, H. H., and Gaddum, J. H. (1930). Reactions of denervated voluntary muscle, and their bearing on the mode of action of parasympathetic and related nerves. *J. Physiol., 70*:109-144.

Dale, H. H., and Laidlaw, P. P. (1910). The physiologic action of β-imidazolyl-etylamine, *J. Physiol., 41*:318.

Dawson, W., Boot, J. R., Cockerill, A. F., Mallen, D. N. B., and Osborne, D. J. (1976). Release of novel prostaglandins and thronboxanes after immunological challenge of guinea-pig lungs. *Nature, 262*:699-707.

Douglas, J. S., Ridgway, P., and Brink, C. (1977). Airway response of the guinea-pig *in vivo* and *in vitro. J. Pharmacol. Exper. Ther., 201*:116-124.

Drazen, J. M., and Austen, K. F. (1974). Effects of intravenous adminstration of slow-reacting substance of anaphylaxis, histamine, bradykinin, and prostaglandin F2α on pulmonary mechanicsin the guinea pig. *J. Clin. Invest., 53*:1679-1685.

Drazen, J. M., and Schneider, M. W. (1978). Comparative responses of tracheal spirals and parenchymal strips to histamine and carbachol *in vitro. J. Clin. Invest., 61*:1441-1447.

Drazen, J. M., Schneider, M. W., and Venugopalan, C. S. (1979). Bronchodilator activity of dimaprit in the guinea pig *in vitro* and *in vivo. Eur. J. Pharmacol., 55*:233-239.

Drazen, J. M., Venugopalan, C. S., and Soter, N. A. (1978). H_2-mediated inhibition of immediate type of hypersensitivity reactions *in vivo. Am. Rev. Respir. Dis., 117*:479-484.

Drazen, J. M., Lewis, R. A., Wasserman, S. I., Orange, R. A., and Austen, K. F. (1979). Differential effects of a partially purified preparation of slow-reacting substance of anaphylaxis on guinea pig tracheal spirals and parenchymal strips. *J. Clin. Invest., 63*:1-5.

Drazen, J. M., Austen, K. F., Lewis, R. A., Clark, D. A., Goto, G., Marfat, A., and Corey, E. J. (1980). Comparative airway and vascular activities of leukotrienes C-1 and D *in vivo* and *in vitro. Proc. Natl. Acad. Sci. USA, 77*:4354-4358.

Dunlop, L. S., and Smith, A. P. (1977). The effect of histamine antagonists on antigen-induced contractions of sensitized human bronchus *in vitro. Br. J. Pharmacol., 59*:475 p.

Durant, G. J., Ganellin, C. R., and Parsons, M. E. (1975). Chemical differentiation of histamine H_2- and H_2-receptor agonists. *J. Medicinal Chemistry, 18*:905-909.

Evans, J. (1979). Mechanical properties of isolated bronchioles. *Am. Rev. Respir. Dis., 119* (Suppl):306.

Evans, J. N., Previti, R. A., Adler, K. B., and Vallyathan, V. N. (1978). Contractile properties of peripheral lung tissue. *Physiolgist, 21*:35.

Eyre, P. (1975). Histamine H_2-receptors in the sheep bronchus and cat trachea; the action of burimamide. *Br. J. Pharmacol., 48*:321-323.

Eyre, P. (1977). Pulmonary histamine H_1 and H_2 receptor studies. In *Asthma II; Physiology, Immunopharmacology and Treatment.* Edited by L. Lichtenstein and K. F. Austen. New York, Academic Press, 170-175.

Fleisch, J. H., and Calkins, D. J. (1976). Comparison of drug-induced responses of rabbit trachea and bronchus. *J. Appl. Physiol., 41*:62-66.

Ganellin, C. R., Durant, G. J., and Emmett, J. C. (1976). Some chemical aspects of histamine H_2-receptor antagonists. *Fed. Proc., 35*:1924-1930.

Golla, F. L., and Symes, W. L. (1913). The reversible action of adrenaline and some kindred drugs on the bronchioles. *J. Pharmacol. Exp. Therap., 5*: 87-103.

Gryglewski, R. J., Dembinska-Kiec, A., Grodzinska, L., and Panczenko, B. (1976). Differential generation of substances with prostaglandin-like and thromboxane-like activities by guinea-pig trachea and lung strips. In

Lung Cells in Disease. Edited by A. Bouhuys. Amsterdam, North-Holland Publ., pp. 289-307.

Hamberg, M., and Samuelsson, B. (1976). Detection and isolation of an endoperoxide intermediate in prostaglandin biosynthesis. *Proc. Natl. Acad. Sci. USA, 73*:899-903.

Hanna, C. J., and Roth, S. H. (1978). The guinea pig tracheobronchial spiral strip: responses to selected agonists. *Can. J. Physiol. Pharmacol., 56*:823-827.

Jakschik, B. A., Falkenstein, S., and Parker, C. W. (1977). Precursor role of arachidonic acid in release of slow-reacting substance from rat basophillic leukemia cells. *Proc. Natl. Acad. Sci. USA, 74*:4577-4581.

Kapanci, Y., Assimacopoulos, A., Irle, C., Zwahlen, A., and Gabbiani, G. (1974). Contractile interstitial cells in pulmonary alveolar septa: A possible regulator of ventilation/perfusion ratio? *J. Cell. Biol., 60*:375-392.

Kelleway, C. H., and Trethewie, E. R. (1940). The liberation of a slow-reacting smooth-muscle-stimulating substance in anaphylaxis. *Q. J. Exp. Physiol., 30*:121-145.

Kliment, V. (1973). Similarity and dimensional analysis, evaluation of aerosol deposition in the lungs of laboratory animals and man. *Folia Morphologica, 21*:59-64.

Krell, R. D. (1978). Pharmacologic characterization of isolated canine bronchial smooth muscle. *Eur. J. Pharmacol., 49*:151-155.

Lewis, R., and Austen, K. F. (1981). Mediators of mast-cell dependent local homeostasis and information: Perspective on the leukotrienes. *Nature*, (In Press).

Lewis, R. A., Austen, K. F., Drazen, J. M., Clark, D. A., Marfat, A., and Corey, E. J. (1980a). Slow-reacting substance of anaphylaxis: identification of leukotrienes C-1 and D from human and rat sources. *Proc. Natl. Acad. Sci. USA, 77*:3710-3714.

Lewis, R. A., Drazen, J. M., Austen, K. F., Clark, D. A., and Corey, E. J. (1980b). Identification of the C(6)-S-conjugate of leukotriene A with cysteine as a naturally occurring slow-reacting substance of anaphylaxis (SRS-A): Importance of the 11- *cis* -geometry for biological activity, *Biochem. Res. Comm., 96*:271-277.

Lichtenstein, L. M., and Gillespie, E. (1975). The effects of the H_1 and H_2 antihistamines on "allergic" histamine release and its inhibition by histamine. *J. Pharmacol. Exp. Therap., 192*:441-450.

Lulich, K. M., Mitchell, H. W., and Sparrow, M. P. (1976). The cat lung strip as an *in vitro* preparation of peripheral airways: a comparison of β-adenoreceptor agonists, autacoids and anaphylactic challenge on the lung strip and trachea. *Br. J. Pharmacol., 58*:71-79.

Maengwyn-Davies, G. D. (1978). The dual mode of action of histamine in the cat isolated tracheal chain. *J. Pharm. Pharmacol., 20*:572-573.

Mathé, A. A., and Standberg, K. (1971). Antagonism of slow reacting substance by polyphloretin phosphate on isolated human bronchi. *Acta Physiol. Scand., 82*:460-465.

Michoud, M. C., Paré, P. D., Orange, R. P., and Hogg, J. C. (1979). Airway sensitivity to slow-reacting substance of anaphylaxis, histamine, and antigen in *Ascaris* sensitive monkeys. *Am. Rev. Respir. Dis., 119*:419-424.

Miller, W. S. (1921). The musculature of the finer divisions of the bronchial tree and its relation to certain pathological conditions. *Am. Rev. Tuberc., 5*:689-704.

Mirbahar, K. B., and Eyre, P. (1980). Bovine lung parenchyma strip has both airway and vascular characteristics. (Pharmacological comparisons with bronchus, pulmonary artery and vein.), *Res. Comm. Chem. Pathol. Pharmacol., 29*:15-25.

Mitchell, H. W., and Denborough, M. A. (1979). Anaphylaxis in guinea-pig peripheral airways *in vitro. Eur. J. Pharmacol., 54*:69-78.

Morris, M. R., Taylor, G. W., Piper, P. J., Sirois, P., and Tippens, J. R. (1978). Slow-reacting substance of anaphylaxis purification and characterization. *FEBS lett, 87*:203-206.

Murphy, R. C., Hammarstrom, S., and Samuelsson, B. (1979). Leukotriene C: A slow-reacting substance from murine mastocytoma cella. *Proc. Natl. Acad. Sci. USA, 76*:4275-4279.

Okpako, D. T., Chand, N., and Eyre, P. (1978). The presence of inhibitory histamine H_2-receptors in guinea-pig tracheobronchial muscle. *J. Pharm. Pharmacol., 30*:181-182.

Orange, R. P., and Austen, K. F. (1969). Slow reacting substance of anaphylaxis. *Adv. Immunol., 10*:105-144.

Orange, R. P., Murphy, R. C., Karnovsky, M. L., and Austen, K. F. (1973). The physicochemical characteristics and purification of slow-reacting substance of anaphylaxis. *J. Immunol., 110*:760-770.

Orange, R. P., Murphy, R. C., and Austen, K. F. (1974). Inactivation of slow-reacting substance of anaphylaxis (SRS-A) by arylsufatases. *J. Immunol., 113*:316-321.

Orehek, J., Douglas, J. S., and Bouhuys, A. (1975). Contractile responses of the guinea-pig trachea *in vitro*; modification by prostaglandin synthesis-inhibiting drugs. *J. Pharm. Exp. Therap., 194*:554-564.

Orning, L., Hammarstrom, S., and Samuelsson, B. (1980). Leukotriene D: A slow reacting substance from rat basophilic leukemia cells. *Proc. Natl. Acad. Sci. USA, 77*:2014-2017.

Patterson, R. (1958). The tracheal strip: Observations on the response of tracheal muscle. *J. Allergy, 29*:165.

Persson, C. G. A., and Eckman, M. (1976). Contractile effects of histamine in large and small respiratory airways. *Agents Actions, 6*:389-393.

Russell, J. A. (1978). Responses of isolated canine airways to electric stimulation and acetylcholine. *J. Appl. Physiol., 45*:690-698.

Schultz, W. H. (1910). Physiological studies in anaphylaxis. I. The reaction of smooth muscle of the guinea pig sensitized with horse serum. *J. Pharmacol. Exp. Therap., 1*:549-567.

Somlyo, A. P., and Somlyo, A. V. (1970). Biophysics of smooth muscle excitation and contraction. In *Airway Dynamics: Physiology and Pharmacology.* Edited by A. Bouhuys. Springfield, Thomas, pp. 209-227.

Souhrada, J. F., and Loader, J. (1979). Role of glucose in contractility of airway smooth muscle. *Respir. Physiol., 36*:231-247.

Stephens, N. L., and Kroeger, E. A. (1980). Ultrastructure, biophysics, and biochemistry of airway smooth muscle. In *Physiology and Pharmacology of the Airways.* Edited by J. A. Nadel. New York, Marcel Dekker, pp. 31-121.

Stephens, N. L., and Van Niekerk, W. (1977). Isometric and isotonic contractions in airway smooth muscle, *Can. J. Physiol. Pharmacol., 55*:833-838.

Stephens, N. L., Kroeger, E. A., and Menta, J. A. (1969). Force-velocity characteristics of respiratory airway smooth muscle. *J. Appl. Physiol., 26*:685-692.

Strandberg, K., and Uvnas, B. (1971). Purification and properties of the slow reacting substance formed in the cat paw perfused with compound 48/80. *Acta Physiol. Scand., 82*:358-374.

Thulesius, O., Boe, J., and Berlin, E. (1978). Physiological and pharmacological studies on isolated human bronchial preparations. *Scand. J. Respir. Dis., 59*:66-74.

Ushinski, S. C., Mansmann, H. C., Jr., and Roberts, J. (1971). The influence of initial tension on the reactivity of guinea-pig tracheal preparations to histamine. *Arch. Int. Pharmacodynam. 190*:61-66.

Windaus, A., and Vost, W. (1907). Synthese des imidazolyl-Athylamins. *Ber., 40*:3691-3695.

Yamatake, Y., Sasagawa, S., and Yanaura, S. (1978). Drug responses of canine trachea, bronchus and bronchiole. *Chem. Pharmacol. Bull., 26*:318-320.

12

Immunopharmacology of the Mucociliary System

ADAM WANNER

Mount Sinai Medical Center
and University of Miami
School of Medicine
Miami Beach, Florida

TAHIR AHMED*

Mount Sinai Medical Center
Miami Beach, Florida

I. Introduction

The primary function of the airway mucociliary system is its contribution to host defenses. This is accomplished by physical removal of inhaled foreign material from the ciliated airways by mucous transport and by biochemical and immunologic processes that protect against the invasion of the mucosa by infectious agents. Normal respiratory secretions contain certain enzymes and immunoglobulins (secretory IgA) which have antimicrobial properties. While the control of the chemical composition of respiratory secretions under normal and pathologic conditions is poorly understood, the alterations in mucociliary function and the mechanisms underlying such alterations have been studied extensively, and several widely accepted concepts have evolved. With respect to immunologic reactions, sufficient data have now been accumulated to justify a review of the effects of airway anaphylaxis on mucociliary function, particularly in relation to allergic bronchial asthma. The purpose of this chapter is to present pathologic and physiologic evidence of mucociliary dysfunction in airway anaphylaxis, to summarize its pathogenesis, and to establish a link between basic observations and some of the clinical aspects of allergic bronchial asthma.

**Present Affiliation*: University of Miami School of Medicine; Mount Sinai Medical Center, Miami Beach, Florida

II. Demonstration of Abnormal Mucociliary Function in Airway Anaphylaxis

A. Structure

Structure/function relationships are difficult to establish in bronchial asthma for at least two reasons. First, airflow obstruction in bronchial asthma is episodic by definition and the associated morphologic abnormalities may follow the same dynamic pattern and hence not be present at autopsy. Second, endoscopic or bronchographic studies of in vivo structure/function relationships are rarely carried out because of the morbidity associated with these procedures in patients with bronchial asthma. Most morphologic examinations have been carried out in patients who died during or from status asthmaticus. However, it has been recently demonstated that the pathologic changes in patients with stable asthma or nonfatal exacerbations of asthma differ only quantitatively from those in status asthmaticus.

Material for pathologic studies of the lungs in patients with bronchial asthma have been derived from three sources: expectorated sputum, bronchial biopsy, and autopsy material. The typical microscopic features of sputum such as Curschman's spirals, Charcot-Leyden crystals, and Creola bodies (clumps of epithelial cells) suggest the presence of narrowed airways, abnormal airway secretions, and epithelial damage, respectively. This is confirmed by the gross appearance of the lung at autopsy (Dunnill et al., 1969). Characteristically, the lungs appear overdistended and fail to collapse in a normal fashion. The cut surface reveals numerous grey plugs in large and small airways; small areas of cystic bronchiectasis may also be seen. Despite the presence of hyperinflation, the microscopic examination shows no evidence of destructive parenchymal changes and the alveolar walls appear normal. Thus, distention of the lung is the result of either changes in lung elastic recoil (Gold et al., 1967) and/or "air trapping" due to bronchial obstruction by excessive airway secretions (or mucosal edema) which persist after death. These mucosal and submucosal abnormalities form the basis of the following discussion. To better appreciate their significance, the normal anatomy will also be reviewed.

Normal Anatomy

Mucosa

The respiratory mucosa from the proximal trachea to the terminal bronchioles consists of a pseudostratified columnar epithelium with cilia protruding from the luminal surface of columnar cells. The major cell types found in the respiratory epithelium are basal cells, intermediate cells, nonciliated columnar cells, ciliated columnar cells, and goblet cells. In the larger airways, the major part of the epithelial surface is ciliated. The ratio of ciliated columnar cells to goblet cells is

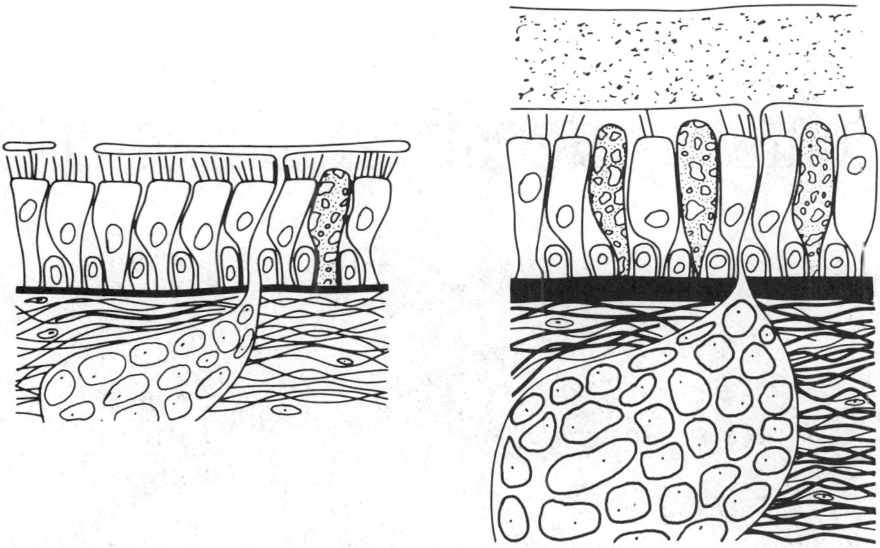

Figure 1 Schematic representation of the bronchial mucosa. Layers from top to bottom are the mucous layer, the periciliary fluid layer, the columnar epithelial cells with goblet cells, the basement membrane and the submucosal gland. *Left panel,* normal. Note abnormalities in asthma (*right panel*). (From Wanner, 1979b.)

5-10:1 in the trachea with a relative decrease in the number of both cell types toward the peripheral airways. The surface of each ciliated columnar cell contains approximately 200 cilia with an average length of 6 μm and diameter of 0.2 μm. The thickness of the normal basement membrane is approximately 7 μm. Tight junctions between adjacent epithelial cells provide a protective barrier against the transport of inhaled agents across the epithelium.

Submucosa

This is defined as the tissue space between the basement membrane of the mucosa and the cartilage. It contains submucosal glands, smooth muscle in longitudinal and circular arrangements, and connective tissue which is well vascularized. The cholinergic nervous system and probably also the sympathetic nervous system supply branches to the bronchial wall, and for the cholinergic nervous system both afferent and efferent fibers have been demonstrated. However, the exact anatomic distribution of nerve endings within the airway wall has not been completely described.

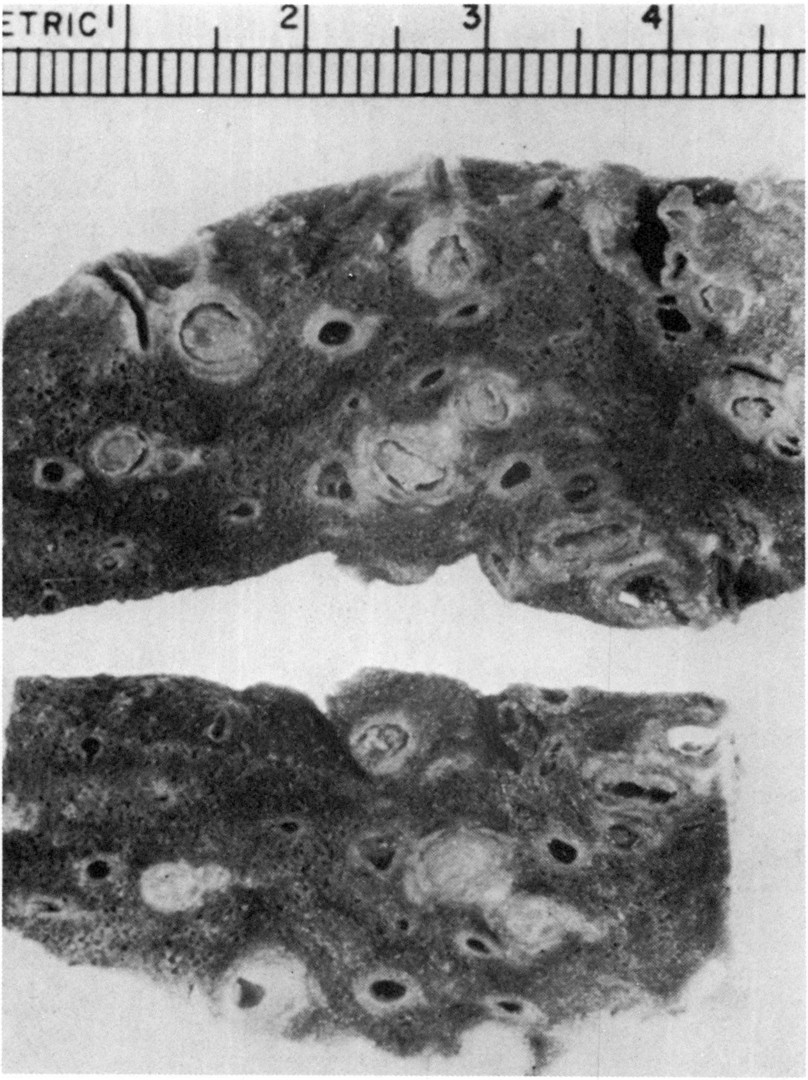

Figure 2 Widespread bronchial obstruction by mucous plugs in a fatal case of bronchial asthma. Scale in centimeters. (From Rezek and Millard, 1963).

Submucosal glands constitute most of the total volume of mucus-producing structures in human airways, and has been estimated to be approximately 4 ml (Reid, 1965). The relative volume of the submucosal gland layer in relation to the total volume of the bronchial wall between the cartilage and the luminal surface of the epithelium is less than 15-20% under normal circumstances with a mean value of 13% in one study (Dunnill et al., 1969). A two-layer concept of respiratory secretions is currently widely accepted (Fig. 1). It visualizes a periciliary fluid layer (sol) covered by a mucous layer (gel) which interacts with the tips of the cilia (Lucas and Douglas, 1934). Some investigators believe that the mucous layer represents a continguous blanket of 5-10 μm thickness covering the luminal surface of the tracheobronchial tree (Hilding, 1957), whereas others suggest that mucus is discontinuous, with foci of mucus floating like lilypads on the periciliary fluid (Van As, 1974). It is possible to reconcile these two concepts in that the normal amount of mucus decreases from the central airways towards the peripheral airways. Thus, the continuity of the mucous layer that is present in central airways cannot be maintained in peripheral airways.

Abnormalities in Bronchial Asthma

Mucosa

In status asthmaticus, the mucosa is characterized by edema, separation of mucosal cells, a decrease in the number of ciliated cells, and an increase in the number of goblet cells along with goblet cell metaplasia in peripheral airways (Fig. 1). Detachment of superficial epithelial cells can be seen in some areas. Widespread mucous plugging of the airways is usually seen (Fig. 2) (Dunnill, 1960; Rezek and Millard, 1963).

In stable bronchial asthma, the destructive changes of the epithelium are not as evident, although it has been recently suggested that the integrity of the tight junction is disrupted. The thickness of the basement membrane is increased to about twice normal. It contains deposits of immunoglogulin G, A, and predominantly M (Callerame et al., 1971a). IgE has not been demonstrated in the basement membrane (Callerame et al., 1971b). However, those studies involved primarily patients with nonallergic asthma. Thickening of the basement membrane is not pathognomonic of bronchial asthma since it can also be observed in patients with chronic bronchitis. Electron microscopy does not provide significant additional information and merely confirms the destructive epithelial changes. Recently, peripheral airway obstruction with mucous plugging has been demonstrated in children with asthma in remission who underwent open lung biopsy (Fig. 3) (Cutz et al., 1978). The intraluminal mucous plugs were mainly present in bronchi greater than 1 mm in diameter, but they were also observed in small peripheral airways.

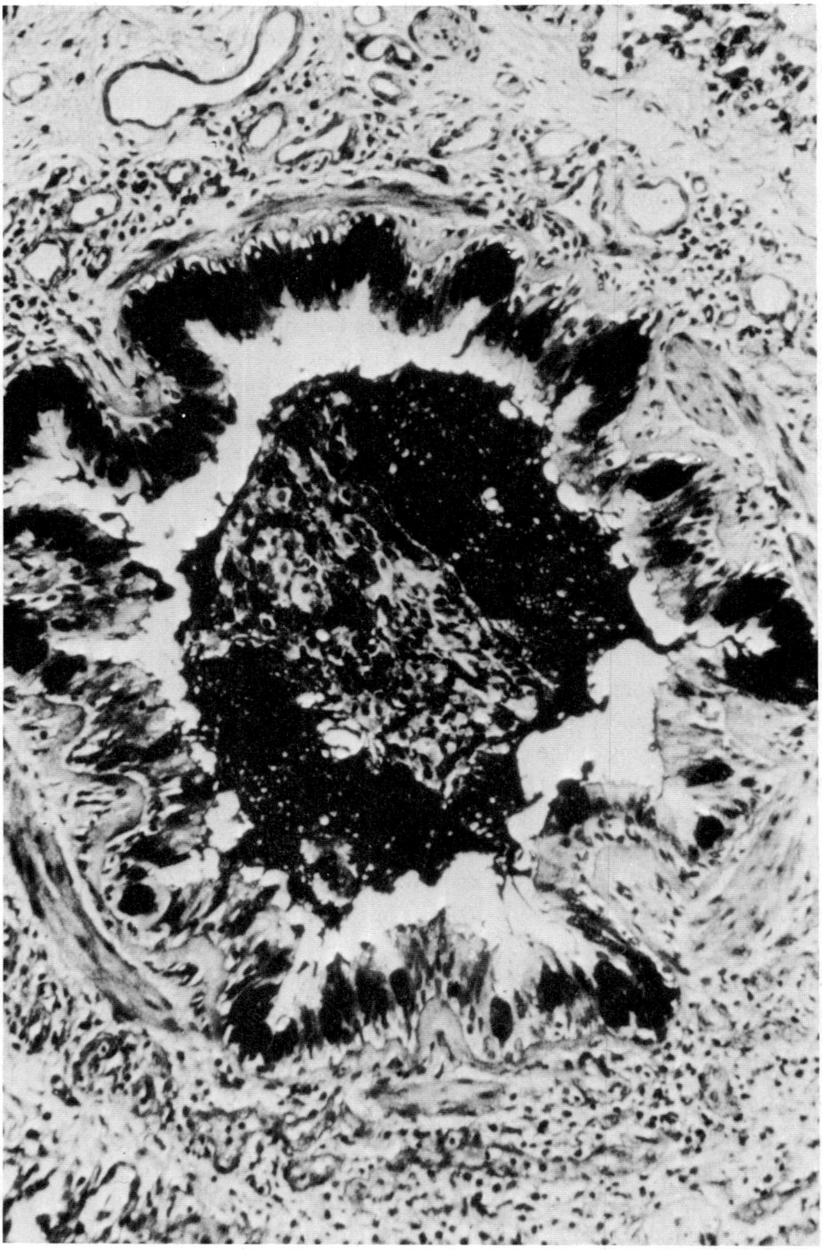

Figure 3 A small airway (ID = 0.15 mm) showing an intraluminal mucous plug in a child with asthma in remission. Numerous macrophages encased in the plug. (Lung biopsy, original magnification 2400 X.) (From Cutz et al., 1978.)

Submucosa

The submucosal tissues show edema, dilated capillaries, and cellular infiltration with eosinophils, lymphocytes, and plasma cells (Dunnill et al., 1969). There is also a decrease in the number of mast cells, with partial degranulation of those remaining. Although IgE has been demonstrated in lymphocytes and eosinophils within the bronchial wall, its presence is not typical of bronchial asthma; it is also seen in patients with nonspecific bronchial inflammation (Callerame et al., 1971b).

Typically, there is hyperplasia and hypertrophy of the submucosal glands. In one study, the mean volume of the submucosal gland layer was 23% in bronchial asthma as compared with 13% in normals (Dunnill et al., 1969). The submucosal gland hypertrophy and hyperplasia are not a specific feature of bronchial asthma. They are also present in chronic bronchitis; indeed, the submucosal gland volume in patients with chronic bronchitis is usually greater than in patients with bronchial asthma.

B. Function

The pathologic abnormalities in patients with stable bronchial asthma or status asthmaticus suggest an abnormality of mucociliary function in the airways, as demonstrated by hyperplasia and hypertorphy of mucus-producing structures, loss of the integrity of the surface epithelium, and the accumulation of mucus in the bronchial lumina. Such mucociliary dysfunction is also demonstrated by the clinical observation of excessive respiratory secretions that are difficult to expectorate, and the endoscopic and radiographic documentation of mucous plugs and atelectasis (Shaw et al., 1957). Recent experiments involving patients with bronchial asthma and animal models of allergic bronchoconstriction have confirmed the presence of abnormal production and elimination of airway mucus. The following discussion summarizes these findings (Table 1).

Several studies have shown abnormal mucociliary transport in patients with bronchial asthma. In elderly patients with stable asthma, tracheal mucous velocity as determined by the radiographic observation of discrete radioopaque particles has been shown to be decreased to 10% of that of young normal controls and to be comparable to that of patients with chronic bronchitis (Santa Cruz et al., 1974). Although an inverse relation seems to exist between mucous transport rate and age (Goodman et al., 1978a), the discrepancy between asthmatics and normals could not be fully accounted for by differences in age, suggesting true impairment of mucous transport mechanisms in bronchial asthma. Another study, using a radioactive particle clearance method in somewhat younger patients with stable asthma, also demonstrated a decrease in both tracheobronchial transport velocity and peripheral mucociliary clearance to about 60% of normal control subjects (Foster et al., 1978). Normal overall clearance of inhaled radioactive aerosols has been observed by Mossberg et al.

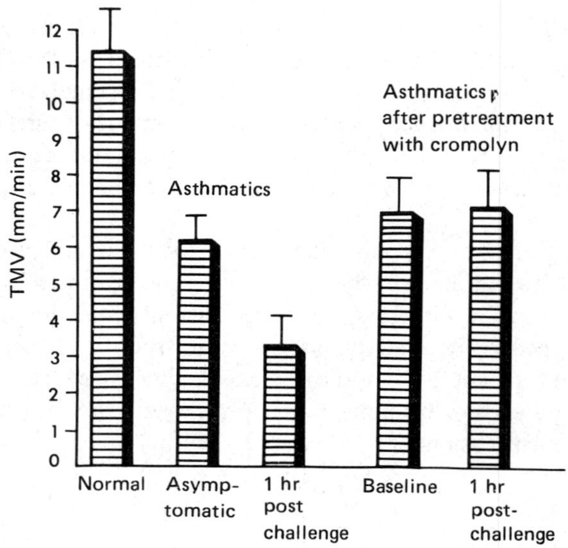

Figure 4 Comparison of tracheal mucous velocity (TMV) between normal subjects and asthmatic patients, before and after bronchial challenge, with and without cromolyn sodium pretreatment. Brackets indicate ± SE. (From Mezey et al., 1978.)

(1976a) in young and middle-aged patients with stable bronchial asthma. However, no corrections were made for abnormal aerosol deposition, which is typically present in patients with airflow obstruction. Therefore, the preferential deposition of particles in central airways, where clearance rates are naturally faster, could have compensated for a possible decrease in overall clearance rates. Finally, a reduction in tracheal mucous velocity to 55% of the velocity of age-matched healthy nonsmokers has also been observed in young asymptomatic patients with allergic asthma (Fig. 4) (Mezey et al., 1978). Pulmonary function in most of these patients showed minimal residual airway dysfunction consistent with asthma in remission.

Abnormal mucociliary transport could result from a primary disorder of ciliary function (decreased number or impaired motility of cilia), or an abnormal interaction of cilia with mucus due to alterations in the quantity or rheologic properties of mucus or periciliary fluid.

Ciliary Function

Alterations or primary ciliary motility are difficult to assess by in vivo techniques which measure ciliary beat frequency or by in vitro techniques using

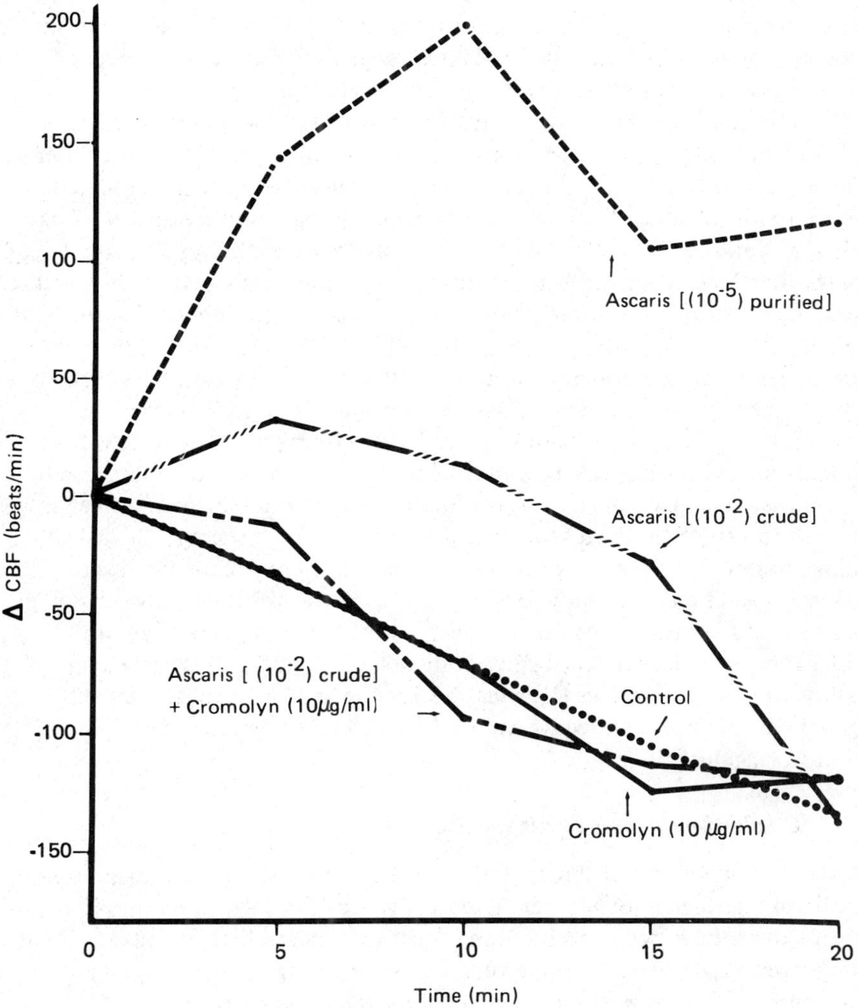

Figure 5 Effects of *Ascaris suum* antigen in the absence and presence of cromolyn sodium on mean ciliary beat frequency of tracheal epithelial cells contained in tracheal brush material (also containing mast cells). △ CBF = change in ciliary beat frequency over time. The slopes of *Ascaris suum* without cromolyn sodium are significantly different from the control slope (effect of time alone).

airway segments because of the presence of mucus, which has an effect on ciliary beat frequency. As a stimulus is applied to the system, it cannot be determined to what extent that stimulus affects ciliary motility directly or indirectly by altering the physical properties of mucus. To study the direct effects of airway anaphylaxis on ciliary function, Maurer et al. (1981) therefore used an in vitro technique by taking advantage of the presence of mast cells in the cellular material obtained by bronchial brushing through a fiber-optic bronchoscope. The recovered cells were suspended in Hank's balanced salt solution, which removed most of the airway mucus, injected into a chamber, and maintained at physiologic conditions. Ciliary activity was viewed through a differential interference-contrast microscope and recorded by a television camera on a videotape recorder for subsequent analysis at slow motion. Ciliary beat frequency of tracheal epithelial cells obtained from sheep with *Ascaris suum* hypersensitivity and previously documented bronchospastic responses to inhaled *Ascaris suum* aerosols, increased upon in vitro exposure to various concentrations of *Ascaris suum* antigen (Fig. 5). This effect was completely blocked by cromolyn sodium and an antagonist of slow-reacting substance (SRS-A), which by themselves had no effect on ciliary beat frequency. One can conclude from this observation that the release of chemical mediators of anaphylaxis from luminal mast cells has a stimulating effect on ciliary beat frequency. This mechanism, therefore, can not be invoked to explain the impairment of mucociliary transport during allergic bronchoconstriction. In vitro dose-response curves with histamine showed a stimulatory effect at very high concentrations only, while those with leukotriene C_4 and prostablandin E_1 and E_2 showed a dose-dependent stimulation of ciliary beat frequency. One explanation for the blocking effects of an SRS-A antagonist on antigen-induced ciliostimulation combined with the ciliostimulatory effect of leukotriene C_4 is that SRS-A released in airway anaphylaxis causes ciliostimulation directly, and possibly by activating other mediators such as prostaglandin E.

Qualitative Changes of Airway Secretions

A variety of biochemical abnormalities characterize airway secretions in bronchial asthma. Glycoproteins seem to determine the rheologic properties to a great extent. Increased concentration of unusual polysaccharides and cross-binding between transudated serum protein and secretary IgA have been found in the sputum of patients with bronchial asthma (Guirgis and Townley, 1973). Changes in electrolyte concentrations including increases in calcium have also been reported, and serum proteins appear to accumulate in the sol phase of asthmatic sputum (Dennis et al., 1964; von Hoffman and Ebelt, 1968). These distinguishing biochemical characteristics of respiratory secretions in asthma could have an effect on their rheologic properties. Unfortunately, the rheologic properties of respiratory secretion of patients with bronchial asthma have not been adequately studied. The best known observation was made on expectorated sputum that might not be representative of lower airway secretions (Charman and Reid, 1972). In that study, sputum from asthmatic patients tended to be more viscous than that from patients with other types of obstruc-

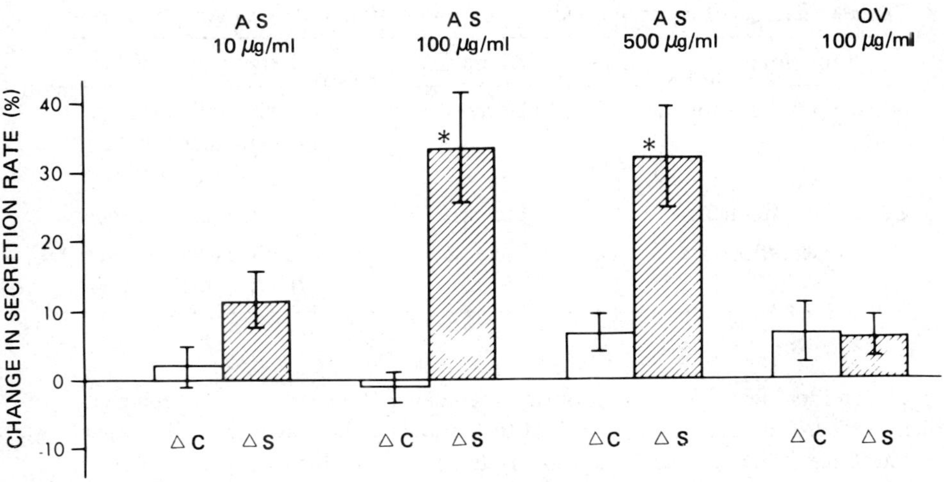

Figure 6 In vitro effects of *Ascaris suum* and ovalbumin on the secretion of [^{35}S] sulfate-labeled macromolecules from tracheal tissues obtained from sheep with *Ascaris suum* hypersensitivity. The histograms represent the percent change in secretion during control periods (△C) and during addition (△S) of different concentrations of *Ascaris suum* (AS) or ovalbumin (OV). Data are means ± SE. Asterisks indicate significant difference between △S and △C ($p < .05$).

tive airway disease; a marked increase in viscosity at low shear rates was particularly characteristic of the sputum obtained from asthmatic patients (Charman and Reid, 1972). If mucus in the lower airways indeed possesses abnormal rheologic properties, then such abnormalities may well alter transport rates. Both theoretical predictions (Miller, 1968; Ross and Corrsin, 1974) and actual measurements of the transportability of viscoelastic substances and sputum on the frog palate (Dulfano et al., 1971; Chen and Dulfano, 1978) suggest basically an inverse relation between transport rate and viscosity, and a direct relation between transport rate and the elastic modulus (elastic recoil) for a range of values that was typical for sputum from patients with chronic bronchitis.

Quantitative Changes of Airway Secretions

Mucociliary interaction also depends upon the respective thicknesses of the periciliary fluid layer and the mucous layer. The "normal" thickness of the periciliary fluid layer is less than, or at most equal to the length of the ciliary shafts, which measure approximately 6 μm in the central airways. It is not known how the thickness of the periciliary fluid layer compares with ciliary length in the smaller airways. It is also uncertain whether respiratory secretions separate into a sol and gel layer in the peripheral airways. Periciliary fluid has not been isola-

Table 1 Effects of Antigen on Mucociliary Function in Airway Anaphylaxis

Function	Alteration	Experimental Design
Mucociliary transport rate	Decreased	In vivo (allergic dog, allergic sheep, patient with allergic asthma)
Ciliary beat frequency	Increased	In vitro (allergic sheep)
Mucous secretion rate	Increased	In vitro (allergic sheep) In vivo (allergic dogs)

ted, and its chemical composition and rheologic properties have not been characterized. A decrease in the depth of the periciliary fluid layer would be expected to result in a decreased mucociliary transport rate due to a reduction of energy transferred from the cilia to the mucous layer (Litt and Eng, 1970; Ross and Corrsin, 1974). Conversely, if the thickness of the periciliary fluid layer exceeds the length of cilia, the cilia cannot interact with mucus. The thickness of the periciliary fluid layer has not been measured in patients with airway disease. However, active transport of chloride and hence water across the tracheal epithelium from the submucosal to the luminal side of the trachea has been reported in dogs (Olver et al., 1975). It is conceivable, although not proven, that this chloride and water transport is a major source of, or contributor to, periciliary fluid. It is also possible that the ionic strength of this fluid influences the rheologic properties or the structure of the overlying mucous layer. Histamine has been shown to stimulate chloride and water transport, and this may relate to abnormal periciliary fluid production in bronchial asthma (Marin et al., 1977).

The thickness of the mucous layer also appears to determine mucociliary transport rate (Litt and Eng, 1970; Ross and Corrsin, 1974). Stewart (1948) investigated the weight-carrying capacity of ciliated epithelium. He found that up to a weight of 20 mg/mm^2 there was no decrease in test particle transport and that no acceleration of particle transport occurred with lighter weight. This indicates that the marked increase in the depth of the mucous layer will not result in a decreased transport rate. Despite the presence of normal ciliary function, however, an extremely thick mucous layer could theoretically decrease the velocity of surface particles due to uncoupling within the mucous layer. Indeed, theoretical predictions suggest an inverse relation between the thickness of the mucous layer and mucous transport rates (Litt and Eng, 1970; Ross and Corrsin, 1974).

Dr. Kim Balfre in our laboratory (Balfre et al., 1980) examined the effect of antigen challenge on in vitro airway mucin secretion in isolated sections of ovine tracheal tissue mounted in Ussing-type chambers containing Hank's balanced salt solution. [^{35}S] sulfate, a mucous glycoprotein precursor, was initially added to both the luminal and submucosal chambers and then removed from the luminal chamber. The subsequent appearance of bound radio-sulfate into the luminal chamber was used as an indication of mucine secretion, which reached a steady-state after several hours. The addition of purified *Ascaris suum* antigen to tracheal tissue preparations obtained from sheep previously sensitized to this antigen increased secretion by a mean of 34% (Fig. 6). Ovalbumin, a control protein, had no effect on secretion. Subsequently, Dr. Roger Phipps showed that the *Ascaris suum* effects could be partially blocked by cromolyn sodium and an SRS-A antagonist (Phipps et al., 1982). These findings suggest that antigen challenge can stimulate secretion of sulfated macromolecules from the sheep trachea through immunologic pathways. The macromolecules presumably represent mucous glycoproteins. These in vitro observations are in keeping with the demonstration of increased amounts of tracheal secretions in allergic dogs after aerosol challenge with antigen (Yamatake et al., 1977).

III. Pathogenesis of Mucociliary Dysfunction

While increased production and impaired transportability of mucus seems to be responsible for the accumulation of airway secretions in patients with nonallergic and allergic asthma, the question of what causes these abnormal functions has thus far only been examined in relation to allergic asthma. The basic hypothesis underlying these experiments is that the immunologic mechanisms involved in bronchoconstriction can also be applied to mucociliary dysfunction.

A. Observations in Animal Models

Our recent experiments involving antigen-induced bronchoconstriction in animal models strongly suggest an important pathogenetic role of chemical mediators of anaphylaxis in allergic asthma. In sheep with *Ascaris suum* hypersensitivity, inhalation of an aerosol of this antigen causes transient bronchoconstriction which is characterized by typical changes in respiratory mechanics, including increases in pulmonary resistance and functional residual capacity and a decrease in arterial oxygen tension (Wanner et al., 1979a). The measurement of tracheal mucociliary transport rate in these animals using a radiographic technique (Friedman et al., 1977) revealed a decrease to 55% of baseline at 1 hr and to 51% of baseline at 2 hr after antigen challenge (Weissberger et al., 1981) (Fig. 7). This decrease in mucociliary transport was not observed in the same animals when they were challenged with a control antigen (ragweed), and could be completely prevented by prior inhalation of cromolyn sodium. Assuming that the primary effect of inhaled cromolyn sodium is inhibition of mediator release, one can conclude from these observations that the acute impairment of mucociliary

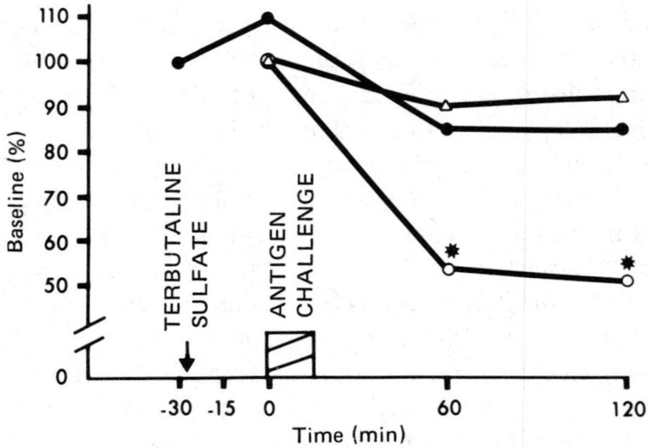

Figure 7 Relative changes of mean mucous velocity in the trachea of sheep with *Ascaris suum* hypersensitivity after *Ascaris suum* challenge (—o—), after control challenge with ragweed (—△—) and after terbutaline sulfate pretreatment (0.25 mg s.c.) with subsequent *Ascaris suum* challenge (—●—). Time zero represents measurements immediately prior to antigen challenge. Asterisks indicate significant ($p < .05$) difference from measurement at time zero. (From Weissberger et al., 1981.)

transport associated with allergic bronchoconstriction is effected by mast cell degranulation. It is of interest that pretreatment with a β-adrenergic agonist also prevented *Ascaris suum*-induced mucociliary dysfunction in these animals (Fig. 7). The administration of 0.25 mg terbutaline sulfate by subcutaneous injection prior to *Ascaris suum* challenge did not produce a significant change in baseline tracheal mucociliary transport rates, but prevented the expected decrease after subsequent *Ascaris suum* challenge in a fashion similar to sodium cromolyn. That this was not a direct stimulatory effect on muciliary transport was suggested by the fact that baseline tracheal mucous transport rates were not altered by terbutaline sulfate, which when given in the presence of impaired mucociliary function causes a significant stimulation at the same time interval (Sackner et al., 1979). Thus, the protective effect of terbutaline sulfate may have been by inhibition of mast cell degranulation (Pepys and Hutchcroft, 1975).

Since several chemical mediators released from mast cells during anaphylaxis could be responsible for mucociliary dysfunction, we carried out additional experiments that focused on histamine and SRS-A, two major chemical mediators which have been characterized with respect to their effects on airway smooth muscle. In addition, we also addressed the question whether the effect of these mediators on the mucociliary apparatus was direct or involved a cholinergic reflex which may represent an important mechanism in allergic bronchoconstriction (Gold et al., 1972). Dogs with *ascaris suum* hypersensitivity were

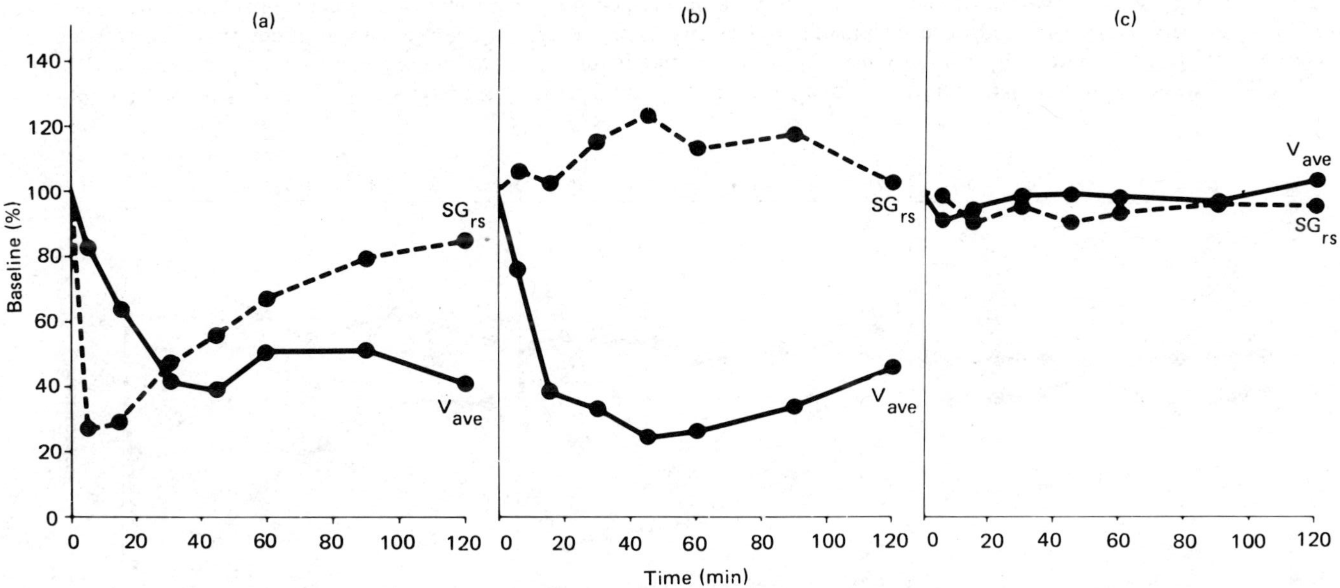

Figure 8 Relative changes in specific respiratory conductance (SG_{rs}) and average tracheal mucous velocity (V_{ave}) after antigen challenge in dogs sensitized to Ascaris suum but not to ragweed extracts. Time zero represents baseline values. (*a*) Dogs that responded to *Ascaris suum* challenge with bronchospasm. (*b*) Dogs without a bronchospastic response to *Ascaris suum* challenge. (*c*) Control dogs that inhaled ragweed extract. (From Wanner et al., 1975.)

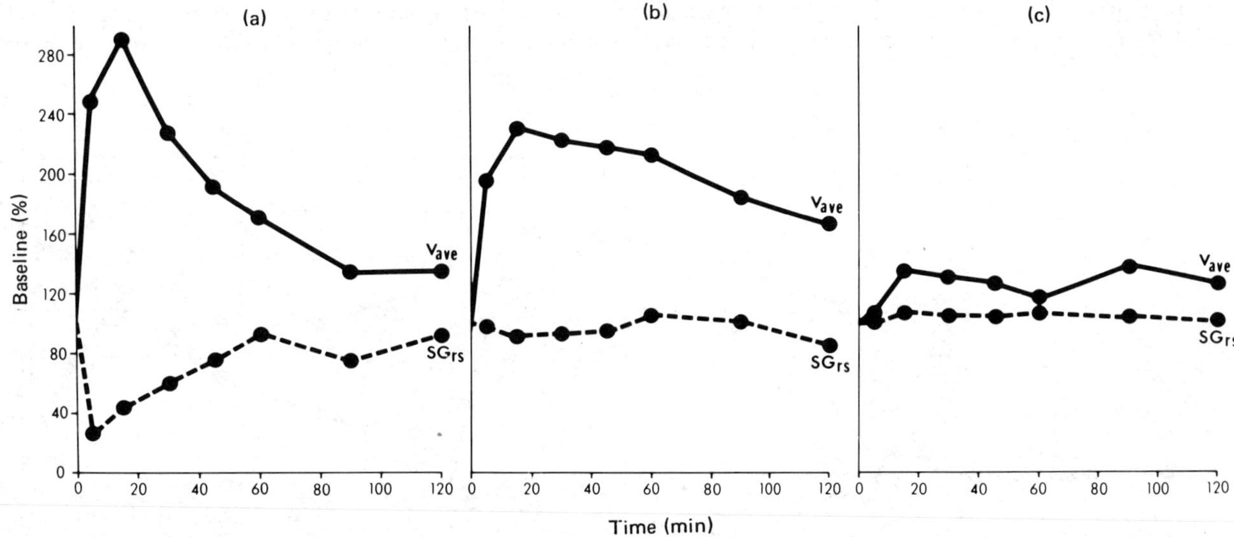

Figure 9 Relative changes in specific respiratory conductance (SG_{rs}) and average tracheal mucous velocity (V_{ave}) in dogs sensitized to *Ascaris suum* antigen following inhalation of both *Ascaris suum* antigen and FPL-55712, an antagonist of slow-reacting substance of anaphylaxis (*a*) Dogs that responded with bronchospasm. (*b*) Dogs without bronchospastic response. (*c*) Control dogs that inhaled FPL-55712 alone. For further explanation, see Figure 8. (From Wanner et al., 1975.)

used (Wanner et al., 1975). Although only 50% of the dogs responded with *Ascaris suum* extract, tracheal mucociliary transport rates decreased in all animals by a mean of 70% within 30-45 min of antigen challenge regardless of whether bronchospasm occurred; tracheal mucociliary transport rate was still significantly decreased at the end of 2 hr (Fig. 8). No changes occurred in controls that inhaled ragweed extract. These results were quite similar to those obtained in the allergic sheep with the exception that an increase in airflow resistance was not invariably present after antigen challenge in contrast to the decrease in tracheal mucociliary transport rates. Inhalation of histamine or acetylcholine solution in concentrations that produced a degree of bronchospasm comparable to that observed in the antigen-challenged dogs resulted in a transient increase in tracheal mucociliary transport rates, thereby excluding them as mediators of the observed mucociliary impairment after antigen challenge. On the other hand, nebulization of *Ascaris suum* antigen together with compound FPL-55712, a relatively selective antagonist of SRS-A, produced a transient, nearly threefold increase in tracheal mucous velocity regardless of whether bronchospasm was elicited (Fig. 9). FPL-55712, when given alone or together with a control antigen (ragweed) had no effect on tracheal mucociliary transport rate, thereby excluding a nonspecific inhibiting action. We concluded that (1) mucociliary transport at least in central airways is impaired in allergic dogs after inhalation of specific antigen, thereby extending the findings in allergic sheep to another species, (2) the change in mucociliary transport is unrelated to bronchospasm, (3) mucociliary dysfunction is not mediated by a vagal reflex, and (4) mucociliary dysfunction may be related to the release of SRS-A. The mechanisms by which FPL-55712 caused an increase in tracheal mucous transport rates when administered together with specific antigen is not clear. One might speculate that inhibition of the depressor mediator SRS-A unmasked the stimulatory effects of other mediators such as histamine.

B. Observations in Patients with Asthma

Recent human investigations tend to support the observations in the experimental canine asthma model (Wanner et al., 1975). Mezey et al. (1978) measured tracheal mucous velocity in six asymptomatic patients with a history of bronchial asthma and ragweed hypersensitivity. Tracheal mucous veolocity was measured before, immediately after and 1 hr after bronchial challenge with ragweed extract. Mean tracheal mucous velocity, which was moderately decreased in comparison with normal nonsmokers, was further reduced by 28% at the end of bronchial provocation, with a further decrease by 53% after 1 hr when specific airway conductance had returned it to its baseline value (Fig. 10). These changes in mucous transport were prevented by pretreatment with a mast cell

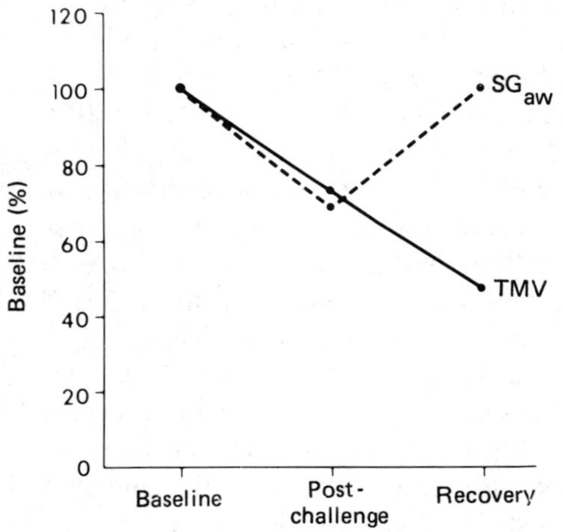

Figure 10 Mean relative changes in mean tracheal mucous velocity (TMV) and specific airway conductance (SG_{aw}) induced by bronchial challenge with ragweed in six asthmatic patients allergic to this antigen. TMV significantly different from baseline at postchallenge and recovery. SG_{aw} at postchallenge only. (From Mezey et al., 1978.)

membrane stabilizing agent, that is sodium cromolyn (Fig. 4). Similar to the findings in the canine asthma model, these human investigations suggested that in patients with allergic asthma and antigen-induced bronchospasm, the tracheal mucous transport is decreased independent of bronchospasm, presumably related to airway anaphylaxis and the release of chemical mediators.

In an attempt to identify the putative chemical mediator, additional experiments were carried out in another group of patients with allergic asthma (Ahmed et al., 1981) (Fig. 11). In this study, tracheal mucous velocity returned to or towards the baseline values at 1 and 2 hr post antigen challenge (Rezek and Millard, 1963). This pattern of response was different from that in the patients of Mezey et al. (1978) in that their patients showed a further decline in tracheal mucous velocity 2 hr post antigen challenge. The discrepancy may have been the result of different experimental designs. The second investigation (Ahmed et al., 1981) required inhalation of bacteriostatic water (placebo) both before and after antigen challenge, and this might have had an irritant effect on mucociliary transport and thus stimulated tracheal mucous velocity after antigen challenge (Foster et al., 1976). However, the siginificance of these observations was not invalidated by the possible placebo effect. By employing the slow-reacting substance antagonist FPL-55712, in conjunction with antigen challenge, we found that the decrease in tracheal mucous velocity after the antigen challenge was not only prevented by prior inhalation of FPL-55712, but reversed to a 30% increase above the baseline (Fig. 11). This effect was observed with both 0.5% and 1% solution of FPL-55712, and there was no difference between the two doses. Similarly, inhalation of FPL-55712 immediately after the antigen challenge also prevented

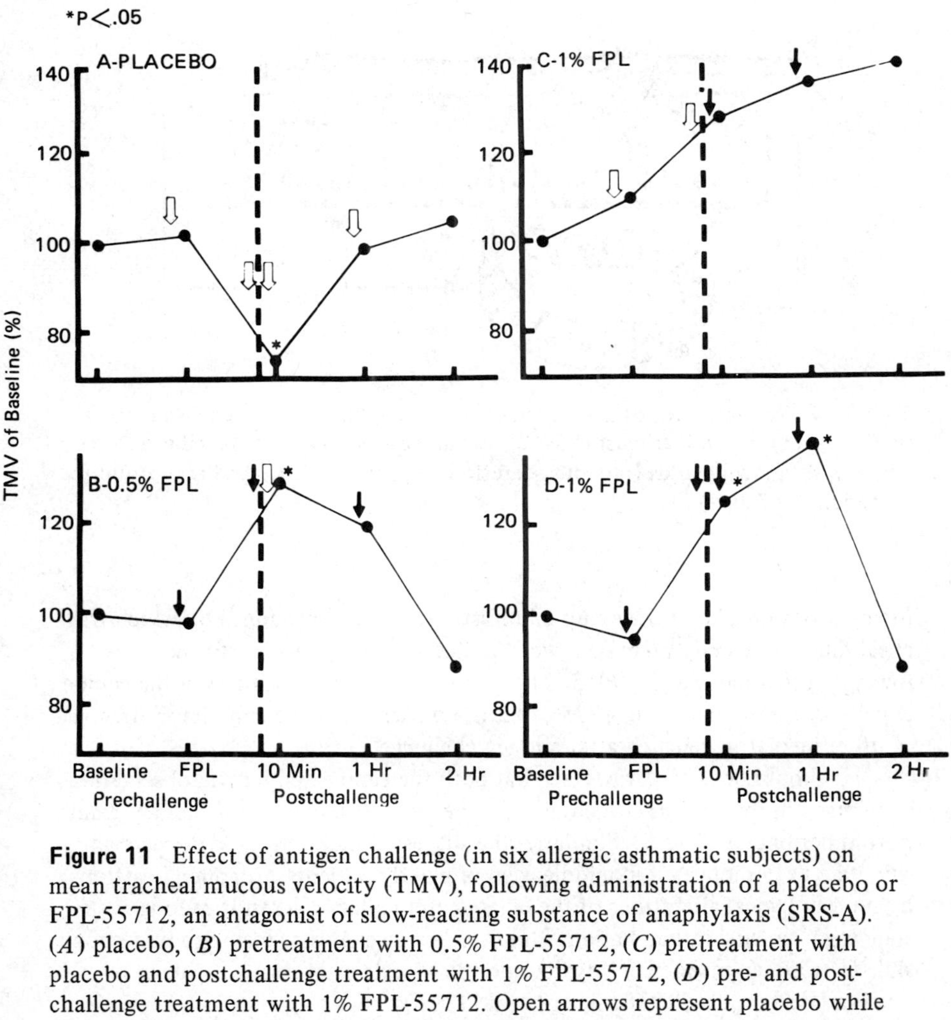

Figure 11 Effect of antigen challenge (in six allergic asthmatic subjects) on mean tracheal mucous velocity (TMV), following administration of a placebo or FPL-55712, an antagonist of slow-reacting substance of anaphylaxis (SRS-A). (*A*) placebo, (*B*) pretreatment with 0.5% FPL-55712, (*C*) pretreatment with placebo and postchallenge treatment with 1% FPL-55712, (*D*) pre- and postchallenge treatment with 1% FPL-55712. Open arrows represent placebo while closed arrows represent administration of FPL-55712 before and/or after antigen challenge. Vertical interrupted line represents time zero at the end of antigen challenge. (From Ahmed et al., 1981.)

the expected decrease in tracheal mucous velocity. As compared with the canine experiments, the observed increase in tracheal mucous velocity in subjects with allergic asthma was of smaller magnitude, probably because of the smaller dose and shorter duration of administration in the canine study of both the antigen and the FPL-55712, a drug which has been shown to have a short plasma half-

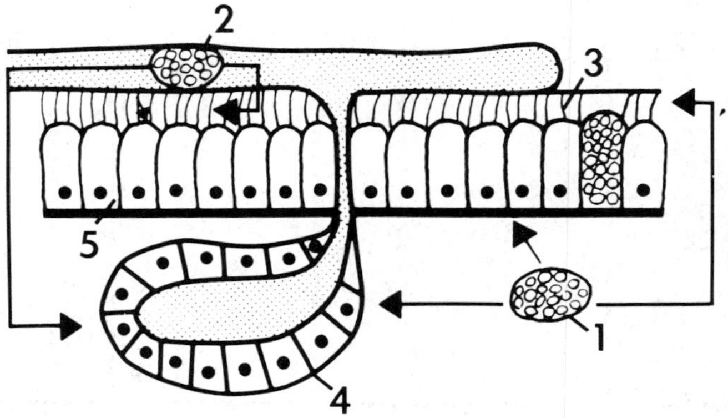

Figure 12 Possible sites of action for chemical mediators released from tissue mast cells (1) or luminal mast cells (2) during airway anaphylaxis: cilia (motility) (3), submucal glands (mucous secretion) (4), and epithelial cells (production of periciliary fluid?) (4).

life of 5-10 min after intravenous administration. The mechanism by which tracheal mucous velocity increased, when antigen challenge was performed following pretreatment with FPL-55712, was presumably the same as in the canine experiments (Wanner et al., 1975), that is, unmasking of the stimulator effects of other mediators released after antigen challenge.

It should be noted, however, that both the canine and human observations were made in the trachea, which may not be representative of mucociliary transport in peripheral airways. Similarly, the suggested pathophysiologic relationship may be complicated in middle-aged or elderly patients with allergic asthma by morphological alterations of the ciliated epithelium as a result of longstanding bronchial inflammation. This or other mechanisms may also be responsible for residual mucociliary dysfunction in allergic asthmatic patients in remission (Foster et al., 1978; Mezey et al., 1978).

This series of experiments conducted in three species (dog, sheep, man) supports the hypothesis that the release of chemical mediators plays an important pathogenetic role in acute mucociliary dysfunction associated with allergic asthma (Fig. 12).

IV. Clinical Implications

Theoretically, mucociliary dysfunction in bronchial asthma may have three major consequences: cough, airflow obstruction, and increased susceptibility to respiratory infections.

A. Cough

In the presence of impaired mucociliary function, cough appears to be an important substitute pulmonary defense mechanism that removes retained respiratory secretions and thereby inhaled foreign materials that have been deposited in the airways. It is not known to what extent excessive airway mucus, as demonstrated by pathologic studies, contributes to the cough of the patient with bronchial asthma, as the cough reflex may also be triggered by inflammatory changes of the epithelium. However, it is a reasonable assumption that a great amount of airway secretions due to increased production and diminished elimination by mucociliary function leads to increased coughing. This hypothesis regarding the relation between the quantity and rheologic properties of airway mucus on the one hand and cough frequency and efficiency on the other has thus far not been tested but clearly deserves to be examined with proper experimental techniques.

B. Airflow Obstruction

Direct structure/function relations have not been established with respect to the effect of excessive airway mucus on airflow obstruction in bronchial asthma; however, there is circumstantial pathologic and physiologic evidence for such a relationship. The postmortem findings of widespread mucous plugging of the airways in patients who die in status asthmaticus have long been considered to represent the major cause of death (Alexander, 1963; Rezek and Millard, 1963; Dunnill et al., 1969). The severity of bronchial obstruction by these mucous plugs clearly demonstrates their contribution to the increased airflow resistance in these patients and hardly requires experimental proof. To what extent mucous plugging of the intermediate and small airways contributes to airflow obstruction in patients with stable bronchial asthma is not known, but appears to be a real possibility at least in childhood asthma as suggested by the histologic observations of Cutz et al. (1978). Finally, it has been suggested that the residual airway dysfunction found in patients with asthma in remission may be partially related to the presence of excessive mucus in peripheral airways (Mcfadden and Lyons, 1968). Frequency dependence of dynamic lung compliance and altered density-dependence of the maximum expiratory flow-volume curve are frequently observed in asymptomatic asthmatic patients with normal or near normal spirometry and airway resistance (Wollcock et al., 1969; Despas et al., 1972). It has been shown that these and similar functional abnormalities suggestive of peripheral airway obstruction are not reversible or only partially reversible by the administration of bronchodilators (McFadden, 1975; Bullow et al., 1978) suggesting excessive airway mucus and/or mucosal edema rather than increased bronchomotor tone as the causes for airflow obstruction. In this regard, the observations of Foster et al. (1978), which suggested abnormal mucous clearance in peripheral airways of such patients, assumes major significance. In normal individuals, submucosal glands and goblet cells are usually absent in peripheral airways that are free of cartilaginous support. Cilia also diminish in number and possibly in length toward the lung periphery (Serafini and Michaelson, 1977). The mechanisms by which mucus accumulates in the peripheral airways are unknown and can only be inferred from morphologic observations. Goblet cell metaplasia suggests mucus hypersecretion, whereas the structural changes in the cilia, in particular fusion of two or more cilia to form a compound cilium (Cutz et al., 1978), indicates ciliary dysfunction. These ciliary abnormalities, however, probably represent secondary, nonspecific changes, since they have also been reported in association with other types of airway disease. An overwhelming of the poorly developed ciliary apparatus by excessive amounts of mucus in the peripheral airways, where ordinarily little or no mucus is secreted, therefore seems to be the more likely explanation for the development of mucus plugging. Abnormal rheologic properties may contribute to faulty mucous transport.

C. Increased Susceptibility to Respiratory Infection

Although epidemiologic data suggest a relation between asthma and respiratory infections (Trendelenburg, 1970), this has not been tested experimentally. The mucociliary dysfunction of bronchial asthma may predispose to respiratory infections by prolonged residence of infectious agents on the respiratory mucosa after impaired transport, the creation of a favorable milieu for the multiplication of infectious agents in pools of airway secretions, or by an inhibitory effect of airway mucus on cellular defense mechanisms. The latter has been recently suggested by Woodside et al. (1981). In addition to the alveoli, macrophages are also present in the airways and may exist either in the periciliary fluid layer or be embedded in mucus (Gil and Weibel, 1971). Some of these macrophages arrive from the pool of alveolar macrophages and may have reached the airways by means of their own migration, while others may arrive from the bronchial circulation and pass directly to the bronchial epithelium (Brain et al., 1977). Mucous plugs in bronchial asthma contain large numbers of macrophages (Cutz et al., 1978); however, the viability of these cells has until recently not been reported.

As a model for the interaction between airway macrophages and mucus in vivo, sheep alveolar macrophages were incubated in vitro with and without airway mucus from the same animal, and their phagocytic function and rates of protein synthesis were tested (Woodside et al., 1981). Administration of pilocarpine by subcutaneous injection was used to obtain tracheal secretions. Studies were carried out without additions, or with mucus 10% by volume or 0.05 mol pilocarpine. Protein synthesis was measured by [^{14}C] phenylalanine incorporation in the presence of 1 mmol L-phenylalanine (Woodside and Massaro, 1979).

Table 2 Effect of Airway Mucus on Protein Synthesis and Phagocytosis of Sheep Alveolar Macrophages[a]

	Protein synthesis (μmol min^{-1}μg^{-1})	Phagocytosis at nonsaturating levels of particles (A_{540})[b]	Phagocytosis at saturating levels of particles (A_{540})[b]
Control (no additions)	0.187 ± 0.013 (6)	1.56 ± 0.17 (3)	4.08 ± 0.33 (6)
Control (pilocarpine 0.05 mM)	0.183 ± 0.018 (6)	1.35 ± 0.05 (3)	3.69 ± 0.18 (6)
Mucus (10% by volume)	0.091 ± 0.009 (6)[c]	0.34 ± 0.08 (5)[c]	2.15 ± 0.23 (6)[c]

[a]Mean values ± SE with number of experiments in parenthesis.
[b]Absorbance at 540 nm.
[c]Significant inhibition ($p < 0.001$).

The rates of phagocytosis were measured with 1.09 μm polystyrene latex particles in the linear portion of the concentration engulfment curve and also at saturating levels of particles (Vassalli et al., 1976). Mucus inhibited protein synthesis significantly by 57%, and phagocytosis at nonsaturating levels of particles by 75% and at saturating levels of particles by 47% (Table 2). Pilocarpine had no effect on protein synthesis and phagocytosis. These results suggest that macrophage function in the tracheobronchial tree may be impaired, particularly in airway diseases associated with mucous hypersecretion including bronchial asthma. How this might alter the susceptibility to respiratory infections remains to be shown.

Despite the scarcity of experimental data relating mucociliary dysfunction to increased susceptibility to respiratory infections in bronchial asthma, the likelihood of such a relation is great and this question therefore deserves further attention. This could be examined by using experimental lung infection in animal models of allergic bronchoconstriction.

D. Treatment and Prevention of Mucociliary Dysfunction in Bronchial Asthma

Based on the physiology and pathophysiology of mucociliary transport in bronchial asthma, physical or pharmacologic intervention might beneficially alter faulty mucociliary function by exerting a mechanical effect on secretions present in the airway lumen, by improving ciliary activity, or by changing the volume and physical properties of periciliary fluid and mucus, thereby improving mucociliary interaction. By using experimental designs that allow separate assessment of individual functions in vitro and in vivo, mechanisms of action have been partially elucidated for some pharmacologic agents. Drugs that are known to increase intracellular cAMP typically stimulate mucociliary transport, but it is not quite clear how exactly cAMP interrelates with ciliary energetics. Of the numerous agents studied, only a few have been reproducibly shown to increase mucous transport rates: adrenergic agonists, cholinergic agonists, and methyl xanthines. In vitro experiments suggest direct stimulation of ciliary activity (Bulbring et al., 1953) and mucus secretion (Sturgess and Reid, 1972) by cholinergic agents, and an increase in chloride and water flux across the airway epithelium by the β-adrenergic agonist terbutaline sulfate (Davis et al., 1975). Stimulation of mucociliary transport by adrenergic agents does not appear to be related to their bronchodilator effect (increase in airway circumference) or increased blood flow to the bronchial mucosa (Foster et al., 1976; Sackner et al., 1976).

With respect to the treatment and prevention of mucociliary dysfunction in patients with airway disease including bronchial asthma, sufficient information has been gathered to draw preliminary conclusions on the effectiveness of the following four measures: (1) stimulation by pharmacologic agents, (2) prevention by pharmacologic agents, (3) physical therapy and bland aerosols, and (4) exercise.

Stimulation by Pharmacologic Agents (Table 3)

β-adrenergic agonists in the dosages recommended for the treatment of bronchospasm have been shown to stimulate mucociliary transport in patients with chronic bronchitis (Santa Cruz et al., 1974; Konietzko et al., 1975), cystic fibrosis (Wood et al., 1975), and asthma (Foster et al., 1978; Mossberg et al., 1976a). This beneficial effect of β-adrenergic agonists seems to encompass the peripheral airways as well (Foster et al., 1978). Stimulation has been observed with all forms of administration and with different β-adrenergic agonists including epinephrine, isoproterenol, and agonists with preferential beta-2 action such as fenoterol, salbutamol, carbuterol, and terbutaline (Iravani, 1972; Van As, 1974b; Sackner et al., 1976). In normal dogs, a dose-dependent effect of inhaled isoproterenol and carbuterol delivered by metered-dose aerosol has been demonstrated (Sackner et al., 1976). Doses of 300 μg of isoproterenol and 500 μg of carbuterol produced increases in tracheal mucociliary transport rates by 100%. The peak effect occurred between 10 and 30 min after drug administration.

Table 3 Pharmacologic Stimulation of Mucociliary Function

Agent	Mucociliary transport	Ciliary motility	Mucous secretion
β-Adrenergic agonists	Stimulation	Stimulation	?
Methylxanthines	Stimulation	?	?
Cholinergic agonists	Stimulation	Stimulation	Stimulation
Prostaglandin E_1	Stimulation	Stimulation	Stimulation

Although the observed increases in mucous transport rates after treatment with β-adrenergic agonists have reached 100% in normal animals (Sackner et al., 1976) and patients with decreased baseline mucous transport rates (Santa Cruz et al., 1974; Wood et al., 1975), the clinical significance of such an effect must be evaluated in light of the baseline values. The doubling of mucous transport rates in a normal individual may represent a substantial increase, whereas a doubling from 10% of normal to 20% of normal in a patient may be of little benefit. In addition, the observations of Mossberg et al. (1976b, 1977) suggest that the stimulatory effect of β-adrenergic agonists is greater in normal individuals than in patients with chronic bronchitis, and in the latter group greater in patients with mild to moderate disease than in patients with severe disease as determined by the forced expiratory volume 1 sec (FEV_1). The concomitant administration of β-adrenergic agonists and methyl xanthines which in themselves stimulate mucous transport (Nelson and Wright, 1974; Serafini et al., 1976) may have an additive or synergistic effect. The exact mechanism by which β-adrenergic agonists stimulate mucociliary transport is not clear but seems to involve ciliary stimulation (Verdugo et al., 1980). They also stimulate mucous secretion from submucosal glands (Sturgess and Reid, 1972; Phipps et al., 1980) as well as the transport of chloride and water across the tracheal wall into the lumen (Davis et al., 1975). This has been supported by the demonstration of increased amounts of respiratory secretions after the administration of terbutaline sulfate in the intact dog tracheal pouch preparation (Giordano et al., 1978).

Prostaglandin E_1 has been shown to stimulate mucociliary transport, mucous secretion, and ciliary motility in vivo and in vitro (Iravani et al., 1976; Maurer et al., 1981). However, these potentially beneficial effects have not been tested in intact humans.

Cholinergic agents, although potent stimulators of mucous transport, cannot be administered to patients with airway disease because of their bronchoconstrictor effect. They stimulate ciliary activity directly (Bulbring et al., 1953), cause hypersecretion of mucus (Sturgess and Reid, 1972), alter the rheologic properties of respiratory secretions (King and Viires, 1979), and stimulate mucociliary clearance in vivo (Camner et al., 1974; Berger et al., 1978). Inhaled mucolytic agents, although effective in reducing the viscosity of mucus in vitro, may be quite irritating to the airway mucosa when administered by inhalation and can promote bronchospasm. In addition, the beneficial effect of inhaled (*N*-acetylcysteine) or oral (*S*-carboxymethylcysteine) mucolytic agents have not been clearly demonstrated, and their use remains controversial (Carson et al., 1968; Thomson et al., 1975; Giordano et al., 1978; Goodman et al., 1978b; Iravani et al., 1978). If mucous hypersecretion is an important factor in mucociliary function, the administration of anticholinergic agents may be of benefit. Unfortunately, atropine has been shown to impair mucociliary transport by most investigators, and it seems to increase the viscoelasticity of respiratory secretions (Wanner, 1977). Ipratropium bromide, a newly introduced atropine analog with a clear-cut bronchodilator effect, seems to lack a depressant effect of mucociliary transport in normal subjects and patients with airway disease (Francis et al., 1977; Sackner et al., 1977). Its effect on mucous secretion has not been evaluated.

Prevention of Mucociliary Dysfunction

The protective actions of cromolyn sodium and the stimulating effects of compound FPL-55712, a relatively selective antagonist of SRS-A in antigen-induced mucociliary dysfunction suggest that they could play a beneficial role in patients with allergic asthma. The clinical trials necessary to substantiate the beneficial role of these agents have not been carried out.

Physical Therapy and Bland Aerosols

A number of recent studies involving actual measurements of mucociliary transport rates seem to support the clinical impression that chest clapping, postural drainage, and systemic hydration are beneficial measures in patients with retained tracheobronchial secretions. In normal subjects, the inhalation of water aerosol seems to be without effect on overall pulmonary mucociliary clearance, whereas hypotonic saline has been reported to stimulate tracheal mucociliary transport rates by 30%. This suggests an effect in central airways. However, this effect was not observed in patients with cystic fibrosis. In patients with chronic bronchitis, a significant stimulation of mucociliary clearance has been observed after inhalation of normal or hypertonic saline aerosols. It has not been determined whether inhalation of the hypertonic saline aerosol improved mucociliary clearance by enhancing mucociliary transport or by rendering cough more effective at removing secretions from the airways. Further studies will be needed to assess the exact role of bland aerosols in the treatment of mucociliary dysfunction associated with airway disease, including bronchial asthma.

Exercise

Intermittent excerise for approximately 1 hr by healthy nonsmokers has been shown to produce slight stimulation of mucociliary clearance which became significant after 2 hr (Wolff et al., 1977). Intermittent eucapnic hyperventilation was less effective. This has not been studied in patients with airway disease. The demonstration of similar or greater effects of exercise on mucociliary transport in patients with airway disease could have interesting therapeutic implications, realizing the adverse effects of exercise on bronchomotor tone in many patients with bronchial asthma.

References

Ahmed, T., Greenblatt, D. W., Birch, S., Marchette, B., and Wanner, A. (1981). Abnormal mucociliary transport in allergic patients with antigen-induced bronchospasm: Rose of SRS-A. *Am. Rev. Respir. Dis., 124*:110-114.

Alexander, H. L. (1963). A historical account of death from asthma. *J. Allergy, 34*:305-322.

Balfre, K., Yerger, L. D., Woodside, K. H., and Wanner, A. (1980). Effect of purified *Ascaris suum* antigen on secretion of sulfated macromolecules in sensitized sheep trachea. *Fed. Proc., 39*:707.

Berger, J., Albert, R. E., Sanborn, K., and Littman, M. (1978). Effects of atropine and methacholine on deposition and clearance of inhaled particles in the donkey. *J. Toxicol. Environ. Health, 4*:587-604.

Brain, J. D., Sorokin, S. D., and Godleski, J. J. (1977). In *Respiratory Defense Mechanisms.* Edited by J. D. Brain, D. F. Proctor, and L. M. Reid. New York, Marcel Dekker, Inc., pp. 849-892.

Bulbring, E., Burn, J. H., and Shelley, H. J. (1953). Acetylcholine and ciliary movement in the gill plates of Mytilus edulis. *Proc. R. Soc. Lond. (Biol.), 141*:445-466.

Bullow, K., Arborelius, M., Christensson, P., and Lilja, B. (1978). Changes in volume of trapped gas in the lungs during provoked asthma followed by beta-2 receptor stimulation. *Respiration, 36*:19-27.

Callerame, M. L., and Condemi, J. J., Bohrod, M. G., and Vaughan, J. H. (1971a). Immunologic reactions of bronchial tissues in asthma. *N. Engl. J. Med., 284*:459-464.

Callerame, M. L., Condemi, J. J., Ishizaka, K., Johansson, S. G. O., and Vaughan, J. H. (1971b). Immunoglobulins in bronchial tissues from patients with asthma, with special reference to immunoglobulin E. *J. Allergy, 47*:187-197.

Camner, P., Strandberg, K., and Philipson, K. (1974). Increased mucociliary transport by cholinergic stimulation. *Arch. Environ. Health, 29*:220-224.

Carson, S., Goldhamer, R., and Carpenter, R. (1968). Responses of ciliated epithelium to irritants: mucus transport in the respiratory tract. *Am. Rev. Respir. Dis., 97*:86-92.

Charman, J., and Reid, L. (1972). Sputum viscosity in chronic bronchitis, bronchiectasis, asthma, and cystic fibrosis. *Biorheology, 9*:185-199.

Chen, T. M., and Dulfano, M. J. (1978). Mucus viscoelasticity and mucociliary transport rate. *J. Lab. Clin. Med., 91*:423-431.

Cutz, E., Levison, H., and Cooper, D. M. (1978). Ultrastructure of airways in children with asthma. *Histopathology, 2*:407-421.

Davis, B., Marin, M. G., and Nadel, J. A. (1975). B-adrenergic receptor in canine tracheal epithelium. *Am. Rev. Respir. Dis., 112*:57.

Dennis, E. G., Hornbrook, M. M., and Ishizaka, K. (1964). Serum proteins in sputum of patients with asthma. *J. Allergy, 34*:464-471.

Despas, P. J., Leroux, M., and Macklem, P. T. (1972). Site of airway obstruction in asthma as determined by measuring maximal expiratory flow breathing air and a helium oxygen mixture. *J. Clin. Invest., 51*:3235-3243.

Dulfano, M. J., Adler, K., and Philippoff, W. (1971). Sputum viscoelasticity in chronic bronchitis. *Am. Rev. Respir. Dis., 104*:88-98.

Dunnill, M. S., Massarella, G. R., and Anderson, J. A. (1969). A comparison of the quantitative anatomy of the bronchi in normal subjects, in status asthmaticus, in chronic bronchitis, and in emphysema. *Thorax, 24*:176-179.

Dunnill, M. S., (1960). The pathology of asthma, with special reference to changes in the bronchial mucosa. *J. Clin. Pathol., 13*:27-33.

Foster, W. M., Langenback, E., Bohning, D., and Bergofsky, E. H. (1978). Quantitation of mucus clearance in peripheral lung and comparison with tracheal and bronchial mucus transport velocities in man: Adrenergics return depressed clearance and transport velocities in asthmatics to normal. *Am. Rev. Respir. Dis., 117* (Suppl):337.

Foster, W. M., Bergofsky, E. H., Bohning, D. E., Limann, M., and Alberut, R. E. (1976). Effect of adrenergic agents and their mode of action on mucociliary clearance in man. *J. Appl. Physiol., 41*:146-152.

Francis, R. A., Thomson, M. L., Pavia, D., and Douglas, R. B. (1977). Ipratropium bromide: mucociliary clearance rate and airway resistance in normal subjects. *Br. J. Dis. Chest, 71*:173-178.

Friedman, M., Stott, F. D., Poole, D. O., Dougherty, R., Chapman, G. A., Watson, H., and Sackner, M. A. (1977). A new roentgenographic method for estimating mucous velocity in airways. *Am. Rev. Respir. Dis., 115*:67-72.

Gil, J., and Weibel, E. R. (1971). Extracellular lining of bronchioles after fixation of rat lungs for electron microscopy. *Anat. Rec., 169*:185-199.

Giordano, A., Holsclaw, D., and Litt, M. (1978). Effects of various drugs on canine tracheal mucociliary transport. *Ann. Otol. Rhinol. Laryngol., 87*: 484-490.

Gold, W. M., Kaufman, H. S., and Nadel, J. A. (1967). Elastic recoil of the lung in chronic asthmatic patients before and after therapy. *J. Appl. Physiol., 23*:433-438.

Gold, W. M., Kessler, G. F., Yu, D. Y. C., and Frick, O. L. (1972). Pulmonary physiologic abnormalities in experimental asthma in dogs. *J. Appl. Physiol., 33*:496-501.

Goodman, R. M., Yergin, B. M., Landa, J. F., Golinvaux, M. A., and Sackner, M. A. (1978a). Relationship of smoking history and pulmonary function tests to tracheal mucous velocity in non-smokers, young smokers, ex-smokers and patients with chronic bronchitis. *Am. Rev. Respir. Dis., 117*: 205-214.

Goodman, R. M., Yergin, B. M., and Sackner, M. A. (1978b). Effects of S-carboxymethylcysteine on tracheal mucus velocity. *Chest, 74*:615-618.

Guirgis, H. A., and Townley, R. G. (1973). Biochemical study on sputum in asthma and emphysema. *J. Allergy Clin. Immunol., 51*:86.

Hilding, A. C. (1957). Ciliary streaming in the lower respiratory tract. *Am. J. Physiol., 191*:404-410.

Iravani, J. (1972). Wirkung einiger bronchodilatierender Substanzen auf die Flimmeraktivitat unter besonderer Berucksichtigung von Berotec. *Int. J. Clin. Pharmacol. Biopharm., 4* (Suppl):20-27.

Iravani, J., Melville, G. N., and Horstmann, G. (1978). *N*-acetylcysteine and mucociliary activity in mammalian airways. *Arzneim Forsch, 28*:250-254.

Iravani, J., Melville, G. N., and Richter, H. G. (1976). Mucus production influenced by drugs: an electron microscopic study. *Pneumonologie*, Suppl.: 267.

King, M., and Viires, N. (1979). Effect of methacholine chloride on rheology and transport of canine tracheal mucus. *J. Appl. Physiol., 47*:26-31.

Konietzko, N., Klopfer, M., Adam, W. E., and Matthys, H. (1975). Die mukociliare Klarfunktion der Lunge unter B-adrenerger Stimulation. *Pneumonologie, 152*:203-209.

Litt, M., and Eng, D. (1970). Mucus rheology: Relevance to mucociliary clearance. *Arch. Intern. Med., 126*:417-423.

Lucas, A. M., and Douglas, L. C. (1934). Principles underlying ciliary activity in respiratory tract. *Arch. Otolaryngol., 20*:518-541.

Marin, M. G., Davis, B., and Nadel, J. A. (1977). Effect of histamine on electrical and ion transport properties of tracheal epithelium. *Am. J. Physiol., 42*: 735-738.

Maurer, D. R., Sielzak, M., Oliver, W., Abraham, W. M., and Wanner, A. (1982). Role of ciliary motility in acute allergic mucociliary dysfunction. *J. Appl. Physiol., 52*:1018-1023.

Maurer, D. R., Schor, J., Sielzak, M., Wanner, A., and Abraham, W. M. (1982). Ciliary motility in airway anaphylaxis. *Cell Motility, 1*:67-70.

McFadden, E. R., Jr. (1975). Exertional dyspnea and cough as precludes to acute attacks of bronchial asthma. *N. Engl. J. Med., 29*:555-559

McFadden, E. R., Jr., and Lyons, H. A. (1968). Airway resistance and uneven ventilation in bronchial asthma. *J. Appl. Physiol., 25*:365-370.

Mezey, R. J., Cohn, M. A., Fernandez, R. J., Januszkiewicz, A. J., and Wanner, A. (1978). Mucociliary transport in allergic patients with antigen-induced bronchospasm. *Am. Rev. Respir. Dis., 118*:677-684.

Miller, C. E. (1968). The kinematics and dynamics of ciliary fluid system. *J. Exp. Biol., 49*:617-629.

Mossberg, B., Strandberg, K., and Camner, P. (1977). Stimulatory effect of beta-adrenergic drugs on mucociliary transport. *Scand. J. Respir. Dis.* (Suppl.), *101*:71-78.

Mossberg, B., Strandberg, K., Philipson, K., and Camner, P. (1976a). Tracheobronchial clearance in bronchial asthma: Response to beta-adrenoreceptor stimulation. *Scand. J. Respir. Dis., 57*:119-128.

Mossberg, B., Strandberg, K., Philipson, K., and Camner, P. (1976b). Tracheobronchial clearance and beta-adrenoceptor stimulation in patients with chronic bronchitis. *Scand. J. Respir. Dis., 57*:281-289.

Nelson, D. J., and Wright, E. M. (1974). The distribution, activity and function of the cilia in the frog brain. *J. Physiol., 243*:63-77.

Olver, R. E., Davis, B., Marin, M. G., and Nadel, J. (1975). Active transport of Na^+ and Cl^- across the canine tracheal epithelium in vitro. *Am. Rev. Respir. Dis., 112*:811-815.

Pepys, J., and Hutchcroft, B. T. (1975). Bronchial provocation tests in etiologic diagnosis and analysis of asthma. *Am. Rev. Respir. Dis., 112*:829-859.

Phipps, R. J., Nadel, J. A., and Davis, B. (1980). Effect of alpha-adrenergic stimulation on mucus secretion and on ion transport in cat trachea in vitro. *Am. Rev. Respir. Dis., 121*:359-365.

Phipps, R., Denas, S., and Wanner, A. (1982). Antigen alters tracheal glycoprotein secretion and ion fluxes in allergic sheep. *Fed. Proc., 41*:1509.

Reid, L. (1965). Natural history of mucus in the bronchial tree. *Arch. Environ. Health, 10*:265-273.

Rezek, P. R., and Millard, M. (1963). Autopsy Pathology. Springfield, IL., Charles E. Thomas, pp. 364.

Ross, S. M., and Corrsin, S. (1974). Results of an analytical model of mucociliary pumping. *J. Appl. Physiol., 37*:333-340.

Sackner, M. A., Chapman, G. A., and Dougherty, R. D. (1977). Effect of nebulized ipratropium bromide and atropine sulfate on tracheal mucous velocity and lung mechanics in anesthetized dogs. *Respiration, 34*:181-185.

Sackner, M. A., Epstein, S., and Wanner, A. (1976). Effect of beta adrenergic agonist aerosolized by Freon propellant on tracheal mucous velocity and cardiac output. *Chest, 69*:593-598.

Sackner, M. A., Yergin, B. M., Brito, M., and Januszkiewicz, A. (1979). Effect of adrenergic agonists on tracheal mucous velocity. *Bull. Eur. Physiopathol. Respir., 15*:505-511.

Santa Cruz, R., Landa, J., Hirsch, J., and Sackner, M. A. (1974). Tracheal mucous velocity in normal man and in patients with chronic obstructive lung disease: Effects of terbutaline. *Am. Rev. Respir. Dis., 109*:458-463.

Serafini, S. M., and Michaelson, E. D. (1977). Length and distribution of cilia in human and canine airways. *Bull. Eur. Physiopathol. Respir., 13*:551-559.

Serafini, S. M., Wanner, A., and Michaelson, E. D. (1976). Mucociliary transport in central and intermediate size airways: effect of aminophylline. *Bull. Eur. Physiopathol. Respir., 12*:415-418.

Shaw, R. R., Paulson, D. L., and Kee, J. L. (1957). Mucoid impaction of the bronchi: A study of thirty-six cases. *Am. Rev. Tuberc. Pulm. Dis., 76*:970-982.

Stewart, W. C. (1948). Weight-carrying capacity and excitability of excised ciliated epithelium. *Am. J. Physiol., 152*:1-5.

Sturgess, J., and Reid, L. (1972). An organ culture study of the effect of drugs on the secretory activity of the human bronchial submucosal gland. *Clin. Sci., 43*:533-543.

Thomson, M. L., Pavia, D., Jones, C. J., and McQuinston, A. C. (1975). No demonstrable effect of S-carboxy-methylcysteine on clearance of secretions from the human lung. *Thorax, 30*:669-673.

Trendelenburg, F. (1970). Bacteriology of chronic lung disease. *Respiration* (Suppl.), *27*:199-211.

Van As, A. (1974). The role of selective B_2-adrenoreceptor stimulants in the control of ciliary activity. *Respiration, 31*:146-151.

Van As, A., and Webster, I. (1974). The morphology of mucus in mammalian pulmonary airways. *Environ. Res., 7*:1-8.

Vassalli, J-D., Hamilton, J., and Reich, E. (1976). Macrophage plasminogen activator: Modulation of enzyme production by anti-inflammatory steroids, mitotic inhibitors, and cyclic nucleotides. *Cell, 8*:271-281.

Verdugo, P., Johnson, N., and Tam, P. (1980). B-adrenergic stimulation of respiratory ciliary activity. *J. Appl. Physiol., 48*:868-871.

von Hoffman, H., and Ebelt, H. (1968). Der elektrolytgehalt des sputums und des serums bei patienten mit asthma bronchiale und bei patienten mit chronischer bronchitis. *Allerg Asthmaforsch, 14*:227-239.

Wanner, A., (1977). State of the Art: Clinical aspects of mucociliary transport. *Am. Rev. Respir. Dis., 116*:73-125.

Wanner, A. (1979b). The role of mucociliary dysfunction in bronchial asthma. *Am. J. Med., 67*:477-485.

Wanner, A., and Rao, A. (1980). Clinical indications for and effects of bland, mucolytic and antibiotic aerosols. *Am. Rev. Respir. Dis., 122*:79-87.

Wanner, A., Mezey, R. J., Reinhart, M. E., and Eyre, P. (1979a). Antigen-induced bronchospasm in conscious sheep. *J. Appl. Physiol., 47*:917-922.

Wanner, A., Zarzecki, S., Hirsch, J., and Epstein, S. (1975). Tracheal mucous transport in experimental canine asthma. *J. Appl. Physiol., 39*:950-957.

Weissberger, D., Oliver, W., Jr., Abraham, W. M., and Wanner, A. (1981). Impaired tracheal mucous transport in allergic bronchoconstriction: effect of terbutaline pretreatment. *J. Allergy Clin. Immunol., 67*:357-362.

Wolff, R. K., Dolovich, M. B., Obminski, G., and Newhouse, M. T. (1977). Effects of exercise and eucapnic hyperventilation on bronchial clearance in man. *J. Appl. Physiol., 43*:46-50.

Wood, R. E., Wanner, A., Hirsch, J., and Di Sant'Agnese, A. (1975). Tracheal mucociliary transport in patients with cystic fibrosis and its stimulation by terbutaline. *Am. Rev. Respir. Dis., 111*:733-738.

Woodside, K. H., and Massaro, D. (1979). Degradation of endogenous protein by rabbit pulmonary macrophages. *J. Appl. Physiol., 47*:79-86.

Woodside, K. H., Denas, S. M., Smith, K. L., and Wanner, A. (1983). Inhibition of pulmonary macrophage function by airway mucus. *J. Appl. Physiol.,* in press.

Woolcock, A. J., Vincent, N. J., and Macklem, P. T. (1969). Frequence dependence of compliance as a test for obstruction in the small airways. *J. Clin. Invest., 48*:1097-1106.

Yamatake, Y., Sasagawa, S., Yanaura, S., and Kobayashi, N. (1977). Involvement of histamine H_1- and H_2-receptors in induced asthma in dogs. *Japan. J. Pharmacol., 27*:791-797.

13

Immunopharmacology of Complement Anaphylatoxins in the Lung

NORMA P. STIMLER*

Scripps Clinic and Research Foundation
and University of California School of
Medicine at San Diego
La Jolla, California

COLIN M. BLOOR

University of California
School of Medicine at San Diego
La Jolla, California

TONY E. HUGLI

Scripps Clinic and Research Foundation
La Jolla, California

I. Introduction

A. Anaphylatoxins: Historical Perspective

The first observation of a pathophysiologic response to the complement anaphylatoxins is credited to Friedberger (1910). He found that guinea pigs developed anaphylactoid responses when injected with immune precipitates suspended in homologous serum. The toxicity of this substance produced by mixing antigen-antibody complexes with serum was thus named "anaphylatoxin" and led Friedberger to formulate a humoral theory of anaphylaxis. He believed the active substance was a fragment released from the complexes and that it acted directly on the tissue. Subsequent analysis of the hypothesis that a union of

---

Present Affiliation

*Loyola University Stritch School of Medicine, Maywood, Illinois

This work was supported by grants HL07104, HL25658, and HL16411 from the National Heart Lung and Blood Institute of the National Institutes of Health. This publication #2408 from the Research Institute of Scripps Clinic.

antibody and antigen in serum causes release of a toxic fragment that is responsible for anaphylaxis gave rise to the eventual realization that the complement system was involved. This fact has been fully appreciated only within the past two decades; as recently as 1959, the existence of anaphylatoxins as molecular entities in complement-activated human serum was still in doubt (Florey, 1960).

The research of Schultz (1910) and Dale (1913) raised serious doubts as to the validity of Friedberger's humoral theory by showing that tissues taken from animals that had been presensitized to selected antigens exhibit in vitro anaphylactic responses in the absence of plasma. In a typical experiment, guinea pigs were sensitized by injection of ovalbumin over a period of several weeks. The animals were then sacrificed and segments of either the ileum or the estrous uterus were removed and washed free of blood. These sensitized tissues were shown to undergo contraction when exposed to the antigen, ovalbumin (Dale, 1913). Such experiments, carried out in vitro in media devoid of plasma, led to the development of a cellular theory of anaphylaxis. Additionally, these studies provided a basis for evaluating potentially anaphylactoid substances in vitro. Schultz and Dale described a procedure whereby the ability of isolated factors that induce contraction of isolated tissues may be assessed.

It is now well established that the classical anaphylactic response is largely dependent on immunoglobulins of the IgE class. The physiologic manifestations of the response of sensitized tissues are mediated primarily by histamine, by various products of arachidonic acid metabolism including slow-reacting substance of anaphylaxis (SRS-A) and certain prostaglandins, and by phospholipid mediators such as platelet-activating factor (PAF). The characteristics of many of these mediators and their actions have been extensively reviewed by Austen and Orange (1975), McCoombs (1972), and Johnson et al. (1979).

A second line of investigation that refutes Friedberger's original humoral theory of anaphylaxis concerns the mode of anaphylatoxin generation. Bordet (1913a,b) and Nathan (1913) showed that immune precipitates are not exclusively required for anaphylatoxin production, but that certain polysaccharides such as agar or starch can effectively generate anaphylatoxin activity in normal, unsensitized serum. Novy and DeKruif (1917) demonstrated potent anaphylatoxin activity in rat serum that had simply been diluted with distilled water. Thus, these investigators showed that the precursor or precursors of anaphylatoxin activity are normal constituents of serum and are not introduced by exogenous activators such as antigens.

Hahn and Oberdorf (1950) and Hahn (1954) studied in vivo responses to the anaphylatoxin by injecting activated serum into guinea pigs. They observed that anaphylatoxin acted as a histamine liberator in these animals, with the greatest amount being released from the lung. Pretreatment of guinea pigs with antihistaminics prior to injection of anaphylatoxin afforded protection against the lethal shock reaction (Hahn, 1960). Simultaneously, Rocha e Silva and

Aronson (1952) and Rocha e Silva (1954) characterized the contractile response of isolated guinea pig ileum induced by a partially purified form of the C5a anaphylatoxin. Like Hahn, they demonstrated that contraction of smooth muscle by anaphylatoxin was inhibited by antihistamines. They also observed that the tissue became refractory or was desensitized to subsequent anaphylatoxin-induced contractions upon repeated exposure to the mediator. Thus, the response of guinea pig ileum to anaphylatoxin must involve interaction with specific cellular receptors that in turn promote histamine release.

Until the 1960s, anaphylatoxin was little more than a pharmacologic curiosity, a substance that could be produced by appropriate manipulation of certain animal sera, but whose activity was not observed in human serum and whose origin was speculated to be associated with the then ill-defined complement system. Demonstration that anaphylatoxin formation in serum was indeed commensurate with complement activation was first provided by the work of Osler et al. (1959). In light of the suspected phlogistic potential of these activation products, and a recognition that substantial quantities are formed during complement activation, new and concerted investigations of the anaphylatoxins were begun. Bodammer (1966) and Bodammer and Vogt (1967) presented physiologic data indicating that the purified C5a anaphylatoxin caused acute bronchospasm when injected intravenously into guinea pigs. This response was caused partly by histamine liberation and partly by another unexplained mechanism, which they though might be evidence for a direct action on smooth muscle. Bodammer and Vogt (1970) have subsequently provided more indirect evidence that histamine release may not be the sole mechanism by which anaphylatoxin promotes contraction of the guinea pig ileum, but they failed to identify the nature of the secondary mechanism.

At approximately the same time, Dias da Silva et al. (1967) showed that anaphylatoxin activity was generated when several of the purified human complement proteins were combined, specifically C1 esterase, C4, C2, and component C3. This anaphylatoxin was characterized as a low molecular weight polypeptide derived from the C3 molecule. A very important finding was that the C3-derived anaphylatoxin, although capable of eliciting a contractile response in guinea pig ileum, was apparently unrelated to the "classical anaphylatoxin"* of guinea pig serum since cross-tachyphylaxis did not occur between these two factors. Simultaneously, Jensen (1967), working with guinea pig

---

*Complement components are named in accordance with the World Health Organization Committee on Complement Nomenclature (1968). Classical anaphylatoxin is defined as the des Arg form of the C5a molecule and is obtained by activation of complement in the absence of inhibitors of endogenous serum carboxypeptidase N.

complement components, observed that component C5 also served as a precursor for anaphylatoxin. Furthermore, the C5-derived anaphylatoxin described by Jensen was tachyphylactic to the guinea pig classical anaphylatoxin as judged by the guinea pig ileal assay. The controversy and confusion over the true origin of the classical anaphylatoxin was seemingly resolved by the work of Cochrane and Müller-Eberhard (1968) and Lepow et al. (1968), when they showed that both purified human C3 and C5 released an anaphylatoxin after cleavage by trypsin or by the approrpiate purified complement convertase. These studies clearly demonstrated the existence of not one but two distinct anaphylatoxins, now identified as C3a and C5a.*

By 1970 the polypeptide nature and origin of the anaphylatoxins were established, however considerable puzzlement remained. Although the purified human complement proteins generated active anaphylatoxic fragments in vitro, it was not possible to detect corresponding activities in whole human serum. Only sera from certain animal species possessed the activity, and then only the classical anaphylatoxin activity was evident. This paradox was somewhat clarified when Lepow et al. (1969) and Bokisch et al. (1969) found that human C3a anaphylatoxin generated in vitro from purified C3 rapidly lost activity upon mixing with normal human serum. Thus an "anaphylatoxin inactivator" exists in serum (Bokish and Müller-Eberhard, 1970), and this realization afforded an explanation for the inability to demonstrate C3a activity in complement-activated serum. Human C5a also appears to be inactivated by serum, and it was concluded that a similar, if not identical, enzymatic mechanism was operative on this mediator. C5a from animal species is only partially inactivated by the serum enzyme, thus a residual activity is discerned. The anaphylatoxin inactivator is the same enzyme as that previously described as kininase I (Erdös et al., 1964; Yang and Erdös, 1967), and it is now known as serum carboxypeptidase N (E.C. 3.4.12.7). This enzyme removes the carboxyterminal arginine residue from the anaphylatoxins resulting in a total inactivation of C3a and a partial inactivation of C5a. The fact that sera from animals such as guinea pigs, pigs, and rats contain levels of serum carboxypeptidase comparable to those in man, but only the sera from lower animals have detectable C5a activity, has remained a paradox until very recently.

The apparent absence of residual C5a anaphylatoxin activity in human serum has now been clarified by Gerard and Hugli (1981). These investigators demonstrated that the molecular form of the "classical anaphylatoxin" in porcine serum is indeed $C5a_{des\ Arg\text{-}74}$ but that the corresponding $C5a_{des\ Arg\text{-}74}$

*Gorski et al. (1979) have recently demonstrated the existence of a third anaphylatoxin, C4a, derived from cleavage of C4.

molecule in man possesses a much weaker spasmogenic acitivty. Consequently, human $C5a_{des\ Arg\text{-}74}$ appears inactive when assayed at levels that are generated in serum. In addition, they established that an oligosaccharide group associated with the human, but not the porcine molecule, is partially responsible for human $C5a_{des\ Arg\text{-}74}$ having significantly lower activity compared with the corresponding animal molecule.

In summary, the anaphylatoxin originally detected in animal sera is identified as a polypeptide fragment that is released from the fifth component of complement during activation of the complement cascade. Chemically similar anaphylatoxins are released from complement components C3 and C4 during activation; however, their biological properties are distinct from those of C5a. All of these factors are susceptible to the action of serum carboxypeptidase N. In some animal sera, a significant residual activity is detected after degradation of C5a by serum carboxypeptidase indicating the relative activity of the des Arg form of C5a differs between animal species. It is now accepted that the toxic effects of the classical anaphylatoxin, when injected into guinea pig results largely from the release of secondary mediators. Furthermore, it was early recognized that these peptides have multiple activities. The anaphylatoxins stimulate a multitude of cellular reactions in various tissues underlining the potential of these bioactive complement fragments in host defense and disease processes.

B. Anaphylatoxin: Involvement in Disease

Approximately the same time that the foregoing data were accumulating, separate evidence indicated that the complement system plays a role in allergic reactions of both immediate and delayed hypersensitivity. In studies of cutaneous anaphylaxis, a reaction characterized by enhanced vascular permeability occurring at the site of an antigen-antibody reaction, Osler et al. (1957) found that heterologous noncomplement-fixing antibody gave a minimal reaction in normal rats and that no reaction occurred in rats depleted of serum complement. The cutaneous reaction was recovered by the injection of fresh serum. Similar results dealing with the effect of complement depletion on cutaneous anaphylaxis have been reported in the mouse (Christian and Thurber, 1962). The extensive work of Ishizaka (1963) with heterologous antibody and aggregated γ-globulin also suggests that complement plays a role in cutaneous anaphylaxis.

The role of complement in allergic reactions involving acute damage to vascular structures in the skin, large vessels, and renal glomeruli has also been the subject of extensive investigation. As a result of these studies, there is now reasonable evidence that complement activation is involved in the development of immunologic vasculitis (Linscott and Cochrane, 1964; Ward and Cochrane, 1965), nephrotoxic nephritis (Hammer and Dixon, 1963; Cochrane et al., 1965), and the vasculitis and glomerulitis associated with serum sickness (Kniker and

Cochrane, 1965). There is evidence that IgG and C3 are frequently localized in renal glomeruli of patients with poststreptococcal nephritis and lupus nephritis (Feldman, 1964), suggesting that complement may be involved in the pathogenesis of these lesions. Observations that experimental immunologic vasculitis or glomerulonephritis can be blocked by depletion of either circulating neutrophils (Humphrey, 1955; Cochrane et al., 1965) or complement (Hammer and Dixon, 1963; Cochrane et al., 1965; Ward and Cochrane, 1965) indicate that neutrophils as well as complement are necessary for development of the tissue lesions. The potent chemotactic activity of C5a for neutrophils (Ward et al., 1965, 1966) seems to indicate that at least one of complement's functions is manifest in these processes. Based on the foregoing evidence, anaphylatoxins are presumed to be important mediators in certain types of immediate hypersensitivity reactions, as well as in inflammation.

Detailed chemical descriptions of C3a and C5a obtained from both human and animal sources have recently been reported (Hugli, 1975; Fernandez and Hugli, 1978; Jacobs et al., 1978; Gerard and Hugli, 1980) and these data provide a firm molecular basis for examining relationships between structure and physiologic action. Information concerning the biologic nature of these molecules, particularly their ability to interact with blood leukocytes and stimulate a number of cellular release reactions (reviewed by Hugli, 1978), further supports our hypothesis that the anaphylatoxins play a major role in immunologic disease. Such advances now make it possible to examine the role of purified anaphylatoxins in pathologic processes. In particular, recent work concerning the role of the complement anaphlatoxins in pulmonary lesions stems from a number of reports that acute and chronic pulmonary inflammation may somehow be linked to complement turnover. Circulating antibodies directed against lung tissue have been identified in patients with chronic bronchitis and bronchial asthma (Wagner et al., 1965; Hall et al., 1966; Leopold and Leicht, 1969), emphysema and pulmonary tuberculosis (Hennes et al., 1961), penumoconiosis (Burrell, 1963; Hagadorn and Burrell, 1968), and interstitial fibrosis (McKay and Ritchie, 1965). This facet of research as it pertains to the anaphylatoxins is elaborated in the discussion to follow.

II. Effects of Anaphylatoxins on Pulmonary Function In Vivo

Experimental models of immune complex disease in which rats were injected intravenously with anti-lung globulins revealed two distinct types of reactions (Hagadorn et al., 1969; Vazquez, 1970). A large dose of anti-tissue globulins killed the rats in a few minutes, after they developed severe cyanosis, dyspnea, and pulmonary edema. However, sublethal doses caused less severe physiologic manifestations, and the pulmonary lesions that appeared were transient. In surviving animals occasional interstitial and perivascular lymphocytic infiltrations were observed. A review of other experimental models of immune complex disease (Dixon, 1971; Cochrane and Koffler, 1973) revealed the following events: (1) Basophils and mast cells release PAF, which in turn stimulates release of vasoactive amines from platelets (Henson, 1971); (2) complement becomes activated by the immune complexes with concurrent release of C3a and C5a anaphylatoxins; (3) anaphylatoxin generation results in an additional histamine release from mast cells, and recent evidence suggests that leukotrienes are released from leukocytes and/or macrophages stimulated by these same humoral factors (Stimler et al., 1980a); (4) increased vascular permeability is induced by the anaphylatoxins, histamine, PAF, and the leukotrienes leading to the hemorrhage and edema that are observed; and (5) chemotactic responses of leukocytes stimulated by C5a or by cellular mediators released by C5a result in an accumulation of cells at the site of immune complex deposition followed by the release of hydrolytic enzymes and associated tissue injury (Dixon, 1971; Cochrane and Dixon, 1978). This sequence of events has become a familiar scenario for tissue injury in the lung and may be the hallmark of pulmonary injury induced by humoral mediators.

Investigations of immunologic injury in pulmonary tissue (Scherzer and Ward, 1978a,b; Ward, 1979) show a direct correlation of lung damage with the complement-fixing activity of preformed immune complexes infused intrabronchially into rats. Their studies demonstrate a diffuse, confluent, hemorrhagic reaction in the alveolar spaces, vessel walls, and interstitia of the lungs in these animals. The predominant cell type is the neutrophil and, as expected, the reaction is dependent upon both complement and neutrophils. Chronic formation of immune complexes within the vasculature leads to an interstitial fibrotic reaction and a thickening of basement membranes.

Demonstration by Shin et al. (1968) and others that C5a is the predominant chemoattractant in complement-activated serum led Kreutzer et al. (1979) and Desai et al. (1979) to instill purified human C5a intratracheally into hamsters. They observed an acute inflammatory reaction characterized by large numbers of intraalveolar neutrophils. The extravasation of plasma protein and accumulation of neutrophils were quantified by the use of specific radiolabels, and they found the response to be dependent on the dose of C5a given (Desai et al., 1979). Similar results were observed by Henson et al. (1979) and Larsen et al. (1980) in rabbit lung, although in their studies human $C5a_{des\ Arg\text{-}74}$ seemed to be more potent than intact C5a. (The reader is referred to Chap. 9 in this volume for a comprehensive review of chemotaxis in the lung.)

In a similar series of experiments, porcine C3a and C5a anaphylatoxins were instilled intrabronchially into guinea pigs (Stimler et al., 1980b). We observed acute pulmonary injury characterized by marked tachypnea beginning after 30 sec and lasting for 20 min or longer (Table 1). Histologic examination

Table 1 Physiologic Response of Guinea Pigs to Intrabronchial Infusion of Complement Anaphylatoxins[a]

	Number of animals	Dose (ng/kg)	Respiratory distress[b]	Pulmonary extravasation[c]	Lethal
Porcine C5a	10	8–10	+	ND[d]	0
Porcine $C5a_{des\ Arg\text{-}74}$	10	8–17	+	1.75	5
Porcine C3a	14	200–500	+	1.61	0
Guinea Pig $C5a_{des\ Arg}$[e]	3	3–5	+	ND	1
Guinea Pig ZAS[e]	3	3–4 μg C5a +50–100 μg C3a	+	ND	1
Porcine $C3a_{des\ Arg}$	6	200–500	–	ND	0
Saline	10		–	1.0	0

[a]Anaphylatoxins were dissolved in 0.3 ml of normal saline and administered intrabronchially into anesthetized guinea pigs via a small catheter.
[b]Onset 30 sec after infusion with a 20-30 min duration.
[c]^{125}I-BSA extravasated into the lungs following administration of C3a or C5a relative to saline-treated controls.
[d]Not determined.
[e]Guinea pig serum was activated with zymosan in the presence or absence of IM EACA to give ZAS or $C5a_{des\ Arg}$, respectively. Activated serum was partially purified and concentrated. The quantity administered to each guinea pig was the equivalent of 1 ml serum.
Source: Stimler et al. (1980b).

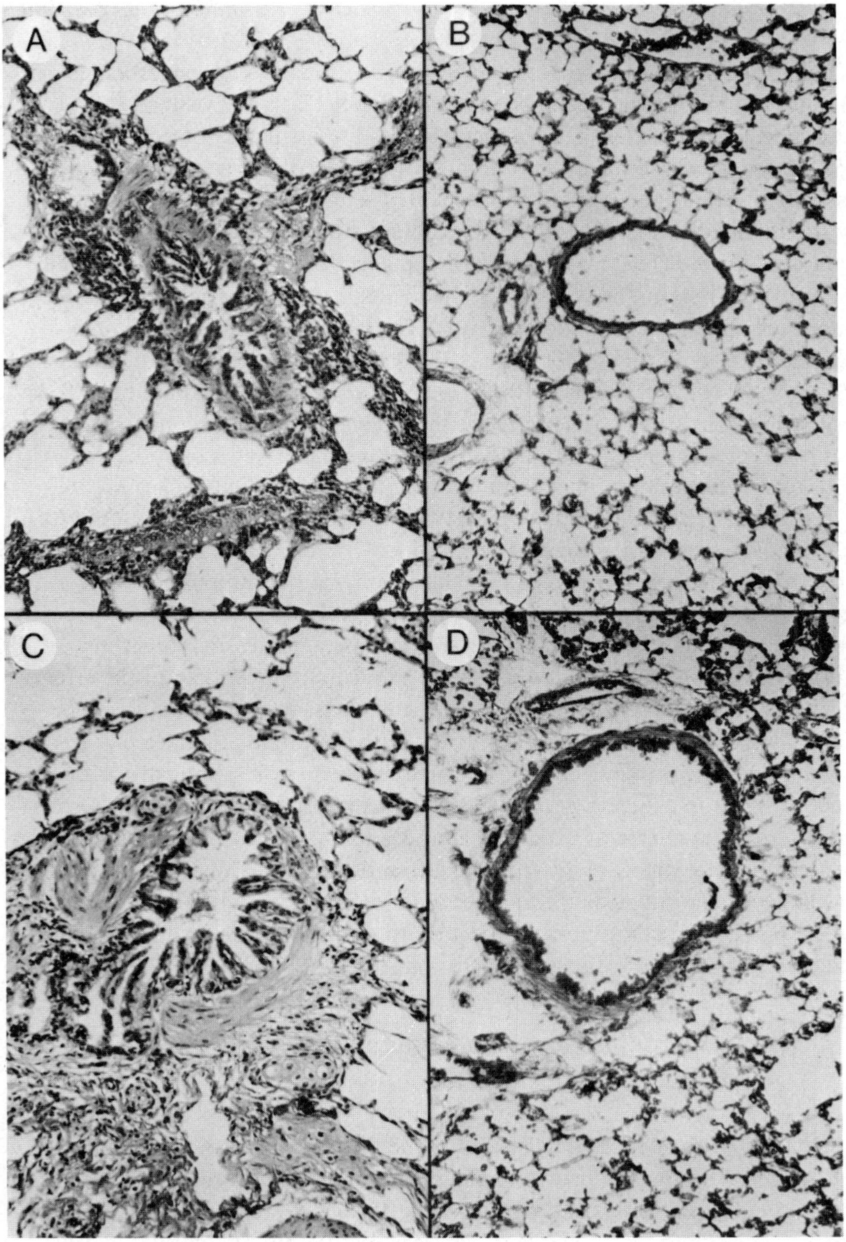

Figure 1 (*A*) Section from the lung of a guinea pig injected intrabronchially with 15 μg/kg porcine C5a (H & E). (*B*) Section from saline-treated control lung (H & E). (*C*) Section from the lung of a guinea pig pretreated ip with 20 mg/kg diphenhydramine followed by intrabronchial instillation of 10 μg/kg porcine C5a (H & E). (*D*) Section from control lung of guinea pig pretreated with 20 mg/kg diphenhydramine followed by 1 μg/kg histamine (H & E).

of guinea pig lung tissue exposed to C3a or C5a showed extensive bronchial and vascular smooth muscle thickening with focal atelectasis and visible intravascular aggregates of platelets and leukocytes (Fig. 1). Instillation of porcine $C5a_{des\ Arg\text{-}74}$ was lethal in some animals within the first few minutes, as was partially purified guinea pig anaphylatoxin (Table 1). Lethal shock was averted by pretreating the animals with antihistamines; however, the bronchospasms were not affected (Fig. 1). We have also reported that anaphylatoxin-induced bronchoconstriction in vivo correlates with a contractile response of isolated guinea pig peripheral airway preparation. The latter response is largely independent of histamine (Stimler et al., 1981a) and recent evidence (Stimler et al., 1980a, 1982b) indicates that SRS-A release from lung tissue exposed to C5a is responsible for tissue contraction. The in vivo responses (i.e., bronchospasm and lethal shock) correspond to effects that Bodammer and Vogt observed (1967) after intravenous injection of porcine anaphylatoxin ($C5a_{des\ Arg\text{-}74}$) into guinea pigs and Hagadorn et al. (1969) observed following injection into rats of antibodies directed against lung.

It is perhaps not surprising that the anaphylactoid response of acute bronchospasm occurs notably only in guinea pigs. Early studies on the bioactivity of the anaphylatoxins established that these peptides are potent mediators of histamine release. Guinea pigs are exquisitely susceptible to the effects of histamine, whereas rats and rabbits are not. Consequently, histamine is believed to play a central role in the severity of the response of guinea pigs to anaphylatoxins. The prophylactic effect of antihistamines on anaphylatoxin-induced shock in guinea pigs strongly suggests that the lethal syndrome results largely from the release of histamine as a secondary mediator. Since the complement anaphylatoxins have different manifestations in individual animal species, it will be of major importance to determine whether C5a-induced histamine and SRS-A release contribute significantly to the clinical manifestations of acute and chronic pulmonary disease in man.

III. In Vitro Studies of Anaphylatoxins on Pulmonary Tissue

In an effort to more quantitatively study the bronchospasms observed in guinea pigs treated with the complement anaphylatoxins, several groups have employed in vitro methods of investigation. The work of Dale (1913) established that contraction of isolated guinea pig ileum serves as a criterion for assessing the anaphylatoxic activity of a substance. It is well documented that C3a and C5a anaphylatoxins stimulate contraction of ileal smooth muscle, a reaction that is mediated, at least in this tissue, primarily by histamine release (Rocha e Silva, 1954; Hahn, 1954). The newly described anaphylatoxin, C4a shows a similar activity, however this factor is much less potent than C3a or C5a (Gorski, et al.,

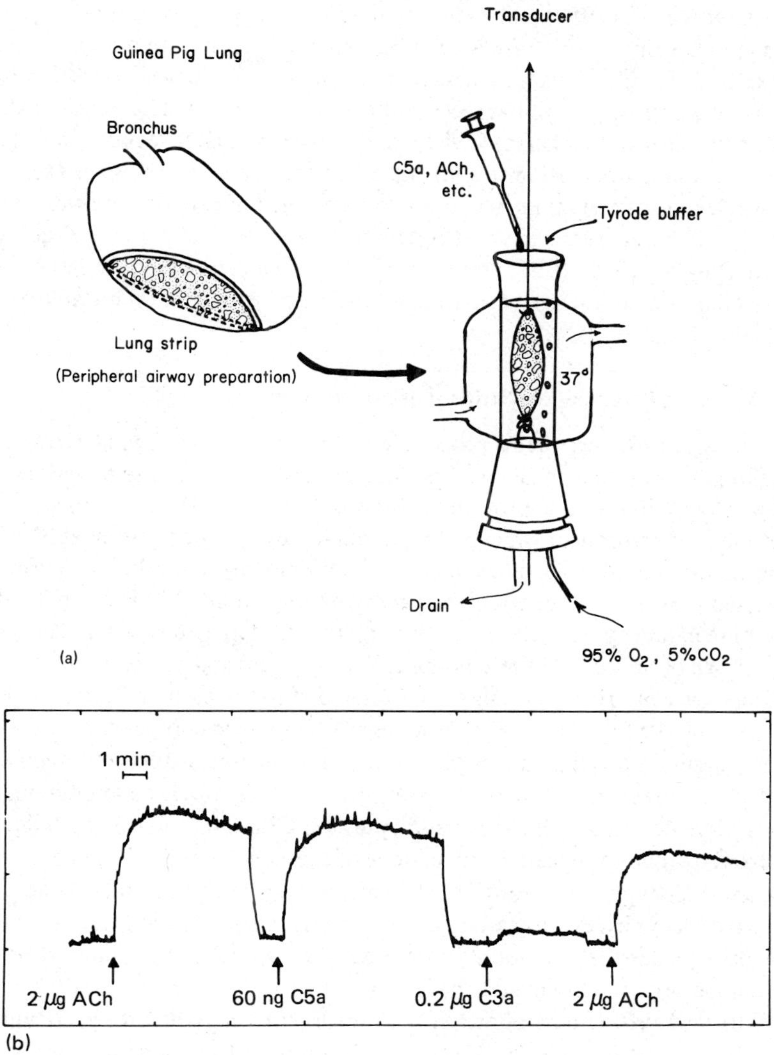

Figure 2 (*A*) Schematic diagram of apparatus used for quantitating responses of isolated guinea pig lung strips. Preparations of peripheral airway tissue from guinea pig lung are tested for the contractile activity of the anaphylatoxin peptides as illustrated. (*B*) Typical kymograph tracing of contractile responses of guinea pig lung strips exposed to 2μg/ml ACh, 60 ng/ml C5a, 0.2 μg/ml C3a, and 2 μg/ml ACh are shown. After each contractile response was recorded the chart was stopped; then the tissue was washed with fresh Tyrode buffer and allowed to relax for 15 min before subsequent challenge.

1979). Greeff et al. (1959) and Kleine et al. (1970) have reported that anaphylatoxins induce contraction of isolated guinea pig tracheal smooth muscle and of other smooth muscle-containing tissues. The response of tracheal smooth muscle to guinea pig $C5a_{des\ Arg\text{-}74}$ has recently been studied in detail by Regal et al. (1980) and Regal and Pickering (1981), as discussed in a later section. In spite of the overwhelming temptation to generalize that the anaphylatoxins act exclusively as releasers of histamine, based on data obtained in experiments with the ileum, several observations in vivo (Bodammer, 1966; Bodammer and Vogt, 1967; Sackeyfio, 1971, 1975; Stimler et al., 1980b) indicate that the response of pulmonary tissue to these mediators is much less dependent on histamine than is the ileum.

A. Lung Parenchymal Strips (Peripheral Airways)

Lulich et al. (1976) described a procedure for mounting parenchymal strips of cat lung to assess the behavior of peripheral airways in response to various pharmacologic stimuli. The procedure involves attaching tissue strips to a smooth muscle transducer while bathing them in physiologic solution at 37°C. In this manner the pharmacologic behavior of pulmonary smooth muscle can be assessed in relatively quantitative terms. We have modified Lulich's method to examine parenchymal strips of guinea pig lung, as depicted schematically in Figure 2. We observed that these peripheral airway preparations contract immediately after purified C3a, C4a, or C5a is added to the bathing fluid (Stimler et al., 1980b, 1981a). This in vitro response of lung tissue correlates with the bronchospasm observed in guinea pigs after intrabronchial instillation of anaphylatoxin. Moreover, the anaphylatoxins produce tachyphylaxis in pulmonary tissue as they do in the guinea pig ileum; purified C3a, C4a, and C5a each desensitize the tissue to repeated applications of the same peptide. C3a and C4a are not tachyphylactic for C5a, or vice versa; however, C3a and C4a do show cross-tachyphylaxis toward one another. The anaphylatoxins are not toxic to the tissue, since they do not affect subsequent responses of the lung strips to histamine or acetylcholine (ACh).

The lung tissue preparations contain small pulmonary blood vessels and contractile cells of the alveolar interstitium in addition to peripheral airways. Therefore, changes in length or tension of the strips reflect the combined responses of this heterogeneous mixture of contractile elements. Which of these elements or how many are responsible for anaphylatoxin-induced contraction (or in fact for contractions induced by other agonists) is not yet clear. However, based on the photomicrographs of lungs treated in vivo (Fig. 1), all of the contractile elements are probably affected to some degree. Regardless, the responses of isolated lung strips represent peripheral airway responses in vivo, and we believe the importance of these observations is reflected in the physiologic

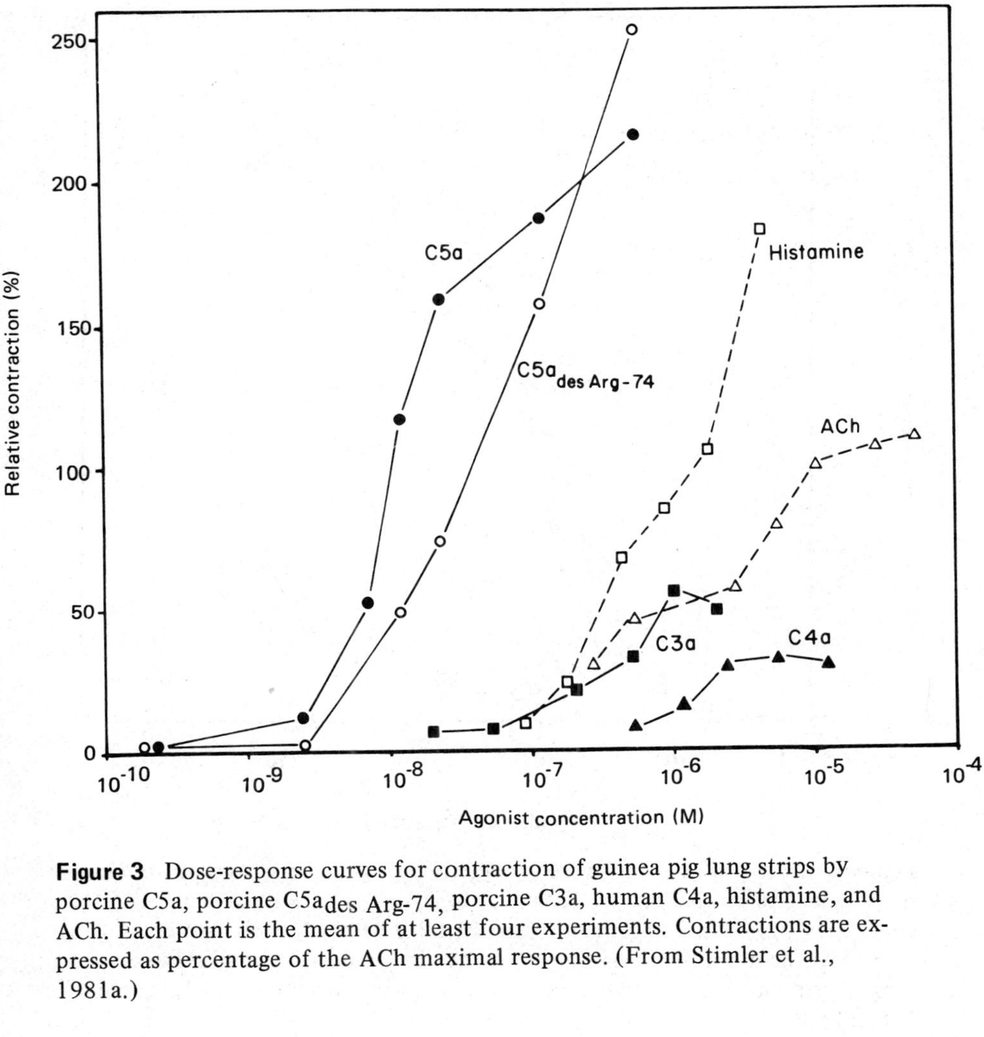

Figure 3 Dose-response curves for contraction of guinea pig lung strips by porcine C5a, porcine C5a$_{\text{des Arg-74}}$, porcine C3a, human C4a, histamine, and ACh. Each point is the mean of at least four experiments. Contractions are expressed as percentage of the ACh maximal response. (From Stimler et al., 1981a.)

manifestations of pulmonary dysfunction. Unfortunately, complete evaluation of the model system will be realized only when the individual cellular mechanisms are understood.

The use of homogeneous anaphylatoxins (C3a, C4a, and C5a) obtained from human or porcine serum has permitted us to generate dose-response curves on isolated guinea pig lung strips. These data are shown in Figure 3 in which the anaphylatoxins are compared with the standard agonists histamine and ACh. C5a obtained from porcine or human serum is by far the most potent of the

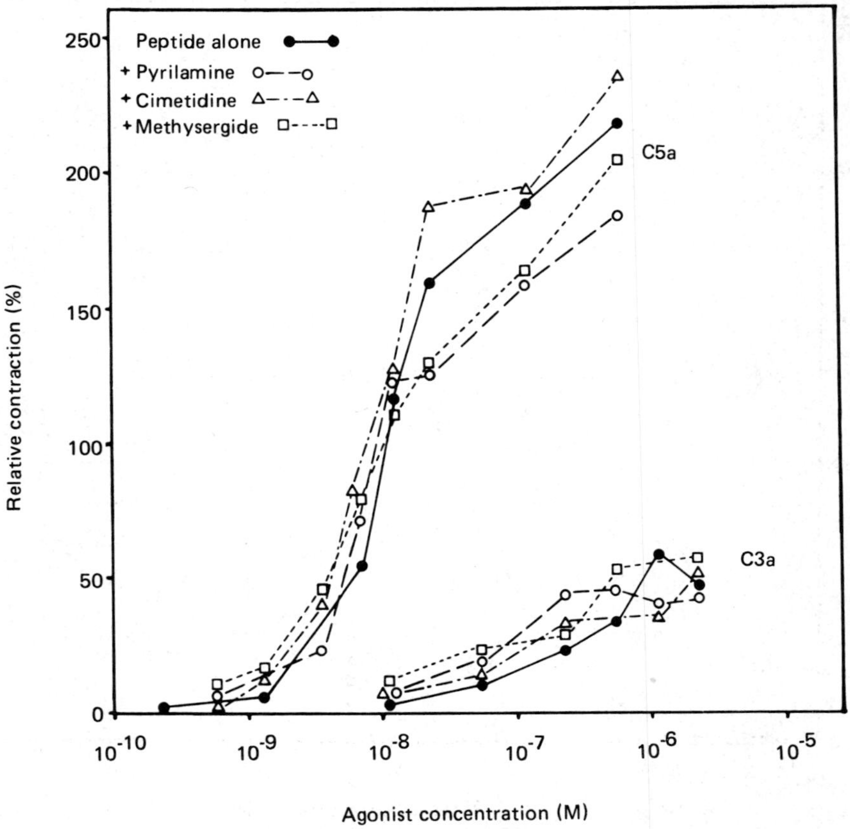

Figure 4 Dose-response curves for contractions of guinea pig lung strips induced by porcine C5a or C3a, in Tyrode buffer alone, in Tyrode + pyrilamine, 10^{-6} M, cimetidine, 1.2×10^{-5} M, or methysergide, 1.1×10^{-5} M. Each data point represents the mean of at least four separate experiments. Contractions are expressed as the percentage of the ACh maximal response. (From Stimler et al., 1981a.)

substances examined, requiring concentrations of only 1-2 $\times 10^{-9}$ M to stimulate appreciable contraction. Human or porcine C3a at 10^{-7} M and human C4a at 10^{-6} M induce threshold contractile responses of lung strips. Both histamine and ACh initiate contractions at a level of 1-2 $\times 10^{-7}$ M. The des Arg derivative of porcine C5a, a physiologic form of C5a resulting from the action of serum carboxypeptidase, is slightly less potent than intact C5a with a roughly parallel dose-response curve. Human or porcine $C3a_{des\ Arg\text{-}77}$ was not active at 10^{-6} M.

Human $C5a_{des\ Arg\text{-}74}$ was not active at concentrations up to 10^{-7} M and higher concentrations have not been tested in this system. However, human $C4a_{des\ Arg\text{-}74}$ was recently shown to exhibit weak intrinsic activity, contracting the guinea pig ileum at 10^{-6} M (Gerard and Hugli, 1981). These investigators presented evidence that the oligosaccharide portion of the human peptide, which is not present on porcine C5a, is at least partially responsible for inhibiting the contractile activity of human $C5a_{des\ Arg\text{-}74}$. In general, the anaphylatoxins elicit contraction of pulmonary tissues at approximately the same concentrations as are required to contract the ileum, therefore we expect that human $C5a_{des\ Arg\text{-}74}$ at 10^{-6}M would contract lung strips as well.

Both porcine C5a and $C5a_{des\ Arg\text{-}74}$ induce maximal contractions of guinea pig lung strips that are more than twice the magnitude of the contraction produced by ACh. In contrast, the magnitude of the contraction induced by C3a is only one-half, and by C4a only one-third, that of the maximal ACh-induced contraction. The magnitude of the tissue response to histamine is roughly parallel to that induced by C5a however, 100-fold higher concentrations of histamine are required to produce an equivalent response.

Investigations of the pharmacology of the anaphylatoxins on isolated lung strips (Stimler et al., 1981a) indicated that antagonists of histamine, of either H_1 or H_2 blocking types, were incapable of inhibiting the responses induced by C5a (Fig. 4). Only at the highest levels of C5a tested (> 0.5 μg/ml) did the antihistamines consistently exert an inhibitory effect. The C3a response was not inhibited at all by these drugs (Fig. 4). Likewise, the contractions of lung strips induced by the anaphylatoxins were not inhibited by the 5-hydroxytryptamine antagonist methysergide. From these studies, we conclude that the anaphylatoxins induce contraction of pulmonary tissue independently of vasoamine release.

The possibility that lipid mediators such as leukotrienes or SRS-A are released by the anaphylatoxins encouraged us to test the effect of FPL-55712*, a specific antagonist of SRS-A (Augstein et al., 1973), on the response of lung tissue to C3a and C5a. We observed no change in the response when 5×10^{-6} M FPL-55712 was present (data not shown). However, when the H_1 antagonist, pyrilamine (10^{-6} M), was added in combination with the FPL-55712 (10^{-6} M) significant inhibition of the tissue response to C5a was observed (Fig. 5). The tissue response to C3a was not affected by these inhibitors. The C5a response was inhibited to a similar degree in the presence of pyrilamine and nordihydroguiaretic acid (NDGA)† (10^{-5} M), an inhibitor of leukotriene biosynthesis

*FPL-55712 was shown by Augstein et al. (1973) to be a specific inhibitor of the contractile activity of SRS-A on smooth muscle tissue.

†Nordihydroguiaretic acid is described as an inhibitor of leukotriene biosynthesis (Tappel et al., 1953).

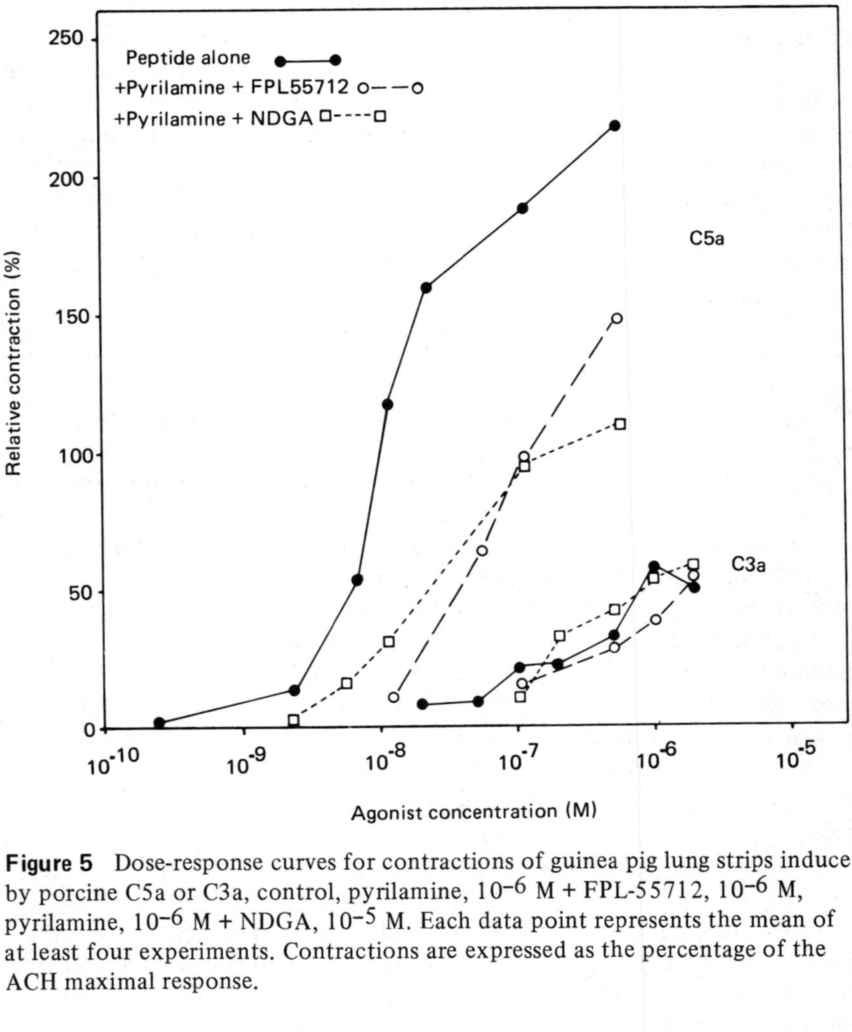

Figure 5 Dose-response curves for contractions of guinea pig lung strips induced by porcine C5a or C3a, control, pyrilamine, 10^{-6} M + FPL-55712, 10^{-6} M, pyrilamine, 10^{-6} M + NDGA, 10^{-5} M. Each data point represents the mean of at least four experiments. Contractions are expressed as the percentage of the ACH maximal response.

(Tappel et al., 1953). As before, no effect was observed on the C3a response (Fig. 5). These data strongly suggest that SRS-A as well as histamine are released from lung tissue stimulated by the C5a anaphylatoxin, whereas C3a appears to act by an independent and unidentified pathway. Whether C3a induces contraction of pulmonary tissue by stimulating the biosynthesis of prostaglandins or acts through yet another mechanism is unclear.

Isolated tracheal rings from guinea pig have also been reported to undergo contraction when exposed to homologous C5a anaphylatoxin (Regal et al.,

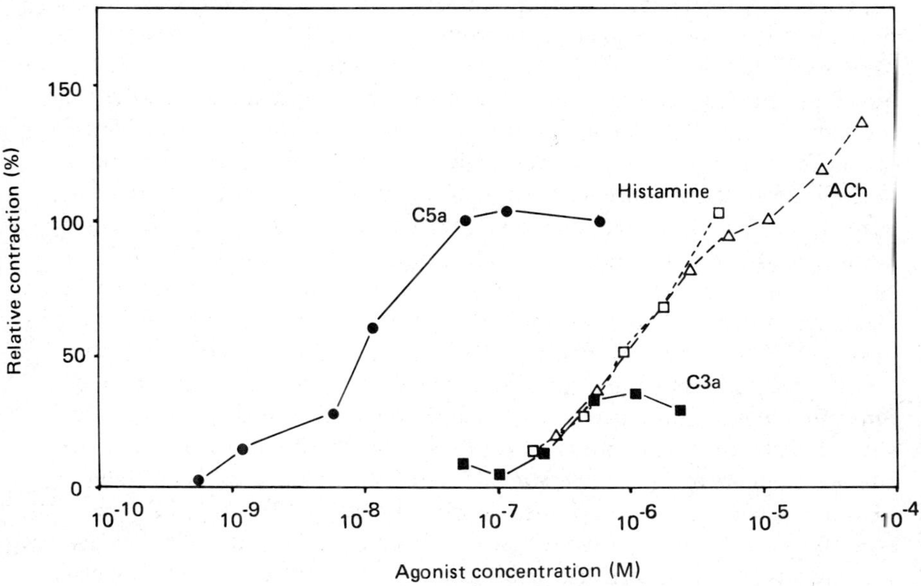

Figure 6 Dose-response curves for contraction of guinea pig tracheal strips induced by porcine C5a, C3a, histamine, and ACh. Each data point represents the mean of at least four experiments. Contractions are expressed as a percentage of the contraction induced by 2×10^{-5} M ACh.

1980). These investigators used a partially purified preparation of the des Arg form of guinea pig C5a, consequently their observations were qualitative rather than quantitative in nature. Nevertheless, these investigators observed that contractions of the trachea induced by C5a was insensitive to the antihistamine, diphenhydramine; however, contractions induced by compound 48/80 or ovalbumin in sensitized animals were significantly reduced in the presence of the antihistamine. More recent studies suggest that it is SRS-A and not histamine that mediates C5a-induced contraction of guinea pig trachea (Regal and Pickering, 1981).

B. Relative Sensitivity of Large versus Small Airways

Drazen et al. (1979) have used partially purified SRS-A to derive evidence that arachidonic acid-derived mediators have a more pronounced effect on peripheral airways than on central airways. They observed threshold contractions of parenchymal strips at a 100-fold lower concentration of SRS-A than was required to contract tracheal tissue. In light of this observation, the relative efficacy of C5a was compared on isolated trachea and on lung parenchymal strips. The data are shown in Figure 6 where quantitative tissue responses to C3a and C5a are compared to the response elicited by 10^{-5} M ACh. Clearly, the concentrations required for threshold contractions of trachea and peripheral airways are the same for both C3a and C5a (compare with Fig. 3). There are, however, several important differences in the overall responses in these tissues. First, in tracheal rings, the ACh curve does not reach a maximum at 10^{-5} M as it does in lung strips. Second, the C5a response in trachea reaches a maximum at 6×10^{-8} M, and the magnitude of this contraction is equivalent to that elicited by 10^{-5} M ACh. In contrast, the contractile response in lung strips does not reach a well-defined maximum even at 6×10^{-7} M, and the magnitude of this contraction is approximately 250% of the ACh response at 10^{-5} M. Third, the slopes of curves generated by plotting the magnitude of C5a- or histamine-induced contraction as a function of concentration are not as steep for the trachea as they are for lung strips. Finally, the C3a response curves are virtually indistinguishable from one another on the two tissue preparations. Whether the differences reflect variations in response capabilities of the two tissue types stimulated by the same agonists or are the result of the release of a dissimilar population of secondary mediators is not yet known. The micrographs of anaphylatoxin-treated guinea pig lungs (Fig. 1) show clear evidence of vascular constriction as well as airway contraction. It is not certain what contribution this vascular component of the lung makes to the overall contraction induced by the anaphylatoxins. Furthermore, until the tissue and cellular responses to the humoral mediators are fully evaluated in terms of the secondary mediators released, the reason for the observed differences in tissue responses remains obscure.

IV. Mediators Released from Lung Tissue by the Anaphylatoxins

A. Histamine

As described earlier, the histamine-releasing activity of the complement anaphylatoxins has been recognized for many years. Hahn and Oberdorf (1950) reported that the bronchospastic and lethal effects of anaphylatoxin preparations (i.e., C5a derivatives) injected into guinea pigs were inhibited by pretreatment with antihistamines. Rocha e Silva et al. (1951) showed that the anaphylatoxin released histamine from guinea pig tissues. Evidence for histamine release induced by the anaphylatoxins was further substantiated by Dias da Silva et al. (1967) and Cochrane and Müller-Eberhard (1968), who observed that anaphylatoxin-induced contraction of guinea pig ileum was effectively inhibited by antihistamines. These combined observations led to the hypothesis that smooth muscle contractions induced by the anaphylatoxins resulted exclusively from release of histamine by tissue mast cells. This theory was further supported by the demonstration of Lepow et al. (1970) and Wuepper et al. (1972) that intradermal injection of C3a produced degranulation of skin mast cells. Subsequently, ter Laan et al. (1974) showed by an immunofluorescence technique, that human C3a binds to rat mast cells and Johnson et al. (1975) observed that isolated rat mast cells release histamine when exposed to either purified C3a or C5a.

Since mast cells from guinea pigs and man are exquisitely sensitive to the anaphylatoxins, it is not surprising that vasoamines are detected in circulation following induced complement activation (Knicker and Cochrane, 1965). Other animals do not share the same sensitivity to the anaphylatoxins; for example, the rat mast cell is particularly insensitive to purified C3a and C5a. This is perhaps the reason that ileal tissue obtained from the rat appears relatively unresponsive to the anaphylatoxins. In certain tissues of the guinea pig, such as the intestine, histamine is clearly the major mediator of anaphylatoxin action. In pulmonary tissue, histamine release from resident mast cells is clearly a component of the response, however the role of this mediator appears much less pronounced than in the gut.

Recent evidence indicates that a class of mediators distinctly different from vasoamines are released from pulmonary tissue by anaphylatoxin action and thereby contribute to the overall contractile response. Stimler et al. (1980a, 1982b) and Regal and Pickering (1981) have shown that spasmogenically active products of arachidonate metabolism are generated as well. Consequently, the effects of the anaphylatoxins on pulmonary tissue are sufficiently complex that it may now be assumed that histamine contributes only a part of the total response. Clearly histamine is released from lung by C5a andC3a, but its role in the tissue response can not be accurately assessed without first eliminating other components of the response contributed by non-vasoamine mediators.

B. Prostaglandins

Evidence was first provided by Greef et al. (1959) that nonhistamine pathways of anaphylatoxin-induced smooth muscle contraction exist. These investigators showed that the uterus of a rat in estrus, a tissue preparation that is insensitive to histamine, contracted when exposed to the anaphylatoxin C3a. More recently, Bodammer and Vogt, (1967) reported that antihistamines prevent the lethal shock reaction in guinea pigs induced by injecting the des Arg form of C5a anaphylatoxin, but do not block the associated bronchospasms. Similar observations were reported by Stimler et al. (1980b) after intrabronchial instillation of purified C3a or C5a anaphylatoxins in vivo. Sackeyfio (1972) showed that contractile substances other than histamine are released from isolated guinea pig lungs perfused with anaphylatoxin. He postulated that these substances were prostaglandins. Subsequently, Stimler et al. (1980b, 1981a) and

Regal et al. (1980) showed that antihistamines do not inhibit anaphylatoxin-induced contractions of isolated lung parenchymal strips or tracheal smooth muscle.

Circumstantial evidence of an involvement of prostaglandins in the pulmonary response to anaphylatoxins derives from studies by Sackeyfio (1972, 1975). He showed that the histopathological effects of anaphylatoxin on guinea pig lung could be mimicked entirely by prostaglandin $F_{2\alpha}$ ($PGF_{2\alpha}$) but not by histamine or several of the other prostaglandins. He postulated therefore that $PGF_{2\alpha}$ was released following C5a stimulation. Additional indirect evidence for involvement of $PGF_{2\alpha}$ has recently been provided by Regal and Pickering (1981) who showed that the SRS-A inhibitor FPL-55712 also inhibits the action of $PGF_{2\alpha}$ on isolated guinea pig trachea. Thus, these investigations suggest that C5a-induced contraction of guinea pig trachea is partially caused by $PGF_{2\alpha}$.

Williams and Jose (1981) recently reported the potentiating effects of vasodilator prostaglandins, PGE_1, PGE_2, or PGI_2 on vascular permeability in rabbit skin induced by C5a. When these investigators combined rabbit $C5a_{des\ Arg}$ with PGE_1 and injected the mixture cutaneously into rabbits, plasma exudation was potentiated 50- to 100-fold over histamine or bradykinin. In human and guinea pig skin, C5a from human or porcine serum enhances vascular permeability in the absence of prostaglandins (Lepow et al., 1970; Vallota and Müller-Eberhard, 1973). To our knowledge, no other studies of potentiation of the effects of anaphylatoxins by prostaglandins have been reported, so it is not clear whether this reflects a species difference or a general interaction between C4a and vasodilator prostaglandins. Further investigations of this phenomena will be of great interest.

Evidence that challenges the proposed involvement of prostaglandins in C5a-induced smooth muscle contraction derives from studies by Jensen (1972) who showed that aspirin, an inhibitor of cyclooxygenase (Vane, 1971), failed to block the respiratory changes induced by injection of porcine C5a into cats. Regal and Pickering (1981) also found that acetylsalicylate failed to inhibit C5a-induced contraction of isolated guinea pig trachea. In addition, we have preliminary evidence that C5a-induced contraction of guinea pig lung strips is not inhibited by indomethacin; however, the C3a response of this tissue was significantly altered in the presence of the drug (data not shown). Taken together, these data neither refute nor confirm that C5a-induced smooth muscle contractions depend on prostaglandin production. Careful studies of the synthesis and/or release of these arachidonic acid metabolites of the cyclooxygenase pathway are needed to prove whether or not prostaglandins participate in the pulmonary constrictor response to anaphylatoxins.

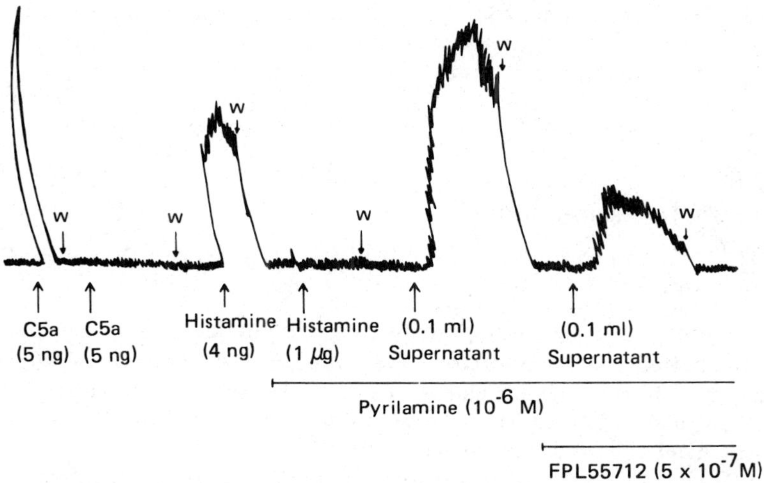

Figure 7 Kymograph tracing of the contractile response of guinea pig ileum induced by substances released from guinea pig lung by porcine C5a. Guinea pig lung fragments (approximately 0.2 mm thick) were incubated in Tyrode buffer (1 g lung/5 ml) for 10 min at 37°C in the presence of 1 μg/ml porcine C5a. The supernatant fluid was decanted and assayed for histamine and SRS-A content. The ileum was first desensitized by pretreatment with C5a to eliminate this component of the spasmogenic reaction. Ileal strips are contracted by 4 ng histamine in the absence of antihistamine. Addition of 10^{-6} M pyrilamine to the Tyrode solution blocks the effect of 1 μg histamine. Supernatant (0.1/ml) from C5a-stimulated lung was then added to the organ bath in the presence of the antihistamine and caused substantial contraction of the ileum (this volume of supernatant was previously determined to containe 20-35 ng histamine). Addition of FPL-55712 at a final concentration of 5×10^{-7} M, 5 min before a second challenge with 0.1 ml of the lung supernatant resulted in a 70% decrease in the contractile response.

C. Slow-Reacting Substance of Anaphylaxis (SRS-A)

Based on earlier work with the anaphylatoxins, we know that they stimulate histamine release from pulmonary tissue. However, no significant change in the anaphylatoxin-induced contractions of guinea pig lung strips are detectable in the presence of antihistamines (Stimler et al., 1980b, 1981a), indicating that histamine may not be important in this reaction. To address this apparent paradox, we examined the supernatant fluid from fragments of guinea pig lung previously exposed to C5a (Stimler et al., 1982b). Lung fragments incubated for 10 min at 37°C with 1 μg/ml porcine C5a released 1.4 ± 0.4 μg histamine/g tissue into the bathing fluid. This quantity of histamine represents 15-20% of

Table 2 SRS-A and Histamine Released from Guinea Pig Lung Stimulated by C5a[a]

	SRS-A[b] (U/g lung)	Histamine (μg/g lung)
C5a (1 μg/ml)	110 ± 8	1.4 ± 0.4
C5a (1 μg/ml) + indomethacin (5 μg/ml)[c]	175 ± 23	1.1 ± 0.4
Control	0	1.1 ± 0.1

[a]Fragments of guinea pig lung (approximately 0.2 mm thick) were incubated in Tyrode buffer (1 g lung/5 ml) for 10 min at 37°C in the presence of 1 μg/ml porcine C5a. The supernatant fluid was decanted and assayed for contractile activity on guinea pig ileum. The concentrations of histamine and SRS-A released were determined as the mean of three experiments ± SD.
[b]One unit (U) of SRS-A is defined as the amount that produces a contraction equivalent to 5 ng histamine.
[c]Tissue was incubated with indomethacin for 5 min at 37°C before addition of C5a.

the total content in such tissue. Based on the dose-response curve for histamine-induced contractions of lung strips, the amount of histamine released from a single strip of tissue is not sufficient to account for the contractions induced in lung strips by C5a. As indicated by the kymograph tracing shown in Fig. 7, in the presence of antihistamine, pyrilamine (10^{-6} M), the contractile response of the ileum is completely blocked when exposed to levels of histamine equivalent to those released from 1 g of lung. However, considerable spasmogenic activity remained in the supernatant fluid from the C5a-stimulated lung tissue. This residual activity is characterized as a substance that contracts the ileum more slowly than either anaphylatoxin or histamine, in a time course that mimics the action of SRS-A. The nonhistamine activity was inhibited by 60-70% in the presence of low concentrations of the SRS-A inhibitor, FPL-55712 (5×10^{-7} M), and at 10^{-6} M FPL-55712, the spasmogenic activity was completely abolished.

The active substance released from lung tissue by C5a was further characterized by the effect of indomethacin on the level of activity released (Table 2). This drug inhibits the cyclooxygenase pathway of arachidonic acid metabolism and stimulates the lipoxygenase pathway. Consequently, the synthesis of SRS-A, now recognized as a mixture of products of the lipoxygenase pathway (Jakschik et al., 1977; Borgeat and Samuelsson, 1979; Parker et al., 1979), is enhanced in the presence of indomethacin. Lung fragments pretreated with indomethacin and stimulated with C5a released approximately 50% more SRS-A activity than was released in the absence of the drug.

Further support for our contention that this material is SRS-A was provided by chromatography on Sephadex LH-20. The smooth muscle contracting activity was not eluted by nonpolar organic solvents that are known to elute other arachidonate derivatives such as prostaglandins. However, activity was eluted by 80% ethanol, a solvent that elutes the complex lipopeptides, SRS-A, and the leukotreines (Watanabe-Kohno and Parker, 1980). In addition, the spasmogenically active material was more than 70% inactivated by incubation with aryl sulfatase for 60 min at 37°C (30 U/100 U SRS-A), conditions which are known to inactivate SRS-A (Orange et al., 1974). Based on these results and the pharmacologic data discussed earlier, we conclude that the anaphylatoxin C5a induces specific release of significant quantities of SRS-A from guinea pig lung tissue in addition to relatively small amounts of histamine.

The C3a anaphylatoxin contracts peripheral airways from the guinea pig by a mechanism that is also apparently independent of histamine release (Stimler et al., 1980b, 1981a), as was found for C5a. However, we have been unable to detect SRS-A activity in supernatant fluids from chopped lung stimulated with C3a. Furthermore, the C3a dose-response curve is not inhibited in the presence of combinations of pyrilamine and FPL-55712 or NDGA. In contrast, the C5a dose-response curve is inhibited at least 10-fold in the presence of either pyrilamine and FPL-55712 or pyrilamine and NDGA (Fig. 5).

Preliminary evidence indicates that the SRS-A antagonist FPL-55712 alone is not sufficient to inhibit the C5a-induced contractions of guinea pig lung strips. Somewhat surprisingly, if an antihistamine is included with FPL-55712 a significantly greater inhibition is observed. The reason for this effect is not immediately clear because the amount of histamine released is apparently not sufficient to account for the contractions observed, unless SRS-A and histamine exhibit synergistic action on smooth muscle. Furthermore, Regal et al. (1980) showed inhibition of C5a-induced contractions of isolated guinea pig trachea by FPL-55712 alone. Although the role of prostaglandins and thromboxanes in the pulmonary constrictor response induced by C5a are indeterminate at this time, the leukotrienes are clearly predominant mediators of this response.

D. Platelet Activating Factor (PAF)

Recent investigations have shown that PAF forms rapidly in the blood of sensitized rabbits undergoing antigen-induced anaphylaxis (Pinckard et al., 1979). This factor characterized chemically as 1-*O*-alkyl-2-acetyl-*sn*-glycero-3-phosphorylcholine (Demopoulas et al., 1979; Benveniste et al., 1979; Hanahan et al., 1980), is produced by leukocytes and mast cells of several species including

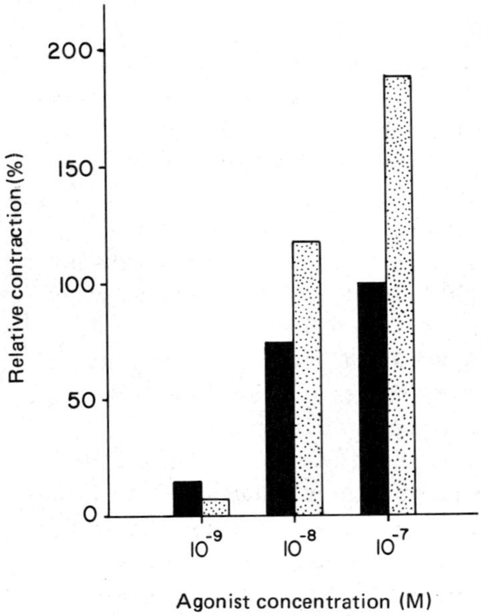

Figure 8 Contraction of guinea pig lung strips in response to PAF (solid bars) is compared with porcine C5a (stipled bars). The extent of contraction represents the mean of at least four experiments, and the data is expressed as the percentage of the ACh maximal response.

guinea pig (Benveniste et al., 1977; Clark et al., 1980). Injected into rabbits, the phospholipid causes a typical anaphylactoid reaction (McManus et al., 1980; O'Flaherty et al., 1981a). Furthermore, C5a has been shown to stimulate release of PAF from leukocytes in vitro (Camussi et al., 1977, 1981; Lynch et al., 1979), a predictable result based on the analogy that anaphylatoxins induce similar mediator release from cell types that undergo surface IgE-antigen reactions (Hugli, 1979).

We recently reported that PAF is capable of contracting smooth muscle and of enhancing vascular permeability as determined by classical anaphylatoxin assays (Stimler et al., 1981b). Since this phospholipid is also a potent mediator of these actions, its release by the anaphylatoxins would contribute significantly to the acute pulmonary injury associated with complement activation.

Contraction of guinea pig lung strips as a function of PAF concentration is illustrated in Fig. 8. PAF is the only mediator tested in our system that is as potent as C5a in contracting lung strips, with threshold contractions occurring at concentrations of 10^{-9} M. At 5×10^{-7} M the maximum contraction induced by PAF is approximately half that of C5a. The PAF dose-response curve levels off at approximately 100% of the ACh maximum. PAF induces selective tachyphylaxis; lung tissue stimulated with PAF is refractory to repeated additions of this factor but still contracts after exposure to C3a, C5a, and the standard agonists histamine and ACh. The mechanism of contraction induced by

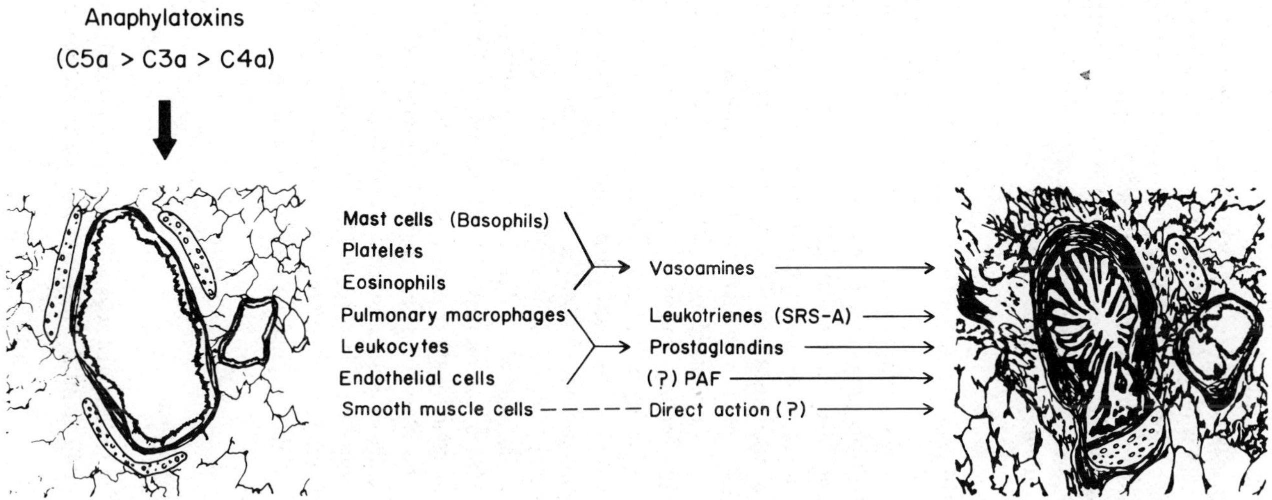

Figure 9 Schematic representation of the proposed mechanism for anaphylatoxin-induced contraction of pulmonary tissue through release of secondary mediators and direct action.

PAF is independent of histamine both in the ileum and in lung strips. The PAF response is also apparently unrelated to SRS-A since FPL-55712 is not inhibitory (Stimler et al., 1981c). PAF is also well known to be a potent mediator of aggregation of platelets (Benveniste et al., 1975; Henson, 1977) and neutrophils (Goetzel et al., 1980; O'Flaherty et al., 1981b). A prominent feature observed in the tissue after intrabronchial instillation of purified anaphylatoxins in guinea pigs is formation of intravascular aggregates of platelets and neutrophils. Since C3a does not cause aggregation of these cell types in vitro, although C5a does (Stimler et al., 1980b), release of PAF from mast cells in pulmonary tissue by the anaphylatoxins could explain these findings.

V. Conclusion

The observation that slow-reacting substances and possibly PAF, in addition to histamine, are released from lung tissue on exposure to C5a suggests a much wider role for the complement anaphylatoxins in lung pathophysiology than has previously been recognized. It would appear that C5a, and possibly C4a and C3a, are capable of eliciting qualitatively similar responses in target cells as are observed in immediate hypersensitivity reactions that involve IgE, because the variety of mediators that are released are virtually identical. A schematic representation of the cellular reactions known to be mediated by the anaphylatoxins in lung tissue is depicted in Figure 9. Consequently, we postulate that complement anaphylatoxins make a significant contribution to the clinical symptoms of numerous airway-constricting diseases that show evidence of complement activation or involvement. These include autoimmune diseases in which primary immunologic injury is occurring elsewhere in the organism. Recent interest in the role of the leukotrienes, and particularly SRS-A, in asthma must now also be extended to include the anaphylatoxins as causative agents.

The concept that evolves from our recognition that anaphylatoxins are multifunctional molecules capable of releasing numerous mediators is that such factors may play an important role as initiators of a cascade of cellular release mechanisms. Estimating the contributions of anaphylatoxins in mediating cellular release in organs such as the lung defines a worthy goal for pharmacologic studies in the 1980s.

Acknowledgments

The authors would like to thank Dr. Craig J. Gerard for providing the anaphylatoxins used in these studies, and Dr. Walter E. Brocklehurst for valuable discussions.

References

Augstein, J., Farmer, J. B., Lee, T. B., Sheard, P., and Tattersall, M. L. (1973). Selective inhibitor of slow reacting substance of anaphylaxis. *Nature New Biol., 245*:215-217.

Austen, K. F., and Orange, R. P. (1975). Bronchial asthma: The possible role of the chemical mediators of immediate hypersensitivity in the pathogenesis of subacute chronic disease. *Am. Rev. Respir. Dis., 112*:423-436.

Benveniste, J., Camussi, J., and Polonsky, J. (1977). Platelet-activating factor. *Monogr. Allergy, 12*:138-142.

Benveniste, J., Kamoun, P., and Polonske, J. (1975). Aggregation of human platelets by purified platelet activating factor from human and rabbit basophils. *Fed. Proc., 34*:985.

Benveniste, J., Tence, M., Varenne, P., Bidault, J., Boullet, C., and Polonsky, J. (1979). Semi-synthèse et structure proposèe du facteur activant es plaquettes (PAF): PAF-acether, unalkyl ether analog de la lysophosphatidylcholine. *C.R.L. Acad. Des. Sci., 289*:1037-1040.

Bodammer, G. (1966). Krieslauf-und atemwirkung gereingter AT-Praparate. *Naunyn-Schmiedebergs Arch. Pharmakol. Exp. Pathol., 255*:4

Bodammer, G., and Vogt, W. (1967). Actions of anaphylatoxin on circulation and respiration of the guinea pig. *Int. Arch. Allergy Appl. Immunol., 32*: 417-428.

Bodammer, G. and Vogt, W. (1970). Contraction of the guinea pig ileum induced by anaphylatoxin independent of histamine release. *Int. Arch. Allergy, 39*:648-657.

Bokisch, V. A., Müller-Eberhard, H. J. (1970). Anaphylatoxin inactivator of human plasma: Its isolation and characterization as a carboxypeptidase. *J. Clin. Invest., 49*:2427-2436.

Bokisch, V. A., Müller-Eberhard, H. J., Cochrane, C. G. (1969). Isolation of fragment (C3a) of the third component of human complement containing anaphylatoxin and chemotactic activity and description of an anaphylatoxin inactivator of human serum. *J. Exp. Med., 129*:1109-1130.

Bordet, J. (1913a). Le Mecanisme de L'anaphylaxie. *C.R. Soc. Biol.* (Paris), *74*:225-227.

Bordet, J. (1913b). Le Mecanisme de L'anaphylaxie II. *C. R. Soc. Biol.* (Paris), *74*:877-880.

Borgeat, P., and Samuelsson, B. (1979). Arachidonic acid metabolism in polymorphonuclear leukocytes: Unstable intermediate in formation of dihydroxy acids. *Proc. Natl. Acad. Sci. USA, 76*:3213-3217.

Burrell, R. G. (1963). Autoantibodies in pulmonary disease. *Am. Rev. Respir. Dis., 87*:389-394.

Camussi, G., Mencia-Huerta, J. M., and Benveniste, J. (1977). Release of platelet-activating factor and histamine. I. Effect of immune complexes, complement and neutrophils on human and rabbit mastocytes and basophils. *Immunology, 33*:523-533.

Camussi, G., Tetta, C., Bussolino, F., Calgaris Cappio, F., Coda, R., Masera, C., and Segoloni, G. (1981). Mediators of immune-complex-induced aggregation of polymorphonuclear neutrophils. II. Platelet-activating factor as the effector substance of immune-induced aggregation. *Int. Arch. Allergy Appl. Immunol., 64*:25-41.

Christian, C. L., and Thurber, R. J. (1962). Studies of anaphylaxis: Effect of decomplementation with aggregated γ-globulin. *J. Immunol., 88*:93-99.

Clark, P. O., Hanahan, H. J., and Pinckard, R. N. (1980). Physical and chemical properties of platelet-activating factor obtained from human neutrophils and monocytes, and rabbit neutrophils and basophils. *Biochem. Biophys. Acta, 628*:69-75.

Cochrane, C. G., and Dixon, F. J. (1978). Immune complex injury. In *Immunological Diseases,* vol. 1. Edited by M. Samter, Boston, Little Brown, pp. 210-229.

Cochrane, C. G., and Koffler, D. (1973). Immune complex disease in experimental animals and man. *Adv. Immunol., 16*:185-264.

Cochrane, C. G., and Müller-Eberhard, H. J. (1968). The derivation of two distinct anaphylatoxin activities from the third and fifth components of human complement. *J. Exp. Med., 127*:371-386.

Cochrane, C. G., Unanue, E. R., and Dixon, F. J. (1965). A role of polymorphonuclear leukocytes and complement in nephrotoxic nephritis. *J. Exp. Med., 122*:99-116.

Dale, H. H. (1913). The anaphylactic reaction of plain muscle in the guinea pig. *J. Pharmacol. Exp. Ther., 4*:167-222.

Demopoulas, C. A., Pinckard, R. N., and Hanahan, D. J. (1979). Platelet-activating factor: Evidence for 1-0-alkyl-sn-glyceryl-3 phosphorylcholine as the active component (a new class of lipid chemical mediators). *J. Biol. Chem., 254*:9355-9358.

Desai, U., Kretuzer, D. L., Showell, H., Arroyave, C. V., and Ward, P. A. (1979). Acute inflammatory pulmonary reactions induced by chemotactic factors. *Am. J. Pathol., 96*:71-84.

Dias da Silva, W., Eisele, J. W., and Lepow, I. H. (1967). Complement as a mediator of inflammation. III. Purification of the activity with anaphylatoxin properties generated by interaction of the first four components of complement and its identification as a cleavage product of C3. *J. Exp. Med., 126*:1027-1048.

Dixon, F. J. (1971). The immunopathology of glomerulonephritis. In *Immunological Diseases.* Edited by M. Samter. New York, Little Brown, pp. 1125-1133.

Drazen, J. M., Lewis, R. A., Wasserman, S. I., Orange, R. P., and Austen, F. (1979). Differential effects of a partially purified preparation of slow-reacting substance of anaphylaxis on guinea pig tracheal spirals and parenchymal strips. *J. Clin. Invest., 63*:1-5.

Erdös, E. G., Sloane, E. M., and Wohler, I. M. (1964). Carboxypeptidase in blood and other body fluids. I. Properties, distribtuion, and partial purification of the enzyme. *Biochem. Pharmacol., 13*:893-905.

Fedlman, J. D. (1964). Ultrastructure of immunologic processes. In *Advances in Immunology,* vol. 4. Edited by F. J. Dixon and J. H. Humphrey, New York, Academic Press, pp. 175-284.

Fernandez, H. N., and Hugli, T. E. (1978). Primary structural analysis of the polypeptide portion of human C5a. *J. Biol. Chem., 253*:6955-6964.

Florey, H. (1960). In Polypeptides Which Affect Smooth Muscles and Blood Vessels. *Proc. symp.* Bristol, Pergamon Press, p. 293.

Friedberger, E. (1910). Weitere untersuchungen uber einweissanaphylaxie. IV. Mitteilung. *Z. Immunitaetsforsch Exp. Ther., 4*:636-689.

Gerard, C., and Hugli, T. E. (1980). Amino acid sequence of the anaphylatoxin from the fifth component of porcine complement. *J. Biol. Chem., 266*: 4710-4715.

Gerard, C., and Hugli, T. E. (1981). Identification of the classical anaphylatoxin as $C5a_{des\ Arg}$: Evidence of a modulator role for the oligosaccharide unit in human C5a. *Proc. Natl. Acad. Sci. USA, 78*:1833-1837.

Goetzel, E. J., Derian, C. K., Tauber, A. I., and Valone, F. H. (1980). Novel effects of 1-*O*-hexadecyl-2-acyl-*sn*-glycero-3-phosphorylcholine mediators on human leukocyte function: Delineation of the specific roles of the acyl substituents. *Biochem. Biophys. Res. Commun., 94*:881-888.

Gorski, J. P., Hugli, T. E., and Müller-Eberhard, H. J. (1979). C4a: The third anaphylatoxin of the human complement system. *Proc. Natl. Acad. Sci.* USA, *76*:5299-5302.

Greeff, K., Benfey, B. G., and Bokelmann, U. A. (1959). Anaphylaktische reaktionen am isolierten herzorhof praparat des meerschweinchens und ihre beeinflussung durch antihistaminica, BOL, dihydroergotamin und reserpin. *Naunyn-Schmiedebergs Arch. Exp. Pathol. Pharmak., 236*:421-434.

Hagadorn, J. E., and Burrell, R. G. (1968). Lung-reactive antibodies in IgA fractions of sera from patients with pneumoconiosis. *Clin. Exp. Immunol., 3*: 263-267.

Hagadorn, J. E., Vazquez, J. J., and Kinney, T. R. (1969). Immunopathologic studies of an experimental model resembling Goodpasture's Syndrome. *Am. J. Pathol., 57*:17-30.

Hahn, F. (1954). Zur anaphylatoxinfrage. *Naturwissenshaften* (Berlin), *41*: 465-470.

Hahn, F. (1960). Anaphylatoxin: Formation, actions and role of anaphylaxis. In Polypeptides Which Affect Smooth Muscles and Blood Vessels. *Proc. Symp.* Bristol, Pergamon Press, pp. 275-292.

Hahn, F., and Oberdorf, A. (1950). Antihistaminica and anaphylaktoid reaktionen. *Z. Immununitaetsforsch Exp. Ther., 107*:528-538.

Hammer, D. K., and Dixon, F. J. (1963). Experimental glomerulonephritis. II. Immunologic events in the pathogenesis of nephrotoxic serum nephritis in the rat. *J. Exp. Med., 117*:1019-1034.

Hall, R., Turner-Warwick, M., and Doniach, D. (1966). Autoantibodies in iodide goitre and asthma. *Clin. Exp. Immunol., 1*:285-296.

Hanahan, D. J., Demopoulas, C. A., Liehr, J., and Pinckard, R. N. (1980). Identifcation of platelet activating factor isolated from rabbit basophils as acetylglyceryl ether phosphorylcholine. *J. Biol. Chem., 255*:5514-5516.

Hennes, A. R., Moore, M. Z., and Carpenter, R. L. et al. (1961). Antibodies to human lung in patients with obstructive emphysema and pulmonary tuberculosis. *Am. Rev. Respir. Dis., 83*:354-358.

Henson, P. M. (1971). Interaction of cells with immune complexes: Adherence, release of constituents of tissue injury. *J. Exp. Med., 134*:114s-133.

Henson, P. M. (1977). Activation of rabbit platelets by platelet-activating factor derived from IgE-sensitized basophils: Characteristics of the aggregation and its dissociation from secretion. *J. Clin. Invest., 60*:481-493.

Henson, P. M., McCarthy, K., Larsen, G. L., Webster, R. O., Giclas, P. C., Dreisen, R. B., King, T. E., and Shaw, J. O. (1979). Complement fragments, alveolar macrophages, and alveolitis. *Am. J. Pathol., 97*:93-105.

Hugli, T. E. (1979). Complement anaphylatoxins as plasma mediators, spasmogens, and chemotaxins. In *The Chemistry and Physiology of Human Plasma Proteins.* Edited by D. H. Bing. New York, Pergamon Press, pp. 225-280.

Hugli, T. E. (1975). Human anaphylatoxin (C3a) from the third component of complement. *J. Biol. Chem., 250*:8293-8301.

Hugli, T. E. (1978). Chemical aspects of the serum anaphylatoxins. In *Contemporary Topics in Molecular Immunology,* vol. 7. Edited by R. A. Reisfeld and F. P. Inman. New York, Plenum Press, pp. 181-214.

Humphrey, J. H. (1955). The mechanism of arthus reactions. I. The role of polymorphonuclear leukocytes and other factors in reversed passive arthus reactions in rabbits. *Br. J. Exp. Pathol., 36*:268-282.

Ishizaka, K. (1963). Gammaglobulin and molecular mechanisms in hypersensitivity reactions. *Progr. Allerg., 7*:32-106.

Jacobs, J. W., Rubin, J. S., Huglie, T. E., Bogardt, R. A., Mariz, I. K., Daniels, J. S., Doughaday, W. H., and Bradshaw, R. A. (1978). Purification, characterization and amino acid sequence of rat anaphylatoxin (C3a). *Biochemistry, 17*:5031-5038.

Jakschik, B. A., Falkenhein, S., and Parker, C. W. (1977). Precursor role of arachidonic acid in release of slow reacting substance from rat basophilic leukemia cells. *Proc. Natl. Acad. Sci. USA, 74*:4577-4581.

Jensen, J. A. (1967). Anaphylatoxin in its relation to the complement system. *Science, 155*:1122-1123.

Jensen, J. A. (1972). Anaphylatoxin(s). In *Biological Activities of Complement.* Edited by D. G. Ingram. Basel, Karger, pp. 136-157.

Johnson, K. J., Chapman, W. E., Ward, P. A. (1979). Immunopathology of the lung. *Am. J. Pathol., 95*:794-844.

Johnson, A. R., Hugli, T. E., and Müller-Eberhard, H. J. (1975). Release of histamine from rat mast cells by the complement peptides C3a and C5a. *Immunology, 28*:1067-1080.

Kleine, I., Poppe, B., and Vogt, W. (1970). Functional identity of anaphylatoxin preparations obtained from different sources and by different activation procedures I. *Eur. J. Pharmacol., 10*:398-403.

Knicker, W. T., and Cochrane, C. G. (1965). Pathogenic factors in vascular lesions of experimental serum sickness. *J. Exp. Med., 122*:83-98.

Kreutzer, D. L., Desai, U., Orr, W., Showell, H., and Ward, P. A. (1979). Induction of acute inflammatory reactions in lung following intrapulmonary instillation of preformed chemotactic peptides and purified complement components. *Chest, 75*:259-261.

Larsen, G. L., McCarthy, K., Webster, R. O., Henson, J., and Henson, P. M. (1980). A differential effect of C5a and $C5a_{des\ Arg}$ in the induction of pulmonary inflammation. *Am. J. Pathol., 100*:179-192.

Leopold, H. C., and P. Leicht (1969). Autoimmune antibodies to human lung in bronchial asthma. *Ann. Allergy 27*:377-383.

Lepow, I. H., Dias Da Silva, W., and Eisele, J. W. (1968). Nature and biological properties of human anaphylatoxin. In *Biochemistry of the Acute Allergic Reactions.* Edited by K. F. Austen and E. L. Becker. Oxford, Blackwell, pp. 265-282.

Lepow, I. H., Willms-Kretschmer, K., Patrick, R. A., and Rosen, F. S. (1970). Gross and ultrastructural observations on lesions produced by intradermal injection of human C3a in man. *Am. J. Pathol., 61*:13-23.

Linscott, W. E., and Cochrane, C. G. (1964). Guinea pig β1c-globulin: Its relationship to the third component of complement and its alteration following interaction with immune complexes. *J. Immunol., 93*:972-984.

Lulich, K. M., Mitchell, M. W., and Sparrow, M. P. (1976). The cat lung strip as an *in vitro* preparation of peripheral airways: A combination of β-adrenoceptor agonists, autocoids and anaphylactic challenge on the lung strip and trachea. *Br. J. Pharmacol., 58*:71-79.

Lynch, J. M., Lotner, G. Z., Betz, S. J., and Henson, P. M. (1979). The release of a platelet-activating factor by stimulated rabbit neutrophils. *J. Immunol., 123*:1219-1226.

McCoombs, R. P. (1972). Diseases due to immunologic reactions in the lungs. *N. Engl. J. Med., 286*:1186-1194, 1245-1252.

McKay, I. R., and Ritchie, B. (1965). Diffuse fibrosing alveolitis (diffuse interstitial fibrosis of the lungs): Two cases with autoimmune features. *Thorax, 20*:200-205.

McManus, L. M., Hanahan, D. J., Demopoulos, C. A., and Pinckard, R. N. (1980). Pathobiology of the intravenous infusion of acetylglyceryl ether phosphorylcholine (AGEPC), a synthetic platelet-activating factor (PAF), in the rabbit. *J. Immunol., 124*:2919-2924.

Nathan, E. (1913). Ueber anaphylatoxin bildung durch agar. *Z. Immunitaetsforsch, 17*:478-495.

Novy, F. G., and DeKruif, P. H. (1917). Specific anaphylatoxin shock. *J. Infect. Dis., 20*:776-802.

O'Flaherty, J. T., Miller, C. H., Lewis, J. C., Wykle, R. L., Bass, C. E., McCall, C. E., Waite, M., and DeChatelet, L. R. (1981a). Neutrophil responses to platelet activating factor. *Inflammation 5*:193-201.

O'Flaherty, J. T., Wykle, R. L., Miller, C. H., Lewis, J. C., Waite, M., Bass, D. A., McCall, C. E., and DeChatelet, L. R. (1981b). 1-*O*-alkyl-*sn*-glyceryl-3-phosphorylcholines: A novel class of neutrophil stimulants. *Am. J. Pathol., 103*:70-77.

Osler, A. G., Randall, G. H., Hill, B. M., and Ovary, Z. (1959). Studies on the mechanism of hypersensitivity phenomena. III. The participation of complement in the formation of anaphylatoxin. *J. Exp. Med., 110*:311-339.

Osler, A. G., Hawrisiak, M. M., Ovary, Z., Siqueria, M., and Bier, O. G. (1957). Studies on the mechanisms of hypersensitivity phenomena. II. The participation of complement in passive cutaneous anaphylaxis of the albino rat. *J. Exp. Med., 106*:811-834.

Orange, R. P., Murphy, R. C., and Austen, K. F. (1974). Inactivation of slow reacting substance of anaphylaxis (SRS-A) by arylsulfatases. *J. Immunol., 113*:316-322.

Parker, C. W., Jakschik, B. A., Huber, M. G., and Falkenhein, S. F. (1979). Characterization of slow reacting substance as a family of thiolipids derived from arachidonic acid. *Biochem. Biophys. Res. Commun., 89*:1186-1192.

Pinckard, R. N., Farr, R. S., and Hanahan, D. J. (1979). Physicochemical and functional identity of rabbit platelet-activating factor (PAF) released in vivo during IgE anaphylaxis with PAF released in vitro from IgE sensitized basophils. *J. Immunol., 123*:1847-1857.

Regal, J. F., and Pickering, R. H. (1981). C5a-induced tracheal contractions: Effect of an SRS-A antagonist and inhibitors of arachidonate metabolism. *J. Immunol., 126*:313-316.

Regal, J. F., Eastman, A. Y., and Pickering, R. J. (1980). C5a induced tracheal contraction: A histamine independent mechanism. *J. Immunol., 124*:2876-2878.

Rocha e Silva, M. (1954). Anaphylatoxin and histamine release (1954). *Rev. Allergy, 8*:220-238.

Rocha e Silva, M., and Aronson, M. (1952). Histamine release from the perfused lung of the guinea pig by serotoxin. *Br. J. Exp. Pathol., 33*:577-586.

Rocha e Silva, M., Bier, O., and Aronson, M. (1951). Histamine release by anaphylatoxin. *Nature, 168*:465-466.

Sackeyfio, A. C. (1971). Definition of the histaminic component of the bronchoconstrictor and cardiovascular effects of anaphylatoxin in the guinea pig. *Br. J. Pharmacol., 43*:424-425.

Sackeyfio, A. C. (1972). Anaphylatoxin-induced release of a substance with prostaglandin-like activity in isolated perfused guinea-pig lungs. *Br. J. Pharmacol., 46*:544-545.

Sackeyfio, A. C. (1975). A comparison of the histopathological effects of anaphylatoxin (AT) and prostaglandins E_2 (PGE_2) and $F_{2\alpha}$ ($PGF_{2\alpha}$) in guinea pig lungs. *Br. J. Pharmacol., 55*:240-421.

Scherzer, H., and Ward, P. A. (1978a). Lung and dermal vascular injury produced by preformed immune complexes. *Am. Rev. Respir. Dis., 117*: 551-557.

Scherzer, H., and Ward, P. A. (1978b). Lung injury produced by immune complexes of varying composition. *J. Immunol., 121*:947-952.

Schultz, W. H. (1910). Physiological studies in anaphylaxis. I. The reaction of smooth muscle of the guinea pig sensitized with horse serum. *J. Pharmacol. Exp. Ther., 2*:221-229.

Shin, H. S., Synderman, R., Friedman, E., Mellors, A., and Mayer, M. M. (1968). Chemotactic and anaphylatoxic fragment cleaved from the fifth component of guinea pig complement. *Science, 162*:361-363.

Stimler, N. P., Brocklehurst, W. E., Bloor, C. M., and Hugli, T. E. (1980a). Complement anaphylatoxins C5a stimulates release of SRS-A-like activity from guinea pig lung fragments. *J. Pharm. Pharmacol., 32*:804.

Stimler, N. P., Hugli, T. E., and Bloor, C. M. (1980b). Pulmonary injury induced by C3a and C5a anaphylatoxins. *Am. J. Pathol., 100*:327-348.

Stimler, N. P., Brocklehurst, W. E., Bloor, C. M., and Hugli, T. E. (1981a). Anaphylatoxin mediated contraction of guinea pig lung strips: A nonhistamine tissue response. *J. Immunol., 126*:2258-2261.

Stimler, N. P., Bloor, C. M., Hugli, T. E., Wykle, R. L., McCall, C. E., and O'Flaherty, J. T. (1981b). Anaphylactic actions of platelet activating factor. *Am. J. Pathol., 105*:64-69.

Stimler, N. P., Bach, M. K., Bloor, C. M., and Hugli, T. E. (1982). Release of leukotrienes from guinea pig lung stimulated by $C5a_{desArg}$ anaphylatoxin. *J. Immunol., 128*:2247-2252.

Tappel, A. L., Lundberg, W., Boyer, P. D. (1953). Effect of temperature and antioxidants on the lipoxidase-catalyzed oxidation of sodium linoleate. *Arch. Biochem. Biophys., 42*:293-304.

ter Laan, B., Molenaar, J. L., Feltkamp-Vroom, T. M., and Pondman, K. W. (1974). Interaction of human anaphylatoxin C3a with rat mast cells demonstrated by immunofluorescense. *Eur. J. Immunol., 4*:393-395.

Vallota, E. H., and Müller-Eberhard, H. J. (1973). Formation of C3a and C5a anaphylatoxins in whole human serum after inhibition of the anaphylatoxin inactivator. *J. Exp. Med., 137*:1109-1123.

Vane, J. R. (1971). Inhibition of prostaglandin synthesis as a mechanism of action for aspirin-like drugs. *Nature New Biol., 231*:232-235.

Vazquez, J. J. (1970). Immunopathologic aspects of lung disease. *Arch. Int. Med., 126*:471-474.

Wagner, V., Tomsikova, A., and Sach, J. et al. (1965). Autoimmune mechanism in diseases of the respiratory tract. *Acta. Allergol., 20*:1-9.

Ward, P. A. (1979). Immune complex injury of the lung. *Am. J. Pathol., 97*:85-92.

Ward, P. A., and Cochrane, C. G. (1965). Bound complement and immunologic injury of blood vessels. *J. Exp. Med., 121*:215-234.

Ward, P. A., Cochrane, C. G., and Müller-Eberhard, H. J. (1965). The role of serum complement in chemotaxis of luekocytes *in vitro. J. Exp. Med., 122*:327-346.

Ward, P. A., Cochrane, C. G., and Müller-Eberhard, H. J. (1966). Further studies on the chemotactic factor of complement and its formation *in vivo. Immunology, 11*:141-153.

Watanabe-Kohno, W., and Parker, C. W. (1980). Role of arachidonic acid in the biosynthesis of slow reacting substance of anaphylaxis (SRS-A) from sensitized guinea pig lung fragments: Evidence that SRS-A is very similar or identical structurally to non-immunologically induced forms of SRS. *J. Immunol., 125*:946-955.

Williams, T. J., and Jose, P. J. (1981). Mediation of increased vascular permeability after complement activation: Histamine-independent action of rabbit C5a. *J. Exp. Med., 153*:136-153.

Wuepper, K. D., Bokisch, V. AA., Müller-Eberhard, H. J., and Stoughton, R. B. (1972). Cutaneous responses to human C3a anaphylatoxin in men. *Clin. Exp. Immunol., 11*:13-20.

Yang, H. Y. T., and Erdös, E. G. (1967). Haematology: Second kininase in human blood plasma. *Nature* (Lond.), *215*:1402-1403.

14

Neutrophil Dysfunction and Lung Disease

HAIG DONABEDIAN* and JOHN I. GALLIN

National Institute of Allergy and Infectious Diseases
National Institutes of Health
Bethesda, Maryland

I. Characteristics of Neutrophils

A. Introduction

The neutrophil is uniquely adapted for defense against infectious invasion from the external environment. Its ability to detect evidence of an infection, adhere to, and traverse the vascular endothelium and to move in a directed fashion to the site of an infection makes it the primary defender of the mucosal and dermal surfaces. As such, intact neutrophil function is critical to the protection of the lung from infection. It is no surprise then that abnormalities of neutrophil function often manifest themselves as pulmonary pathology. The neutrophil is not the sole defender of the lung against infection. The lung has numerous alveolar macrophages which have a primary role in lung defenses but which also interact with the neutrophil system. An important part of the alveolar macrophage's role is to recruit neutrophils to the site of an infection and thus take advantage of

Present Affiliation
*Medical College of Ohio, Toledo, Ohio

the neutrophils' motility, efficiency in killing, and enormous numbers. The ability of the neutrophil to kill efficiently depends on its oxidative and nonoxidative bactericidal components. Both of these components may be a two-edged sword which, under certain circumstances, may become destructive agents of the very lung tissue they protect. Thus, it is important to understand normal neutrophil function, neutrophil interactions with other cells in the lung, and the neutrophil's toxic potential in order to understand the lung pathology that occurs when there are abnormalities in neutrophil function.

B. Adherence, Motility, and Chemotaxis

Chemotaxis is directed migration towards an increasing gradient of an attractant substance. The function of neutrophil chemotaxis is to deliver circulating neutrophils from the blood stream and marginated neutrophils from the vascular endothelium to the tissues where they can kill invading organisms.

The details of this process have been well reviewed by Klebanoff and Clark (1978a) and Gallin and Quie (1978) and in the chapter by Ward et al. in this volume. The circulating neutrophil, when exposed to a chemoattractant substance, will adhere to the vascular endothelium (MacGregor, 1980), crawl between the endothelial cells (exhibit diapedesis) (Cramer et al., 1980), and enter the interstitial space. This process requires cell orientation along the chemoattractant gradient, using the microtubular apparatus to provide stability (Malech et al., 1977) and an intact actin and myosin microfilament network which provides the contractile forces for locomotion (Stossel, 1978). The neutrophil crawls on the substratum of the interstitial space as fast as 5 μm/min along the increasing gradient of the chemoattractant substance.

The major chemoattractant substances in the human are probably products of the complement activation—predominantly C5a and C5a des arg (Fernandez et al., 1978) and bacterial products (Ward et al., 1968). A wide variety of substances such as arachidonic acid pathway products (Goetzl and Pickett, 1980), kallikrein (Kaplan et al., 1972), fibrin-split products (Kay et al., 1974), elastin-derived peptides (Senior et al., 1980), and products from virally infected tissues (Ward et al., 1972) may also be of importance to neutrophil chemotaxis in the lung. Of special relevance to the lung are the chemotactic factors produced by the human alveolar macrophage (Kazmierowski et al., 1973; Merrill et al., 1980; Hunninghake et al., 1980).

When neutrophils have followed the chemotactic gradient to the point of infection or inflammation, they may then phagocytize invading organisms or foreign matter and also secrete the contents of their intracellular granules. Phagocytosis of invading organisms is often facilitated by opsonization by antibodies and/or complement (Frank, 1980). The phagocytized particle is enveloped by a membrane derived from the cell membrane of the neutrophil to form the phagolysosome. Upon stimulation, the plasma membrane produces toxic oxygen-derived products which are released to the extracellular environment and into the phagolysosome. The toxic oxygen-derived products include singlet oxygen, superoxide anion, the hydroxyl radical, and hydrogen peroxide. These are capable of oxidizing and thus disrupting living systems (Klebanoff and Clark, 1978b). The products of oxidative metabolism produced in response to chemoattractants may modulate the inflammatory process by generating (Petrone et al., 1980) or inactivating (Clark et al., 1980; Clark, 1981) chemoattractants as well as causing direct damage to the lung tissue.

The lysosomal granules of the neutrophil fuse with the phagolysosome and release into it various proteases, lysozymes, and iron-binding (lactoferrin) and B_{12}-binding proteins as well as myeloperoxidases which contribute to the destruction of the ingested organisms (Klebanoff and Clark, 1978c). In the process of chemotaxis and ingestion, these granule contents are secreted extracellularly as well, where they may act as antimicrobial agents as well as modulators of the inflammatory reaction by generating and destroying chemotactic factors (Wright and Gallin, 1977, 1979).

Both oxidative and nonoxidative mechanisms are important to the killing of ingested organisms. Neutrophils can thus kill aerobically and anaerobically, although bacterial killing is much more efficient in the presence of oxygen. Thus, in order to have an effective neutrophil component of the body's defense system, the neutrophils must be able to sense a chemoattractant, adhere to a vessel wall, exhibit diapedesis through the wall of the vessel, and crawl along a gradient of a chemoattractant to the area of infection or inflammation. Once at the site of injury, they may phagocytize the invading organism. The neutrophil may then fuse its granule contents with the phagolysosome and release toxic O_2 products into the phagolysosome, or it may secrete those toxic oxygen products and granule contents extracellularly. If the neutrophil has a significant defect in one or more of these processes, then the lung's defenses will be diminished accordingly. The variety of neutrophil defects is large and the defects may be inherited or acquired. The effect on the lung is often a large part of the clinical presentation of these defects, as a review of these defects will show.

II. Inherited Disorders of Neutrophil Function

A. Chronic Granulomatous Disease

One of the most intensively studied and dramatic inherited neutrophil defects is chronic granulomatous disease (CGD). It was first clearly described in 1957 as a disease of four male children with chronic suppurative lymphadenitis, pulmonary infiltrates, splenomegaly, and eczematoid dermatitis (Berendes et al., 1957). The pathology of this disease is characterized by scattered abscesses with a predominant neutrophilic response; however, granulomata are evident. The abscesses may have multinucleated giant cells and may caseate. The noninfected tissues may also reveal lipid-laden macrophages of variable number. The basic defect of this syndrome was revealed when Holmes et al. (1966) showed that neutrophils from patients with this syndrome fail to kill ingested bacteria. It was rapidly shown that CGD neutrophils have a severe defect in oxidative metabolism (Holmes et al., 1967). Studies by many groups in the ensuing 13 years have shown that both neutrophils and macrophages obtained from patients with this disease are incapable of producing superoxide (O_2^-) anion upon stimulation by soluble or particulate factors. This lack of stimulation may be due to the absence of an enzyme which catalyzes the oxidation of reduced nicotinamide adenine nucleotides (NADPH or NADH) and the reduction of O_2 to O_2^- (Curnutte et al., 1974); or, it may be due to the inability of CGD cells to couple the stimulus with the activation of the NADPH oxidase enzyme, as suggested by recent reports implicating abnormal elicited membrane-potential changes in CGD neutrophils (Seligmann and Gallin, 1980; Whitin et al., 1980).

The formation of O_2^- is critical in the oxidative killing of ingested organisms. O_2^- is involved with the subsequent formation of toxic O_2 intermediates and hydrogen peroxide (H_2O_2) through the mechanism:

$$2\,O_2^- + 2\,H^+ \rightarrow H_2O_2 + O_2 \tag{1}$$

The inability to form hydrogen peroxide severely hampers the killing efficiency of the neutrophil and explains the bacteriological spectrum of the agents that infect patients with this disease. Most bacteria and fungi produce H_2O_2 in the course of their own metabolism. Since H_2O_2 is toxic to these organisms, it must be either secreted extracellularly or detoxified. Those organisms which have the enzyme catalase can detoxify the hydrogen peroxide to water and oxygen; those without catalase must secrete it. When a CGD neutrophil ingests an organism without catalase, such as *Streptococcus penumoniae,* the bacterium's own secreted H_2O_2 can be used by the bactericidal system of the neutrophil to destroy the digested bacterium. Therefore, it is the catalase-positive bacteria (such as those of the genera *Staphylococcus, Escherichia, Klebsiella, Serratia, Pseudomonas, Nocardia,* and *Mycobacterium*) and catalase-positive fungi (such as *Aspergillus* and *Candida*), which infect CGD patients.

The inability of CGD neutrophils to produce O_2^- when stimulated is the basis of the most commonly used clinical test in the diagnosis of CGD, the nitroblue tetrazolium (NBT) test. Normal neutrophils, when stimulated by the presence of bacteria, endotoxin, or a soluble agent such as phorbol myristate acetate, will reduce NBT to formazan, an insoluble blue dye which appears in the stimulated neutrophils. CGD neutrophils (and those with other, more rare, abnormalities in oxidative metabolism) will not do so. Other more sensitive tests (such as the luminol-chemiluminescence test [Rosen and Klebanoff, 1976]) and more specific tests (such as monitoring O_2 consumption or production of O_2^- [O_2^- dismutase-inhibitable cytochrome *c* reduction] [Curnette et al., 1975]) are useful. We have found recently that monitoring elicited changes in the fluorescence of a lipophilic membrane-potential-sensitive fluorescent cyanine dye, di-*O*-C(5)3, is an easy way to detect patients with CGD or heterozygote carriers of the disease (Seligmann and Gallin, 1980).

The inheritance of CGD is predominantly X-linked. As such, the great majority of patients are hemizygous males. The disease does occur in females and these patients may have an autosomal recessive form. It has recently been shown that females may be heterozygous for the abnormal X chromosome but show clinical evidence of the disease, presumably through variable inactivation of the normal X chromosome according to the Lyon hypothesis (Mills et al., 1980).

The clinical presentation of CGD often begins in the first years of life and continues with severe, persistent, and recurrent infections throughout life. Most patients die of infection by age 30. Some pertinent clinical characteristics of 10 patients we have been following at the National Institutes of Health (NIH) are shown in Table 1. Since the respiratory tract is a major surface interfacing with the outside world and its infectious agents, one would expect a major defect in neutrophil function to have pulmonary manifestations. Indeed, in a review of 168 patients with CGD, 134 had pneumonitis at one time in their history (Johnston and Newman, 1977). Pulmonary disease was the primary cause of death in 30 of the 52 reported patients in whom the cause of death was stated. The disease may present relatively late in life and have a relatively mild course. Balfour et al. (1971) reported a case of a 23-year-old man who was asymptomatic until age 12, when he developed bilateral *Aspergillus* pneumonia. He was subsequently treated for three more pneumonias but had been asymptomatic for a 22-month follow-up period. His neutrophils had a marked inability to kill *Staphylococcus aureus* in vitro and to reduct NBT. The great majority of cases present with recurrent infections by 2 years of age, however. Another review of 92 patients reported that 80 of them had pulmonary infiltrates on x-ray (Johnston and Baehner, 1971).

American and British reviews of the radiological findings in the chests of CGD patients are in general agreement (Wolfson et al., 1968; Sutcliffe and Chrispin, 1970) about the frequency and extent of pulmonary involvement in CGD. The study of Wolfson et al. (1968) reported that 14 or 18 patients had a bronchopneumonia pattern on x-ray examination with patchy infiltrates frequently in the bases of the lungs that at times presented as a fine haze. The infiltrates typically resolve slowly with antibiotic therapy, or they can go on to massive consolidation, despite therapy. Lobar pneumonia developed in four patients presenting with a bronchopneumonic pattern. Enlarged hilar and/or mediastinal nodes were seen in ten of those with pneumonia and in two without pneumonia. Eight of the patients developed what the authors felt was a distinctive infiltrate, which they call "encapsulated" and which showed a

Table 1 Characteristics of Patients with CGD Seen at NIH[a]

Patient	Sex	Age (years)	Pertinent clinical history
CH	F	18	Nocardiosis (osteomyelitis)
			Recurrent staphylococcal infections, including hepatic abscess
DH	M	27	*Mycobacterium fortuitum* pneumonia (brother of CH)
LH	F	4	Recurrent staphylococcal pneumonias (niece of CH)
PR	M	21	Pulmonary aspergillosis
			Recurrent staphylococcal infections
			Pseudomonas cepacia pneumonia
			Staphylococcal hepatic abscess
BP	M	14	Disseminated aspergillosis
			Recurrent staphylococcal infections
SS	M	4.5	Recurrent staphylococcal infections
			Ureteral granulomas
EH	M	2½	Recurrent staphylococcal infections
			Serratia marcescens sepsis and osteomyelitis
			Granulomas of the pylorus
HP	M	9	Pulmonary aspergillosis
			Recurrent staphylococcal infections
LO	F	18	Recurrent staphylococcal pneumonia, chronic sinusitis
			Pseudomonas cepacia pneumonia
MJ	M	23	Right pneumonectomy for recurrent pneumonias, predominantly staphylococcal

[a]Patients CH, PR, and BP have been followed by Dr. A. S. Fauci at NIH.

discrete and rounded contour. Cavitation, empyema, and pleural thickening were also seen. The British radiologists Sutcliffe and Chrispin (1970) also stress that a patient's bronchopneumonic picture may progress on antibiotics to consolidation. They also noted widening of the mediastinal shadow and enlargement of mediastinal nodes as evidence of mediastinitis, a diagnosis supported by autopsy or surgery in four cases. An interesting report (Fleming et al., 1975) suggests that repeated bronchopneumonic infections in CGD may lead to diffuse interstitial fibrosis with honeycombing, as seen at autopsy in an 18-year-old boy who had steadily decreasing vital capacities during his life. Autopsy revealed Langhans giant cells, lipid-laden histiocytes, and diffuse alveolar septal thickening.

The presentation of widespread foci of infection, which progresses to consolidation and possible cavitation, correlates with the understanding that CGD neutrophils cannot efficiently kill invading organisms. There is the possibility that ingested organisms may persist in the neutrophil in a viable state and may thus be spread in the tissues as well as escape antibiotic action sequestered in the neutrophil. The chronic inflammatory reaction often seen in the setting of apparent sterilization of the infection with antibiotics suggests the abnormal elimination of toxic antigens or abnormal "turnoff" of inflammatory reactions. The recent demonstration that O_2^--related products inactivate (deformylate) chemoattractants may be particularly relevant in this regard (Clark et al., 1980; Clark, 1981). The protracted course of pneumonias in patients with CGD, even with appropriate antibiotics, attests to the importance of the neutrophil oxidative killing mechanisms in lung defenses.

The decrease in lung defenses makes more unusual pathogens more likely. Note the presence of unusual agents of pneumonia, such as *Pseudomonas cepacia* and *Aspergillus* in Table 1. The literature contains reports of a diffuse pneumonia and osteolyelitis of a rib in an 8-year-old boy with CGD. The only pathogen found on biopsy was a catalase-positive *Aspergillus nidulans* (Bujak et al., 1973). Three of ten patients we have seen (Table 1) have had *Aspergillus* infection. One patient (PR) is a 17-year-old CGD patient who presented with *Aspergillus fumigatus* pneumonia, probably from inhalation of contaminated marijuana (Chusid et al., 1975b). Another patient (DH) was a 27-year-old man with CGD presented with a right lower lobe infiltrate and empyema. The pleural fluid grew only *Mycobacterium fortuitum* (Chusid et al., 1975a). Infection with protozoa is not usually reported with CGD, so a report from a Danish group (Pedersen et al., 1979) of an 11-year-old girl with *Pneumocystis* pneumonia and CGD, which only responded to sulfamethoxazole-trimethoprim and granulocyte transfusions, is significant.

The above reports indicate the importance of oxidative killing by neutrophils and macrophages in infection that are thought to be combatted primarily by cell-mediated immunity. CGD lymphocytes do not appear to have any in vitro defects (Good et al., 1968) in their ability to respond to antigens. However, it has recently been shown (Katz et al., 1980) that CGD neutrophils, lymphocytes, and monocytes display abnormal antibody-dependent cellular cytotoxicity towards antibody-coated human erythrocytes. This defect may be important in dealing with mycobacterial, fungal, and protozoal infections. These unusual infections also serve to remind the clinician to consider the diagnosis of CGD in similarly unusual pneumonitides.

The treatment of CGD patients is at present unsatisfactory. Acute infections are managed with conventional antibiotic or amphotericin therapy, which must be continued longer than would be the case for a normal host. It is not unusual for a pneumonia to persist for more than 4 weeks on therapy. Frequently, patients with CGD are placed on daily oral sulfisoxazole prophylaxis, based on sulfa drugs' broad spectrum of activity, low cost, and inability to create bacterial resistance to commonly used therapeutic antibiotics. Johnston et al. (1975) found a decrease in severity and frequency of infections in five patients with CGD who were studied prospectively using their pretreatment years as a control. Patients in this study received from 500 mg to 4 g of sulfisoxazole daily. There was modest improvement of in vitro staphylococcal killing when CGD neutrophils were preincubated with sulfisoxazole at 7 μg/ml. The mechanism of this increased killing is not clear. There was no significant increase in oxygen uptake or glucose oxidation in sulfisoxazole-treated normal or CGD cells. The use of prophylactic antistaphylococcal oral antibiotics has been suggested by some investigators. However, infection with antibiotic-resistant organisms has occurred in patients on antibiotics. Therefore, prophylactic antibiotics should be used with caution.

The use of granulocyte transfusion for severely infected CGD patients may be of value. A previously cited case (Pedersen et al., 1979) reported clinical failure of antibiotics alone when used in a CGD patient with *Pneumocystis* pneumonia. When the same antibiotics were reinstituted with granulocyte transfusion, there was rapid improvement. Granulocyte transfusions were also used in conjunction with amphotericin B in an 8-year-old male with CGD and *Aspergillus* pneumonia (Raubitshek et al., 1973). It was found that 5 min after transfusion the patient's white cells could kill *E. coli* as effectively as the donor's cells. Using HLA-matched donors, Chusid and Tomasulo (1978) reported that circulating transfused granulocytes could be detected up to 24 h after transfusion of 7.5×10^9 neutrophils into a 16-kg boy with CGD and a hepatic abscess. As with all patients receiving white cell transfusions, the development of antineutrophil antibodies and the difficulty of providing adequate numbers of cells render this mode of therapy still experimental.

B. Chediak-Higashi Syndrome

The Chediak-Higashi syndrome (CHS) is an autosomally linked recessive abnormality of intracellular granules. Its most dramatic manifestations involve granulocytes and the pigment-containing cells, but the disorder seems to involve granules of most cell types. The patients present with recurrent infections of the respiratory tract and skin. They have a partial albinism of their hair and retinas due to abnormal pigment granule formation. Some patients progress to develop both peripheral and central neurologic deficits as well as hemorrhagic problems. Some die from an "accelerated phase" of lymphoid infiltration, which may be neoplastic. Interestingly enough, the syndrome has its equivalent in Hereford cattle, Aleutian mink, killer whales, and beige mice (Windhorst and Padgett, 1973).

The basis of the disease is not clear. All the patients are neutropenic and CHS neutrophils contain giant granules which seem to be abnormal variants of the primary or azurophil granules. The fact that the giant granules contain abnormal pleomorphic figures (Davis and Douglas, 1972; White and Clawson, 1980) has led some investigators to suggest that they are the result of abnormal fusions between the primary granules and other neutrophil components. Recent evidence for this theory comes from the work of Rausch et al. (1978), who found that the giant granules of CHS neutrophils contained enzymes which are normally seen only in the secondary granules. Furthermore, they note that no normal primary granules could be found, although normal secondary granules were present in CHS cells. The CHS neutrophils contain significantly less of certain lysosomal enzymes (Kimball et al., 1975), but there is no enzyme which is deficient. There is evidence that a basic defect of lipid metabolism underlies the formation of giant granules. Sphingolipid turnover is abnormal in CHS neutrophil membranes (Kanfer et al., 1968), and the membranes of CHS cells are reported to be more fluid than those of normal controls (Haak et al., 1979). Beige mice have been found to have significantly more surface active materials in their lungs than normal mice, and they have significantly more phospholipid and disaturated phosphatidylcholine (Prueitt et al., 1978). An abnormality in membrane lipid dynamics could explain aberrant fusions of intracellular granules, but there is no direct evidence for this.

There is also a body of evidence which incriminates faulty microtubule function in CHS cells. Normal and CHS neutrophils bind fluorescein-labeled concanavalin A, but CHS cells more readily display "capping" of this label similar to normal cells treated with the microtubule-disrupting drug colchicine. Capping involves movement of the originally diffusely membrane-bound label to one pole of the cell. Normal cells will display CHS-like behavior if they are treated with colchicine, an agent that inhibits microtubule assembly. Morphologic studies indicated a deficiency of microtubules in neutrophils from some but not all patients with CHS, although this was not seen in the beige mouse model of this disease (Frankel et al., 1978). Recent studies of human cells indicate that there is an abnormality in the tyrosylation of the α-chain of tubulin

(Nath et al., 1980), providing the first biochemical evidence of a microtubule defect in this disease.

CHS neutrophils display poor chemotaxis through nitrocellulose filters in an in vitro assay and in an in vivo skin window assay (Clark and Kimball, 1971). This defect in chemotaxis is also seen in the CHS mononuclear cells (Gallin et al., 1979a). The cause of decreased chemotactic activity is unclear, but it may be due to decreased deformability of the cells. Clark and Kimball (1971) report that the extent of the defect diminishes as the pore size of the nitrocellulose filters through which the neutrophils must travel is increased, suggesting a defect in cell deformability. This idea is supported by the later work of Clawson et al. (1978), who postulated that the physical size of the giant granules prevented effective deformation through small filter pore openings. However, recent studies by Miller (1979) indicate that deformability of CHS is normal and the basis of chemotactic abnormalities may be more subtle.

Phagocytosis appears to be normal, and O_2 metabolism is greater than normal in resting CHS neutrophils; but the ability to degranulate enzyme contents extracellularly and to fuse intracellular granules with the ingested organism is diminished (Root et al., 1972). Thus, CHS neutrophils display diminished chemotaxis and delayed granule fusion. The resultant clinical picture is predictable. CHS patients have increased upper and lower respiratory tract infections with a variety of bacteria. *Staph. aureus* predominates as the most common etiologic agent, but *Streptococcus pyogenes, Hemophilus influenzae,* and *E. coli* are also prevalent.

Cholinergic and other agents which increase guanosine 3′, 5′-cyclic monophosphate (cGMP) in relation to adenosine 3′, 5′-cyclic monophosphate (cAMP) in the neutrophil will block the increased capping of concanavalin A in CHS neutrophils and colchicine-treated normal cells (Oliver and Zurier, 1976). cGMP is a promoter of microtubule assembly, and the ratio of cGMP/cAMP is thought to affect the polymerization of tubulin into microtubules. Addition of dibutyryl cGMP and cholinergic agents also normalized chemotaxis and enzyme release in human CHS neutrophils (Boxer et al., 1977). These findings may be primary or secondary abnormalities in CHS. The basic defect in CHS which results in abnormal neutrophil function is not yet clear. It is this abnormal function together with the neutropenia that is critical to the CHS patients' increased incidence of infection, an increased incidence seen in the animal homologs of this syndrome.

A definitive review by Blume and Wolff (1972) described four patients followed at the NIH and cites 59 other reported cases of CHS in humans. In 53 patient-months, there were 29 pyogenic infectious episodes of which 3 were bronchitis, 2 were bronchopneumonia, and 4 were lobar pneumonia. The organisms implicated in these pulmonary infections were all *Staph. aureus* or members of the *Hemophilus* genus. These organisms encompass both catalase-positive and catalase-negative varieties of bacteria. These bacteria predominate in other neutrophil dysfunction syndromes as well, implying that lung defense against these organisms is dependent on effective, motile neutrophils. There was a notable absence of *Strep. pneumoniae* infections. A review of the literature reveals 34 bronchopneumonias and empyemas out of 113 reported infections. The remainder were predominantly skin and nasopharyngeal infections. Out of the 34 isolations of causative agents reported 21 were *Staph. aureus,* two were *Aspergillus* and one was *Candida.* CHS, unlike CGD, does not seem to predispose overly to fungal or unusual infections. It is almost as if the infection with a common agent were due to the quantitative disorder involving the comparatively late arrival and slower killing mechanism of the CHS neutrophils, while infection with an unusual agent depends on a qualitative disorder, such as the lack of oxidative killing in CGD.

It is interesting that the increased susceptibility to pneumonia in the human CHS is mirrored in the beige mouse model of CHS. In fact, the increased susceptibility to pneumonia, which has been subjected to careful genetic analysis, is a phenotypic marker for these mice (Lane and Murphy, 1972).

The treatment of CHS patients is controversial with respect to prophylaxis. Previously cited studies have implicated agents that raise neutrophil cGMP and the cGMP/cAMP ratio as possible effective therapeutic or prophylactic agents. Ascorbic acid, which raises leukocyte cGMP levels (Sandler et al., 1975) and increases normal neutrophil microtubule assembly (Boxer et al., 1979), has been used in patients with CHS. Boxer et al. (1976) found that administering 200 mg of ascorbic acid daily to a 9-month-old CHS girl weighing about 3 kg increased her neutrophils' ability to kill *Staph. aureus* and to degranulate. The posttreatment CHS neutrophils had an increased cGMP/cAMP ratio, but no increase in cGMP. Chemotaxis was markedly improved in vitro. However, Gallin et al. (1979b) could not corroborate these results with two CHS brothers in their twenties who were given 6 g of ascorbic acid a day, although the latter authors noted that ascorbic acid improved neutrophil function and provided protection from lethal infection with *Candida* in the beige mouse model. The role of ascorbic acid therapy is not clear and a prospective double-blind crossover study to look at the incidence of infection in patients receiving ascorbate versus placebo has not been done.

Such a prospective study has been done using prophylactic oral antibiotic cloxacillin in four CHS patients followed at the NIH (Dale et al., 1972). This study revealed no significant effect of cloxacillin in preventing clinically apparent infection when the study was terminated at 20 months. There was a significant decrease specifically in staphylococcal infection, however. Due to the generally serious nature of staphylococcal infections, there may well be a place for oral antistaphylococcal prophylactic therapy, and we have used this approach in two patients we have followed with this disease (Fauci and Gallin, unpublished data).

Antibiotic therapy may have to be prolonged in the treatment of infection in CHS (Blume and Wolff, 1972). Pneumonias and other infections frequently require several weeks of antibiotic therapy. They may be due to suboptimally effective killing of bacteria by the CHS neutrophils.

There is good experimental evidence that bone marrow transplant cures the susceptibility to infection in CHS mice (Kazmierowski et al., 1976), but this drastic therapeutic maneuver has yet to be attempted in humans. There is still hope of pharmacologic amelioration of this disorder with cholinergic agents; but until the real basis of CHS is known, therapeutic advances may well be haphazard.

C. Hyperimmunoglobulin E and Recurrent Infection Syndrome

In 1966 Davis et al. (1966) reported two young red-haired girls with recurrent staphylococcal abscesses since birth, eczema, recurrent sinusitis, and otitis media. The abscesses were characteristically free of inflammatory heat and were therefore called "cold." The syndrome was named after the Biblical character Job who was struck with "sore boils from the sole of his foot unto his crown." One of these two patients had recurrent pneumonias and *Staph. aureus* was repeatedly isolated from her sputum. The characteristic laboratory abnormalities of this syndrome were not noted at that time. A clearer picture of this syndrome was drawn by Buckley et al. (1972) when they reported two adolescent boys with chronic recurrent skin, pulmonary, and joint infections with staphylococcus as well as chronic dermatitis, course facies, and increased serum levels of immunoglobulin E (IgE).

These patients did not have strong atopic histories and were not infected with parasites. By the age of 3.5 years, one patient had had eight separate pneumonias with frequent cyst formation on x-ray. The second case had recurrent pneumonias starting at the age of 3 months. He also had chronic mucosal and nailbed involvement with *Candida.* Immunological evaluation revealed diminished lymphocyte responses to typhoid and keyhole limpet hemocyanin antigens in vivo. Both patients had normal immunoglobulin levels except for IgE, which was at least 10 times higher than normal and in one instance was 200 times higher than normal. The patients' neutrophils reduced NBT and killed staphylococci normally. Both patients had strong immediate hypersensitivity testing to various common antigens; but delayed hypersensitivity to dinitrochlorobenzene, *Staph. aureus, Candida,* and others was poor. One patient died and was found to have a normal thymus gland at autopsy. The picture of this syndrome was enhanced by Clark et al. (1973) and by Hill et al. (1974a) and Hill and Quie (1976), who detected the presence of a chemotactic defect in these patients' neutrophils. They reported four patients (two from the original report of Davis et al. [1966]). They all had a low-grade eosinophilia (250-860/mm^3). All had IgE levels greater than 10 times normal, and they all had a chemotactic abnormality as measured by a chemotactic index less than one-half that of normal controls. They found that the chemotactic abnormality could not be recreated by suspending normal neutrophils in the patients' plasma. Likewise, the patients' serum generated normal chemotactic activity when it was exposed to zymosan.

The major feature of this syndrome therefore appears to be recurrent infections of the skin and lung (frequently due to *Staph. aureus*), very high levels of circulating IgE in the absence of atopy or parasitism, and a chemotactic defect of the circulating neutrophils at some time in the course of the disease.

The predominance of staphylococci as infecting organisms and the frequent involvement of the skin and respiratory tract are compatible with the chemotactic defect in the HIE syndrome. The peculiar presence of "cold" abscesses remains a mystery, but the phenomenon is real. In the authors' experience deep-seated abscesses of the skin and soft tissue may contain several hundred milliliters of pus, yet often the skin is not hot and the patient is not febrile.

In their review, Buckley and Becker (1979) reported 20 patients with the hyper-IgE-recurrent infection (HIE) syndrome. They state that these patients invariably have recurrent pneumonia, often with pneumatoceles. The predominant infecting organism was *Staph. aureus*; but *H. Influenzae,* pneumococci, group-A streptococci, and Gram-negative and fungal infections were seen. There is no consistent association with red hair and fair skin. The patients seem to have coarse facies, and many have scars of thoracic operations. Males and females were affected in a 13/7 ratio in this review, but there is no sex predominance when all the reported cases are reviewed. There was a familial clustering of some but not a majority of cases, a finding supported by others (Van Scoy et al., 1979). Buckley and Becker also found an invariable blood and sputum eosinophilia, a finding that Hill et al. (1974a) and the authors' clinical experience does not support. Buckley and Becker also found only three of nine patients tested had consistent depressions of neutrophil and mononuclear cell chemotaxis. This variability in the chemotactic abnormality over a period of time is supported by others (Gallin, 1980; Mawhinney et al., 1980).

The basic defect in the HIE syndrome is not known nor is the cause of the variable chemotactic defect. Because of the high amounts of IgE present and because of cell-bound IgE's role in releasing histamine and other mediators, Hill and Quie (1976) suggested that increased exposure to histamine could account for the chemotactic defect. This hypothesis is supported by the findings of two groups (Schopfer et al., 1979; Berger et al., 1980) that there are antistaphylococcal IgE's in these patients. It is possible that staphylococcal infection could release basophil and mast cell products via an antistaphylococcal IgE trigger mechanism and that these products could inhibit the chemotaxis of circulating neutrophils. Further support for this comes from improvement of HIE neutrophils' chemotaxis when histamine H_2 blockers are added in vitro (Hill et al., 1976) or administered in vivo (Mawhinney et al., 1980). The foregoing explanation really does not account for the absence of chemotactic defects in atopy or parasitism, both of which have IgE that reacts with environmental or parasitic antigens. Nor does it explain the lack of a predisposition to infection in patients with systemic mastocytosis who have frequent and massive release of mast cell mediators.

The basis of the increased IgE levels may well be a defect in a class of T lymphocytes, which regulates IgE synthesis (Katona et al., 1980). Donabedian and Gallin (1982a) recently presented evidence that a product from mononuclear cells of HIE patients may inhibit the chemotaxis of normal cells. A defect involving lymphocyte-neutrophil and lymphocyte-lymphocyte interactions or a more basic membrane abnormality has thus not been ruled out.

A review of the radiographic features of the HIE syndrome stresses the indolent and recurrent nature of the staphylococcal pneumonias typically found in those patients (Merten et al., 1979). Eleven patients varying from 4 to 39 years old were reviewed. All lobes were involved with pneumonia, and four patients had multiple lobe involvement. All were lobar or segmental pneumonias caused predominantly by *Staph. aureus.* Seven of the eleven developed pulmonary cysts, not necessarily related to the initial bout of pneumonia. The cysts were single or multiple, having variable thickness of the wall. They would occasionally have an air-fluid level. The cysts usually disappeared on therapy but would sometimes take up to 2 years to resolve. Five patients required lobectomy or pneumonectomy for persistent infection. Bronchiectasis was seen in one patient on plain radiograph.

The authors' experience with lung disease in the HIE syndrome is similar to the reported findings. The pneumonia may be quite extensive and the patient may have minimal symptoms and fever, almost the pulmonary counterpart of the cold abscess. We also not frequent chronic bronchitis as defined by chronic productive cough. Occasionally, only *H. influenzae* can be grown from the sputum, but the predominant organism is usually *Staph. aureus.*

The treatment of the HIE patient with pneumonia may require prolonged intravenous antibiotics. The patient typically looks better than the x-ray, and there is a temptation to curtail therapy due to a paucity of symptoms. However, prolonged antibiotic therapy is required to clear the infection. The possibility of using systemic H_2 blockers such as cimetidine (Mawhinney et al., 1980) has been raised in an effort to improve neutrophil chemotaxis. There is also evidence that the immunostimulant drug levamisole can improve HIE neutrophils when administered to the patient or added in vitro the the patient's neutrophils (Wright et al., 1977). An open-ended clinical trial at the NIH indicated levamisole's possible efficacy in this syndrome (Gallin, 1980). A prospective double-blind trial recently completed at the NIH (Donabedian and Gallin, 1982b) did not show levamisole to be efficacious in preventing infections in the HIE syndrome.

D. Other Inherited Abnormalities of Neutrophils

Myeloperoxidase is an enzyme located in the primary or azurophil granules of the neutrophil. It catalyzes the oxidation of a halide ion by hydrogen peroxide. In doing so it transforms chloride and possibly iodide into the hypochlorite or hypoiodite ions. These are powerful oxidants and antibacterial agents in vitro. Sodium hypochlorite is the active agent in laundry bleach and swimming pool algicides.

Deficiency of neutrophil myeloperoxidase may be a relatively common neutrophil dysfunction. Parry et al. (1980) found that 15 out of approximately 60,000 patients screened had complete neutrophil myeolperoxidase deficiency and 13 had partial deficiency. They and others (Lehrer and Cline, 1969) agreed that this seemingly important enzyme deficiency has little in vitro effect in the killing of staphylococci but that it does significantly affect the killing of fungi. Most of the patients with this deficiency are asymptomatic, but a patient reported by Lehrer and Cline (1969) and one by Parry et al. (1980) had serious lung infections; both of these patients had diabetes as well. The latter patient had a chronic *Candida* pneumonia. Myeloperoxidase deficiency may also be acquired in severe infections and preleukemic and leukemic states (Klebanoff and Clark, 1978e).

Kartagener's syndrome is an autosomally and recessively transmitted disorder involving chronic, recurrent infection of the sinuses, middle ears, and respiratory tract in the presence of situs inversus. The predominant abnormality in this syndrome may well be immotile cilia due to the absence of the dynein component of the cilial energy transduction system. However there is evidence that the neutrophils from patients with Kartagener's syndrome have decreased motility (Malech, 1980; Afzelius et al., 1980). Time-lapse photography of neutrophils from patients with Kartagener's syndrome show that compared with normal neutrophils, the cells moved more slowly and more frequently crossed over their own paths, indicating that their net translational movement was decreased. The importance of this neutrophil movement defect in Kartagener's syndrome in relation to the absence of effective ciliary action has not been determined. Certainly a diminished ability to recruit neutrophils to a site of infection could only increase the incidence of infection. No information is published on pharmacological interventions with a drug such as levamisole in Kartagener's syndrome. However, ascorbic acid has been shown not to be efficacious when tested in vitro with neutrophils from Kartagener's syndrome patients (Afzelius et al., 1980).

Five patients have been reported who lack neutrophil-specific granules (reviewed in Breton-Gorius et al., 1980). These granules contain lactoferrin and B_{12}-binding protein, which are thought to be important in bacterial killing. Other specific granule products activate the complement system which further modulates the inflammatory response (Wright and Gallin, 1977). In addition, neutrophil specific granules are thought to be an important source of new plasma membrane during neutrophil migration. These five patients have recurrent bacterial pneumonias and skin infections. Defects in killing and chemotaxis have been reported in some but not all of these patients. This disorder is apparently quite a valuable model for studying the importance of specific granules in host defenses and in the regulation of inflammation.

III. Acquired Neutrophil Defects and Lung Disease

The list of acquired neutrophil defects is large. Many systemic diseases produce neutrophil dysfunction and are associated with an increased incidence of respiratory diseases. However, these systemic diseases affect a myriad of other aspects of anatomy, physiology, and immunology. Thus, an increased incidence of infection can be explained by numerous factors that do not relate to neutrophils. In this chapter, we have decided to discuss a selection of acquired diseases that involve interesting effects on the neutrophil. We will also mention acquired diseases in which the neutrophil's role has not been adequately recognized.

A. Diabetes

Diabetics may have an increased incidence of infection or the severity of their infections may be greater than that of nondiabetics. There appears to be a neutrophil dysfunction in both juvenile and adult onset diabetes, which may contribute to the frequency of the diabetes and severity of infections. Nonketotic diabetic children were shown to have abnormal neutrophil recruitment in vivo using the skin window technique (Koutras and Bodenbender, 1968). The skin window responses of 35 diabetic children were both delayed in the appearance of neutrophils and monocytes at the skin site of inflammation and decreased in final number at the skin window site. Since these patients were children under the age of 20, vascular insufficiency as a cause of decreased inflammation was unlikely. Another study confirmed these results and added that diabetic acidosis did not significantly further reduce neutrophil migration to the skin window site (Brayton et al., 1970). The patients in this latter study had serum glucoses of less than 250 mg/dl and were classified as being in good to fair control. Mowat and Baum (1971a) studied the in vitro chemotaxis of neutrophils in 21 diabetics and found it to be depressed and uncorrelated with the patients' fasting blood glucose, plasma insulin level, or whether the patient was taking oral hypoglycemics or insulin. Incubation of diabetics' cells with insulin and glucose decreased the defect. Incubation of normal cells with added glucose up to 900 mg/dl did not produce a chemotactic defect. This amelioration of the chemotactic defect by added insulin was also seen by Hill et al. (1974c) in juvenile diabetics. There appears to be no microbiocidal defect in diabetes per se, although Muller and Baker showed a marked decrease in the ability of serum of juvenile diabetics to generate chemotactic factors when incubated with staphylococci or antigen-antibody complexes (Miller and Baker, 1972).

The research on neutrophil function in diabetes points to a cellular defect in chemotaxis, which is unexplained by the presence of extracellular glucose or keto acids. The amelioration with insulin indicates that diabetics have a significant alteration in their neutrophils' metabolism which is reversible. This conclusion leads to hope for decreased infectious complications by better control of serum glucose and insulin in these patients.

B. Alcoholism

Alcoholics have many reasons to get recurrent infections, especially respiratory infections. The research on acute alcohol ingestion shows no consistent in vivo or in vitro effect of ethanol on neutrophil function (Spagnuolo and MacGregor, 1975), unless levels of greater than 800 mg/dl are reached in vitro. There is consistent evidence that Laënnec's cirrhosis is associated with the presence of serum factors, which decrease the generation of chemotactic factors in the cirrhotic patient's serum and which inhibit the function of both serum and bacterially derived chemotactic factors (Anderson, 1975; Maderazo et al., 1975). There were no such abnormalities in three patients tested by Maderazo et al. (1975) with hepatitis from alcohol, halothane, or methimazole. The neutrophils of cirrhotic patients seem to function normally in the absence of the serum containing the inhibitory factors. No comparison was made with neutrophils from patients with cirrhosis derived from other causes.

The presence of these inhibitory factors would lead to a predicted poor inflammatory response to an infection both by inhibiting the efficacy of an invading bacterium's chemotactic factors and by limiting the amount of complement-derived chemotactic factors generated by activation of the complement cascade by bacteria in the presence or absence of antibodies. This prediction is supported by the well-known picture of the cirrhotic patient presenting with a life-threatening pneumonia and little systemic toxicity.

C. Infection

The presence of one infective agent can induce changes in neutrophil function that may predispose to a second infection. The picture of bacterial pneumonia after infection with influenza virus is a classical example of this paradigm.

Studies on the neutrophils of acutely or chronically infected patients do not reveal a consistent pattern. There does not appear to be any particular factor that enables the prediction of the chemotactic function of the infected patients' neutrophils. Some investigators find predominantly enhanced neutrophil chemotaxis in bacterially infected patients (Hill et al., 1974b), others find significant enhancement or inhibition (Link et al., 1979), and a third group found a decrease in chemotactic function in more acute infections and an increase in more chronic infections (Mowat and Baum, 1971b). The bactericidal activity of neutrophils from bacterially infected patients may also be decreased, but the evidence for this is not overwhelming. McCall et al. (1971) reported that neutrophils with toxic granulations (basophilic cytoplasmic granules) seen in infection (all but one of their patients had Rocky Mountain Spotted Fever) have decreased chemotaxis and killing. Hellum and Solberg (1977) report that decreased killing capacity of neutrophils from infected patients correlates with the percentage of juvenile forms present in the blood of the patients.

There is evidence that subpopulations of neutrophils as determined by their ability to rosette IgG-sensitized erythrocytes change in endotoxemia (Klempner, 1980). The nonrosetting cells display less chemotactic and bactericidal activity than rosetting cells. Rosetting neutrophils may also be important in regulating myelopoiesis (Broxmeyer et al., 1980). Normally about 80% of neutrophils in peripheral blood are capable of rosetting sensitized erythrocytes. Under conditions of complement activation, such as endotoxemia or hemodialysis, there may be preferential margination of rosette-forming neutrophils and relative enrichment of circulating nonrosetting cells. This enrichment of relatively less active cells may account for some of the observed defects of neutrophil function during infection. Thus, the defect may reflect an alteration of circulating subpopulations of cells rather than an acquired abnormality of all circulating neutrophils.

There is good evidence that the neutrophils from patients with herpes simplex (Rabson et al., 1977) and measles (Anderson et al., 1976) show a chemotactic defect. In the case of measles, the defect was shown in vitro and in vivo, and the defect reversed itself by the 11th day after the onset of rash. Monocyte chemotaxis is depressed in those infected with influenza A (Kleinerman et al., 1979); however, neutrophil chemotaxis was not measured. There is evidence that the exposure of human neutrophils to influenza virus in vitro can inhibit neutrophil chemotactic and phagocytic function (Larson and Blades, 1976; Schlesinger et al., 1976). It can be speculated that influenza virus could inhibit the normal function of alveolar macrophages and perhaps could secondarily affect those cells' ability to recruit neutrophils.

Many bacteria and viruses produce materials which are in themselves toxic to neutrophils. These microbial products are well reviewed by Wilkinson (1981).

Obviously, neutrophils exposed to toxic products of one infective agent would theoretically be unable to combat any other, less virulent agent that might superinfect the patient.

Thus, there is a basis for increased susceptibility to infection in infected hosts due to neutrophil dysfunction. The evidence, however, is stronger for viral infections than for bacterial infections.

D. Thermal Injury

The thermally injured patient has lost a significant barrier to infection, an intact epidermis. These patients frequently succumb to sepsis and pneumonia. There is probably a role in decreased neutrophil function in this susceptibility to infection.

Burned patients have a neutrophil chemotactic defect, the extent of which correlates with the surface area of the burn. Furthermore, the extent of the chemotactic defect can be used to predict the survival of the burn patient (Warden et al., 1974a). Two common topical agents used in burn patients, silver sulfadiazine and mafenide acetate, both inhibit leukocyte chemotaxis at levels found in the serum of burn patients (Warden et al., 1974b). The chemotactic defect has also been found to correlate to a decreased specific (secondary) granule enzyme content in the circulating neutrophils of burn patients (Davis, 1980) and in this regard may represent an acquired form of specific granule deficiency. A decreased ability of neutrophils from thermally injured patients to kill *Staph. aureus* and *Pseudomonas* has also been reported (Alexander et al., 1971; Grogan, 1976). This bactericidal defect has been shown to correlate with the extent of burn and to be reversible in convalescence.

These defects in neutrophil chemotaxis and bactericidal activity, when combined with a compromised physical barrier to infection, can explain the high incidence of infection in these patients, as well as the finding of pneumonia in the absence of sepsis.

E. Neoplasia

The best data for chemotactic defects in neoplasia refer to monocyte chemotactic defects (Klebanoff and Clark, 1978d). The discussion of Snyderman et al. (1980) of monocyte chemotactic abnormalities in neoplasia indicates that various tumor cell lines produce substances that inhibit monocyte chemotaxis in vitro and in vivo. There is less extensive information on neutrophil chemotactic defects in patients with cancer. Twenty patients with carcinoma were studied by Ward et al. (1976), who found that 18 of the 24 patients had a serum factor that inhibited normal chemotaxis of the patients' neutrophils. This inhibition disappeared when the neutrophils were exposed to normal serum and their chemotaxis tested in vitro.

A more specific ability of a neoplasm to inhibit neutrophil function was elucidated by Van Epps and Williams (1976). They found that serum from IgA myeloma patients, but not from IgG myeloma or Waldenström's macroblobulinemia, significantly inhibited neutrophil chemotaxis in vitro. This inhibition was lost if the sera were absorbed in an anti-IgA column. Furthermore, the $F(ab)_2$ fragments of monomeric IgA did not produce an inhibition of chemotaxis. The same researchers presented evidence that IgA in alcoholic liver disease also has the ability to inhibit neutrophil chemotaxis (Van Epps et al., 1975). This specific immunoglobulin class seems to inhibit neutrophil chemotaxis when it is polymerized and its Fc portion is intact. The clinical relevance of this fascinating information is unclear. IgA myelomas do not appear to have a higher rate of infection than other myeloma classes (Wintrobe et al., 1974). This type of specific tumor product may be a prototype of cell-directed inhibitory products in neoplasia, infection, and other diseases.

F. Adult Respiratory Distress Syndrome

The final acquired dysfunction of neutrophils to be discussed is the adult respiratory distress syndrome (ARDS). There is considerable evidence that this syndrome is at least initiated by the aggregation of neutrophils in the lung and the subsequent release of toxic and inflammatory substances by the neutrophils. Whether this represents true neutrophil dysfunction or merely a predicted response to abnormal stimuli is a moot point. Jacob et al. (1980) recently reviewed evidence of neutrophil involvement in ARDS.

Lung biopsies of patients with septicemia and ARDS show large amounts of interstitial neutrophils, considerable interstitial edema, and occasional neutrophil migration through the vascular endothelium, but little evidence of intravascular neutrophil aggregation (Bachofen and Weibel, 1977). These biopsies were done at time of the patients' death, however, and all had ARDS for at least 24 hours. A model similar to ARDS is hemodialysis-associated pulmonary insufficiency and neutropenia (Craddock et al., 1977a). Craddock et al. infused cellophane dialyzer membrane-activated rabbit plasma into rabbits and duplicated the syndrome in the rabbit model. The rabbit's lungs during the infusion of the activated plasma showed leukostatic plugs. This activated factor in human plasma is probably C5a or C5a-related (Craddock et al., 1977b). This neutrophil dysfunction is rapidly reversible, while ARDS is not. The dialyzer membrane ceases to generate C5a rapidly, however, and the neutrophil aggregates will dissociate within minutes in vitro (O'Flaherty et al., 1979).

During sepsis, however, the deposition of fibrin and the continued generation of complement products could both lead to prolonged generation of high amounts of chemotactic factors in the lungs. The resulting aggregation of neutrophils and secretion of their granule contents along with toxic oxygen metabolites could worsen the damage to the lung parenchyma caused by the by-products of sepsis. The secreted products of neutrophils are capable of generating new chemotactic factors from lung elastin (Senior et al., 1980), as well as by activating the complement system to amplify the inflammation and establish an interstitial lesion of long duration. Experimental support for this scenario comes from Hosea et al. (1980), who showed that leakage of albumin into the lungs of guinea pigs made septic with pneumococci did not occur if the guinea pigs were deficient in the fifth component of complement or if they were neutropenic. Further evidence for the involvement of neutrophils in ARDS is the recent work of Lee et al. (1981), which shows increased neutrophil-derived elastase enzyme activity in pulmonary lavage fluid of ARDS patients as compared with that in patients with chronic obstructive lung disease.

In the instance of ARDS, there is evidence that normal neutrophil function in response to abnormal stimuli (i.e., generation of large amounts of chemotactic factors in the lung) can lead to serious lung dysfunction. The aggregation and secretion of neutrophils may well occur in other organs in conditions that lead to ARDS, but the delicate relationship of circulation and gas exchange makes the lung especially vulnerable to the inflammatory capacity of the neutrophil.

IV. Conclusion

This chapter has dealt with the major inherited dysfunctions of neutrophil function and selected acquired abnormalities. The basis for these dysfunctions varies from the inability of the neutrophil to generate a specific oxygen metabolite (as in chronic granulomatous disease) to the presence of inhibitory substance in the serum (as in alcoholic cirrhosis).

By studying the various syndromes of neutrophil dysfunction it becomes evident that the neutrophil is a critical part of the lung's defenses against infection. The neutrophil itself may also play a role in inducing lung pathology as in ARDS. Whatever the basis of the neutrophil defect, it is clear that an understanding of lung disease cannot be fully attained without recognition and understanding of the neutrophil's functions.

References

Afzelius, B. A., Ewetz, L., Palmblad, J., Uden, A. M., and Venizelos, N. (1980). Structure and function of neutrophil leukocytes from patients with the immotile-cilia syndrome. *Acta Med. Scand., 208*:145-154.

Alexander, J. W., Dionigi, R., and Meakins, J. L. (1971). Periodic variation in the antibacterial function of human neutrophils and its relationship to sepsis. *Ann. Surg., 173*:206-213.

Anderson, B. R. (1975). Host factors causing increased susceptibility to infection in patients with Laennec's cirrhosis. *Ann. N.Y. Acad. Sci., 252*:348-352.

Anderson, R., Rabson, A. R., Sher, R., and Koornhof, H. J. (1976). Defective neutrophil motility in children with measles. *Pediatrics, 89*:27-32.

Bachofen, M., and Weibel, E. R. (1977). Alteration of the gas exchange apparatus in adult respiratory insufficiency associated with septicemia. *Am. Rev. Respir. Dis., 116*:589-615.

Balfour, H. H., Jr., Shehan, J. J., Speicher, C. E., and Kander, E. (1971). Chronic granulomatous disease of childhood in a 23-year-old man. *J. Am. Med. Assoc., 217*:960-961.

Berendes, H., Bridges, R. A., and Good, R. A. (1957). A fatal granulomatosis of childhood. The clinical study of a new syndrome. *Minn. Med., 40*:309-312.

Berger, M., Kirkpatrick, C. H., Goldsmith, P. K., and Gallin, J. I. (1980). IgE antibodies to *Staphylococcus aureus* and *Candida albicans* patients with the syndrome of hyperimmunoglobulin E and recurrent infections. *J. Immunol., 125*:2437-2443.

Blume, R. S., and Wolff, S. M. (1972). The Chediak-Higashi syndrome: Studies in four patients and a review of the literature. *Medicine, 51*:247-280.

Boxer, L. A., Rister, M., Allen, J. M., and Baehner, R. L. (1977). Improvement of Chediak-Higashi leukocyte function by cyclic guanosine monophosphate. *Blood, 49*:9-17.

Boxer, L. A., Vanderbilt, B., Bonsib, S., Jersild, R., Hsin-Hsin, Y., and Baehner, R. L. (1979). Enhancement of chemotactic response and microtubule assembly in human leukocytes by ascorbic acid. *J. Cell. Physiol., 100*:119-126.

Boxer, L. A., Watanbe, A. M., Rister, M., Besch, H. R., Allen, J., and Baehner, R. L. (1976). Correction of leukocyte function in Chediak-Higashi syndrome by ascorbate. *N. Engl. J. Med., 295*:1041-1045.

Brayton, R. G., Stokes, P. E., Schwartz, M. S., and Louria, D. B. (1970). Effect of alcohol and various diseases on leukocyte mobilization, phagocytosis and intracellular bacterial killing. *N. Engl. J. Med., 282*:123-128.

Breton-Gorius, J., Mason, D. Y., Buriot, D., Vilde, J.-L., and Griscelli, C. (1980). Lactoferrin deficiency as a consequence of a lack of specific granules in neutrophils from a patient with recurrent infections. Detection by immunoperoxidase staining for lactoferrin and cytochemical electron microscopy. *Am. J. Pathol., 99*:413-419.

Broxmeyer, H. L., Ralph, P., Bognacki, J., Kincade, P. W., and DeSousa, M. (1980). A subpopulation of human polymorphonuclear neutrophils contains an active form of lactoferrin capable of binding to human monocytes and inhibiting production of granulocyte-macrophage colony stimulatory activities. *J. Immunol., 125*:903-909.

Buckley, D. H., Wray, B. B., and Belmaker, E. Z. (1972). Extreme hyperimmunoglobulinemia E and undue susceptibility to infection. *Pediatrics, 49*: 59-70.

Buckley, R. H., and Becker, W. G. (1978). Abnormalities in the regulation of human IgE synthesis. *Immunol. Rev., 41*:288-314.

Bujak, J. S., Kwon-Chung, K. J., and Chusid, M. J. (1973). Osteomyelitis and pneumonia in a boy with chronic granulomatous disease of childhood caused by a mutant strain of *Aspergillus nidulans. Am. J. Clin. Pathol., 61*:361-367.

Chusid, M. J., and Tomasulo, P. A. (1978). Survival of transfused normal granulocytes in a patient with chronic granulomatous disease. *Pediatrics, 61*:556-559.

Chusid, M. J., Parrillo, J. E., and Fauci, A. S. (1975a). Chronic granulomatous disease. Diagnosis in a 27 year old man with *Mycobacterium fortuitum. J. Am. Med. Assoc., 233*:1295-1296.

Chusid, M. J., Gelfand, J. A., Nutter, C., and Fauci, A. S. (1975b). Pulmonary aspergillosis, inhalation of contaminated marijuana smoke, CGD. *Ann. Intern. Med., 82*:682-683.

Clark, R. A. (1981). Chemotactic peptides trigger their own oxidative inactivation by neutrophils. *Clin. Res.*, (In Press).

Clark, R. A., and Kimball, H. R. (1971). Defective granulocyte chemotaxis in the Chediak-Higashi syndrome of man. *J. Clin. Invest., 50*:2645-2652.

Clark, R. A., Root, R. K., Kimball, H. R., and Kirkpatrick, C. H. (1973). Defective neutrophil chemotaxis and cellular immunity in a child with recurrent infections. *Ann. Intern. Med., 78*:515-519.

Clark, R. A., Szot, S., Venkatasubramanian, K., and Schiffmann, E. (1980). Chemotactic factor inactivation by myeloperoxidase-mediated oxidation of methionine. *J. Immunol., 124*:2020-2026.

Clawson, C. G., White, J. G., and Repine, J. E. (1978). The Chediak-Higashi syndrome. Evidence that defective leukotaxis is primarily due to an impediment by giant granules. *Am. J. Pathol., 92*:745-751.

Craddock, P. R., Fehr, J., Dalmasso, A. P., Brigeram, K. L., and Jacob, H. S. (1977a). Hemodialysis leukopenia. Pulmonary vascular leukostasis resulting from complement activation by dialyzer cellophane membranes. *J. Clin. Invest., 59*:879-888.

Craddock, P. R., Hammerschmidt, D., White, J. G., Dalmasso, A. P., and Jacob, H. S. (1977b). Complement (C5a)-induced granulocyte aggregation in vitro. A possible mechanism of complement-mediated leukostasis. *J. Clin. Invest., 60*:260-264.

Cramer, E. B., Milks, L. C., and Ojakian, G. K. (1980). Transepithelial migration of human neutrophils: An *in vitro* model system. *Proc. Natl. Acad. Sci. USA, 77*:4069-4073.

Curnutte, J. T., Kipnes, R. S., and Babior, B. M. (1975). Defect in pyridine nucleotide dependent superoxide production by a particulate fraction from the granulocytes of patients with chronic granulomatous disease. *N. Engl. J. Med., 293*:628-632.

Curnutte, J. T., Whitten, D. M., and Babior, B. M. (1974). Defective superoxide production by granulocytes from patients with chronic granulomatous disease. *N. Engl. J. Med., 290*:593-597.

Dale, D. C., Alling, D. W., and Wolff, S. M. (1972). Cloxacillin chemoprophylaxis in the Chediak-Higashi syndrome. *J. Infect. Dis., 129*:393-397.

Davis, J. M. (1980). Thermal injury (p. 529). In Disorders of phagocyte chemotaxis (NIH Combined Clinical Staff Conference, J. I. Gallin, moderator). *Ann. Intern. Med., 92*:520-538.

Davis, S. D., Schaller, J., and Wedgwood, R. J. (1966). Job's syndrome. Recurrent, "cold," staphylococcal abscesses. *Lancet, i*:1013-1015.

Davis, W. C., and Douglas, S. D. (1972). Defective granule formation and function in the Chediak-Higashi syndrome. *Semin. Hematol., 9*:431-450.

Donabedian, H., and Gallin, J. I. (1982a). Mononuclear cells from patients with hyper IgE-recurrent infection syndrome (HIE) produce an inhibitor of leukocyte chemotaxis. *J. Clin. Invest., 69*:1155-1163.

Donabedian, H., and Gallin, J. I. (1982b). Levamisole is inferior to placebo in the hyperimmunoglobulin E-recurrent infection (JOB's) syndrome. *N. Engl. J. Med., 307*:290-292.

Fernandez, H. M., Henson, P. M., Otani, A., and Hugli, T. E. (1978). Chemotactic response to human C3a and C5a anaphylatoxins. I. Evaluation of C3a and C5a leukotaxis *in vitro*, and under simulated *in vivo* conditions. *J. Immunol., 120*:109-115.

Fleming, G. M., Kleinerman, J., Doershuk, C. F., and Perrin, E. V. (1975). Chronic granulomatous disease of childhood. An unusual cause of honeycomb lung. *Chest, 68*:834-837.

Frank, M. M. (1980). Complement mediated defense mechanisms in the immune compromised host. In *Infections in the Immunocomprised Host–Pathogenesis, Prevention and Therapy.* Edited by J. Verhoef, P. K. Peterson, and P. G. Quie. New York, Elsevier/North Holland, pp. 23-36.

Frankel, F. R., Tucker, R. W., Bruce, J., and Steinberg, R. (1978). Fibroblasts and macrophages of mice with the Chediak-Higashi syndrome have microtubules and actin cables. *J. Cell Biol., 79*:401-408.

Gallin, J. I. (1980). Therapeutic considerations. In Disorders of phagocyte chemotaxis (NIH Combined Clinical Staff Conference, J. I. Gallin, moderator). *Ann. Intern. Med., 92*:520-538.

Gallin, J. I., and Quie, P. G. (1978). *Leukocyte Chemotaxis: Methods, Physiology, and Clinical Implications.* New York, Raven Press.

Gallin, J. I., Klimerman, J. A., Padgett, G. A., and Wolff, S. M. (1979a). Defective mononuclear leukocyte chemotaxis in Chediak-Higashi syndrome of humans, mice and cattle. *Blood, 45*:863-870.

Gallin, J. I., Elin, R. J., Hubert, R. T., Fauci, A. S., Kaliner, M. A., and Wolff, S. M. (1979b). Efficacy of ascorbic acid in Chediak-Higashi syndrome (CHS): Studies in humans and mice. *Blood, 53*:226-234.

Goetzl, E. J., and Pickett, W. C. (1980). The human PMN leukocyte chemotactic activity of complex hydroxy-eicosatetraenoic acids (HETES). *J. Immunol., 125*:1789-1791.

Good, R. A., Quie, P. G., Windhorst, D. B., Page, A. R., Rodey, G. E., White, J., Wolfson, J. J., and Holmes, B. H. (1968). Fatal (chronic) granulomatous disease of childhood: A hereditary defect of leukocyte function. *Semin. Hematol., 5*:215-254.

Grogan, J. B. (1976). Altered neutrophil phagocytic function in burn patients. *J. Trauma, 16*:734-738.

Haak, R. A., Ingraham, L. M., Baehner, R. L., and Boxer, L. A. (1979). Membrane fluidity in human and mouse Chediak-Higashi leukocytes. *J. Clin. Invest., 64*:138-144.

Hellum, K. B., and Solberg, C. O. (1977). Granulocyte function in bacterial infections in man. *Acta Pathol. Microbiol. Scand.* [*C*], *85*:1-9.

Hill, H. R., and Quie, P. G. (1976). Raised serum IgE levels and defective neutrophil chemotaxis in three children with eczema and recurrent bacterial infections. *Lancet, i*:183-187.

Hill, H. R., Estensen, R. D., Hogan, N. A., and Quie, P. G. (1976). Severe staphylococcal disease associated with allergic manifestations, hyperimmunoglobulinemia E and defective neutrophil chemotaxis. *J. Lab. Clin. Med., 88*:796-806.

Hill, H. R., Gerrard, J. M., Hogan, N. A., and Quie, P. G. (1974b). Hyperactivity of neutrophil leukotactic responses during active bacterial function. *J. Clin. Invest., 53*:996-1002.

Hill, H. R., Sauk, H. S., Dettloff, J. L., and Quie, P. G. (1974c). Impaired leukotactic responsiveness in patients with juvenile diabetes mellitus. *Clin. Immunol. Immunopathol., 2*:395-403.

Hill, H. R., Quie, P. G., Pabst, H. F., Dochs, H., Clark, R. A., Klebanoff, S. J., and Wedgwood, R. J. (1974a). Defect in neutrophil granulocyte chemotaxis in Job's syndrome of recurrent "cold" staphylococcal abscesses. *Lancet, ii*:617-619.

Holmes, B., Quie, P. G., Windhorst, D. B., and Good, R. A. (1966). Fatal granulomatous disease of childhood. An inborn abnormality of phagocytic function. *Lancet, i*:1225-1228.

Holmes, B., Page, A. R., and Good, R. A. (1967). Studies of the metabolic activity of leukocytes from patients with a genetic abnormality of phagocytic function. *J. Clin. Invest., 46*:1422-1432.

Hosea, S., Brown, E., Hammer, C., and Frank, M. (1980). Role of complement activation in a model of adult respiratory distress syndrome. *J. Clin. Invest., 66*:375-382.

Hunninghake, G. W., Gadek, J. E., Fales, H. M., and Crystal, R. G. (1980). Human alveolar macrophage-derived chemotactic factor for neutrophils. Stimuli and partial characterization. *J. Clin. Invest., 66*:473-483.

Jacob, H. S., Craddock, P. R., Hammerschmidt, D. E., and Moldow, C. F. (1980). Complement-induced granulocyte aggregation. An unsuspected mechanism of disease. *N. Engl. J. Med., 302*:789-794.

Johnston, R. B., Jr., and Baehner, R. L. (1971). Chronic granulomatous disease: Correlation between pathogenesis and clinical findings. *Pediatrics, 48*:730-739.

Johnston, R. B., Jr., and Newman, S. L. (1977). Chronic granulomatous disease. *Pediatr. Clin. North Am., 24*:365-376.

Johnston, R. B., Wilfert, C. M., Buckley, R. H., Webb, L. S., DeChatelet, L. R., and McCall, C. E. (1975). Enhanced bactericidal activity of phagocytes from patients with chronic granulomatous disease in the presence of sulphisoxazole. *Lancet, i*:824-827.

Kanfer, J. N., Blume, R. S., Yankee, R. A., and Wolff, S. M. (1968). Alteration of sphingolipid metabolism in leukocytes from patients with the Chediak-Higashi syndrome. *N. Engl. J. Med., 279*:410-413.

Kaplan, A. P., Goetzl, E. J., and Austen, K. F. (1972). A prealbumin activator of prekallikrein. III. Appearance of chemotactic activity for human neutrophils by the conversion of human prekallikrein to kallikrein. *J. Exp. Med., 135*:81-97.

Katona, I. M., Tata, G., Scanlon, R. T., and Bellanti, J. A. (1980). Hyper-IgE syndrome: A disease with suppressor T cell deficiency. *Ann. Allergy, 45*:295-300.

Katz, P., Simone, C. B., Henkart, P. A., and Fauci, A. S. (1980). Mechanisms of antibody-dependent cellular cytotoxicity. The use of effector cells from chronic granulomatous disease patients as investigative probes. *J. Clin. Invest., 65*:55-63.

Kay, A. B., Pepper, D. S., and McKenzie, R. (1974). The identification of fibrinopeptide B as a chemotactic agent derived from human fibrinogen. *Br. J. Haematol., 27*:669-677.

Kazmierowski, J. A., Gallin, J. I., and Reynolds, H. Y. (1973). Mechanism for the inflammatory response in primate lungs. *J. Clin. Invest., 59*:273-281.

Kazmierowski, J. A., Elin, R. J., Reynolds, H. Y., Durbin, W. A., and Wolff, S. M. (1976). Chediak-Higashi syndrome: Reversal of increased susceptibility to infection by bone marrow transplantation. *Blood, 47*:555-559

Kimball, H. R., Ford, G. H., and Wolff, S. M. (1975). Lysozomal enzymes in normal and Chediak-Higashi blood leukocytes. *J. Lab. Clin. Med., 86*:616-630.

Klebanoff, S. J., and Clark, R. A. (1978a). *The Neutrophil: Function and Clinical Disroders.* New York, North-Holland Publ. Co., pp. 73-162.

Klebanoff, S. J., and Clark, R. A. (1978b). *The Neutrophil: Function and Clinical Disorders.* New York, North-Holland Publ. Co., pp. 283-368.

Klebanoff, S. J., and Clark, R. A. (1978c). *The Neutrophil: Function and Clinical Disorders.* New York, North-Holland Publ. Co., pp. 408-466.

Klebanoff, S. J., and Clark, R. A. (1978d). *The Neutrophil: Function and Clinical Disorders.* New York, North-Holland Publ. Co., p. 532.

Klebanoff, S. J., and Clark, R. A. (1978e). *The Neutrophil: Function and Clinical Disorders.* New York, North-Holland Publ. Co., pp. 725-728.

Kleinerman, E. S., Synderman, R., and Daniels, C. A. (1979). Depressed monocyte chemotaxis during acute influenza infection. *Lancet, ii*:1063-1066.

Klempner, M. S. (1980). Neutrophil heterogeneity as a possible basis for abnormal chemotaxis (NIH Combined Clinical Staff Conference, J. I. Gallin, moderator), pp. 529-531. *Ann. Intern. Med., 92*:520-538.

Koutras, S. B., and Bodenbender, J. G. (1968). Studies of the inflammatory cycle in juvenile diabetes. *Am. J. Dis. Child., 116*:130-134.

Lane, P. W., and Murphy, E. D. (1972). Susceptibility to spontaneous pneumonitis in an inbred strain of beige and satin mice. *Genetics, 72*:451-460.

Larson, H. E., and Blades, R. (1976). Impairment of human polymorphonuclear leukocyte function by influenza virus. *Lancet, i*:283.

Lee, C. T., Fein, A. M., Lippmann, M., Holtzman, H., Kimbel, P., and Weinbaum, G. (1981). Elastolytic activity in pulmonary lavage fluid from patients with Adult Respiratory-Distress syndrome. *N. Engl. J. Med., 304*: 192-196.

Lehrer, R. I., and Cline, M. J. (1969). Leukocyte myeloperoxidase deficiency and disseminated candidosis: The role of myeloperoxidase in resistance to *Candida* infection. *J. Clin. Invest., 48*:1478-1488.

Link, A. S., Bass, D. A., and McCall, C. E. (1979). Altered neutrophil migration during bacterial infection associated with a serum modulator of cellular motility. *J. Infect. Dis., 140*:517-526.

MacGregor, R. R. (1980). Granulocyte adherence. In *The Cell Biology of Inflammation.* Edited by G. Weissman. New York, Elsevier/North Holland, pp. 267-298.

Maderazo, E. G., Ward, P. A., and Quintiliani, R. (1975). Defective regulation of chemotaxis in cirrhosis. *J. Lab. Clin. Med., 85*:621-630.

Malech, H. L. (1980). Abnormal neutrophil migration in Kartagener's syndrome (pp. 527-529). In Disorders of phagocyte chemotaxis (NIH Combined Clinical Staff Conference, J. I. Gallin, moderator). *Ann. Intern. Med., 92*: 520-538.

Malech, H. L., Root, R. K., and Gallin, J. I. (1977). Structural analysis of human neutrophil migration centriole, microtubule, microfilament orientation and function during chemotaxis. *J. Cell. Biol., 75*:666-693.

Mawhinney, H., Killen, M., Fleming, W. A., and Roy, A. D. (1980). The hyperimmunoglobulin E syndrome. A neutrophil chemotactic defect reversibility histamine H_2 receptor blockade? *Clin. Immunol. Immunopathol., 17*: 483-491.

McCall, C. E., Caves, J., Cooper, R., and DeChatelet, L. (1971). Functional characteristics of human toxic neutrophils. *J. Infect. Dis., 124*:68-75.

Merrill, W. W., Naegel, G. P., Matthay, R. A., and Reynolds, H. Y. (1980). Alveolar macrophage-derived chemotactic factor kinetics of in vitro production and partial characterization. *J. Clin. Invest., 65*:268-276.

Merten, D. F., Buckley, R. H., Pratt, P. C., Effmann, E. L., and Grossman, H. (1979). Hyperimmunoglobulinemia E syndrome: Radiographic observations. *Radiology, 132*:71-78.

Miller, M. E. (1979). Cell elastimetry in the study of normal and abnormal movement of human neutrophils. *Clin. Immunol. Immunopathol., 14*:502-510.

Miller, M. E., and Baker, L. (1972). Leukocyte function in juvenile diabetes mellitus. Humoral and cellular aspects. *Pediatrics, 81*:979-982.

Mills, E. L., Rholl, K. S., and Quie, P. G. (1980). X-linked inheritance in females with chronic granulomatous disease. *J. Clin. Invest., 66*:332-340.

Mowat, A. G., and Baum, J. (1971a). Chemotaxis of polymorphonuclear leukocytes from patients with diabetes mellitus. *N. Engl. J. Med., 284*:621-627.

Mowat, A. G., and Baum, J. (1971b). Polymorphonuclear leukocyte chemotaxis in patients with bacterial infection. *Br. Med. J., 3*:617-619.

Nath, J., Flavin, M., and Gallin, J. I. (1980). Tubulin tyrosylation in normal and Chediak-Higashi syndrome neutrophils (part 2). *J. Cell Biol., 87*:256.

O'Flaherty, J. T., Showell, H. J., Ward, P. A., and Becker, E. L. (1979). A possible role of arachidonic acid in human neutrophil aggregation and degranulation. *Am. J. Pathol., 96*:799-809.

Oliver, J. M., and Zurier, R. B. (1976). Correction of characteristic abnormalities of microtubule function and granule morphology in Chediak-Higashi syndrome with cholinergic agonists. *J. Clin. Invest., 57*:1239-1247.

Parry, M., Root, R. K., Metcalfe, J. A., and Delaney, K. (1980). Myeloperoxidase deficiency: The most common neutrophil functional defect? *Clin. Res., 28*:549A.

Pedersen, F. K., Johansen, K. S., Rosenkvist, J., Tygstrup, I., and Valerius, N. H. (1979). Refractory *Pneumocystis carinii* infection in chronic granulomatous disease: Successful treatment with granulocytes. *Pediatrics, 64*: 935-938.

Petrone, W. F., English, D. K., Wong, K., and McCord, J. M. (1980). Free radicals and inflammation: Superoxide-dependent activation of a neutrophil chemotactic factor in plasma. *Proc. Natl. Acad. Sci. USA, 77*:1159-1163.

Prueitt, J. L., Chi, E. Y., and Lagunoff, D. (1978). Pulmonary surface-active materials in the Chediak-Higashi syndrome. *J. Lipid Res., 19*:410-415.

Rabson, A. R., Whiting, D. A., Anderson, R., Gloves, A., and Koornhof, H. J. (1977). Depressed neutrophil motility in patients with recurrent herpes simplex virus infections: In vitro restoration with levamisole. *J. Infect. Dis., 135*:113-116.

Raubitshek, A. A., Levin, A. S., Stites, D. P., Shaw, E. B., and Fudenberg, H. H. (1973). Normal granulocyte infusion therapy for aspergillosis in chronic granulomatous disease. *Pediatrics, 51*:230-233.

Rausch, P. G., Pryzwansky, K. B., and Spitznagel, J. K. (1978). Immunocytochemical identification of azurophilic and specific granule markers in the giant granules of Chediak-Higashi neutrophils. *N. Engl. J. Med., 298*:693-698.

Root, R. K., Rosenthal, A. S., and Balestra, D. J. (1972). Abnormal bactericidal, metabolic and lysosomal function of Chediak-Higashi syndrome leukocytes. *J. Clin. Invest., 51*:649-665.

Rosen, H., and Klebanoff, S. J. (1976). Chemiluminescence and superoxide production by myeloperoxidase-deficient leukocytes. *J. Clin. Invest., 58*:40-50.

Sandler, J. A., Gallin, J. I., and Vaughn, M. (1975). Effects of serotonin, carbamylcholine and ascorbic acid on leukocyte cyclic GMP and chemotaxis. *J. Cell Biol., 67*:480-484.

Schlesinger, J. J., Ernst, C., and Weinstein, L. (1976). Inhibition of human neutrophil chemotaxis by influenza virus. *Lancet, i*:650-651.

Schopfer, K., Baerlocher, K., Proce, P., Krech, U., Quie, P. G., and Douglas, S. D. (1979). Staphylococcal IgE antibodies, hyperimmunoglobulinemia E and *Staphylococcus aureus* infections. *N. Engl. J. Med., 300*:835-838.

Seligmann, B. E., and Gallin, J. I. (1980). Use of lipophilic probes of membrane potential to assess human neutrophil activation. Abnormality in chronic granulomatous disease. *J. Clin. Invest., 66*:493-503.

Senior, R. M., Griffin, G. L., and Mecham, R. P. (1980). Chemotactic activity of elastin-derived peptides. *J. Clin. Invest., 66*:859-862.

Snyderman, R., Pike, M. C., and Cianciolo, G. J. (1980). An inhibitor of macrophage accumulation produced by neoplasms: Its role in abrogating host resistance to cancer. In *Mononuclear Phagocytes, Functional Aspects.* Part I. Edited by R. van Furth. Boston, Martinus Nijhoff, pp. 569-590.

Spagnuolo, P. J., and MacGregor, R. R. (1975). Acute ethanol effects on chemotaxis and other components of host defense. *J. Lab. Clin. Med., 86*:24-31.

Stossel, T. P. (1978). Mechanism of chemotaxis. In *Leukocyte Chemotaxis: Methods, Physiology, and Clinical Implications.* Edited by J. I. Gallin and P. G. Quie. New York, Raven Press, pp. 143-160.

Sutcliffe, J., and Chrispin, A. R. (1970). Chronic granulomatous disease. *Br. J. Radiol., 43*:110-118.

Van Epps, D. E., and Williams, R. C., Jr. (1976). Suppression of leukocyte chemotaxis by human IgA myeloma components. *J. Exp. Med., 144*: 1227-1242.

Van Epps, D. E., Strickland, R. G., and Williams, R. C., Jr. (1975). Inhibitors of leukocyte chemotaxis in alcoholic liver disease. *Am. J. Med., 59*:200-207.

Van Scoy, R. E., Hill, H. R., Pitts, P. E., Jr., and Quie, P. G. (1979). Familial neutrophil chemotaxis defect, recurrent bacterial infection, mucocutaneous candidiasis and hyperimmunoglobulin E. *Ann. Intern. Med., 82*: 766-771.

Ward, P. A., Anton, T., and Maderazo, E. (1976). Defective leukotaxis in cancer patients. *Clin. Res., 24*:463A.

Ward, P. A., Cohen, S., and Flanagan, T. D. (1972). Leukotactic factors elaborated by virus-infected tissues. *J. Exp. Med., 135*:1095-1103.

Ward, P. A., Lepow, I. H., and Newman, L. J. (1968). Bacterial factors chemotactic for polymorphonuclear leukocytes. *Am. J. Pathol., 52*:725-736.

Warden, G. D., Mason, A. D., Jr., and Pruitt, B. A., Jr. (1974a). Evaluation of leukocyte chemotaxis in vitro in thermally injured patients. *J. Clin. Invest., 54*:1001-1004.

Warden, G. D., Mason, A. D., Jr., and Pruitt, B. A., Jr. (1974b). Suppression of leukocyte chemotaxis in vitro by chemotherapeutic agents used in the management of thermal injuries. *Ann. Surg., 181*:363-369.

White, J. G., and Clawson, C. C. (1980). The Chediak-Higashi syndrome: The nature of the giant granules and their interactions with cytoplasm and foreign particulates. *Am. J. Pathol., 98*:151-196.

Whitin, J. C., Chapman, C. E., Simons, E. R., Chovaniec, M. E., and Cohen, H. J. (1980). Correlation between membrane potential change and superoxide production in human granulocytes stimulated by phorbol myristate acetate. Evidence for defective activation in chronic granulomatous disease. *J. Biol. Chem., 255*:1874-1878.

Wilkinson, P. C. (1981). Leukocyte locomotion and chemotaxis: Effects of bacteria and viruses. *Rev. Infect. Dis.,* (In Press).

Windhorst, D. B., and Padgett, G. (1973). The Chediak-Higashi syndrome and the homologous trait in animals. *J. Invest. Dermatol., 60*:529-537.

Wintrobe, M. M., Lee, G. R., Boggs, D. R., Bithell, T. C., Athens, J. W., and Foerster, T. (1974). *Clinical Hematology.* Philadelphia, Lea & Febiger, p. 1613.

Wolfson, J. J., Quie, P. G., Laxdal, S. D., and Good, R. A. (1968). Roentgenologic manifestations in children with a genetic defect of polymorphonuclear leukocyte function. *Radiology, 91*:37-48.

Wright, D. G., and Gallin, J. I. (1977). A functional differentiation of human neutrophils granules: Generation of C5a by a specific (secondary) granule product and inactivation of C5a by azurophil (primary) granule products. *J. Immunol., 119*:1068-1076.

Wright, D. G., Kirkpatrick, C. H., and Gallin, J. I. (1977). Effects of levamisole on normal and abnormal leukocyte locomotion. *J. Clin. Invest., 59*:941-950.

Wright, D. G., and Gallin, J. I. (1979). Secretory responses of human neutrophils: Exocytosis of specific (secondary) granules by human neutrophils during adherence *in vitro* and during exudation *in vivo*. *J. Immunol., 123*: 285-293.

AUTHOR INDEX

Italic numbers give the page on which the complete reference is listed.

B

D

F

H

L

Mc

M

N

P

Q

S

T

U

V

W

SUBJECT INDEX

T

V

W

Y